Cognitive psychologists and neuropsychologists are moving beyond the laboratory and attempting to understand human cognitive abilities as they are manifested in natural contexts. This book offers, for the first time, a comprehensive overview of research on everyday cognition in the adult phases of the life course.

The book addresses the basic conceptual issues regarding the trade-offs between the naturalistic approach compared to the traditional laboratory approach, and it thoroughly analyzes the problems of generalizability on the one hand and rigor on the other. The authors present relevant data that point to new directions for those studying cognition over the adult life span, considering clinical and educational applications.

Researchers, clinicians, and students will find *Everyday Cognition in Adulthood and Late Life* an invaluable resource.

Everyday cognition in adulthood and late life

Everyday cognition in adulthood and late life

Edited by

LEONARD W. POON
University of Georgia

DAVID C. RUBIN
Duke University

BARBARA A. WILSON
University of Southampton

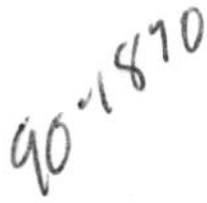

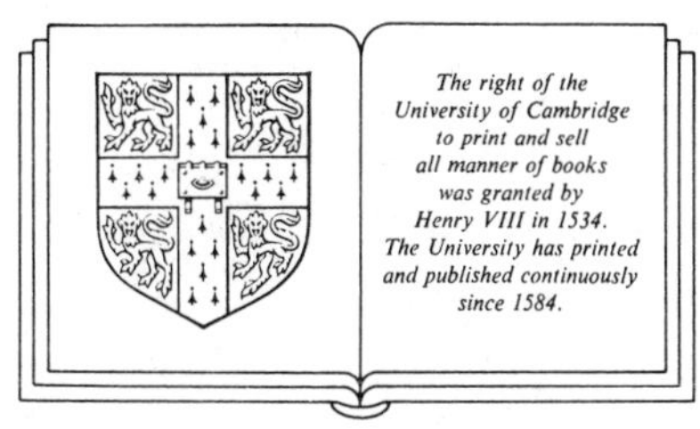

CAMBRIDGE UNIVERSITY PRESS

Cambridge
New York Port Chester Melbourne Sydney

Published by the Press Syndicate of the University of Cambridge
The Pitt Building, Trumpington Street, Cambridge CB2 1RP
40 West 20th Street, New York, NY 10011, USA
10 Stamford Road, Oakleigh, Melbourne 3166, Australia

First published 1989

Printed in the United States of America

Library of Congress Cataloging-in-Publication Data

Poon, Leonard, 1942–

Everyday cognition in adulthood and late life / Leonard W. Poon,
David C. Rubin, Barbara A. Wilson.

p. cm.

ISBN 0-521-37148-1

1. Cognition – Age factors. 2. Memory – Age factors. 3. Cognition –
Research. 4. Memory – Research. 5. Aging – Psychological aspects.
I. Rubin, David C. II. Wilson, Barbara A. III. Title
BF724.55.C63P66 1989
155.6–dc19 88–29974
CIP

British Library Cataloguing in Publication Data
Everyday cognition in adulthood and late life.

1. Man. Cognition
I. Poon, Leonard W. II. Rubin, David C.
III. Wilson, Barbara A.
153.4

ISBN 0 521 37148 1

Contents

Contributors

Lars Bäckman, Department of Psychology, University of Umea, Umea, Sweden

Alan Baddeley, Medical Research Council Applied Psychology Unit, Cambridge, England

Harry P. Bahrick, Department of Psychology, Ohio Wesleyan University, Delaware, Ohio

Nancy L. Bowles, Veterans Administration Outpatient Clinic, Boston, Massachusetts

Darryl Bruce, Department of Psychology, Florida State University, Tallahassee, Florida

Cameron J. Camp, Department of Psychology, University of New Orleans, New Orleans, Louisiana

John C. Cavanaugh, Department of Psychology, Bowling Green State University, Bowling Green, Ohio

Neil Charness, Psychology Department, University of Waterloo, Waterloo, Ontario, Canada

Gillian Cohen, Psychology Department, The Open University, Milton Keynes, England

Herbert F. Crovitz, Psychology Department, Duke University, Durham, North Carolina

Nancy Wadsworth Denney, Psychology Department, University of Wisconsin, Madison, Wisconsin

Roger A. Dixon, Psychology Department, University of Victoria, Victoria, British Columbia, Canada

Dorothy Faulkner, Psychology Department, The Open University, Milton Keynes, England

Alan A. Hartley, Department of Psychology, Scripps College, Claremont, California

Joellen T. Hartley, Department of Psychology, California State University, Long Beach, California

Donald H. Kausler, Department of Psychology, University of Missouri, Columbia, Missouri

Kathleen C. Kirasic, Department of Psychology, University of South Carolina, Columbia, South Carolina

Thomas K. Landauer, Bell Communications Research, Inc., Morris Research and Engineering Center, Morristown, New Jersey

Danielle Lapp, Geriatric Research Educational and Clinical Center, Veterans Administration Medical Center, Palo Alto, California, and Department of Psychiatry and Behavioral Sciences, Stanford School of Medicine, Stanford, California

Nadina B. Lincoln, Stroke Unit, General Hospital, Nottingham, England

Bonnie J. F. Meyer, Department of Educational Psychology, University of Washington, Seattle, Washington

Nicholas J. Moffat, District Psychology Service, Branksome Clinic, Poole, England

Richard A. Monty, U.S. Army Human Engineering Laboratory, Aberdeen Proving Ground, Aberdeen, Maryland

Douglas G. Mook, Department of Psychology, University of Virginia, Charlottesville, Virginia

Loraine K. Obler, Speech and Hearing Sciences Graduate Center, City University of New York, New York, New York

Lawrence C. Perlmuter, Memory Clinic, Veterans Administration Outpatient Clinic, Boston, Massachusetts

Lewis Petrinovich, Department of Psychology, University of California, Riverside, California

Leonard W. Poon, Gerontology Center and Department of Psychology, University of Georgia, Athens, Georgia

Patrick Rabbitt, Department of Psychology, University of Manchester, Manchester, England

G. Elizabeth Rice, Department of Anthropology, Arizona State University, Phoenix, Arizona

David C. Rubin, Psychology Department, Duke University, Durham, North Carolina

Javaid I. Sheikh, Geriatric Research Educational and Clinical Center, Veterans Administration Medical Center, Palo Alto, California, and Department of Psychiatry and Behavioral Sciences, Stanford School of Medicine, Stanford, California

Jan D. Sinnott, GRC/NIA Francis Scott Key Hospital, Baltimore, Maryland, and Psychology Department, Towson State University, Baltimore, Maryland

Elizabeth Lotz Stine, Department of Psychology, Brandeis University, Waltham, Massachusetts

Robin L. West, Department of Psychology, University of Florida, Gainesville, Florida

Sherry L. Willis, College of Human Development, Pennsylvania State University, University Park, Pennsylvania

Barbara A. Wilson, Psychology Department, University of Southampton, Southampton, England

Arthur Wingfield, Department of Psychology, Brandeis University, Waltham, Massachusetts

Jerome A. Yesavage, Geriatric Research Educational and Clinical Center, Veterans Administration Medical Center, Palo Alto, California, and Department of Psychiatry and Behavioral Sciences, Stanford School of Medicine, Stanford, California

Preface

Increasing numbers of cognitive psychologists and neuropsychologists are moving beyond the laboratory and attempting to understand human cognitive abilities as they are manifest in natural contexts. This volume offers a comprehensive overview of research on "everyday" cognition in the adult phases of the life course by integrating theoretical and methodological issues in everyday-cognition research with findings in real-life situations. In this manner, this book will outline for the reader theoretical and methodological trade-offs and dilemmas along the continuum between laboratory research and naturalistic or real-world research.

The book is divided into three parts. Part I addresses fundamental conceptual issues in everyday-cognition research. The first five chapters outline competing theoretical reasons for choosing different approaches in cognitive studies. The next four chapters provide examples of research combining laboratory and real-world strategies.

Part II reviews findings on everyday cognitive behaviors. These chapters concentrate on the everyday cognitive behaviors of adults from early to late adulthood. The first eleven chapters in Part II review and summarize findings from a wide assortment of everyday cognitive activities, and the last six chapters examine the major concomitant factors that could influence the observed outcomes. Whenever possible, generalizations between classic experimental and real-world stimuli and techniques are contrasted.

Part III concentrates on applications of findings in everyday cognition to cognitive-enhancement procedures in everyday and clinical situations. The first two chapters after the introduction review models and theories associated with compensation and remediation. The next two chapters examine enhancement and mnemonic techniques, and the last four chapters examine data and outcomes in cognitive and memory rehabilitation programs.

Each of the three parts can be used independently for reviewing the substantive issues addressed. However, the three parts are designed to flow integratively from theoretical frameworks to findings to applications. For the convenience of the reader, the first chapter in each part of the book provides an introduction, and the last chapter a synthesis.

This book is the third and last in a series of books and conferences dedicated to the memory of George A. Talland, who made significant contributions to the field of memory and aging prior to his premature death in 1968 at the age of 51. Dr. Talland spent his entire research career at the Department of Psychiatry, Massachusetts General Hospital and the Harvard Medical School. He brought experimental psychology techniques into the clinical arena, specifically in regard to examination of amnestic syndromes in normal aging, Korsakoff's syndrome, and other brain abnormalities. His creative research and clinical talents will be long remembered by his many colleagues, admirers, and students.

The first book in the Talland memorial series, *New Directions in Memory Aging,* was published in 1980 and was devoted to exploration of basic theoretical issues related to cognition and aging. The second book, *Handbook for Clinical Memory Assessment of Older Adults,* published in 1986, focused on bridging laboratory findings and clinical diagnostic issues specific to cognitive and memory impairment. This final book highlights laboratory and naturalistic techniques in cognitive study.

I would like to acknowledge the many individuals who made the conference and this edited volume possible. I wish to acknowledge the continuous encouragement of Thomas G. Hackett, chair, Department of Psychiatry, Massachusetts General Hospital and Harvard Medical School; Leonard Jakubczak, project officer, National Institute on Aging; and M. Louise McBee, vice-president for academic affairs, University of Georgia. The conference and the publication were made possible by conference grant 1R13 AG 04032 from the National Institute on Aging. During the editing process, support from the University of Georgia Gerontology Center and the Mental Performance and Aging Laboratory made the final publication steps possible. Also, the patience of the contributors and my fellow editors during my move from Boston to Athens, Georgia, during the editing process is appreciated.

I am grateful to David C. Rubin and Barbara A.Wilson, my coorganizers of the conference and coeditors of the book. They helped to set the high standards for all the contributors. More important, they persevered with me to bring this publication into print. Support for Dr. Rubin for editing this book was provided by NSF grant BNS-8410124, NIA grant AG04278, and a Raymond McKeen Cattell Fund Sabbatical Award.

Reviewers, who spent a considerable amount of time in shaping Part II of the book, were Doug Herrmann, David Hultsch, Leah Light, Denise Park, Marion Perlmutter, Tim Salthouse, George Spilich, Alan Welford, and Art Wingfield. Susan Milmoe and Sophia Prybylski of Cambridge University Press worked closely with me to shape the book and its contents into publishable form. Finally, my wife, Billie Poon, deserves a significant portion of the credit for taking charge of all three Talland Memorial Conferences and carrying out many of the editorial responsibilities for all three publications.

Leonard W. Poon

Athens, Georgia

Part I

Adult cognitive abilities in the laboratory and in real-life settings: Basic theoretical and methodological issues

1 Introduction to Part I: The how, when, and why of studying everyday cognition

David C. Rubin

As a scientific enterprise, the study of memory is relatively new and fairly successful. The methods set out by Ebbinghaus only a century ago are adequate to demonstrate that the psychological study of memory can be scientific. As we progress and try to demonstrate that psychology can also increase our practical and theoretical understandings, Ebbinghaus's laboratory methods often seem insufficient. Our own progress and confidence have led us to broaden the research we do.

One aspect of this progress has been the call for cognitive and experimental psychologists to move out of the laboratory. Recent examples include this book, Neisser's attacks on the kind of laboratory studies he carried out in 1967, numerous *American Psychologist* articles on basic methodological issues, and even the "Call for Papers" of the Psychonomic Society. Possibly independent of all of this, academic and research psychologists are spending a greater proportion of their time studying practical, complex, real-world problems in the name of science. Is this really a good idea, or just the latest fad? Psychology is fond of the theory of pendulum swings. Can a little forethought dampen the pendulum?

Part I of this book provides a rationale, or, more accurately, a set of rationales, for studying cognition in the "real world" rather than in the laboratory. Unlike Parts II and III, Part I does not provide reviews of the literature, but rather provides arguments for pursuing science in various ways. Each chapter in Part I addresses one or more of the following three questions: *How, when,* and *why* should a scientist interested in aging, memory, or, for that matter, any psychological issue prefer working in real-world situations instead of working in the laboratory? The *how* is a methods question. The *when* asks when conditions are favorable for each type of work. The *why* asks what would be gained by each type of work. The chapters vary in the emphasis they place on these questions, and some chapters even argue that the entire matter of such a choice is a poor question. Taken together, the chapters provide researchers with a set of possible guidelines and directions to ponder.

In asking the individual contributors to prepare chapters for Part I, I did not ask them to write the most reasonable, middle-of-the-road views that they could; rather, I asked them to present the most extreme views they cared to defend. That is, the goal of Part I is not to reach a compromise position but rather to provide a set of views that researchers and students can use to challenge and improve their own thinking.

Scientists are high-stakes gamblers. They gamble much of their careers trying to get nature to reveal its secrets. There are rules to the game, but most of the important bets are based on art or intuition. Gerontologists and psychologists are no exception. If anything, the state of knowledge in their fields leads them to gamble more than most. From the perspective of the gambling metaphor, Part I is a collection of hot tips as to where several leading psychologists and the editor think the best odds lie. The tips are honest, in that the people offering them follow their own advice. As a group, the tips show as much agreement as most competitive gambling situations involving intelligent players (e.g., horse racing or the stock market). All the tips have some value. The odds are, however, that no one tip will maximize one's chances of winning if it is taken without consideration of the alternatives.

The eight chapters in Part I are divided into two sections. The first section provides theoretically motivated reasons for a choice between the laboratory and the real world. The second section provides the views of psychologists who have conducted research in both contexts. In the following overview of the two sections of Part I, no attempt is made to cover all the main points of each chapter or to resolve the sometimes uncomfortable differences among them. The purpose of the overview is simply to provide a context in which to read the individual chapters.

Theoretical reasons to study everyday cognition

Petrinovich presents the first theoretical argument for changing the way we do research. Based on Brunswik's principles of representative design, Petrinovich argues that our current methods of laboratory science are not sufficient to develop a general theory of behavior. If we are to understand the behaviors of organisms in their natural environments, we cannot continue simply to perform experiments that control for all but a few variables. Approaches are needed that will sample situations as well as subjects, that will consider individual differences as more than error variance, and that will not arbitrarily select stimulus values and response measures. Petrinovich suggests one such approach based on representative design using multiple regressions and demonstrates how it works in his own research.

In arguing against what he fears will become the new orthodoxy of real-world research, Mook claims that research conducted outside of laboratory controls is neither needed nor desirable for most questions we ask. In doing so, he argues that artificial situations, as well as arbitrary stimulus values and response measures, are adequate in most investigations. The reader who follows standard methods of laboratory research and experimental design should, however, not take comfort in Mook's argument. The same logic that Mook applies to sampling situations, he applies to sampling subjects; in neither case is sampling needed. Thus, the common orthodoxy some of us teach in introductory statistics is called into question on a par with Petrinovich's call for the sampling of stimuli. If we want to generalize our results to new people and new situations, we need to sample people and situations accordingly. It is Mook's contention, however, that we hardly ever want to do either. Mook does more than argue against the rationale for current practices and suggests some possible replacements. He offers guidelines on how to do research in order to increase our understanding of behavior.

To the extent that the chapters by Petrinovich, Mook, and others presented here constitute debates, the reader should return to them after a first reading and weigh their merits carefully.

Bruce argues the need for and the benefits of functional explanations of memory. Cognitive psychologists have long avoided the implications of Darwinian theory for human cognition, and not without cause. It is easy for the uninitiated researcher to err in this subtle form of argumentation. Yet this is no excuse for our collective avoidance of Darwinian theory. Bruce demonstrates the benefits of including concepts such as *ultimate causation* and *population thinking* in our attempts to understand human cognition. Laboratory research is not enough to answer all the questions a Darwinian perspective raises, and we are forced to study cognition in its natural context. Bruce's arguments lead to points of agreement and disagreement with Petrinovich and Mook, as well as to specific recommendations on how the study of memory should proceed.

Sinnott's chapter on general systems theory is the last of the four chapters that provide theoretical reasons for considering real-world research. Her approach is in many ways the most foreign to those of us trained in cognitive and experimental psychology. Like those of Petrinovich and Bruce, Sinnott's approach requires psychologists to consider real-world situations.

General systems theory analyzes the world in terms of interacting systems at different levels. For example, a person is a system embedded in a family system, which is itself embedded in a cultural system. The person can be considered to contain a memory system, a motivational system, a perceptual system, and other systems that all interact with each other and that all contain other component systems. Systems at all levels try to maintain continuity over time, but they must change to accommodate changes in the systems with which they interact. Systems must have a way to create and maintain boundaries, but these boundaries must be permeable enough to allow for transfer of energy and information between systems. Viewed this way, memory must be studied in a context that encompasses the systems at its own level with which it interacts as well as the systems embedded within it and the systems in which it is embedded; memory cannot be understood without reference to the natural environment of the memory system. Sinnott describes not only the advantages of a general-systems-theory approach to the study of human cognition but also the advantages in studying how cognition changes over the life span.

Combining laboratory and real-world research

In the second half of Part I, Bahrick, Rubin, Baddeley, and Landauer discuss their views and experiences in pursuing cognitive research in and out of the laboratory. Bahrick begins his chapter with a historical review. He traces the trends in research out of, into, and back out of the laboratory. Psychologists study cognition where they think they can make the most progress and where social forces outside of their discipline lead them. Next, Bahrick turns to the question of why some research should be conducted without the benefit of laboratory controls. His answer is simple and forceful: There are domains, such as the learning and retention of academic subjects, that cannot be studied in any other way. Failure to study these domains not only will leave us unable to give sound practical advice but also will leave us with inadequate theories of cognitive processes. Bahrick ends his chapter with a discussion of the multiple-regression methods used in his pioneering studies of the retention and maintenance of knowledge.

Rubin argues that at our present state of knowledge, it is more important to uncover and quantify the regularities present in complex cognitive tasks than it is to exert experimental control. This state of affairs should change as our theories become more sophisticated and we begin to understand the regularities found. The real world is chosen over the laboratory as a place to study cognition because, counter to what most researchers seem to expect, people display more regular behavior in less controlled situations. The rationale for this argument and its statistical implications are explored. Rubin then describes three heuristics to increase the chances of finding regular data and demonstrates their value using examples from research on long-term memory.

Baddeley begins by noting that British studies of memory, traced from Galton through Bartlett to contemporary work, have always maintained an interest in real-world problems. It is probably no accident that the major center for the study of memory in the United Kingdom, of which Baddeley is the director, is called the *Applied* Psychology Unit. Baddeley illustrates the benefits and difficulties of pursuing an approach based in large part on the functional role of cognition by citing examples from his own studies of working memory, memory questionnaires to assess loss after closed-head injury, and a new standardized test to probe everyday memory loss in amnesic patients. Baddeley then considers ways in which naturalistic memory studies can be used to advance theory. Again using an example from his own work, he shows how one of the most practical of everyday-memory questions (Where did I park the car?) can be used to throw light on laboratory theories of forgetting based on decay, interference, and trace discrimination.

Landauer completes Part I by reviewing some good and bad reasons for choosing to study cognition outside of the laboratory. The list of bad reasons that have been advanced by some researchers includes claims that laboratory studies produce erroneous results (he shows that they do not) and that laboratories do not generate enough ideas (he shows that they do). The list of good reasons to move outside of the laboratory has to do with the availability of tests of adequacy, setting the problems for research, and the support of invention. This last good reason holds fascinating possibilities. The introduction of writing and, later, printing technologies greatly changed the way in which people performed cognitive tasks. The introduction of computer technologies probably will do the same. If only we knew enough about what cognitive prosthetics would be useful, we probably would have the technology to develop them. Landauer provides examples from his own work and the work of others to illustrate his points and to suggest paths to follow.

The eight chapters in Part I should provide the reader with a collection of well-articulated, well-reasoned, and often contradictory rationales and plans regarding how to proceed with research. With luck, they may improve the way future research is done. At the least, they should lead to less naive and less arbitrary rationales for choosing the setting of that research.

Part IA

Systematic approaches to laboratory and real-world research

2 Representative design and the quality of generalization

Lewis Petrinovich

I consider the title of this section of the conference, "Theoretical Reasons for a Choice" (between the laboratory and everyday life), to be a bit misleading because, really, there is no necessity for choice. The issue should be considered from the perspective of adopting sampling strategies that will support the scientific generalization to be drawn: Do the sampling procedures support the inference from the particular samples chosen to the universes of interest?

Brunswikian representative design

To begin, I shall briefly describe some Brunswikian views regarding research strategies and develop these ideas within a sampling framework. Brunswik (1952, 1956) argued that we should build a science adequate to understand the behavior of organisms in their environment and should adopt research strategies appropriate to that undertaking. Because behavior takes place in a semichaotic medium that contains cues of limited trustworthiness, expressed vicariously, a research strategy different from those usually advocated will be necessary to realize this understanding. This strategy is called probabilistic functionalism; it utilizes representative design and is adequate to the task of conceptualizing and understanding complex behavior (Petrinovich, 1979). Unfortunately, it is not a simple conceptualization, nor is it easy to implement.

The Brunswikian argument can be conceived as an exercise in sampling theory. First, there is agreement between proponents of representative design and systematic design that it is essential to obtain a representative sample of subjects on which to base theoretical conclusions of general applicability. Brunswik insisted that it is equally important to obtain an adequate sample of distal stimuli, part of what many people mean when they speak of situational or contextual sampling.

The ideas expressed in this chapter have benefited from many discussions I have had with Dr. Keith Widaman. The bird research was supported by grants from the University of California, the National Institutes of Health (grants HD 04343 and MH 38782), and the National Science Foundation (grants BNS 7914126 and BNS 8004540).

This conception of distal stimuli also demands representative sampling of objects within representative samples of situations.

I have argued that psychology has a reigning paradigm, in the Kuhnian sense, and this paradigm is that of systematic design. This classic view is that an investigator should systematically include and exclude factors and manipulate variables systematically as the investigator deems useful and appropriate. I have documented the steps of this argument elsewhere (Petrinovich, 1979, 1980, 1981) and shall not pursue it here, except to say that it is nomothetic (seeks general laws), it carefully samples subjects, it ignores situation sampling, it ignores object sampling by arbitrarily selecting stimulus values to be manipulated, it arbitrarily selects responses to be measured, and, both conceptually and statistically, it considers individual differences to be unwanted error variance.

The alternative paradigm that has long been available is that of representative design. This design is based on the assumption that it is necessary not only to study the organism and its adjustment capacities but also to understand the situations in which stimuli are encountered, and then representatively sample stimuli from that population of situations.

Brunswik cautioned against the tendency to succumb to the nomothetic bias: a tendency to develop general laws by using analytic strategies that ignore individual differences through the simple expediency of consigning them to an error term. The usual interest in the search for general theoretical laws is to see through individual differences to arrive at overriding principles. Usually, there is little concern for the niceties of measurement in this enterprise. For how many experimental tasks are the reliabilities known, and how often in the experimental literature is concern shown for such things as method variance when making trait attributions? There is also a lack of concern regarding the focus of generalizations. Often, a generalization is made to conditions; yet the degrees of freedom for significance tests are based on subjects (Hammond, 1954).

One should always be alert to the behavioral regularities of the individual case: the idiographic approach. Estes (1956) and Sidman (1960) argued convincingly that it is a risky business to derive laws of behavior from averaged group data, because the general laws might not typify a single one of the subjects. Estes (1956) pointed out that if learning takes place completely in one trial, and if different individuals make the association on different trials, and if these individual differences are normally distributed, one will get the typical S-shaped acquisition curve, although every subject will display a zero-one step function.

Only after a number of individual cases have been studied is it proper to aggregate data into general expressions. The laws for the individual should be determined, and then classes of individuals can be identified. Petrinovich and Widaman (1984) evaluated the operating characteristics of different analytic strategies using both computer simulations and some real data from a study of the behavior of birds hearing the playback of song. It was found, as Estes warned, that there might be more than one universe involved in terms of the factors regulating response changes. Group analyses (repeated measures ANOVA or regression) of data obtained in situations in which all subjects were treated alike indicated overall significant effects, because the results for the majority of the cases were large enough to swamp the effects of the minority who did not behave in the majority manner. When individuals were classified into response types (using statistical criteria), it was possible to identify systematic effects that abridged what appeared to be a general nomothetic law. It was then possible to cast a family of laws: Different subgroups displayed completely different regularities.

The meaning of ecological and functional validity

I shall now develop an argument that I believe offers a different kind of "anything goes" than that of either the revisionist laboratoryists (Mook, 1983) or the epistemological anarchists (Feyerabend, 1975). First of all, variables differ in the degree to which they are related to behavioral events, and these relationships should be objects of study. This quality of relationship between distal events and proximal stimulation is their ecological validity: the degree of trustworthiness of proximal stimulus elements to mediate distal events. Some stimuli, for example, are unfailing indicators of an event (they have a high ecological validity), whereas others are present only some of the times the event occurs (they have a low ecological validity).

There is an almost universal misunderstanding of Brunswik's concept of ecological validity; it does *not* refer to the naturalness of a research setting, but is a technical, specialized term within the Brunswikian system. "Ecological validity" refers to the potential *utility* of various cues for organisms in their ecology, and "representative design" refers to the quality of naturalness, or lifelikeness, of the research.

Ken Hammond (1978) pointed out that the Brunswikian meaning of "ecological validity" was established for three decades (1947–77), but that its meaning has been eroded. People now speak in terms of the ecological validity of an experiment when they really mean the representativeness of the design (Bandura, 1978; Bronfenbrenner, 1977; Erickson, Poon, & Walsh-Sweeney, 1980; Lachman & Lachman, 1980; Neisser, 1976; Parke, 1976; Perlmutter, 1980).

Misconstruing the technical meaning of ecological validity, and its distinction from functional validity, can lead to a misunderstanding of Brunswik's conceptions. Thus, Stokols (1982) stated that Brunswik construed the environment only in terms of its objective, material features and neglected consideration of the objective and subjective elements of the environment within the same analysis. This misconception is based on a failure to appreciate the difference between ecological validity and functional validity.

"Ecological validity" refers to the structure of the environment, and "functional validity" to the organism's use of that structure. An organism might not use a stimulus (it is assigned a low functional validity) even though it is a good stimulus (has a high ecological validity). Conversely, a stimulus with low ecological validity can have a high functional reliability: The organism employs it constantly in spite of its lack of usefulness—at a cost to the organism's success.

Perhaps it is enough that people are now concerned with the problem of representativeness, and the technical Brunswikian term should be surrendered. The distinction between ecological validity and functional validity is, however, a valuable one and should not be obscured.

Characteristics of controlled experimentation

The traditional single-variable experiment is not suited to the task of constructing a complete behavioral science, because of its capacity to magnify the size of the effect of one variable through control of others. This does not mean that traditional single-variable laboratory research is of no use. It can be used to determine the *possibility* that a variable is important and to investigate the processes through which the variable's action is mediated, but it falls short of being adequate to determine the *probability* that a variable controls any given proportion of the variance.

If I am a sufficiently good experimenter, and I have an independent variable that controls only a thousandth of 1% of the total variance, I should be able to make the dependent variable jump hoops (or null-hypothesis barriers) with consummate ease. The very strength of the true experiment results in an inherent limitation to the quality of generalization, especially regarding causal events.

One method, be it contextualism or laboratoryism, cannot provide the royal road to truth. The key to understanding involves a clear conceptualization of the generalization to be made. I can study the nictitating membrane of the rabbit, can condition it, and can write a treatise of the psychology of learning, conditioning, and memory of the rabbit nictitating membrane. There is no problem with this; it can be a valuable and valid scientific enterprise. The preparation is explicitly described, and the boundaries of the theoretical concerns and generalizations are explicit.

A problem occurs if I extend the meaning and talk of rabbits, of learning, or of conditioning. If I want to talk of rabbit learning, I have to demonstrate that the nictitating-membrane preparation provides an adequate basis for theoretical generalization. If I want to talk of the laws of conditioning, I have to demonstrate that the principles I have derived can be used to encompass the subject of conditioning. I cannot merely rely on the assumption that there is a continuous uniformity across nature in terms of such things as the basic associative building blocks, as did James Mill, Thorndike, and Hull, for example. Such an assumption of uniformity should not be a conclusion, but should be an entirely new hypothesis that merits investigation.

Indeed, if the focus is on physiological mediation, or on the responses of sensory systems to defined classes of stimulation, the laboratory is the preferred arena for such study. Whenever a generalization is made to complex behavior, the study must move to a representative sample of the contexts in which those behaviors are displayed. We know that the expression of a variable can be completely suppressed, or even reversed, when variables other than the one we have considered are present in representative situations.

The universe of generalization

Cronbach, Gleser, Nanda, and Rajaratnam (1972) have developed a multivariate view of reliability that sharpens the concept of the universe of generalization for a given observation. An observed score can be considered to be a representative of a universe of conditions (e.g., raters, tasks, stimuli presented, day and hour, settings) and of subjects and can be generalized well to some universe of scores, and poorly to others.

"The decision maker is almost never interested in the response given to the particular stimulus objects or questions, to the particular tester, at the particular moment of testing. . . . The universe of interest to the decision maker is defined when he tells us what observations would be equally acceptable for his purpose" (Cronbach et al., 1972, p. 15). An observation should be considered to be representative of a number of different universes of generalization; it might provide adequate support for some generalizations and be inadequate for others.

It is also essential that the natural correlations (the intraecological correlations) among variables be preserved to permit meaningful generalizations regarding the interaction of variables. When factorial design is used, variables often are set in orthogonal relation to one another, and different cells have equal *n*'s to facilitate computation. Using factorial design in this way obscures an understanding of the relative effects of the different factors and their interactions. The issue becomes, then, one of defining universes of generalization in a clear and detailed fashion and then making observations in such a way that they are representative of those universes.

Reactions to Brunswikian principles

I am pleased that some of the foregoing message is coming to be appreciated, especially by investigators in such fields as environmental psychology, social psychology, health psychology, personality assessment, and cognitive psychology, as well as by many doing research in settings of the kinds discussed at this conference. Most of psychology, like much of sociology (as far as I am aware), had rejected the ideal of representative design and, in the quest for certainty that characterized the postintrospection period, had adopted the Newtonian ideal of the older physical sciences.

I suppose I should take it as a positive sign that the Brunswikian research strategies are not being ignored completely, as was the case for many years. Unfortunately, this recognition often amounts to little more than lip service, sometimes accompanied by misunderstanding, and finally, missing the point of the argument.

For example, in 1983, Mook, like Henshel earlier (1980), argued the merits of the artificiality of the laboratory setting on the grounds that generalizations to the real world may not necessarily be intended. Mook (1983, p. 382) maintains that findings in the laboratory have added force because of the artificiality of the setting: "We may demonstrate the power of a phenomenon by showing that it happens even under unnatural conditions that ought to preclude it." Mook appeals to the importance of theory development because it is "theories that generalize to the real world if anything does," and "research findings are interesting because they lead to theory."

Mook (Chapter 3, this volume) is the victim of two serious misconstruals: One is the conflation of the Brunswikian conception of representativeness with randomness, and the other regards the concept of generalization. Random sampling is only one way to obtain a representative sample. We are all aware that often there are more efficient methods to obtain representative samples, depending on the ethics and economies involved. For example, pollsters effectively use stratified sampling, and cross-cultural studies are focused on one or a few variables of interest (such as breast-feeding practices) with samples of cultures drawn along the dimensions of interest. There is no reason to take leave of our senses and conclude that if we cannot randomly sample cultures, for example, we cannot meaningfully study the question of cross-cultural universals or specificity. The logic requires us only to obtain a representative sample.

In the research on universals in facial expression conducted by Ekman (1973), cultures were chosen for study because of varying degrees of exposure to modern Western cultural influences. The sampling problems that Ekman identified involved ensuring that a situation was chosen that would arouse the same emotion in each culture and that the chosen situation would not involve the use of different display rules in two cultures. Ekman's generalizations were based on studies in 13 literate cultures and 2 visually isolated preliterate cultures. There was no attempt to obtain a random sample of anything; the attempt was to identify those factors that were important for the theoretical concerns and to control, experimentally or statistically, suspected nuisance parameters. The problem of the distribution of patterns of experimental factors in a study of interactions becomes immensely difficult and complicated, as Meehl (1986) has outlined in a compelling discussion of issues that "social scientists don't understand."

The question "Representative of what?" raises the second misconstrual: that regarding the concept of generalization. I am convinced that everything a research scientist does is intended to be generalized to something. The only possible exception I can conceive arises when one is interested in knowing only about this individual, at this time, and in this place, and I believe that that is seldom, if ever, of interest.

Consider, for example, the study of Brown and Hanlon (1970), which Mook (Chapter 3, this volume) cites as an instance in which there was no interest in representative sampling of children: "The conclusions drawn do not depend on generalizing the results to any population whatever." A careful reading of the

Brown and Hanlon paper, however, makes it clear that subject sampling was of little consequence because of the special nature of the theory being examined.

Their conceptions are based on Chomsky's theory that language development is a performance event mapped onto an innate, universal, underlying competence. Thus, Brown and Hanlon (1970, pp. 160–1) are interested in "children," and the "generative grammar is intended to represent the linguistic knowledge of the native speaker," and because "a grammar formalizes adult knowledge it is reasonable to hypothesize that the child's knowledge of the structure of his language grows from that which is, in the grammar, less complex to that which is derivationally more complex."

It is clear that when conceiving of universals in this way, subject sampling is of no concern, by definition. It is also clear that this assumption could itself be questioned, and a representative sampling of subjects would thereby be in order. Brown and Hanlon (1970, p. 203) conclude that "the fact that some ungrammatical or immature forms have been used by all the children that have been studied shows that all children are alike in the innate knowledge, language processing routines, preferences, and assumptions they bring to the problem of language acquisition."

Brown and Hanlon do take elaborate pains to describe and justify the representativeness of the sample of sentence types on which they base their conclusions. They also speak to the representativeness of their methods of recording parent-child interactions (p. 194), because these, too, could restrict the generality of their conclusions. There was, therefore, great concern in their study for the representativeness of those aspects that would be variable in terms of the theory under consideration.

A theory is always a general statement about some specific set of occurrences. This set of occurrences can be conceived to be universal, to hold widely, to apply only to certain individuals at certain times and places, or to apply only to this individual in this place. A theory always applies to some universe of occurrences, and the question of sampling representativeness always rears its ugly head whenever a theory is about anything.

I agree completely that the development of sound theory is the concern of paramount importance, but I must emphasize again that the inherent power of laboratory procedures to control experimentally all variables except those of interest to the experimenter makes the laboratory an almost impossible place to develop general behavior theory. By "general theory" I mean theory adequate to understand the magnitudes of effects and interactions of different variables in a broader context than that the experimenter has used. If the intraecological correlation of variables influencing the behavior of interest is not maintained, we can examine only possibilities concerning the effects of variables, and we cannot address the central question of probabilities.

It is possible that, when present, a given independent variable will control all of the variance in a dependent variable, but if it is present in only 1% of representative situations, then a theory built on that variable will have no predictive value and will lead to little increase in understanding. If one is interested in understanding the behavior of organisms in their environment, an understanding of only 1% of instances is not enough; one is still 99% ignorant. Further, if standard design procedures are used, and if factors are represented in the experiment with equal densities, there will be no way of ever appreciating the fact that only a limited subset of the phenomena toward which the theory is directed has been investigated.

It is possible to force a change in variables of interest by using the single-variable strategy. However, when variables are isolated, one cannot support a generalization that the observed causal mechanism extends beyond the laboratory and the specific arrangements of variables that have been studied. The identities of causal factors and their relative importances can be inferred only when variables are represented with the distribution and density with which they occur in the universe of generalization.

Mook's argument that correlating any single variable with an outcome will give only false negatives is based on a narrow and restrictive view of correlational methods. Modern methods of causal analysis, such as structural-equation modeling, are consistent with the Brunswikian view that independent variables are organized hierarchically and operate in a vicarious fashion. A full causal model permits the detection and understanding of such multiple causal determinants. Indeed, multivariate correlational methods probably are the only methods that will permit the realization of such redundant, multiple, and vicarious causal networks.

It has been argued that one value of laboratory investigations is that one can test arrangements of variables that are important for theory, even though those arrangements may not frequently occur in nature. Although that is true, the question of generalization surfaces whenever theory is applied beyond the immediate test situation.

If one wishes to understand receptor processes, for example, the laboratory is the best place to be. Problems arise, however, when one moves from the level of receptor processes to perception. The cues for depth perception have been known for many years, and their ecological reliability and validity have been studied in laboratory settings. However, representative studies of depth perception by J. J. Gibson (1979) revealed that none of the classic cues for depth perception predicted the success or failure of student pilots making the depth judgments involved while actually landing an airplane.

The permissible extent of a theoretical generalization is never known until the particular experimental conditions, task variables, and subjects used in a study are transcended. We may, as Mook (1983) points out, care about only an arbitrarily selected set of "processes of interest," and there may be no interest in naturalness. I agree that it is not naturalness we care about—it is representativeness, from a sampling point of view, to the universe of generalization. Representativeness can be obtained only if it is accompanied by an adequate definition of the universe of instances and situations in terms of the intended theoretical generalization.

The laboratory seldom defines the population of generalization, even when that population can be defined. The problem arises when one moves beyond the study of isolated monkeys, for example, and offers a generalization regarding a theory of drive reduction. Drive-reduction theory has been couched in general terms, and its inapplicability in a limited experimental situation does not falsify the theory any more than a deprivation experiment can falsify models of normal behavioral or physiological development (Lorenz, 1935/1965). Failure to find a predicted effect in a specific experimental situation may be due to a bizarre combination of variables that exists only in the laboratory, a combination that might never be encountered in situations to which the theory is generalized. This failure of prediction might lead to additional studies aimed at identifying the reasons for the failure and might thereby limit the scope of generalization.

Thus, Mook's argument is based on a failure to appreciate the requirements of representative sampling from the universe of theoretical generalization. I conclude that laboratoryists such as Mook must fall back to the failed inductivist principles of logical positivism, according to which all theoretical statements must be reduced to a logically equivalent observational statement. This faith in positivism is accompanied by a hope based on the possibility of serendipity and is bolstered by a bit of what Kaplan (1964) called the Drunkard's Search—to be sure, the laws of behavior may not be found here in the laboratory, but the light is better than back there in the universe of generalization.

A research example: Bird-song development

To leave the level of pronunciamentos for a moment, I shall offer a concrete example of the result of overgeneralization in my own research area. I study the development of song in the white-crowned sparrow (*Zonotrichia leucophrys nuttalli*). Hand-raised birds are placed in acoustic isolation at different ages and exposed to tutor songs that have different characteristics (Petrinovich, 1985). One goal of this research is to understand the proximate mechanisms involved in song learning and performance and in relating these to the ultimate evolutionary significance of learned song dialects.

All of the early research bearing on this question had been done using tape-recorded songs as the stimulus material, because the use of tape recordings affords good control of factors involved in stimulus presentation. The generalizations regarding the nature of song development (Marler, 1970, 1976) have been widely accepted: There is a critical period for song learning between 10 and 50 days of age; the song of alien species cannot be learned; conspecific song is always learned in preference to allospecific song; learned song cannot be altered. These generalizations have provided the basis to postulate a physiological auditory gating mechanism and an environmentally influenced, genetically based song template.

It has been found, however, that the foregoing characteristics of song development apply only when song tutoring is done using tape-recorded song. When a live tutor is used, the findings are quite different: The sensitive phase is not from

10 to 50 days, but from 10 to 100 days of age (perhaps becoming less and less sensitive over that time); song of alien species can be learned from a live tutor even if there is loud conspecific song present; song learned between 10 and 50 days of age can be altered when the student bird is more than 50 days of age if the bird is exposed to a live tutor singing a different song (Baptista & Petrinovich, 1984, 1986; Petrinovich & Baptista, 1987). These results have major implications regarding the physiological mechanisms involved in song development (Petrinovich, in press), as well as for the ultimate significance of song (Petrinovich & Baptista, 1984).

Thus, an arbitrary and narrow choice of stimulus objects and situations resulted in a series of faulty generalizations. There is no problem if one is content to study the physiological mechanisms of song development when tape tutoring is used: Because of tight experimental control, questions can be asked regarding such things as the effects of different numbers of song inputs on learning (Petrinovich, 1985). The problem arises when one generalizes to song learning in the field (young birds experiencing only live tutors) and when those results are then offerred as an analogue for human speech development (Marler, 1970, 1975; Petrinovich, 1972).

Arbitrary and unrepresentative sampling of stimuli and situations has led to a theory that is protected by an unsuspected protective belt of auxiliary hypotheses and particular experimental conditions; an almost overwhelming ceteris paribus clause lurks in the theoretical fabric. If investigators had been more alert to the population of generalization and had framed studies with alternative hypotheses bearing on sampling considerations, our progress toward understanding the processes involved in song development might have proceeded more quickly.

The inadequacy of null hypotheses

For some time there has been agreement that the usual statistical procedure of null-hypothesis testing is not adequate to support a progressive scientific program (Morrison & Henkel, 1970). Popper (1962) argued that scientific progress will occur only if there is boldness in conjectures, coupled with a rigorous attempt to refute them. One should not attempt to prove one's position, but rather to specify the precise conditions under which one would be willing to give up that position, something none of us seems to do. At the very least, we should invoke the law of triviality: An experiment that will be meaningful only if it comes out in one way probably is too trivial to conduct.

No theory is true; at best, a theory can be an approximation to the truth (verisimilitude): The best we can do is cast better theories. One problem is that we can never test a theory, because it never stands in isolation, nakedly exposed to a disconfirmatory fact. Theory has what Lakatos (1970) referred to as a protective belt of auxiliary hypotheses, and the consequence of this is that theory will remain unviolated until there is a better theory to take its place.

The protective belt of auxiliary hypotheses (A) and the particular experimental conditions (C) protect the theory (T) from falsification; thus, there is never a pure test of a theory, and no experiment can ever falsify a theory. A test is always a test of the conjunction T-A-C, and usually the investigator has not been so bold as to specify precisely the conditions under which the position will be abandoned. If a prediction has been made that T-A-C will lead to a given observation (O), and if O does not occur, we cannot conclude that T is incorrect. ''Not O'' could mean ''not T,'' ''not A,'' ''not C,'' or any combination. We do not know what is falsified, and this sounds the death knell for what Lakatos (1970) referred to as naive falsification.

When one is faced with a refutation, an ad hoc explanation often is made, and there is the risk of building a degenerating scientific programme, in Lakatos's terminology. We understand and explain less and less the more we do, because each new finding makes it necessary to add another primitive term to the theory. We lose parsimony and gain post-hocness.

Meehl (1967, 1978, 1986), among others, has argued against the reasonableness and adequacy of null-hypothesis procedures on the grounds that the null inherently is false. One can even accept the fact that the null can sometimes be true, but still must reject it as a sufficient model on which to base a progressive science. When reliability of measurement increases, any variable that controls a minuscule proportion of variance in the population will be strong enough to force the rejection of the null hypothesis. We are in a situation in which as our measurement becomes more precise and reliable, and as control becomes better, the empirical criterion for theory to satisfy becomes increasingly weaker. What is needed is a scheme whereby we attempt to fit functions, as is done, for example, with signal-detection models and structural-equation modeling.

Strategies to enhance discovery

The direction of science is determined primarily by human creative imagination, not by the universe of facts that surrounds us. The facts we choose as relevant are arbitrarily selected, and their place in the theoretical fabric often is post hoc in nature. There is no effective falsification before the emergence of a new theory. This all leads me to the conclusion that because justification is logically of minor value, we should emphasize methods that will enhance discovery—the development of risky theories and the embellishment of useful auxiliary hypotheses—and these theories must be subjected to severe tests.

We should develop methods that will enhance the context of discovery—methods that will employ pluralistic yet rigorous methodology. The need is for a logical, rational context of discovery: a methodological system that will allow one to work adequately within the context of justification, while not abandoning all hope of discovery.

Although some have expressed the sentiment that one should not use a ''kitchen-sink'' or ''actuarial'' approach (doing such things as packing variables into a regression equation), I advocate just that approach. It is clear that we have, at the outset, chosen to study those variables we and others consider to be important. The problem with restricting our observations to these things is that we examine only those things we already know or suspect, and we will have a difficult time discovering unsuspected influences. One should include every variable that can be observed without damaging the main thrust of a study, and then step these background variables into the equations. In this way we can enhance the power of serendipity, discover unsuspected influences, and even identify variables that are the real underlying factors influencing those we thought were the primary causal factors. Of course, such exploratory procedures will uncover chance as well as real relationships, but cross-validation on independent samples is all that is necessary to protect against this danger.

Including such a large number of variables in multiple-regression analyses, for example, will violate one of the assumptions underlying the method: There probably will be a disproportionate number of variables compared with the number of subjects. This will be a serious problem only if the analysis is the last step in theory construction and evaluation. The spirit of the strategies suggested here is that of discovery rather than justification; if a variable has an unexpectedly strong effect, that is not the end of the road. The unexpected finding should be taken as a signal for the direction the next study should take; the new variable now should be included as a variable of major focus. In general, my advice is similar to that offered in Fowler's *Modern English Usage* (1944) regarding the split infinitive: "A real split infinitive, though not desirable in itself, is preferable to either of two things, to real ambiguity, and to patent artificiality" (p. 560). Though it may not be desirable to violate an assumption, it is preferable to do so rather than overlook important variables in the service of the automaticity of statistical assumptions.

The aim should be to build better theories, not merely to test existing theories. Analytic procedures should be chosen, not for the purity of p levels, but for the adequacy of their heuristic value. Probability levels can tell us only if there is something other than chance at work; they are *not* sufficient to develop a progressive science. Ideas lead; "facts" are arbitrary and selected and are meaningful only when they can be placed in the context of an explanatory model.

I have developed a research gambit that aims to add particulars to theories with the greatest economy of subjects and time. Emphasis is placed on the elaboration of theory through a series of constructive replications, with the goal of developing a degree of precision that will make it possible to fit curves or structural equations. Space will not permit the development of this research strategy here, and its detailed description will await another forum.

My theme has been that our goal is to develop theory that will help us understand the phenomena in which we are interested. I have maintained that the major hindrance in moving toward this goal is a clear characterization of a universe of events. Lacking this characterization, often we do not gather data that are representative of the proper universe. A major stumbling block in our scientific efforts has been the use of a method of justification that is not adequate to the task, a method that hinders the discovery of new concepts. I suggest we should adopt a pluralistic, yet rigorous, methodology that will permit the creative imagination to contribute as it will, while providing safeguards against the excesses of subjective meanderings.

References

Bandura, A. (1978). On paradigms and recycled ideologies. *Cognitive Therapy and Research, 2,* 79–103.

Baptista, L. F., & Petrinovich, L. (1984). Social interaction, sensitive phases and the song template hypothesis in the white-crowned sparrow. *Animal Behaviour, 32,* 172–181.

Baptista, L. F., & Petrinovich, L. (1986). Song development in the white-crowned sparrow: Social factors and sex differences. *Animal Behaviour, 34,* 1359–1371.

Bronfenbrenner, U. (1977). Toward an expermental ecology of human development. *American Psychologist, 32,* 513–531.

Brown, R., & Hanlon, C. (1970). Derivational complexity and order of acquisition in child speech. In J. R. Hayes (Ed.), *Cognition and the development of language* (pp. 155–207). New York: Wiley.

Brunswik, E. (1952). The conceptual framework of psychology. In *International encyclopedia of unified science* (Vol. 1). Chicago: University of Chicago Press.

Brunswik, E. (1956). *Perception and the representative design of psychological experiments.* Berkeley: University of California Press.

Cronbach, L. J., Gleser, G. C., Nanda, H., & Rajaratnam, N. (1972). *The dependability of behavioral measurements.* New York: Wiley.

Ekman, P. (1973). Cross-cultural studies of facial expression. In P. Ekman (Ed.), *Darwin and facial expression* (pp. 169–222). New York: Academic Press.

Ericson, R. C., Poon, L. W., & Walsh-Sweeney, L. (1980). Clinical memory testing of the elderly. In L. W. Poon, J. L. Fazard, L. S. Cermak, D. Arenberg, & L. W. Thompson (Eds.), *New directions in aging* (pp. 379–402). Hillsdale, NJ: Lawrence Erlbaum.

Estes, W. K. (1956). The problem of inference from curves based on group data. *Psychological Bulletin, 53,* 134–140.

Feyerabend, P. (1975). *Against method.* London: Verso Press.

Fowler, H. W. (1944). *Modern English usage.* Oxford: Oxford University Press.

Gibson, J. J. (1979). *The ecological approach to visual perception.* Boston: Houghton Mifflin.

Hammond, K. (1954). Representative vs. systematic design in clinical psychology. *Psychological Bulletin, 51,* 150–159.

Hammond, K. (1978). *Psychology's scientific revolution: Is it in danger?* Report No. 211. Boulder, CO: Center for Research on Judgment and Policy.

Henshel, R. L. (1980). The purposes of laboratory experimentation and the virtues of deliberate artificiality. *Journal of Experimental Social Psychology, 16,* 466–478.

Jenkins, J. J. (1974). Remember that old theory of memory? Well, forget it! *American Psychologist, 29,* 785–795.

Kaplan, A. (1964). *The conduct of inquiry.* San Francisco: Chandler.

Lachman, R., & Lachman, J. L. (1980). Picture naming: Retrieval and activation of long-term memory. In L. W. Poon, J. L. Fazard, L. S. Cermak, D. Arenberg, & L. W. Thompson (Eds.), *New directions in memory and aging* (pp. 313–343). Hillsdale, NJ: Lawrence Erlbaum.

Lakatos, I. (1970). Falsification and the methodology of scientific research programmes. In I. Lakatos & A. Musgrave (Eds.), *Criticism and the growth of knowledge.* Cambridge University Press.

Lorenz, K. (1965) Companions as factors in the bird's environment. In *Studies in animal and human behaviour* (Vol. I, pp. 101–258). Cambridge, MA: Harvard University Press. (Original work published 1935)

Marler, P. (1970). A comparative approach to vocal learning: Song development in white-crowned sparrows. *Journal of Comparative and Physiological Psychology Monographs, 71* (Pt. 2).

Marler, P. (1975). On the origin of speech from animal sounds. In J. F. Kavanagh & J. E. Cutting (Eds.), *The role of speech in language* (pp. 11–37). Cambridge, MA: M.I.T. Press.

Marler, P. (1976). Sensory templates in species-specific behavior. In J. C. Fentress (Ed.), *Simpler networks and behavior* (pp. 314–329). Sunderland, MA: Sinauer.

Meehl, P. E. (1967). Theory-testing in psychology and physics: A methodological paradox. *Philosophy of Science, 34,* 103–115.

Meehl, P. E. (1978). Theoretical risks and tabular asterisks: Sir Karl, Sir Ronald, and the slow progress of soft psychology. *Journal of Consulting and Clinical Psychology, 46,* 806–834.

Meehl, P. E. (1986). What social scientists don't understand. In D. W. Fiske & R. A. Shweder (Eds.), *Metatheory in social science* (pp. 315–338). Chicago: University of Chicago Press.

Mook, D. G. (1983). In defense of external invalidity. *American Psychologist, 38,* 379–387.

Morrison, D. E., & Henkel, R. E. (1970). *The significance test controversy.* Chicago: Aldine.

Neisser, U. (1976). *Cognition and reality.* San Francisco: W. H. Freeman.

Parke, R. P. (1976). Social cues, social control and ecological validity. *Merrill Palmer Quarterly, 22,* 111–123.

Perlmutter, M. (1980). An apparent paradox about memory aging. In L. W. Poon, J. L. Fazard, L. S. Cermak, D. Arenberg, & L. W. Thompson (Eds.), *New directions in memory and aging* (pp. 345–353). Hillsdale, NJ: Lawrence Erlbaum.

Petrinovich, L. (1972). Psychobiological mechanisms in language development. In G. Newton & A. H. Riesen (Eds.), *Advances in psychobiology* (Vol. 1, pp. 259–285). New York: Wiley.

Petrinovich, L. (1979). Probabilistic functionalism: A conception of research method. *American Psychologist, 34,* 373–390.

Petrinovich, L. (1980). Brunswikian behavioral biology. In K. R. Hammond & N. E. Wascoe (Eds.), *Realizations of Brunswik's representative design; new directions for methodology of social and behavioral science* (Vol. 3, pp. 85–93). San Francisco: Jossey-Bass.

Petrinovich, L. (1981). A method for the study of development. In K. Immelmann, G. Barlow, L. Petrinovich, & M. Main (Eds.), *Behavioral development* (pp. 90–130). Cambridge University Press.

Petrinovich, L. (1985). Factors influencing song development in the white-crowned sparrow (*Zonotrichia leucophrys). Journal of Comparative Psychology, 99,* 15–29.

Petrinovich, L. (in press). The role of social factors in white-crowned sparrow song development. In T. Zentall & B. G. Galef (Eds.), *Social learning: A comparative approach.* Hillsdale, NJ: Lawrence Erlbaum.

Petrinovich, L., & Baptista, L. F. (1984). Song dialects, mate selection, and breeding success in white-crowned sparrows. *Animal Behaviour, 32,* 1078–1088.

Petrinovich, L., & Baptista, L. F. (1987). Song development in the white-crowned sparrow: Modification of learned song. *Animal Behaviour, 35,* 961–974.

Petrinovich, L., & Widaman, K. F. (1984). An evaluation of statistical strategies to analyze repeated measures data. In H. V. S. Peeke & L. Petrinovich (Eds.), *Habituation, sensitization, and behavior* (pp. 17–55). New York: Academic Press.

Popper, K. R. (1962). *Conjectures and refutations: The growth of scientific knowledge.* New York: Harper & Row.

Sidman, M. (1960). *Tactics of scientific research.* New York: Basic Books.

Stokols, D. (1982). Environmental psychology: A coming of age. In A. G. Kraut (Ed.), *The G. Stanley Hall lecture series* (Vol. 2). Washington, DC: American Psychological Association.

3 The myth of external validity

Douglas G. Mook

The explosion of interest in everyday memory over the past few years has enormously enriched the field. Entire areas of investigation that were unknown a few years ago—prospective memory, for instance—are boiling with ideas and findings. The excitement of new horizons has been a large part of what has made this conference a delightful intellectual experience.

The new wave of real-world research in memory is, of course, part of a more general trend toward application and social relevance in psychology. Bahrick (Chapter 6, this volume) discusses the history of this trend as a reflection of social forces that affected the scientific enterprise across the board. Specifically within psychology, it is tempting to see it also as a continuation of our progressive liberation from the "snaffles and curbs" of orthodoxy—first structuralism, then behaviorism, then laboratory rigorism (Baddeley, Chapter 8, this volume). Cognitive scientists breathed a sigh of relief when they were given permission to study the mind. We are breathing another sigh of relief as we find that we are allowed, even encouraged (Neisser, 1976), to study *interesting things* about the mind. We have been turned loose to seek the bloody horse, and we love it.

What is worrisome about this development, however, is that it appears to be hardening into an orthodoxy of its own. Experimenters are being told that their research ought to have real-world relevance, that it must be generalizable to real life, and that a measure of its value is the variance accounted for by its manipulations and measures. This is all summed up in the phrase *external validity* (not to be confused with *ecological validity*) (Petrinovich, Chapter 2, this volume). This we can define for our purposes simply as *the extent to which experimental findings make us better able to predict real-world behavior.*

If this trend has enriched the study of behavior, it has also distorted it. For example, Ostrom (1984) has noted some unfortunate ways in which social

James Deese, Bella DePaulo, David C. Rubin, Sandra Scarr, and Sue Wagner made helpful comments on preliminary versions of this chapter. Needless to say, they do not all agree with what it says.

psychology has been affected by it. First, it has led to rejection of sound and informative laboratory research by journals whose referees reflexively insist on external validity. Second, and as a result, it has led authors in self-defense to invent slice-of-life applications for findings that in fact do not speak to real life and were not intended to. This again invites rejection, on the grounds that the generalizations to real life are not justified. Ostrom's remarks describe an intolerable catch-22: Experimenters are punished if they do not disguise their work as real-world-applicable, and they are punished if the disguise is penetrated. It is as if they were spies in enemy territory during wartime.

In this essay, my ambition is to serve as peacemaker—which probably will mean losing all my friends, in both camps. It does seem to me, though, that the quarrels between experimental scientists and external-validitorians rest on a misunderstanding—nay, a myth. That myth is that the purpose of research is to make direct predictions about real-life behavior. In fact, in the majority of cases, that may not be its purpose at all (Berkowitz & Donnerstein, 1982; Mook, 1983). It does illuminate the real world, but not in that way. And if we recognize that, the controversy disappears.

A short pantheon of myths

The myth consists of several interlocking fables. The best known are probably these: One measures some variable in a "representative sample." One then "generalizes" the findings to the "population," to say that, within a known margin of error, the population will behave as the sample did. Knowing that, we are better able to "predict behavior" in the population—especially if our independent variable "accounts for a whole lot of variance."

Is this what we actually do—or should do? Let us examine some case studies.

Case study 1: Of falling bodies

One wonders how science would have fared if it had accepted that model from the outset. To see what might have happened, consider how a modern reviewer would react to Galileo's experimental research.

Galileo, as we know, held a research grant from the duke of Tuscany, based on the relevance of his work in mechanics to a practical problem: the behavior of cannonballs in flight. But rather than study cannonballs in flight, Galileo dropped little balls straight down, and then he introduced the further distortion of an intrusive and reactive inclined plane. He did obtain lawful functional relations—in that artificial setting—and he put his findings together as the famous *law of falling bodies*, $d = kt^2$, where d is distance fallen, t is time, and k depends on such factors as the units of measurement and what planet one is standing on.

We treat this law as a landmark in the history of science. But the duke's review panel might have said, What of its external validity? Galileo was dealing with a highly biased sample of falling objects—objects heavy enough to make air resistance and air currents negligible. Research using more natural material shows his conclusions to be of terribly limited generality and robustness.

Galileo's equation treats *time* as the independent variable. But in the real world, how much of the variance in distance fallen is accounted for by time? If one deals with cannonballs, a considerable amount. But for falling rain, it is much less; for falling snow, less still; for falling leaves, well. . . . Considering that rain, snow, and leaves surely account for at least 99% of the falling that occurs in nature, it all begins to look pretty restricted.

Worse, Galileo entirely ignored the most important variable of all, the one that accounts for the overwhelming preponderance of the variance in distance fallen: Is there, or is there not, something underneath the object that prevents it from falling? If our objective is to account for variance in natural events, we must fault Galileo seriously for his neglect of support systems.

Now, this is a caricature of the external-validity argument—an unfair one, like all caricatures—and yet there is a serious point secreted here. *A variable that is theoretically trivial can be of overwhelming real-world importance*—and conversely. We shall return to that idea. But first, let us look at examples from psychological research.

Case study 2: The subjects

A central concept of external validity has been with us for a long time, as applied to the sampling of subjects. Thus, Petrinovich (Chapter 2, this volume) says that "there is agreement . . . that it is essential to obtain a representative sample of subjects on which to base theoretical conclusions of general applicability." Yes, there is such agreement, I'm afraid; but what we agree on is wrong, and it has given rise to ferocious confusion. In fact, the notion that we *need* a representative sample of some population is mostly myth. To see why, consider as a case study the investigation of children's speech by Brown and Hanlon (1970).

The study by Brown and Hanlon challenged a powerful theory of syntax acquisition, one that we took for granted for quite a long time. That is reinforcement theory, which says this: Children acquire grammatical sentence structure because parents reinforce grammatically correct speech—by approval, perhaps, or by continuing the dialogue without correcting the child's utterance. But Brown and Hanlon found that that simply is not what happens. If parents consistently reinforce any kind of sentence, it is the *true* sentence, not the grammatical sentence. Thus:

> *Child:* Mama isn't boy, he girl.
> *Parent:* That's right.
> *Child:* There's the animal farmhouse.
> *Parent:* No, that's a lighthouse.

A true, ungrammatical sentence was approved; a grammatical but untrue sentence was disapproved. Such cases were by far the most frequent in Brown and Hanlon's sample of parent–child exchanges.

The sample of subjects in their study was wildly unrepresentative of any interesting population. The subjects were children of affluent, well-educated Bostonian parents who, moreover, were willing to tolerate the intrusive presence of psychologists armed with tape recorders. Any generalizations from the data would have to be restricted to the population of atypical families like these—a severe limitation on generality.

That would be a serious criticism of the study, if generalization to a population had been intended. If Brown and Hanlon had concluded that "*X* percent of children's utterances, plus or minus *Y*, are true and are approved," they would have been in deep trouble. Their biased sample precludes any such generalization to a population even of Bostonian children. But they drew no such conclusion. Their conclusion was not about a population, but about a theory.

The logic went like this: (1) Reinforcement theory tells us that parents selectively reinforce grammatical utterances by their children. If that is so, then *these* parents should behave as the theory specifies. They do not. The prediction is disconfirmed. (2) If the theory is correct, and if *these* parents do not provide appropriate reinforcement for grammatical utterances, then *these* children should not acquire grammatical speech. But they do (at least we shall assume so, though this was not part of the study). Again the prediction is disconfirmed, and the theory is in trouble on two counts.

The important point is that the conclusions drawn do not depend on generalizing the results to any population whatever. They depend on what happened *in the sample*—on what *these* parents and *these* children were observed to do in *these* homes.

What other examples can we give? *The overwhelming majority of published papers in psychology are of this kind.* One usually does not estimate what some population of subjects will do, but rather asks whether or not *these* subjects in *this* setting behave as a theory, hunch, hypothesis, or implication (as described later) says they should. And one draws conclusions, not about a population, but about the theory, hunch, hypothesis, or implication.

As another example, consider the important role of reconstruction and inference in memory. If *these* subjects "remember" a sentence that in fact was never given them (Bransford & Franks, 1971), then it follows at once that memory is not simply the passive registration and storage of experienced events.

But, of course, that conclusion does not rest on one study alone, but on many. In one study, subjects "remembered" that their moods over the days of the preceding week had been correlated with their hours of sleep the night before, when in fact there had been no such correlation (Wilson, Laser, & Stone, 1982). In another study, subjects asked about a stop sign that was not there later "remembered" seeing one (Loftus & Palmer, 1974). John Dean "remembered" a number of things Richard Nixon never said (Neisser, 1982). And so on. Now, *not one* of these investigations took a representative sample from any identified population.

All the samples together do not add up to a representative one; biased samples added to biased samples give us biased supersamples. That is not a weakness of the research, for the issue of generalizing to a population never really arose.

Rather, it is the repeated, replicable occurrences of the effect, *in the samples and settings that were actually studied,* that tell us something about how memory works. The individual studies stand not as samples to population but as examples of a principle to the principle itself (see the later section on the analytic model), and the generality of the principle rests on the diversity—not the representativeness—of subjects and settings in which its instances arise. The external validity of individual studies, or the lack thereof, plays no part in this inductive process.

The same process can reveal the limitations of general conclusions. Over a series of studies, most of which find *X,* some studies will find "not *X.*" Mapping hits and misses over a representative sample of settings and manipulations will not tell us why. Rather, someone must suggest a *variable, Z,* that underlies the discrepancy—*X* if *Z,* "not *X*" if "not *Z*"—and design an experiment to test that idea. Then the findings of that experiment, too, will be tested by further systematic replication and variation, until the limiting conditions for the principle are clear.

Case study 3: The setting

The myth of representative sampling has itself been generalized. We are asked, following Brunswik (Petrinovich, Chapter 2, this volume), to extend it to the research *setting* as well as to the subjects we use.

Neisser's call (1976) for the study of real-life phenomena was widely misinterpreted as a call for an approach of this kind:

> There is still no account of how people act in or interact with the real world. . . . This trend can only be reversed, I think, if the study of cognition takes a more "realistic" turn, in several senses of the word. First, cognitive psychologists must make a greater effort to understand cognition as it occurs in the ordinary environment. . . . Second, it will be necessary to pay more attention to the details of the real world in which perceivers and thinkers live, and the fine structure of information which that world makes available to them. . . . Third, psychology must somehow come to terms with the sophistication and complexity of the cognitive skills that people are really capable of acquiring. . . . A satisfactory theory of human cognition can hardly be established by experiments that provide inexperienced subjects with brief opportunities to perform novel and meaningless tasks. (Neisser, 1976, pp. 7–8)

This good advice has been misunderstood. Neisser asks us to study the complex information the real world provides, given the complex knowledge structures the real-world subject possesses. But he never says that we must study these processes *in* the real world, or in settings drawn from it.

In fact, Neisser's own research, and the research he cites with approval, does nothing of the sort. A few pages later, he describes Johansson's classic study (1973) in which people walked around a darkened room with small light bulbs attached to their joints. Subjects who were shown a movie that showed only the lights reported that they saw people walking. Subjects who looked at still frames saw only meaningless patterns of dots.

Could we find a more blatant case of external invalidity? Does your representative *Homo sapiens* walk around in the dark with light bulbs on his knees? Does he watch other people doing so? Are we going to generalize these findings and attempt to predict how a population will react to ambulant Christmas trees? I do not think so. We are asking a question: How much information is required to support the perception of a person walking? By darkening the room, we remove all visual information. Then, by turning on the little lights and letting the person move—thereby creating a setting and a stimulus never before seen on land or sea—we put a bit of the information back (the counterexperiment, as described later). And we discover that that bit is enough.

Case study 4: The manipulation

Let us turn to a third element in external validity: the naturalness of the manipulation. This will invite us to look at another pervasive myth: that worthwhile manipulations are those that account for real-world variance in the measures we take. We have an excellent counterexample in the experiments of Stine, Wingfield, and Poon (Chapter 13, this volume). In their first experiment, Stine and associates showed that elderly subjects, hearing random words at a speeded-up rate, did very poorly on a test of memory. Then they added *syntactic constraints* to the material; it was still nonsense, but grammatical nonsense. Memory in the aged was much improved; the older subjects did about as well as younger ones with such material.

Now consider this: How much of the variance in real-world discourse is accounted for by syntactic constraints? None. Why not? Because in nature, the presence or absence of constraints is not a variable. All natural discourse embodies such constraints. The great importance of syntactic constraint could never have been discovered by sampling from, or mimicking, the natural world. *Nor does knowing about it help us predict anything about the real world.* It does help us *understand* how real-world speech is processed—a quite different thing.

This example should give us serious pause. How many variables exert powerful real-life effects, and account for a lot of the variance, simply because in nature they vary over a wide range? How many variables or mechanisms are there that are crucial to an understanding of what is going on, but do not account for much variance because, in nature, they do not vary?

If we take that question home and worry about it, we shall find ourselves having second thoughts not only about the myth of "variance accounted for" but also about some of our methods that depend on it, such as multiple-regression methods (Bahrick, Chapter 6, this volume). Do they tap the most important variables, or only the most variable variables? To find out, we must go beyond them.

We also have second thoughts about Brunswik's representative designs (Petrinovich, Chapter 2, this volume). Brunswik's research concerned an organisms's use of environmental cues for such purposes as self-location and navigation within the world. One may determine the ecological validity of a cue (e.g., retinal size) by noting its correlation with a distal variable (e.g., distance). One may determine its functional validity by correlating it with the creature's behavior (e.g., judgments of distance). Ecological validity limits the use a creature can make of a proximal cue; functional validity tells us the use it does make of that cue.

Unfortunately, no variable can have either ecological or functional validity unless it is correlated with something, and it cannot be correlated with anything unless it varies. Thus, representative design, though perfectly suited for the questions Brunswik addressed, is nearly useless for the analysis of mechanism. Important but *invariant* real-world processes fall through its net at the outset.

A final point before moving on. We have focused on "variance accounted for" as the traditional measure of the magnitude of an effect. That measure has come under question, and there may be better measures (Abelson, 1985; Rosenthal & Rubin, 1979). If so, the current argument applies to those, too. The important point is that the real-world *magnitude* of an effect is simply not a good index of its *importance* for our understanding of the system.

A look forward: The problem of generality

This way of looking at the matter does go hard against our grain. That is because—so I argue—we are steeped in mythology. I mentioned earlier our "understanding of the system." But whose system? I have said that the results of Stine and associates tell us something about "how memory works." But whose memory, and when? What if subjects from other cultures had been used? Chimpanzees? Different materials? What if the room had been painted blue? And so on for a thousand what-ifs. To whom and to what do the results apply?

Well, because I am losing friends anyway, let me suggest that these actually are not very interesting questions and are not questions we need to ask—not now. The fact is, we do not really care whether or not the specific results of Stine and associates apply to, say, gondoliers in Venice—unless the *principles* drawn from them turn out not to apply. That would be interesting, for it would suggest that some variable(s) correlated with culture affect how speech is processed and how aging affects this. But if that is so, we can discover the fact in other ways. As our understanding of memory develops, someone sooner or later will ask, perhaps with entirely different experiments, if the same principles apply to Venetians or vervets or in rooms painted violet. If they do not, then the development of theory must take account of the variables so implicated. Direct generalization of the original findings has little to do with the matter.

Prediction or understanding?

We indicated at the outset that notions of representative sampling, generalizing to populations, and accounting for lots of variance are subsidiary fables within the major myth: that the aim of research is to make predictions about the real world. We turn now to a critique of that superordinate myth.

The research enterprise often is treated as a matter of identifying the variables with which behavior covaries. We thus become better and better able to predict behavior by entering values of these independent variables and solving for the value of our behavior measure. The image of a multiple-regression equation comes readily to mind.

From this perspective, a common criticism of experiments is that they inflate the effects of the variable(s) manipulated. They make them seem more predictive than they are. Thus, "if I am a sufficiently good experimenter, and I have an independent variable that controls only a thousandth of 1% of the total variance, I should be able to make the dependent variable jump hoops (or null-hypothesis barriers) with consummate ease" (Petrinovich, Chapter 2, this volume). The remark is quite correct. Is it a criticism of traditional experiments? If *prediction* is our aim, then it is; if not, then it is not.

Behavior is subject to multiple influences, and often there are many reasons, each sufficient and none necessary, for the occurrence of an event. This is especially true where there are *redundant* controls, all designed to promote some important outcome. Such multiple-control systems are fiercely resistant to change (Sinnott, Chapter 5, this volume). As a result, one may have to inflate some important influences in order to see them at all. Again, this can best be made clear with examples.

Consider aging itself. As internally generated memory processes become less competent, the elderly person likely will rely more and more on external aids, as discussed by Moskovitch (1982) and Cohen and Faulkner (Chapter 14, this volume). The effect is that effective memory-controlled performance suffers less than it would if those external props were not available. In some contexts it may not suffer at all (Moscovitch, 1982). The increased use of one kind of support for performance compensates for a deficit in the other. That means, in turn, that laboratory studies of aging, if they deny external memory aids to the elderly, inflate the performance deficits relative to what occurs in real life. They introduce a bias that makes internally driven memory systems look more important than they are in real life. Such laboratory data are, strictly speaking, ungeneralizable! They remove a compensating memory support—the external strategies for remembering—that real life makes available.

A more detailed example is again provided by the wonderful experiments reported by Stine and associates (Chapter 13, this volume). Let us look at them from the current perspective. Look at their Figure 13.1, and focus on the lowest point: the performance of elderly subjects listening to random material at the highest speech rate. We can take this as our reference point. Performance was severely depressed relative to that of subjects who had youth, processing time (the slow rate), and syntactic constraints to work with. By making appropriate comparisons, Stine and her colleagues were able to introduce various influences, one at a time and in combination, against this background. In effect, having taken out a number of memory supports at once, they put them back in, one or a few at a time—the famous counterexperiment of Claude Bernard.

First, Stine and associates put back *syntactic constraints.* Elderly subjects listened to fast but constrained material. Performance improved relative to the background condition. Second, whatever it is that is correlated with *youth* could, in a sense, be put back in. This was done by comparing the young subjects, hearing fast random material, with the background condition (elderly subjects hearing such material). Putting back youth also improved performance, and to about the same extent as putting back syntactic constraints in elderly subjects. Putting back both youth and constraints (by comparing "young fast constrained" with "elderly fast random") improved performance only a little more than did putting back either one of them (note the small differences in the middle panel). These two variables, youth and syntactic constraint, are interchangeable in the multiple-control system; either can compensate for the absence of the other, and their relation to each other is occlusive. (Pop goes another myth. It simply is not true that experimental analysis commits us to a linear, "*a* causes *b* causes *c*" conception of the phenomenon) (McGuire, 1973). Finally, putting back only *processing time* (the slower presentation rate) also led to some improvement, as compared with the fast presentation rate in elderly subjects.

This example makes two important points. First, by introducing each of these aids against a background of depressed performance, one can see the effect of each aid. It is unlikely that we could see these effects in any other way. Removing one or another would tell us little, for the ones remaining would compensate. For the same reason, correlating any one of them with anything else would only give us false negatives; as one support diminishes, performance does not diminish, because another support can substitute.

Indeed, it seems to me that this is the major advantage of a laboratory environment: not that it controls extraneous variables, though it does that, too, but that it permits introduction of variables of interest against a background as blank as we can make it. Within a system of multiple and redundant controls, this may be the only way of making any single influence visible.

The second point is this: The procedure, it is true, exaggerates the effect of each memory support. It makes the predictive value of each one seem much greater than it would be in real life. But that is a criticism only if our intent is real-life prediction. If our aim is an understanding of mechanism, then it is no criticism at all; it is simply irrelevant.

Let us take one more example of the difference between *prediction* and *understanding* as goals of research. We noted earlier that as people age, frequently they depend more heavily on external memory aids, thus compensating for deficits in internally generated memory support. If this is so, then age and dependence on external aids are positively correlated.

The Brunswikian perspective (Petrinovich, Chapter 2, this volume) points out correctly that the real-world predictive value of a variable depends on the effects of other variables with which it covaries (i.e., the "intraecological correlations" between one variable and another). From this perspective, it makes no sense to try to separate the effects of aging from the effects of external-aid dependence. If they vary together in nature, we should let them vary together in our observations and then determine the predictive value of the combination.

This logic cannot be faulted—if *prediction* is our aim. Indeed, the idea can be stated more generally than that. To the extent that any two independent variables are intercorrelated, we gain less predictive power by learning about either one if we already know about the other. But from the point of view of *understanding* how the system works, surely it is important to know that we have a multiple-control system here, in which a deficit in one set of operations is compensated for by another. Surely, if what we see can be produced by either of two covarying independent variables, it is important to know which is actually doing it. This is not because we can make better predictions by knowing that—perhaps we cannot—but because the mechanisms involved are very different in the two cases.

From this perspective, it would seem that Petrinovich and I have no real disagreement, just a difference in aims. When he says that "the identities of causal factors and their relative importances can be inferred only when variables are represented with the distribution and density with which they occur in the universe of generalization," he is quite right, if prediction, within the universe of generalization, is the goal. If the goal is understanding the workings of the system, the remark is quite wrong, as the foregoing examples make clear.

To summarize thus far, we have seen that every one of the canons of external validity (representativeness of subjects, manipulations, and settings; prediction of real life from experimental findings; the aim of accounting for a whole lot of real-world variance) is routinely violated in the research we do. Either we are doing something catastrophically wrong or else we are doing something different from what the external-validity notion implies. I suggest the latter. I suggest that the notions of representativeness, prediction, and external validity itself arise within one conceptual model of the aims of research. Most psychological research fits a quite different model. The next section compares these two models.

Two models for research

In previous sections, I have purposely overdrawn the picture, and now may be a good time to admit it. I do not really want to claim that external validity is *always* irrelevant, or that such requirements as representative sampling and generalizable settings are *always* mythical. Just usually.

Obviously, there are cases in which we do research specifically in order to predict what happens in the real world, or what would happen if such and such were the case. Let us call that the *analogue* model of research. Our research setting, subjects, and manipulations are models, or analogues, of the general case about which we wish to draw conclusions. The concepts and criteria of external validity may apply to research of that kind, if we intend to base a decision on the study in question.

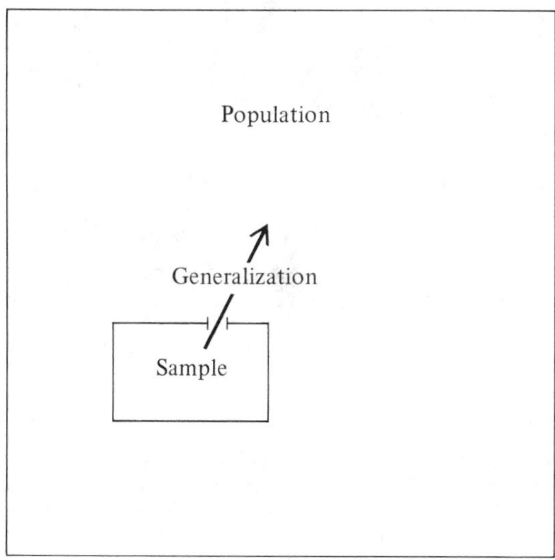

Figure 3.1. Sample, generalization, population.

Then there are the other cases, in which the aim of our research is not to predict real-world events—at least not directly. Rather, we seek to improve our understanding of the workings of a system. Then the understanding will apply to real life—the understanding, not the data, and not through generalization as we understand the term. Let us call this the *analytic* model of research. Here, the concepts and criteria of external validity are irrelevant; the issue simply does not arise.

The analogue model

The analogue model applies whenever we intend our findings to be a guide to real-world prediction or action. It is here that we find the familiar text-book rules for research—representative sampling, generalizing to a population, and the like. And with good reason. The discipline from which we borrowed these concepts—agricultural research—fits this model nicely.

The shape of such research is as shown in Figure 3.1. We draw conclusions about the general case by observing a little bit of it, called the *sample,* and from that we generalize to the population, or the "universe of generalization," from which the sample was drawn. If we are to do that with confidence, we must be assured that the sample (of subjects, settings, and manipulations) is representative of the target population to which generalization is to be made. Usually it is true that the variables that account for most variance are the most important, because they add the greatest increments to our ability to predict.

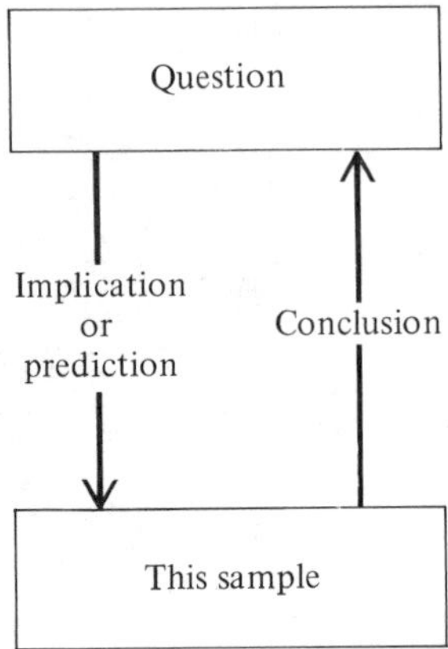

Figure 3.2. Question, implication, sample, conclusion.

One example that fits this model is survey research. Another is outcome research—research designed to try out an intervention technique. A method of memory training in aged persons may be tried in a sample of cases, with an eye to implementing it on a broader scale (i.e., in the population) if the results in the sample make it look promising. We have many excellent examples before us in the last section of this volume.

Finally, the analogue model lays out for us the answers to the tactical questions that were posed in the Introduction to Part I: How do we move from the laboratory to the real world? By generalizing to the population of subjects, settings, and manipulations from which our sample was drawn. When do we do it? In the discussion section. And why? Because that was our intention from the outset; we designed and conducted the experiment in the first place so that we could learn about real life from what the results showed.

I should make it clear that my intent is not to attack this kind of research—only to distinguish it from the other kind. There is absolutely nothing wrong with it; it is a necessary and valuable kind of research. Our mistake has been to treat *all* research as if it fit this mold—which takes us to the other model.

The analytic model

This second model characterizes most of the work done by experimental psychologists, experimental physiologists, cognitive scientists, and others concerned with understanding the behaving organism as a functioning system. The shape of this kind of research is shown in Figure 3.2. I have called this analytic research, but with some discomfort. In writing about this matter earlier (Mook, 1983), I spoke of it as research designed to test theory. That is misleading, because it connotes formal theory testing and the hypotheticodeductive method; it can even be confused with logical positivism. But the word "analytic" is also misleading, for it connotes an exclusive concern with how the system works, as opposed to why (Bruce, Chapter 4, this volume).

Because a good one-word name has eluded me, let me try to explain what is meant. It is a matter of *asking a question,* where the question leads to an implication about what the data should show if the answer is such and such. Examples include the following:

1. Does syntactic structure aid retention? If it does, subjects should remember structured material better than random material (an implication, but hardly a theoretical triumph). We look to see whether or not, in *these* subjects, this is so.
2. Does working memory serve an important function in reading? If so, working-memory performance should be correlated with reading skill. Is it—in *these* subjects? This example, from Bruce (Chapter 4, this volume), shows that functional questions dealing with what memory is for and how it serves us can also fit this question-and-answer model.
3. What is the forgetting curve (Bahrick, 1984) for schoolroom Spanish, in *these* subjects who studied it varying numbers of years ago? That is an exploratory question, in the "context of discovery." The analytic model is not limited to theory testing in the "context of verification," as my earlier discussion may have implied (Mook, 1983).

Looking again at Figure 3.2, we see that the shape of this kind of research is entirely different from that of analogue research (Figure 3.1). There is no *population;* so the notion of *representativeness* simply does not apply. There is no step called *generalization.* We do not measure a sample to estimate what the general case is like. Rather, we ask: How do *these* subjects, in *this* setting, respond to *this* manipulation? Knowing their response, we answer our question.

Of models and settings

The analogue/analytic distinction is orthogonal to the distinction, itself not a sharp one, between laboratory and real-world research. Table 3.1 shows the resulting fourfold division. In cell A, we have laboratory analogue research. Much of medical research is of this kind: One does laboratory tests for therapeutic efficacy or toxicity of a drug, in order to know what to expect of it in real-world application. In psychology, any case in which the laboratory setting is designed to model and predict real-world phenomena falls here. For example, Kurt Lewin's group-dynamics experiments were of this kind. His studies of democratic versus authoritarian group structures, modeled in the laboratory, were intended to be generalized, to illuminate the costs and benefits of each kind of structure in the world of affairs. (Of course, we would now say that Lewin's sampling procedures, for settings and manipulations even more than for subjects, were inadequate to the task. The criteria of external validity apply to this cell, when the research is used for such purposes, and Lewin's experiments did not meet them.)

Table 3.1

Model	Laboratory	Natural environment
Analogue	A: Laboratory analogues or models of real-life phenomena, designed to predict events in, or to estimate the characteristics of, a population of natural events	B: Field observations, experiments, or correlational studies designed to predict or estimate events or characteristics of a population of such events
Analytic	C: Laboratory investigations of the functions or mechanisms of mind or behavior	D: Field observations, experiments, or correlational studies designed to elucidate the functions or mechanisms of mind or behavior

In cell B, we have real-life analogue research. We generalize what happens in the real-world sample to the real-world population. Survey or marketing research is the prototype here, but much outcome research, in which the therapeutic intervention and follow-up occur in the real world, also fits.

Cell C gives us laboratory analytic research. This, of course, is the traditional home of the experimental psychologist. The experiments of Stine and associates and Johansson's walking-lights experiments fit nicely.

Finally, in cell D we have real-life analytic research. Here we place any field experiment or correlational study designed to test a theory or to put a question to *these* subjects under *these* conditions. Examples are the Brown and Hanlon study of children's grammar, Bahrick's study (1984) of retention of Spanish, and many of the studies of reconstructive or theory-driven memory that happen to have been conducted in a natural environment.

It is worth noting that in cell D, the naturalness of the setting has no special virtue. As with laboratory research, field research of this kind chooses its settings and materials for convenience and for relevance to the question. It is true that field conditions are more variable, and if a manipulation cuts through this variability to have a significant effect, one has more confidence in the power of that manipulation because of this (Rubin, Chapter 7, this volume). Then, too, as Rubin points out, more natural materials and settings may actually give us more lawful and regular data than restricted ones. And Rubin chooses natural material because of this greater regularity—not because of its naturalness per se.

The choice of model

As we shall see in a minute, there are cases in which research can fit both models at once—the analytic and the analogue. In other cases, however, one may have to make an either-or decision—whether, on the one hand, to model a real-world phenomenon, in the laboratory or in the real world, or, on the other hand, to ask a question about the system's mechanisms or functions. It comes back to the old question: Are we seeking to predict or to understand?

Let me give a personal example that, though not from memory research, brought the point home vividly. Briefly, my students and I were seeing a peculiar phenomenon in rats' ingestive behavior, and we wondered if the release of insulin might be involved in it. So we looked for ways of eliminating endogenous insulin in the rat, which is not a simple matter. It is easy to *depress* insulin secretion in the rat, but to be certain that we have abolished it entirely, and still have a rat to work with, is a problem. A student pointed out that, in fact, a severe depression of insulin secretion, but without its total abolition, is characteristic of diabetic patients. To make diabetic rats comparable to diabetic people, we *ought* to try to depress insulin secretion without abolishing it.

It struck me at the time that that was an excellent example of the difference between the analogue and analytic approaches. My student was right. If we want a model of human diabetes, then what we want is a preparation in which insulin secretion is down but not out. But if we want to know how the system works—and whether or not insulin plays a part in what we see—then our requirements change. We want a preparation in which there is no insulin whatsoever, unless we put it there. And this is our objective, whether or not such conditions ever occur in nature.

Mixtures of models

As the diabetes example shows, the choice of analogue or analytic model may have to be an either-or decision. On the other hand, it is also possible to work toward both objectives at once—prediction of real-world behavior and understanding of what the system does. That kind of research has a foot in each row of Table 3.1.

Outcome studies again provide an example. If a therapeutic technique looks promising in the sample, we may predict its efficacy on a wider scale in a population (the analogue model). At the same time, its success with these persons may support the theory that gave rise to it (the analytic model). What that means is that in evaluating a study, we may need to identify carefully how its findings are being used at any given time. The study may be called on to meet the standards of external validity if we discuss it in an analogue, generalization-and-prediction mode. When we discuss the same study in an analytic, instance-of-principle mode, those standards may be quite irrelevant.

The problem of provincialism

I have argued that the nature of analytic research lies not in generalizing to a population, but in asking and answering questions put to *these* subjects in *these* settings. Clearly, however, we are not seeking a science only of *these* subjects. We surely want more general conclusions than that! As for *these* settings, especially if they are artificial settings, what about *those* settings in the real world? We do want to get back to them somehow. How do we get to them? Where's the bloody horse?

Part of an answer was suggested earlier: We do not take the data to the real world, but the principles the data reveal, and the generality of principles is established by the diversity of the findings on which they rest. But that raises another problem, and it is this that gives rise to external-validity concerns. How do we ensure sufficient diversity? This is the problem of provincialism—not unrepresentativeness but simple *limitedness* of the data base on which our principles rest.

If we ask our questions by dealing with restricted materials—nonsense syllables, white rats, and college sophomores—may we not end up with principles that apply only to nonsense syllables, white rats, and college sophomores? Will we build theories of conditioning on a data base of nictitating membranes? Will we end up, again, in the tail-chase derby, doing experiments that are about other experiments and not about nature? The danger is real. It was not that long ago that the behavior of rats in experimental chambers was seriously advanced as a model of purposive behavior in animals and humans (Tolman, 1932), or of the behavior of organisms (Skinner, 1938), or of the principles of behavior (Hull, 1943).

Given that danger, the question is what to do about it. Representative sampling offers no solution except the formal models of statistical-sampling theory, but, for reasons given earlier, we would miss far too many important influences that way.

There are other solutions to the problem, solutions that do not treat it as a problem of sampling at all. Let us consider two of them.

The real world as a starting point

First, we can consider what Neisser really said, and we can profit from his good advice: We can take our *questions* from the real world. Rather than looking to theory or to other experiments for a starting point, we can look at the things humans and other animals actually do. If we see something interesting—and we shall—we can move it into the laboratory and take it apart to see what makes it work.

Then, having done that, we may check our understanding by testing predictions in the real world to see if our understanding is complete. Petrinovich's elegant studies of bird song (Chapter 2, this volume) began that way. He has found not (I think) that information from artificial settings is invalid but simply that there is more to be learned.

All this is quite different from generalizing *results* to real life. The results may not generalize at all, either because the setting has no real-life parallel (as with walking lights) or because the relevant variables do not vary there (as with syntactic constraints). What generalizes is the understanding of processes that the answers to our questions provide.

It is true that if we do that, we face the problem of ensuring that the laboratory setting captures the process of interest. There is a nice question there, and a topic for a conference in its own right: How do we move from the real world to the laboratory?

Generality as the question

Another approach to generality is to apply the analytic model to that issue, too. We can treat the question (Is phenomenon *X* limited to only such and such settings or subjects?) as a question about a variable or set of variables. Consider cross-cultural research, for instance. Research psychologists have never, to my knowledge, tried for a random sample even of the world's cultures, much less its inhabitants. Rather, they have wondered if this or that phenomenon is specific to our own culture, especially when there has been reason to think it might be. And they have checked the possibility by seeking a culture very different from our own in the respects that ought to be important.

For instance, Ekman and Friesen (1971) asked if the recognition of emotional expression depended on the conventions of particular cultures (i.e., on schemata placed in semantic memory by the training a particular culture provides) (Birdwhistell, 1963). To answer that question, they did not seek a representative sample of cultures. They chose a culture as isolated from ours as possible—the Fore of New Guinea, who had seen few Westerners, had no movies, and owned no television sets. In other words, they manipulated the *variable* of culture, or its correlates, over as wide a range as they could. In the event, expressions of happiness, for example, as produced by the Fore, were recognized without difficulty by Americans, and conversely.

A similar logic can apply to other specifics of our subjects and settings. For example, Stine and associates (Chapter 13, this volume) pointed out that their subjects were a provincial sample with respect to education level; all had more education than the average. And this might make a difference: Certain skills are overlearned in well-educated subjects. Would less well schooled subjects be different? Well, let us look and find out.

If Stine and associates, or others, should go that route in further research, then they would be sampling across a wider range of education levels than was sampled in the studies reported here. In that sense, the aggregate sample would be a more representative sample than the original. But the purpose of the extension would not be to enhance representativeness, and the formal machinery for doing so (say, random sampling stratified by education) would have no particular advantage. Rather, the shape of the research would remain analytic. Education would be varied explicitly by selection of subjects, perhaps even by selecting extremes high and low. And the conclusion would be about a question (Does education make a difference?), not about a population.

Thus, the problem of provincialism—rats, sophomores, and the nictitating membrane—has more than one solution, and different investigators will prefer different solutions. Perhaps our best bet is to depend on the plurality of methods and concerns that characterizes us today. We shall each of us—we psychologists, linguists, neurologists, and anthropologists—pursue our own problems in our own ways, and sooner or later we shall catch each other's errors and omissions. After all, our ideas do change, and so our preconceptions cannot be as well defended as some writers imply (McGuire, 1973; Petrinovich, Chapter 2, this volume).

That sounds facile, but it is the best I can do. As someone has said of democracy, it is probably the worst possible solution except for all the others.

Some writers call this anarchy. They are probably right. It is not, however, a revolutionary anarchy. In fact, my suggestion—like most of my comments, come to think of it—is really just a description of what we actually do, and a claim that what we are doing is reasonable after all. From this perspective, the only real mistake would be to force research into any single mold—including the representative, real-life-relevant, external-validity mold. That can be a snaffle and a curb, too.

References

Abelson, R. P. (1985). A variance explanation paradox: When a little is a lot. *Psychological Bulletin, 97,* 129–133.

Bahrick, H. P. (1984). Semantic memory content in permastore: Fifty years of memory for Spanish learned in school. *Journal of Experimental Psychology: General, 113,* 1–29.

Berkowitz, L., & Donnerstein, E. (1982). External validity is more than skin deep: Some answers to criticisms of laboratory experiments. *American Psychologist, 37,* 245–257.

Birdwhistell, R. L. (1963). *Kinesics and context.* Philadelphia: University of Pennsylvania Press.

Bransford, J. D., & Franks, J. J. (1971). The abstraction of linguistic ideas. *Cognitive Psychology, 2,* 331–350.

Brown, R., & Hanlon, C. (1970). Derivational complexity and order of acquisition in child speech. In J. R. Hayes (Ed.), *Cognition and the development of language* (pp. 11–54). New York: Wiley.

Ekman, P., & Friesen, W. V. (1971). Constants across cultures in the face and emotion. *Journal of Personality and Social Psychology, 17,* 124–129.

Hull, C. L. (1943). *Principles of behavior.* New York: Appleton-Century-Crofts.

Johansson, G. (1973). Visual perception of biological motion and a model for its analysis. *Perception and Psychophysics, 14,* 201–211.

Loftus, E., & Palmer, J. C. (1974). Reconstruction of automobile destruction: An example of the interaction between language and memory. *Journal of Verbal Learning and Verbal Behavior, 13,* 585–589.

McGuire, W. J. (1973). The yin and yang of progress in social psychology: Seven koan. *Journal of Personality and Social Psychology, 26,* 446–456.

Mook, D. G. (1983). In defense of external validity. *American Psychologist, 38,* 379–387.

Moscovitch, M. (1982). A neuropsychological approach to memory and perception in normal and pathological aging. In F. I. M. Craik & S. Trehub (Eds.), *Aging and cognitive processes.* New York: Plenum Press.

Neisser, U. (1976). *Cognition and reality.* San Francisco: W. H. Freeman.

Neisser, U. (1982). *Memory observed: Remembering in natural contexts.* San Francisco: W. H. Freeman.

Ostrom, T. M. (1984). The role of external invalidity in editorial decisions. *American Psychologist, 39,* 324.

Rosenthal, R., & Rubin, D. B. (1979). A note on percent variance explained as a measure of the importance of effects. *Journal of Applied Social Psychology, 9,* 395–396.

Skinner, B. F. (1938). *The behavior of organisms.* New York: Appleton-Century-Crofts.

Tolman, E. C. (1932). *Purposive behavior in animals and men.* New York: Century.

Wilson, T., Laser, P. S., & Stone, J. I. (1982). Judging the predictors of one's own mood: Accuracy and the use of shared theories. *Journal of Experimental Social Psychology, 18,* 537–566.

4 Functional explanations of memory

Darryl Bruce

For approximately 100 years, psychologists have been conducting scientific research on memory. Such research has been propelled largely by laboratory procedures and data and by theories about laboratory findings. Lately, sentiment has been growing that memory scientists should be more concerned about memory as it operates in natural settings, in other words, about the ecology of memory. A strong advocate of the ecological movement is Ulric Neisser. He has been harshly critical of traditional memory research because it has contributed so little to our understanding of everyday memory (Neisser, 1878). It is not difficult to sympathize with this complaint, but the dilemma is what to do about it. Although most ecologists of memory are rather vague on how to proceed, it is evident that they would like to see more attention to memory problems of the real world and less to procedures and theories resulting from laboratory work (Hirst & Levine, 1985; Neisser, 1978, 1982a). Clearer guidelines are possible, however, if we specify the fundamental questions that memory researchers have asked in the past and show how these could be changed (and indeed already are changing) to yield a broader understanding of memory. In this chapter, I shall describe an ecological orientation that has its roots in Charles Darwin, evolutionary biology, ethology, and the functional psychology of William James. Its objective is to encourage functional explanations of memory. The approach will be illustrated with examples drawn from the current memory literature. I shall also indicate how the framework squares with other views about the study of everyday memory and how it relates to the investigation of memory and aging.

Four fundamental questions for memory research

Four core questions or issues can be specified for the science of memory: immediate causation, development, evolutionary history, and function.

I thank Mike Rashotte and Glayde Whitney for many helpful discussions of the ideas presented in this chapter. Final preparation of the manuscript was supported by a grant from the Alberta Law Foundation to J. Don Read.

These questions were first spelled out by Tinbergen (1963) in his description of ethology (Hinde, 1982), but they apply equally to the domain of memory (Bruce, 1985).

Questions of immediate causation ask about the mechanisms directly responsible for memory phenomena. I use "mechanisms" here in a general way. Investigations of such memory components and processes as short-term and long-term stores, schemas, memory scanning, automatic versus effortful encoding, levels of processing, and episodic versus semantic memory all qualify as studies of immediate causation. So does the search for neurophysiological mechanisms of memory. It should be mentioned, however, that the pursuit of immediate causation does not imply a reductionism of any kind. It means only an effort to uncover the direct causes of memory phenomena.

The question of development refers to the changes in memory performance or mechanisms that occur throughout the life span. For instance, Hasher and Zacks (1979) hypothesize that automatic encoding of information in memory does not vary substantially with age, whereas effortful encoding does. Frequently, the interest is in the roles that memory mechanisms play in developmental memory phenomena. Hence, the distinction between problems of immediate causation and development is sometimes more arbitrary than logical, something that both Hinde (1982) and Tinbergen (1963) admit.

Questions about evolutionary history bear on the evolution of memory mechanisms. Such matters are difficult to resolve; they also require application of the comparative method. It is not surprising, therefore, that students of human memory have rarely raised such issues or paid much attention to the literature on animal memory.

The final question is function, that is, the real-world usefulness or adaptive significance of memory mechanisms. Do they solve any ecological problems for us, and if so, what are they? There is no shortage of statements about function: Echoic memory underlies speech perception (Crowder, 1976) and the appreciation of music (Neisser, 1967). Short-term memory plays an important role in reading (Crowder, 1982). Rapid short-term forgetting is adaptively suited to the constant heavy processing demands placed on working memory (Lachman, Lachman, & Butterfield, 1979). Forgetting from long-term memory is useful because if we remember too much, we will never know where to find something when we want it (James, 1890/1950; Miller, 1962). I could cite many more such assertions. The problem with most of them is that they have never been tested.

Following biologists such as Alcock (1979) and Wilson (1975), I shall lump the four questions just described into two broader categories. Inasmuch as the distinction between immediate causation and development is somewhat arbitrary, these concerns will be grouped together as "how" questions. Evolutionary history and function are related matters and will be called "why" questions. Alternative labels exist for these two categories, namely, proximate causation and ultimate causation. But I shall stick to the how–why terminology because I think it conveys a better idea of the kinds of explanations of memory that are sought within each category. Psychologists interested in the how of memory wish to understand how memory works; that is, they wish to determine the basic mechanisms of memory. Those interested in the why of memory wish to understand why memory came to be the way it is and what ecological functions it serves. A rare example in the field of cognition of an emphasis on why is the Mergler and Goldstein (1983) discussion of the relation between aging and cognitive processes, including memory. In this essay, I shall restrict my consideration of "why" questions to inquiries into the functions of memory. This merely reflects the fact that the evolutionary history of memory is difficult to unravel, whereas questions of function are more tractable. From the perspective of "how" and "why" questions, it may be claimed that in 100 years of scientific research on human memory, we have concentrated on the how of memory. Our objective has been to determine the basic mental components and processes that underlie the operation of memory. By contrast, we have almost entirely avoided tackling "why" questions in any serious scientific way.

Functional explanations of memory

The imbalance just described should be redressed, but it is not simply a matter of shifting from the traditional laboratory overemphasis on the facts of "how" to an equally lopsided concern for memory in natural contexts. Such a shift is unlikely to lead to any genuine understanding of everyday memory. Rather, it seems to me that if any progress is to be made toward this objective, a much greater segment of our research must be devoted to the pursuit of functional explanations of memory. By this I mean an attempt to uncover connections between the how and why of memory. The aim is to take conceptions about how the memory system works and link them to memory as it functions in the environment, to determine what memory problems are solved by what memory mechanisms.

A major step toward functional explanations has been the adoption of what biologists call "population thinking" (Ghiselin, 1969; Mayr, 1982). I have considered this idea at length elsewhere (Bruce, 1985). Therefore, I shall limit the present discussion to its main point and its implication for memory research. "Population thinking" emphasizes the uniqueness of individuals and the differences among members of a group. The population is thus a pool of variations rather than a class of identical things that happen to differ owing to nature's faulty aim, errors of measurement, or training. Such variation is important because it can be acted on by natural selection to produce evolution. From the perspective of population thinking, then, we should pay more attention to individual differences in memory and to cases of exceptionally good or bad memory.

But how, and to what end? One way is correlational (Cronbach, 1957). One can start with individual differences in a proposed mechanism of memory (e.g., echoic memory) and attempt to relate such differences to differences in putative functions that the mechanism supports (e.g., speech perception). Obtaining a significant correlation is not definitive evidence that the mechanism in question has the claimed functional validity, but a negligible correlation undermines such a claim. As for exceptional cases like amnesics and memorists, it is the extremes of their memories that often can paint a clear picture of the mechanisms of memory and their functions. For example, Tulving (1983) argues that some amnesics show deficits indicating a dissociation between episodic and semantic memory and that therefore these are different subsystems of normal memory. As another example, the expert digit recall of the subject S.F. led Chase and Ericssen (1981) to suggest that one important component of skilled memory is rapid storage and retrieval from intermediate knowledge structures. Crowder (1982) refers to individual differences in memory as theoretical wild cards and hopes that they will come to play a leading role in the development of theories of memory. I agree, but such cards can do more than that. They can provide entrée into the uses of memory.

In principle, the quest for functional explanations can proceed in either of two ways: One can begin with the basic memory mechanisms of interest and attempt to determine the ecological functions of the mechanisms; or one can start with the naturalistic functions of memory and try to link these to the mechanisms that play roles in the functions. The next sections illustrate these two approaches with instances drawn from existing memory literature.

Functional explanations: From mechanism to function

There are some promising examples of the first category of functional explanation, and I shall comment on two of them. Both are good illustrations of the application of population thinking. First is the work described by Hunt (1978). He asks if individual differences in certain mechanistic processes are related to performance in different subgroups of the population. Consider the process of scanning immediate memory as assessed by the well-known Sternberg procedure. In this task, one measures a subject's reaction time to indicate whether a probe digit did or did not occur in a just-presented sequence of digits that can be of variable length (the memory set). The rate at which the memory set is mentally scanned is given by the slope of the linear function relating reaction time to size of the memory set. Table 4.1 shows how scanning speeds vary for different subjects, ranging from the mnemonist V.P. (Hunt & Love, 1972), who scans extremely rapidly, to senior citizens, who scan at a much slower pace. How one interprets this relation between short-term memory scanning and different subject groups is, of course, highly problematic. One difficulty is the real-world function that the subject groups in Table 4.1 represent. Hunt intimates that they may constitute a range of intelligence. But even if this is so, one can complain that this is hardly an ecological function. Another problem is that the relation may be due to some other variable correlated with the search rate. But whatever the interpretation placed on the data, one possibility is that short-term memory scanning is directly related to whatever ecological function is repre-

Table 4.1. *Rates of scanning immediate memory by different subject groups*

Subject group	Scan rate (msec/item)
V.P.	10
"Typical" adults	24
High school students	46
Cultural-familial retardates	70
Encephalitic mental retardates	111
Senior citizens	125

Source: The information in this table has been adapted by permission from Figure 3 of Hunt (1978, p.119). Copyright 1978 by the American Psychological Association.

sented by the different subject groups shown in Table 4.1. In this sense, the Sternberg memory-search process, which has been so ardently studied in the laboratory, may be seen as ecologically relevant.

My second example is functional research on the short and long of memory, but mainly the short of it. Many models of memory, beginning in the late 1950s, have distinguished between short-term and long-term stores. Since that time, experimental laboratory studies, ably reviewed by Crowder (1982), have produced many reasons to doubt the distinction, and especially the notion of short-term store as an undifferentiated memory structure. Crowder describes another group of studies that followed in the wake of the experimental work and also questioned early versions of the short–long duality. These studies were functional in the sense that they assessed functional hypotheses about short-term memory. One such hypothesis is that variations in long-term memory, but not short-term memory, are related to measures of intelligence and changes in mental performance with age. Another is that amnesia may be due to an inability to transfer information from short-term store to long-term store or due to a breakdown of short-term store. A third idea is that reading depends on short-term memory to hold a verbatim record of the last few words that have been read; this permits strings of text to be interpreted by higher-level comprehension processes. Hence, good readers should have larger short-term memory capacity than poor readers. Crowder's careful examination of the relevant evidence indicates that none of these functional hypotheses is compelling. In sum, both traditional research on the how of memory and functional research on the uses of memory have led to the demise of early ideas about the short-term store, with the traditional experimental approach leading the way, and the functional approach trailing, the normal order of things, as Crowder has noted.

A footnote on current thinking about short-term memory is apposite. The term of choice nowadays is "working memory," and it is seen as an assemblage of subsidiary stores linked by a central processor (Baddeley, 1983). Something interesting is happening in the development of this concept. Experimental laboratory research is not leading the way. Rather, studies aimed at a functional understanding of working memory are proceeding apace. (The terminology "working memory" strikes me as no accident; it implies a functional orientation.) For example, although the earlier views of the role of short-term memory in reading seem to have been incorrect, there is promising evidence that the more differentiated concept of working memory may be important in reading. Baddeley, Logie, Nimmo-Smith, and Brereton (1985), Daneman and Carpenter (1980), and Masson and Miller (1983) have all found measures of working memory to be strongly correlated with measures of reading comprehension. Presently, it is not certain what these correlations mean. At a minimum, they suggest that working memory is not functionally sterile.

Functional explanations: From function to mechanism

Memory research does not have much of a history of tracing paths from ecological memory functions to mechanisms. There are numerous reasons for this, and some are worth mentioning. As has been pointed out by proponents of an ecological approach, most memory research has been driven by laboratory theories and findings, not by naturalistic considerations about memory. Moreover, if natural contexts have been important, the research typically has been dedicated to the solution of practical memory problems, with little or no interest in the mechanisms mediating the solution. Another difficulty, I suspect, is knowing what qualifies as an important ecological function of memory. Some things seem obvious. I rely on memory to read, to speak and comprehend a language, to teach, to write articles on psychology, to write computer programs, to recognize my family, to interact socially, to know who I am, and, in general, to get me through the day. But what about playing bridge, recalling baseball statistics, doing crossword puzzles, telling jokes, and remembering novels that I have read? Memory undoubtedly supports these actions, but somehow they do not seem as crucial to my survival as the first set I mentioned. Is it a waste of time to attempt to tie such activities to memory mechanisms? No, simply because one never knows whether or not the mechanisms uncovered by investigation of ostensibly trivial memory activities also contribute to those ecological memory phenomena that seem to be more critical to survival. Studies of memory among master chess players and other experts (Charness, Chapter 24, this volume) can be viewed in this light. There is something else that may have daunted us in working from function to mechanism. Many, if not most, ecological memory behaviors probably are determined by more than a single memory mechanism. For instance, playing golf can be claimed to call on episodic, semantic, and procedural components of memory (Schacter, 1983). One solution to clarifying the many determinants of ecological memory is to apply multiple-regression methods (Bahrick, 1984a).

Despite the scarcity of functional studies of memory that have tracked ecological memory phenomena to their underlying mechanisms, some good examples exist. I shall describe three of them. The first is the Brown and Kulik (1977) investigation of flashbulb memories, that is, seemingly indelible memories for personal circumstances surrounding an important event. For instance, those who remember the assassination of John F. Kennedy typically report the following categories of information: how they found out the news, what they were doing at the time, where they were, how they felt, how others around them felt, and some immediate personal aftermath. It is noteworthy that Brown and Kulik were interested not only in the mechanism of flashbulb memories but also in why they occur. Why should we permanently retain such information? Brown and Kulik proposed that a neurophysiological mechanism, evolved for permanently registering biologically crucial and unexpected events, also captures the accompanying circumstances. Such circumstances are recorded because they were either directly or indirectly relevant to fitness at some time in our evolutionary history. Although there may be some truth to this, evolutionary hypotheses of this sort are exceedingly difficult to test. Therefore, an explanation offered by Neisser (1982b) may be more appealing. Neisser invokes the the mechanisms of schemas and constructive recall (Bartlett, 1932). Flashbulb information categories reflect the conventions of a narrative structure or schema for telling stories, and a flashbulb report is a construction within such a framework. As for the why of such memories, Neisser sees them as benchmarks: Their function is to link our own lives to the course of history.

My second example is yet another contribution from Neisser (1981): observations and interpretations of John Dean's memory. Dean testified before a Senate committee about his conversations with President Nixon concerning the Watergate crime. Neisser compared this testimony with transcripts of tape recordings of the conversations. What was Dean's memory like? What mechanisms and functions were involved? To begin with, Dean did not remember as a tape recorder does; his recall was clearly constructive. But it would be misleading to say that his reconstructions retained the gist of his conversations with President Nixon, for sometimes they were completely wrong in this sense. What Dean did remember and report was accurate at a deeper level, at the level of truth, at the level of invariant themes: Nixon was unscrupulous; he knew what was going on; there was a cover-up; Nixon wanted it to succeed; and so on. Neisser refers to Dean's recollection as "repisodic." It represented the repeated characteristics of an entire series of episodes. Repisodic memory is faithful to invariant themes across episodes, but not necessarily faithful to the details of any one episode. On the matter of function, Neisser suggests that the repisodic and constructive features of Dean's memory may have served to place him at the center of a historical event. He may be right. I suspect, however, that persuasion was a more fundamental function. Dean wanted to persuade the members of the Senate committee that Nixon was guilty and perhaps that he himself was not entirely dishonorable. Indeed, persuasion may be an ultimate function of all story-telling memory mechanisms (e.g., schemas, reconstruction, and repisodic memory). As a footnote, this research illustrates population thinking: John Dean's memory probably was abnormal, but it suggests a memory mechanism (repisodic memory) that may be of wide applicability.

A third example of moving from ecological memory observations to a consideration of mechanisms is Bahrick's study (1984a) of long-term memory for Spanish learned in the classroom. Bahrick's surprising finding was that after exponential declines over the first 6 years, retention functions showed no further forgetting across the next 25 years or so. To account for this fact, Bahrick proposed a memory mechanism called "permastore," a semipermanent part of associative semantic memory that depends primarily on the degree to which material is learned. Bahrick's memory mechanism is conservative: It is not far removed from the data, and it adheres to the associative tradition in memory that goes back to Ebbinghaus. Permastore may not be the only determinant of the results, of course, something that Bahrick (1984b) concedes. Nevertheless, his interpretation illustrates that ecological memory phenomena need not always imply the operation of schemas and constructive recall (but see Neisser, 1984, for a schema explanation of Bahrick's results). Where there is a premium on accuracy or on literal recall (as in Bahrick's tests of vocabulary knowledge and recall of idioms), associative connections may contribute substantially to performance. Rubin (1977) makes the same point in his investigation of long-term memory for passages such as the preamble to the U.S. Constitution and the 23rd Psalm.

Functional explanations of memory demarcated

Functional explanations of memory, to repeat, involve tracing connections between the how and why of memory, between memory mechanisms and their ultimate uses or fitness value. The words "function" and "functional" are also used in several other ways, however, and it will be helpful to distinguish my use of these terms from two other common usages. First, "function" may refer not to ultimate but to immediate uses of memory mechanisms. For example, in Atkinson and Shiffrin's original model of memory (1968), rehearsal had the functions of maintaining information in the short-term store and of transferring information to the long-term store. As another example, the function of "iconic memory is to hold information briefly in its original form, so that it can be recognized and passed on in the system" (Klatzky, 1980, p. 32). Such immediate uses of memory mechanisms really have to do with how memory operates and are different from ultimate ecological uses, which concern the why of memory and are the focus of the functional view set forth here.

There is yet a second sense in which those interested in the how of memory emphasize the functional. For instance, Tulving (1983) states that episodic memory and semantic memory are functionally different memory systems. Baddeley (1982) discusses the fractionation of memory into parts and refers to their "functional distinctions," "functional differences," and "functional separability" (p. 60). "Functional," with reference to the parts of memory, means that they operate differently; that is, they "are governed at least partially by different principles" (Tulving, 1984, p. 226). Such functional distinctions, then, concern differences among the components of the memory system. But functional explanations, as I have characterized them, connect the parts of memory to the everyday-memory problems that the parts solve. As a footnote, it may be mentioned that successful functional explanations can also provide support for hypothesized differences among memory mechanisms (Bruce, 1985).

Functional explanations and other research

Approaches to everyday memory

In this section, I contrast the current theoretical stance with selected other perspectives on understanding everyday memory.

Mook on analytic versus analogue research. Mook, in this volume (Chapter 3) and elsewhere (Mook, 1983), distinguishes between analytic and analogue research. With respect to memory, the former aims to find out how the system works; the latter attempts to predict performance in real-life memory situations. As Mook sees it, the crucial step in analogue research is to generalize from research to the everyday work; in analytic research, this step does not exist.

Analytic research is clearly aimed at the how of memory. But is analogue research targeted at the why of memory? I think not. Analogue research is applied research. For example, we wish to predict how pilots will perform in the cockpit under conditions of memory overload, and we use as our predictor their performance on a laboratory perceptual-scanning task as they concurrently carry out a difficult short-term memory test. This is not functional memory research. If, in the pursuit of functional explanations, I ask whether or not a measure of working memory is related to reading and listening comprehension, I do so with the intent not of predicting such comprehension but of finding out if the mechanism called working memory contributes to solving the problems of reading and listening. In short, analogue research and functional interpretations of memory have fundamentally different goals.

Does this mean that Mook and I agree or disagree? We agree in that we are both after external validity of theories and mechanisms, not findings. This is precisely the focus of functional explanations of memory. We disagree to the extent that Mook believes an analytic "how" approach is sufficient to accomplish this goal. The past 100 years of memory research, however, convince me that we also need a well-defined functional orientation. I note that Mook's more recent description of the analytic model (Chapter 3, this volume) contains such an emphasis.

Petrinovich on representative design. Petrinovich (1979; Chapter 2, this volume) contends that the analytic method is inappropriate for determining whether or not scientific constructs apply to environmental situations in which the behavior of interest normally occurs. For this purpose, he argues that we must turn to Egon Brunswik's idea of representative design, in which not only subjects but also situations or the ecology of the individual are randomly sampled. In this way, variables will be studied that will be relevant to the organism's adjustment and survival, not simply to laboratory-generated paradigms and theories.

Petrinovich and I are in substantial agreement about overall objectives: When it comes to memory, we both seek ecologically valid concepts. We differ, I think, in how to achieve this end. I propose that we trace mechanisms suggested by analytic scientific work to their putative environmental functions, or vice versa. By contrast, "the most radical departure involved in the use of representative design is the emphasis on obtaining random samples of the ecology of the organism in order to study behavior in the natural, cultural habitat of organisms" (Petrinovich, 1979, p. 383). Although my reading of this statement may be too narrow, the implication is that the ecology is the exclusive starting point for determining ecological validity. At the risk of sounding monotonous, concepts generated by analytic "how" research can also play this role. One other point of disagreement between us may be largely terminological, but it is no less worth clarifying on that account. Petrinovich is right in stressing that paying attention to the ecology can lead us to study variables that are relevant to an organism's adjustment and survival. But what are directly pertinent to adjustment and survival are not the variables per se, or even the memory mechanisms, but the functions (more accurately, individual differences therein) for which the variables or the mechanisms are responsible. Hence, what are most crucial are mechanism–function relations, rather than the more general organism–environment relationships advocated by Brunswik and Petrinovich.

Neisser on ecological memory theory. In two recent articles, Neisser (e.g., 1986) has begun to reveal his theoretical ideas about the ecology of memory. He believes that the key to the structure of memory is not in the head, but is out there in the environment. It is not memory traces or mental representations that are important, but the characteristics of remembered objects and events. For example, episodic memory and semantic memory are not different mental structures, but different classes of remembered things – not mental categories, but environmental categories. In the same way, such things as memories for motor skills, Spanish learned in the classroom, spatial arrangements, repeated social routines, and autobiographical events should be construed as environmental rather than mental structures. Such structures and categories are registered directly in memory and are not, as traditional information-processing theories would have it, constructed out of the wave of elementary information that meets the senses. Memory construction occurs, but it follows directly encoded structures; it does not create them.

Make no mistake about it, Neisser's ideas mark a radical departure from traditional thinking about memory. Whatever their ultimate correctness, he is surely right about one thing: We do require more complete descriptions of what we remember in various naturalistic contexts. Otherwise, I doubt that we would have arrived at the concept of repisodic memory (Neisser, 1981). On the other hand, structures and categories of the environment should not be the exclusive sources of our theoretical mechanisms. I repeat, memory mechanisms can also be inspired by an analysis of how the system works. Episodic memory and semantic memory may be environmental concepts, but their existence in memory science emerged from "how" considerations (Tulving, 1983). As a final comment, Neisser's current ideas about memory strike me as a retreat from his earlier concern about function (Neisser, 1978). In 1978, he emphasized the natural uses of memory and asked for what purposes we use the past. I detect no such emphasis in the two articles just described. If it is true that function no longer plays a central role in his thinking, then this represents a considerable difference from the functional orientation that I advocate.

Functional explanations, aging, and memory

The pursuit of functional explanations of memory may be comprehensible in the abstract, but vague when it comes to concrete research practice. It may be useful, therefore, to sketch an example of a functional approach. The example will also illustrate the significance of the study of memory and aging for a functional research program.

Consider the framework for investigating memory proposed by Hasher and Zacks (1979). The framework has a number of critical ideas and assumptions, but only a few are relevant for present purposes. The main one is the distinction between automatic and effortful registration of information in memory. I shall focus on the former. Automatic encoding operations use up little of the limited processing resources of the individual. If events are attended to, it is assumed that automatic encoding goes on at an optimal level. A number of criteria must be jointly satisfied to claim that information is automatically coded (Hasher & Zacks, 1984). Two of them are pertinent to the present discussion: First, people differ very little in their abilities to encode this information. Second, there is no variation in the encoding of this information as a function of age. Such invariance follows from the assumption that automatic processes require little of the processing capacity of the individual. So even though processing capacity may decline with increasing age, automatic encoding remains unaffected. Hasher and Zacks (1979) hypothesize that certain automatic processes are processes for which we are genetically prepared. These processes encode fundamental aspects of the flow of information, in particular, spatial, temporal, and frequency-of-occurrence information.

I wish to focus on frequency coding, because it is here that Hasher and Zacks (1984) have stated their position most forcefully. Frequency coding apparently conforms to all the criteria of automaticity. With reference to the two criteria mentioned earlier, it would appear that there are limited individual differences and that frequency coding is developmentally invariant beyond the age of 4 or 5 years. Hasher and Zacks also emphasize the importance of automatically registered frequency information with a lengthy discussion of its wide functional value. I shall limit my comments to the hypothesized utility of frequency coding for event memory.

What does the functional perspective presented in this chapter say about all this? To begin with, it is at odds with Hasher and Zack's claim that there are negligible individual differences in frequency coding. Their claim reflects the view that frequency coding is a process that has evolved to the point that there is no more reliable variability across individuals. This is, of course, quite possible. By contrast, the fundamental postulate of the functional approach is population thinking, that is, diversity within a population. We may each have a frequency registration mechanism, but it should not be the case that there are no (or even limited) reliable individual differences in this respect. The first order of business for a functional approach, then, would be a concerted effort to find such differences using a wide range of subjects and tasks. As it happens, evidence of consistent individual differences has been observed in frequency coding (Underwood, Boruch, & Malmi, 1978), as well as in other automatic memory encoding processes (Cohen, 1984; Zacks, Hasher, Alba, Sanft, & Rose, 1984).

The next step (it could even be the first step) would be to measure performance in a variety of ecological memory situations thought to depend on frequency monitoring. If variability in performance on frequency judgment tasks were found to be related to variability in any of the ecological memory phenomena, then one would have in hand a functional explanation of frequency coding. Otherwise, the case for the utility of such coding would, from a functional standpoint, be suspect. Interestingly, Hasher and Zacks (1984) report data in this vein: The frequency processing of children who were proficient classroom learners did not differ from that of children who were poor classroom learners. Instead of seeing this as a warning signal about the functional value of frequency coding, Hasher and Zacks simply view it as consistent with the idea that such processing shows no individual differences and hence is automatic.

This brings me to the hypothesis that frequency-of-occurrence coding does not decline with age. As Hasher and Zacks (1984) note, episodic or event memory ability, on balance, does decline with age. But if it is to be claimed that automatic frequency monitoring has utility for memory, it would be much more in order to maintain not that the registration of frequency information should remain invariant with age but that it should, like event memory, show some impairment in old age. In fact, persuasive evidence for just such an impairment exists; for reviews of the data, see Kausler (1982) and Salthouse (1982). Moreover, Weingartner, Grafman, Boutelle, Kaye, and Martin (1983) reported that Alzheimer patients were extraordinarily deficient in monitoring the frequency with which events occurred. For the functional orientation expressed here, these data come as no surprise. They simply intimate that frequency coding may well be an adaptive characteristic of memory.

Although my disagreement with the Hasher and Zacks framework is limited, I wish to underscore that that disagreement is at the core of functional explanations and population thinking. Hasher and Zacks argue that frequency coding and other automatic processes for which humans are genetically prepared show negligible individual differences. A functional approach says otherwise; indeed, individual differences are the very stuff of such an approach. And it is just this emphasis that squares so nicely with the study of memory and aging. What the aged and pathology among the aged can provide are the abnormalities and the variability on which functional research capitalizes to couple mechanisms with function. In other words, aging is likely to be related either to variability in laboratory memory performance caused by known or suspected mechanisms or to variability in ecological memory phenomena. Such variability is a first step toward a functional understanding of memory: In the former case, it is then a matter of zeroing in on the ultimate ecological memory behaviors; in the latter case, it is a question of unearthing the mediating memory mechanisms.

References

Alcock, J. (1979). *Animal behavior: An evolutionary approach* (2nd ed.). Sunderland, MA: Sinauer.

Atkinson, R. C., & Shiffrin, R. M. (1968). Human memory: A proposed system and its control processes. In K. W. Spence & J. T. Spence (Eds.), *The psychology of learning and motivation* (Vol. 2, pp. 89–195). New York: Academic Press.

Baddeley, A. D. (1982). Implications of neuropsychological evidence for theories of normal memory. *Philosophical Transactions of the Royal Society of London, B298*, 59–72.

Baddeley, A. D. (1983). Working memory. *Philosophical Transactions of the Royal Society of London, B302*, 311–324

Baddeley, A. D., Logie, R., Nimmo-Smith, I., & Brereton, N. (1985). Components of fluent reading. *Journal of Memory and Language, 24*, 119–131.

Bahrick, H. P. (1984a). Semantic memory content in permastore: Fifty years of memory for Spanish learned in school. *Journal of Experimental Psychology: General, 113*, 1–29.

Bahrick, H. P. (1984b). Associations and organization in cognitive psychology: A reply to Neisser. *Journal of Experimental Psychology: General, 113*, 36–37.

Bartlett, F. C. (1932). *Remembering: A study in experimental and social psychology.* Cambridge University Press.

Brown, R., & Kulik, J. (1977). Flashbulb memories. *Cognition, 5*, 73–89.

Bruce, D. (1985). The how and why of ecological memory. *Journal of Experimental Psychology: General, 114*, 78–90.

Chase, W. G., & Ericsson, K. A. (1981). Skilled memory. In J. R. Anderson (Ed.), *Cognitive skills and their acquisition* (pp. 141–189). Hillsdale, NJ: Lawrence Erlbaum.

Cohen, R. L (1984). Individual differences in event memory: A case for nonstrategic factors. *Memory & Cognition, 12*, 633–641.

Cronbach, L. J. (1957). The two disciplines of scientific psychology. *American Psychologist, 13*, 671–684.

Crowder, R. G. (1976). *Principles of learning and memory.* Hillsdale, NJ: Lawrence Erlbaum.

Crowder, R. G. (1982). The demise of short-term memory. *Acta Psychologica, 50*, 291–323.

Daneman, M., & Carpenter, P. A. (1980). Individual differences in working memory and reading. *Journal of Verbal Learning and Verbal Behavior, 19*, 450–466.

Ghiselin, M. T. (1969). *The triumph of the Darwinian method.* Berkeley: University of California Press.

Hasher, L., & Zacks, R. T. (1979). Automatic and effortful processes in memory. *Journal of Experimental Psychology: General, 108,* 356–388.

Hasher, L., & Zacks, R. T. (1984). Automatic processing of fundamental information: The case of frequency of occurrence. *American Psychologist, 39,* 1372–1388.

Hinde, R. A. (1982). *Ethology: Its nature and relation with other sciences.* New York: Oxford University Press.

Hirst, W., & Levine, E. (1985). Ecological memory reconsidered: A reply to Bruce's "The how and why of ecological memory." *Journal of Experimental Psychology: General, 114,* 269–271.

Hunt, E. (1978). Mechanics of verbal ability. *Psychological Review, 85,* 109–130.

Hunt, E., & Love, T. (1972). How good can memory be? In A. W. Melton & E. Martin (Eds.), *Coding processes in human memory* (pp. 237–260). Washington, DC: Winston-Wiley.

James, W. (1950). *The principles of psychology* (Vol. 1). New York: Dover. (Original work published 1890).

Kausler, D. H. (1982). *Experimental psychology and human aging.* New York: Wiley.

Klatzky, R. L. (1980). *Human memory: Structures and processes* (2nd ed.). San Francisco: Freeman.

Lachman, R., Lachman, J. L., & Butterfield, E. C. (1979). *Cognitive psychology and information processing: An introduction.* Hillsdale, NJ: Lawrence Erlbaum.

Masson, M. E. J., & Miller, J. A. (1983). Working memory and individual differences in comprehension and memory of text. *Journal of Educational Psychology, 75,* 314–318.

Mayr, E. (1982). *The growth of biological thought.* Cambridge, MA: Harvard University Press.

Mergler, N. L., & Goldstein, M. D. (1983). Why are there old people: Senescence as biological and cultural preparedness for the transmission of information. *Human Development, 26,* 72–90.

Miller, G. A. (1962). *Psychology: The science of mental life.* New York: Harper & Row.

Mook, D. G. (1983). In defense of external invalidity. *American Psychologist, 38,* 379–387.

Neisser, U. (1967). *Cognitive psychology.* New York: Appleton-Century-Crofts.

Neisser, U. (1978). Memory: What are the important questions? In M. M. Gruneberg, P. Morris, & R. H. Sykes (Eds.), *Practical aspects of memory* (pp. 3–24). New York: Academic Press.

Neisser, U. (1981). John Dean's memory: A case study. *Cognition, 9,* 1–22.

Neisser, U. (Ed.). (1982a). *Memory observed: Remembering in natural contexts.* San Francisco: Freeman.

Neisser, U. (1982b). Snapshots or benchmarks? In U. Neisser (Ed.), *Memory observed: Remembering in natural contexts* (pp. 43–48). San Francisco: Freeman.

Neisser, U. (1984). Interpreting Harry Bahrick's study: What confers immunity against forgetting? *Journal of Experimental Psychology: General, 113,* 32–35.

Neisser, U. (1985). The role of theory in the ecological study of memory: Comment on Bruce. *Journal of Experimental Psychology: General, 114,* 272–276.

Neisser, U. (1986). Nested structure in autobiographical memory. In D. C. Rubin (Ed.), *Autobiographical memory.* Cambridge University Press.

Petrinovich, L. (1979). Probabilistic functionalism: A conception of research method. *American Psychologist, 34,* 373–390.

Rubin, D. C. (1977). Very long-term memory for prose and verse. *Journal of Verbal Learning and Verbal Behavior, 16,* 611–621.

Salthouse, T. A. (1982). *Adult cognition: An experimental psychology of human aging.* New York: Springer-Verlag.

Schacter, D. L. (1983). Amnesia observed: Remembering and forgetting in a natural environment. *Journal of Abnormal Psychology, 92,* 236–242.

Tinbergen, N. (1963). On aims and methods of ethology. *Zeitschrift für Tierpsychologie, 20,* 410–429.

Tulving, E. (1983). *Elements of episodic memory.* New York: Oxford University Press.

Tulving, E. (1984). Précis of *Elements of episodic memory. The Behavioral and Brain Sciences, 7,* 223–268.

Underwood, B. J., Boruch, R. F., & Malmi, R. A. (1978). Composition of episodic memory. *Journal of Experimental Psychology: General, 107*, 393–419.

Weingartner, H., Grafman, J., Boutelle, W., Kaye, W., & Martin, P. R. (1983). Forms of memory failure. *Science, 221*, 380–382.

Wilson. E. O. (1975). *Sociobiology: The new synthesis.* Cambridge, MA: Harvard University Press.

Zacks, R. T., Hasher, L., Alba, J. W., Sanft, H., & Rose, K. C. (1984). Is temporal order encoded automatically? *Memory & Cognition, 12*, 387–394.

5 General systems theory: A rationale for the study of everyday memory

Jan D. Sinnott

In the course of this chapter, I hope to convince the reader that research methods in cognitive psychology have a great deal to gain by adopting a view of the world based on general systems theory (GST). The study of memory should be no exception. I hope to describe what GST is, how it evolved, and what some core themes and systems functions might be.

The human is a system, I shall argue, and it is nested in social and environmental systems. Memory serves as a control for the availability and flow of information and energy with the human system and between systems, balancing and regulating stimulation. So, I shall argue, memory should be studied keeping in mind its overall purpose, that is, control of the overall daily inner and outer environments in a world in which the present copies the past to some degree.

For memory research, this implies the inclusion of several levels of everyday tasks and the broadening of research questions to include several nested systems. I hope to demonstrate through examples that research questions related to aging make more sense when framed in terms of GST ideas, such as "control of stimulation," "compensatory strategies," "boundary flexibility," and "entropy," because the systems approach is larger than most other models or approaches. I shall be emphasizing David Rubin's "why" question, although "how" and "when" will be touched on.

What is GST

GST is an *amusing* theory. The physicist Wigner, in a lecture, once said that theories can be "interesting" or "amusing." An interesting theory may have merit, but often such theories are quickly forgotten; an amusing theory is a theory that makes one *think*. GST is an amusing theory.

The support of David Arenberg, chief of the Learning and Problem Solving Section, Laboratory of Behavioral Sciences, Gerontology Research Center, National Institute of Aging (NIA), and of Towson State University is gratefully acknowledged, as is the support provided by an NIA postdoctoral fellowship to the author. Thanks to Robin Armstrong for her assistance.

GST, as I shall use the term here, is an attempt to unify science by finding structures and processes common to many entities. Of greatest interest are entities that are complex organizations that have boundaries, that have some continuity over time, and that are able to change in orderly ways over time. Such entities may be called living systems (Miller, 1978), whether they are cells or societies. GST had for its earlier theorists such luminaries as Norbert Weiner (1961) and Ludwig von Bertalanfy (1968). Today it is expressed in the language of quantum physics, chemistry, the family-systems approach in clinical psychology, von Neumann's (von Neumann & Morgenstern, 1947) game theory, biofeedback, sociology (Lockland, 1973), and many other disciplines. The growth of interest in systems views is partly due to the growth of knowledge that prods us to go beyond single-variable studies because we see many more complex components in the expression of any relationship. We also have new ways to analyze such complex systems data (e.g., multivariate analysis), and when tools exist, uses are created. Of course, that statement itself is a systems-theory interpretation of these events over time.

What are some core themes of GST? The first is the concept of a *system,* that is, a network of related components and processes that work as a whole. *Linkage* and *interaction* are key themes, because whatever influences one part or process influences all of the parts and processes (i.e., the entire system). Systems coordinate their activities by means of *feedback,* either from within or from without. Feedback from within leads to homeostasis or equilibrium within; feedback from without leads to balance between two systems. *Equilibrium* is a balance between or among system parts. Given a state of disequilibrium, there will be an energy flow from one part to another. Any number of systems can have common mechanisms – *isomorphic processes* – for doing some task. For example, getting energy from one point to another may occur by means of chemical transmission or glucose metabolism or by moving commuters via subways. Because systems do interact and trade things such as energy, GST recognizes that scientists need to make deliberate decisions to determine system limits or parameters and levels of description. We have not always done this in the past. Thus, there is an awareness of the observer's input on the "reality" observed. For example, if I draw my boundaries of the system at the person level, I may correctly say that an elder's depression is caused by poor coping strategies; if I draw boundaries at the societal level, I may say with equal correctness that the depression is caused by social stigmas attached to aging. I would be correct in both cases and would investigate different things. Systems theory examines multiple causal variables, or at least considers that they may be present, and focuses most on the processes used to go from one state to another. This makes GST a "natural" for developmental psychologists, such as myself, who are interested in the processes behind changes over time as much as in the states of persons at various time points.

What are some systems functions that are commonly present in all systems? First, a "living" (in the broad sense used previously) system operates so as to maintain some continuity over time, some structured wholeness, even while continuing, if appropriate, to grow. Second, systems function to contain and transfer

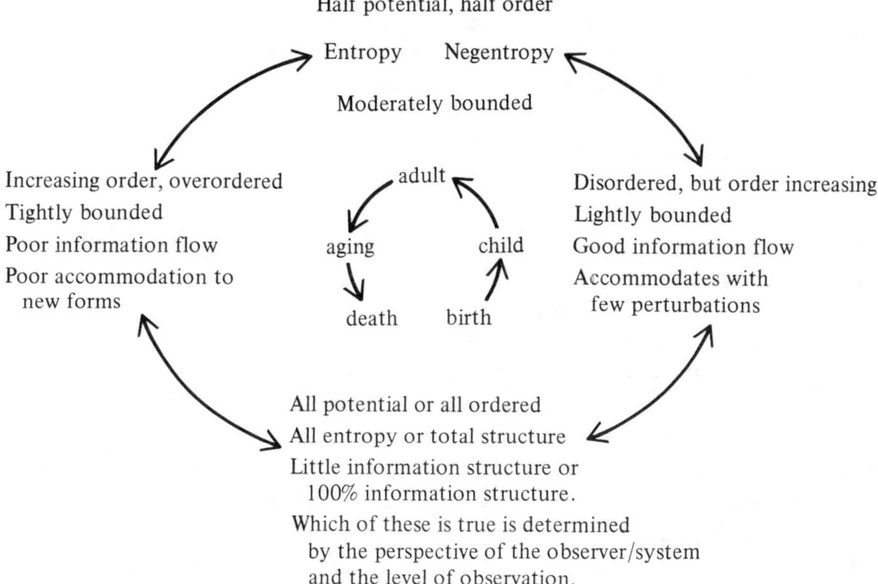

Figure 5.1. A living system: potential/actualized balance.

energy and information from one point to another, within or between them. All systems have some means of boundary creation and maintenance, as well as means of interaction with other systems. This implies that the boundary must be permeable, to some extent, but not so permeable that the system will merge with other systems. Other systems functions are to control other processes, run circular processes, and give feedback. The overall goal is to provide optimum input for continuity and growth, while avoiding pathologic abnormalities and maintaining flexibility.

Change

Systems do change over time. How does this happen? The only way systems can change over time is if some entropy or disorder is present. If this is not readily obvious, consider for a moment what would happen if no disorder were present and all elements were structured into some form; there would be no space available and no raw material to use to make new forms. If a child has used all available blocks and space to make a toy city (all ordered), some disorder must be introduced (push the blocks aside) to make room for the next orderly structure (perhaps a tower) to be built. If my mind is made up on an issue, I must introduce doubt before a change of mind is possible. So disorder – entropy – is not only the catastrophic final state predicted by the second law of thermodynamics but also the beneficial means to a flexible reordering, or growth to a larger order. Figure 5.1 illustrates this further.

When systems change over time, they usually move from complete disorder through increasing order and bounding (a state that may last most of the system's lifetime) to overrigidity. The overly ordered, overly structured rigid state admits no change and will be shattered by any input from outside. An analogy is what happens to a rigid crystal goblet that breaks under high-frequency vibrations, whereas the even thinner skin on the hand holding it does not. Prigogene (1980) notes that it is always possible to create a better structure by shattering a rigid state. From that shattering and the availability it creates will come a more flexible, more complex form. This means the death of the old system, or its reemergence in very altered form.

Imagine a situation in which two systems – societies, for example – come up against each other and try to influence each other (i.e., intrude on each other's boundaries). If the first system is not too rigid and too ordered, the influence and energy of the second will have an impact and alter the first. The reciprocal will also be true. But if the first system is rigid, the second will not be able to influence it. Now, if the energy of the second becomes stronger still, and it cannot influence the first subtly, violent influence may result in a complete shattering of the first. Instead of gradual change occurring, complete change occurs. Thus, defenses sometimes become problems in their own right and destroy rather than protect. The gentler dynamic – mutual influence of semiordered systems – occurs during political dialogue. The second, more catastrophic dynamic – destruction of an old, overly rigid system – occurs during revolutions. Some other examples of the dynamics of change over time in a number of very different systems are given in Tables 5.1, 5.2, and 5.3.

Table 5.1 describes, in column 1, six steps that typically occur over time in any "living" system. Examples of their presence are given for physical systems (column 2), couple or dyad systems (column 3), and cognitive systems (column 4) to show how common and widespread is the evidence for such dynamics over time. Table 5.2 outlines the characteristics of systems that influence whether or not the potential changes over time in Table 5.1 can actually come about in any given case. Table 5.3 relates those characteristics to the challenge of personal change, suggesting that change is a necessary, challenging, natural opportunity that need not be harmful or overly stressful. Intentional personal change, such as that sought in psychotherapy, simply uses these processes efficiently.

System change over time demands more than some degree of entropy. Systems resist disorder on any large scale, and change means the temporary elimination of much order. The resistance to this in the psychological system is evident in the sometimes painful reorganizations during personal change (e.g., in psychotherapy). Any system tries to monitor and control the extent of disorder, but not to resist absolutely, because that would take too much energy. Surviving systems balance their potentials and actualizations, have boundaries (but are not closed), try to fit many contexts flexibly, and attempt to interface with other systems without being engulfed or engulfing. Nonsurviving systems may have the same

Table 5.1. *Patterns of systematic system change over time*

Living system	Physical system	Couple system	Cognitive system
1. Symbiosis, undifferentiated	High entropy, low order	Honeymoon period, finding roles in the marriage	Bottom-up data processing; focused attention; small data base
2. Differentiation	Increasing boundary creation; increasing structure and efficiency	Power struggle	Concrete operations and concept development
3. Temporary homeostasis		Stability	Abstract thought, formal or scientific reasoning; top-down processing now combined with bottom-up processing; spotlight and floodlight attention
4. Dynamic homeostasis		Commitment to the paradox of the other	Selective creation of chosen realities and belief systems
	Balanced, flexible; half-ordered, with moderate boundaries to permit assimilation of new information		
5. Reproduction/synthesis		Co-creation of the relationship and the world	Wisdom; awareness of #4 above; problems usually seen as ill-structured
6. Decay/death	Rigid boundaries, no information flow; any one perturbation can lead to disaster and final entropy		Idiosyncratic top-down imposition of abstract constructs

Table 5.2. *System characteristics that permit change and retard change*

1. The system must permit information to enter; flexibility, but under bounded control.
2. Systems resist disorder.
3. Change means a temporary increase in disorder.
4. Systems monitor and control the amount of disorder.
5. Surviving systems contain the seeds of their own change, are "programmed" to get to the next highest level of order (e.g., puberty is inherent in an infant).
6. Surviving systems balance potentials and activated processes.
7. Surviving systems fit many contexts.
8. Surviving systems are programmed to interfere with each other.
9. Nonsurviving systems have the same parts as surviving systems, but different processes.

Table 5.3. *What systems theory teaches about personal change*

1. All systems change, except those near death; so change is a good sign.
2. Patterns of change are predictable, based on the state of the system and the state of adjacent systems.
3. Change in any one system will influence other systems nearby. Whether this leads to useful or maladaptive changes in those other systems depends on their states.
4. Boundary rigidity in the face of information or energy flow means death; being completely unbounded means dissolution of the system. Systems strive for continuity.
5. Immersion in a new group (i.e., interaction with a new system that is powerful) is a sort of reparenting (transference and imaginal reparenting are other forms) that can efficiently and effectively reorient a system.

structures (e.g., a boundary), but have different processes (e.g., rigidity in a boundary) that are less adaptive.

GST: Next-generation cognitive research?

Systems theory provides a way for us to make sense of a new generation of cognitive research. This volume is addressing one aspect of that new generation of research by examining everyday or naturalistic memory. We are responding to more information that we have allowed to enter our system and disturb it. We have become aware that perceptions of events, and attention, and salience of events, and context, and change over time are important in assessing memory in old age. We have seen that the respondent and the experimenter are not independent of each other, but influence each other at all times. We have seen that what is remembered depends on the vantage point of the rememberer. We have seen that change over time in memory involves compensatory mechanisms that help maintain homeostasis for the person. How do we deal with this complexity? A world view in which causality is linearly dependent on single variables does not do it justice. Simply adopting a multivariate perspective is not adequate either, because such a view often leaves us casting about in the choice of variables to explore. Adoption of a GST view gives us more options regarding ways to talk about process and structure, suggesting variables, dynamics, and even *levels* of study that would be relevant. GST lets us reorder our perturbed system on a more complex level, rather than making our boundaries more rigid in order to ward off the new information.

GST gives cognitive studies access to a relativistic, contextual world view in which subject and object are necessarily related, but in which the scientific method can still be employed and must be. GST is the language of the so-called new physics (relativity theory, quantum mechanics, etc.). In an earlier paper (Sinnott, 1981), I discussed a relativistic model for development. GST is one language that model might use.

What is memory in a GST model?

Memory in a GST model is a storage and organizing function. It can be represented by several different structures, depending on the system in which it operates. Notice that each of the systems can have such a storage mechanism, whose final goal, as stated earlier, is to maintain equilibrium. In each of the systems, there is some structure for storage and some process for storage. The structure might be a short-term bioelectric charge in a cell, or a library, ranging from making associations to storing stone tablets. The same system function is served by many structures and processes.

But what is the purpose of memory in a system? One essential purpose is to preserve equilibrium or to bring it about again by compensations if it is not present or is being threatened. The storage must be storage of information and processes that tend to make peace, so to speak, between the elements within the system or between that system and another system. This means that memory must be able to adjust itself, and to readjust the organism, to events in the ongoing flow of life, and to do so in a way that will lead to real-world survival. Whatever process is involved, real-world survival must be the outcome. What is remembered can be defined only in terms of the real-world success of the living system that *lives.* To the extent that a system has good storage of some element that pushes that system toward abnormality or death, or nonstorage of adaptive information, we can say that it has "memory problems." Systems with problems might be cells that store erroneous information in genes, leading to tumor production, or humans who are obsessive regarding memories from childhood, leading to maladaptive responses today. The problem might be forgetting digits when recall of digits is needed, or remembering digits when anger or love songs are required.

Four GST arguments for natural memory research

Memory-based equilibrium-generating processes determine and result from interactions among systems (e.g., interpersonal interactions). Any study of memory that neglects those other systems is, to some extent, invalid. Memory for digits, then, may not mean that a person-system can stay equilibrated in a survival-oriented sense, a truth that absentminded professors show us. This is one reason that systems theory is an argument for natural memory research.

Another essential purpose of memory in systems theory is to preserve the flexibility of the system. With the passage of time, a system becomes more rigid and ordered (negentropic). Storage includes storage of rules that permit modification of that order to some degree. It also includes basic processes for restructuring the self at points of growing energy and disorder; see Prigogene (1980) and Prigogene and Stengers (1984) for more on this. Material can be stored and accessed when needed in more flexible or less flexible ways. When one system interfaces with another and storage/access is more flexible, the interfacing can go more smoothly. So, when studying memory, the functions of flexible change and interfacing with other systems must be addressed. What are the contexts in which memory is shaped so that the end result is flexible storage and access? What are the storage systems that lead to greater flexibility in real-world handling of information? The fact that we do not know the answers to these questions (questions generated from GST) argues for natural memory studies and a GST approach.

A third essential purpose for memory in systems theory is to control and limit information flow. Memory/storage categories and processes can limit the perceptual filter and thereby decrease the risks of overstimulation or understimulation. They can permit more or less information to be processed, changing, for example, the number of other systems with which one might be capable of interacting meaningfully. Because the purpose of the control of information flow in GST is optimization of multisystem functioning in the real world, the systems view again argues for naturalistic memory studies.

A final major purpose of memory or storage in GST relates to entropy (i.e., disorder). Memory serves to keep disorder at bay and to increase the structuredness or orderedness of the system. This function, over time, increases internal order and efficiency at the expense of external order; in other words, outside the system there is greater and greater entropy, whereas inside there is greater order. If GST tells us that the function of memory is an ordering function, and that this happens over time, natural memory studies are necessary to tease out the nature of that order – with its survival value – and to see the effects on the other systems from increasing the order in one system.

GST generates questions

Memory in a GST model can be storage of energy for cells or storage of concepts for humans or storage of historical data for societies or many other actualities. A GST model is useful, then, for suggesting some further purposes and processes for memory, based on its analogues in the other systems involved. If memory, for a culture, involves relativistically storing many truths and deriving from them a single truth, what is the analogous process for the human system? Is there one? If memory, for a cell, involves energy storage and release in transformed bursts, what might be an analogue process in memory for emotions in humans? Beyond this, the whole of GST teaches us to beware of a memory model that does not reach beyond its own system to the nested systems within and without. Memory studies must deal with the role of memory as a regulation (control, monitor), especially between the person and what Bronfenbrenner (1979) calls the microsystem, mesosystem, macrosystem, and exosystem (i.e., the progressively larger social and cultural worlds). Memory studies must explore the real-world compensatory functions of which storage and retrieval are parts. Blauberg, Sadovsky, and Yudin (1977) and Miller (1978) have suggested many other control-, attention-, and survival-related questions generated by GST.

General implications

What does knowledge of a systems approach imply for the study of memory and aging? We saw some of those implications in the preceding comments. "Memory problems" now must have an expanded definition. Survival value must be considered the criterion for success (Bruce, Chapter 4, this volume). Memory itself must be seen in its much more active role of defender of equilibrium, compensations, flexibility, and control of intrasystem and intersystem forces. The contexts in which system memory develops best and retains its adaptivity under stress need to be examined. How memory operates as a controller needs study. The optimum entropy useful for different memory capacities would be useful to know to make better sense of research results related to aging. And other systems at levels other than the human level need to be examined for storage processes that might give clues to other processing aspects of memory that we have discounted (e.g., the control function for information flow). All this is best examined in some combination of naturalistic and laboratory settings.

The major implication is this: Memory research must include the everyday, the naturalistic, to generate meaningful questions about an ability that is really a survival function for an organism living in a multisystem world. The human system is not operating in a vacuum; it operates in a context and is defined by interactions in that context. Within a systems view, every laboratory study of memory is a study of memory in context, the context of the laboratory. In that context, the analysis and manipulation of other systems levels are minimized to achieve control, but the cost is large. Interactions with other systems are trivialized, and the purpose – survival – is distorted. One can learn very different things about the human heart by dissecting it or by observing it as a functioning part of an intact body. Science need not restrain itself from examining all truths, and GST permits syntheses of many ideas, so that focused analyses can be based on a richer theoretical view.

Some implications suggested by a GST approach, especially the work of Miller (1978), include the following: Storage capabilities may differ between those using *much* or *little* stored information to solve problems. Memory may improve if boundaries become more flexible. Storage may be handled differently by overloaded and understimulated systems. At some *n*th level of load or complexity, individual memory systems may begin to "compensate" by some sharing device. Storage processes in the laboratory and in the natural contexts may or may not be comparable. Several kinds of memories may serve different survival needs. Storage processes may help maintain equilibrium. Because human systems are nested in social systems and hold physical systems within them, changes in physical or social functional parameters may lead to changes in human storage systems. Storage processes of two systems in proximity to one another may influence each other across flexible boundaries; there may be certain systems contexts in which very good storage systems become that good. More entropy may be introduced into an overstructured storage system. Younger systems may compensate for less well ordered storage processes. Other cognitive processes may be influenced by the level of order within storage systems. I could go on, but the point is clear already. A GST approach does enrich our study of memory and implies that much of our work should occur in natural settings.

Applications to aging

Throughout this discussion there have been hints about ways GST thinking might apply to studies of aging memory. In this section, I hope to make several ideas more explicit. It is important first to mention that, for this author, "aging" is defined not so much by years as by degree of rigid structuredness or terminal entropic deterioration. To some degree, of course, age and structuredness correlate. But for the moment, let us remember that a system is old when it is rigid and has strong boundaries that permit little information flow. Our aging studies will include, then, chronologically old persons, some of whom have old systems and some of whom do not.

Aging, then, means slower, more idiosyncratic performance. GST ideas serve aging studies when we address how the degree of stimulation is regulated in such a system. A system has an optimum amount of stimulation (or information, energy) it can process; old systems process less. What information is selected for processing? How? What survival effects result? Can lack of stimulation be modified by modifying boundaries? Explanations for slowing of memory and possibilities for intervention are richer if one thinks in GST terms.

Older persons often perform adequately although seriously lacking in one or more processes. Perhaps they compensate somehow, we say. Using a GST view, we assume that all systems compensate and have regulatory processes to decide when to compensate. They compensate for internal disequilibria and for disequilibria resulting from encounters with other systems. Older systems need to compensate for rigid boundaries and excessive orderedness (and therefore for too little information entering and leaving storage); younger systems need to compensate for too little structuredness and for boundaries that are too porous (and therefore for too few pegs on which to store data, and for too few data overall). The overall system state is the only thing that can predict the kinds of cognitive compensation needed or the outcomes of various compensations. GST would consider how those behaviors serve the system and result from storage problems.

Rigid, cautious performance is characteristic of the declining old, and such performance influences families and society. The overstructured system has little storage available. Another system may encounter it, try to share information, and be rebuffed in self-defense, unheard, making no impact on thicker and thicker boundaries. Perhaps the second system then tries harder to share information. This induces perturbations in the first. If these become strong enough, the structure of the first system may fly apart and be destroyed (this is a sort of terminal disorder), or it may be ordered at a new, more adaptive level (this is the leap to a new order described by Prigogene). At this point, storage either will have ended or will have become more adaptive: one cycle of effects and feedback from an individual to other levels of family and society. Any action influences the entire order of nested systems. So memory can be viewed as an information-processing component that helps keep order in the continually changing multiperson space of the older person.

In Chapter 20, I give an example of one simpleminded approach to employment of GST in memory/aging research, namely, the study of prospective/intentional memory (memory for what one needs to know to do something later). This sort of storage is survival-oriented and links a personal system with other personal systems and with the social system.

In closing, let me point out the key differences between the GST way of thinking about memory and more common models of memory, aware as always that each serves a different but useful purpose. GST has the following characteristics:

1. Change over time is emphasized.
2. The inner and outer contexts of the person-system are crucial.
3. Boundary rigidity, information flow, and equilibrium maintenance are important because they are crucial to survival.

In addressing research questions where systems operations can be assumed to occur, where multiple systems seem to be in effect, where survival-related functioning is present, or where change over time is important, GST suggests that the study of natural memory is needed.

References

Bertalanfy, L. von (1968). *General systems theory.* New York: Braziller.

Blauberg, I. V., Sadovsky, V. N., & Yudin, E. G. (1977). *Systems theory.* Moscow: Progress Publishers.

Bronfenbrenner, U. (1979). *The ecology of human development.* Cambridge, MA: Harvard University Press.

Lockland, G. T. (1973). *Grow or die.* New York: Random House.

Miller, J. G. (1978). *Living systems.* New York: McGraw-Hill.

Neumann, J. von, & Morgenstern, O. (1947). *Theory of games and economic behavior.* Princeton: Princeton University Press.

Prigogene, I. (1980). *From being to becoming*. San Francisco: Freeman.

Prigogene, I., & Stengers, I. (1984). *Order out of chaos: Man's new dialog with nature*. New York: Bantam.

Sinnott, J. D. (1981). The theory of relativity: A metatheory for development? *Human Development, 24*, 293–311.

Weiner, N. (1961). *Cybernetics*. Cambridge, MA: M.I.T. Press.

Part IB

Combining laboratory and real-world research

6 The laboratory and ecology: Supplementary sources of data for memory research

Harry P. Bahrick

Nonexperimental methods have a well-accepted place among the research strategies employed by psychologists. Such methods have long been part of the standard content of textbooks dealing with research methodology (Elmes, Kantowitz, & Roediger, 1985; Festinger & Katz, 1953). In certain areas of the field (e.g., the psychology of personality or abnormal psychology), naturalistic investigations predominate. In other areas (e.g., perception, learning, and memory), the laboratory approach has been preeminent.

Historical perspective

Experimental methods were introduced into psychology during the 19th century, when it was first demonstrated that some psychological questions would yield to a laboratory attack. The success of these first efforts promoted the acceptance of psychology as a science and gave rise to the term "experimental psychology." Although the meaning of that term has changed somewhat during the last 100 years (Danziger, 1985), the emphasis on the laboratory as a place for empirical explorations has remained and has promoted the scientific status of psychology. Exclusive organizations and journals (e.g., the Society of Experimental Psychologists and the *Journal of Experimental Psychology*) helped to establish traditions and define a separate, elitist image for laboratory research and for psychologists who used experimental methods. Memory research has been dominated by these traditions for most of the past century. However, demands for ecological validity have challenged these traditions from time to time, and the challenges have been particularly effective during the last decade. It appears that we are now ready for an objective examination of the kinds of research strategies most likely to advance the field, and I shall attempt such an examination after a brief recapitulation of the developments that have brought on today's more eclectic climate.

This material is based on work supported by the National Science Foundation under grant BNS-8417788.

Twelve years ago, when I submitted a manuscript to the *Journal of Experimental Psychology,* dealing with 50 years of memory for the names and faces of high school classmates, I fully expected the manuscript to be rejected. Up until that time, so far as I know, that journal had published only the results of experiments. To my surprise, the issue was never raised. Obviously, standards had fallen everywhere, and experimental psychology was no exception.

The decade of the 1970s was not the first time the issue of ecological validity was raised in regard to psychological research. Empirical psychology began in Germany by analyzing conscious content down to its elements, and no one in the Humboldtian university would have earned the respect of academic peers by raising questions about the ecological validity of scholarship. Everyone who has read Boring's *History of Experimental Psychology* (1950) knows that the psychology imported from Germany changed radically when it was brought to America. Our philosophy of education was greatly influenced by pragmatism, which in turn reflected the impact of evolutionary theory and an emphasis on the process of adaptation. Functional psychologists studied adjustment in all sorts of settings, including the workplace, the school, and the home. Learning research was influenced by this pragmatic ethos. It will suffice to cite the classic work on learning curves by Bryan and Harter (1897). These pioneers investigated the process of learning to send and receive Morse code, and they collected their data over a period of 40 weeks in an ecological setting.

The pragmatic emphasis had changed completely by the 1940s and 1950s, when I received my psychological education. The new zeitgeist was a reaction to the frustrations of an era in which laissez faire theorizing and inadequate methods of verification had produced irresolvable controversy and an accumulation of untestable theory. The reaction brought the imposition of operationist rules and a determination to follow the model provided by physics. Experimental psychology was characterized by a relentless demand for analytic reductionism in the study of learning and memory and an uncompromising pursuit of laboratory control as the basis for establishing scientific truth. Challenging questions regarding the ecological relevance of the work on eye blinks, nonsense syllables, and rats were brushed aside with the assertion that the pursuit of pure science had priority and that the rest would readily fall into place.

What turned things around again during the iconoclastic 1960s? We all have our own historical perspectives over the recent past. I would cite the involvement of physicists in the development of atomic weapons as a significant stimulus for heightened public awareness of the social responsibilities of scientists. The Vietnam War and the challenges to our institutions that came in its wake also played important roles. The psychological establishment could not remain immune, and questions about the relevance of psychological research to the pressing problems of society could no longer be brushed aside.

The new ecological emphasis has affected all areas of psychology. One need only examine the divisional membership of the American Psychological Association (APA), or the program of an APA convention to be convinced that psychologists now believe that their work must address the needs of society. Although experimental psychologists have not been in the forefront of this change, they have shared in it. Applications of the principles of learning to ecological problems include techniques of behavior modification, desensitization, biofeedback, and programmed instruction, to name but a few. It is my belief that we have had a good start in applying what we know about learning to ecologically important situations, but we have been much less successful in developing applications for our knowledge of memory. Neisser (1982), in the preface to his book *Memory Observed,* concurs with this view. He states that we have lots of data, but the wrong kind of knowledge. Theories of memory, he says, ''are either so closely bound to particular experiments that they are uninteresting, or so vague, that they are intellectually unsatisfying'' (p. xii). There is now a growing realization that the study of memory must deal with problems that are important, rather than with problems that lend themselves to laboratory investigation, and that the gap between memory research and real-life problems requiring an understanding of memory can be closed only if we deal with the problems directly, not if we wait for things to fall into place.

When David Rubin raised the questions of when, why, and how memory researchers collect data in the real world, he may not have had in mind the changes of *Fachgeist* that I have reviewed, but the sociology of science provides a start toward the answers of which we must not lose sight. Researchers will go outside of the laboratory to collect data only if doing so is likely to be accepted by the scientific establishment. Although attitudes regarding the merits of nonlaboratory research on memory still vary widely, there is now sufficient support for this approach to expect it to be pursued by a significant number of investigators.

Why look beyond the laboratory?

Given the circumstances that make ecological memory research an option, we should now ask under what circumstances the decision to go outside the laboratory is sensible.

The laboratory generally offers the greatest control over potentially intrusive conditions, and it permits manipulation of individual variables. This environment is considered optimal for obtaining reliable answers to questions. The trouble, of course, has been that many phenomena of memory that we wish to know more about do not lend themselves to laboratory exploration, and it has become apparent to most memory scholars that we cannot expect to overcome that problem by extrapolating from available laboratory findings. Thus, Kintsch (1974) concluded a decade ago that

> Most of the experimental research concerning memory has never really dealt with problems of the acquisition and retention of knowledge, but with episodic memory which is not

> at all the problem of interest in education. Simply replacing the words with sentences in our experiments will make the research no more relevant to education than it was before. An educational technology squarely based upon psychological research needs research concerned with problems of knowledge. (p. 4)

Neisser (1978) is even more explicit in his critique of the failure of traditional memory research to deal with important naturalistic memory problems. He points out that higher education

> depends heavily on the assumption that students remember something valuable from their educational experience. One might expect psychologists to leap at the opportunity to study a critical memory problem so close at hand, but they never do. It is difficult to find even a single study, ancient or modern, of what is retained from academic instruction. Given our expertise and the way we earn our livings, this omission can only be described as scandalous. (p. 5)

Naturalistic memory research is essential whenever the memory content of interest does not lend itself to laboratory acquisition. Only recently has it been made explicit (Bahrick & Karis, 1982) how many types of memory content are unsuitable for laboratory acquisition, and consequently how limiting the exclusive reliance on laboratory memory research has turned out to be.

Content must generally be acquired in nonlaboratory settings if the acquisition period exceeds a few hours, if long retention intervals are of interest, if the content to be investigated is acquired under conditions that may be dangerous or motivationally or emotionally potent, or if the content is legally, morally, or ethically controversial. Other domains of content are intrinsically unamenable to laboratory control because they are autonomously generated (i.e., they are widely independent of manipulable conditions). Memory content involving fantasy, dreams, and diverse thought processes is an example. Such content can, of course, be experienced in the laboratory, but the advantages of the laboratory are lost to the extent that the content cannot be controlled and objectively assessed. Laboratory memory research is therefore largely limited to the retention of content that is under direct control of an experimenter, that can be presented during a few hours or less, that is emotionally and motivationally neutral, and that is tested for retention within a few days following acquisition. Excluded from laboratory memory research on this basis is virtually all semantic content, including material taught in schools, and most autobiographical content. Semantic content is excluded because acquisition and retention periods are excessive, and most autobiographical content is excluded not only for these reasons but also because it is acquired under a diversity of naturalistic situations unsuitable for laboratory observation or monitoring.

Thus, one answer to the question of why naturalistic memory research needs to be done is quite simple. If we fail to do it, we shall exclude from scientific exploration most of the domains of memory content likely to interest the educator, the psychotherapist, the novelist, the jurist, and so on, and memory research will fail to address the needs of society.

Memory research limited to the laboratory not only will fail to solve applied problems in need of solutions but also will fail to develop general principles governing the functions of memory in a wide range of situations. Naturalistic memory research is the only way, for example, to discover those general characteristics of the memory system that apply to long time periods and therefore cannot be explored in the laboratory. Discovering principles of memory relevant to education not only requires the examination of relevant memory content, as Kintsch (1974) has pointed out, but also requires an understanding of memory functions that extend over decades, rather than minutes, hours, or days. The goals of education extend over the human life span, and effects that are of short duration are trivial. The potential of naturalistic memory research for developing general principles governing very long term memory has already been demonstrated in a study of 50 years of memory for Spanish language learned in school (Bahrick, 1984). This investigation shows that forgetting comes to a halt 3 to 5 years after learning terminates, and the remaining content survives undiminished for at least a quarter of a century. This study of "permastore" memory content has led to the conclusion that there is a discrete change in the prospective life span of information, from a life span of less than 5 years to a life span of more than 25 years, and that this discrete change occurs at a certain point during an extended period of exposure to the same information. The generality of this conclusion is yet to be established, as are the circumstances under which this discrete transition occurs; however, the important point is that such characteristics of the memory system can be established only on the basis of cross-sectional, naturalistic investigations capable of dealing with very long time intervals.

The sacrifice of laboratory control may, of course, involve a loss of scientific rigor, and questions arise regarding the acceptability of such trade-offs. How much loss of rigor can be justified in order to be able to investigate memory content not amenable to laboratory exploration? In a previous publication (Bahrick & Karis, 1982), we argued that it makes little sense to adopt an arbitrary standard of precision that must be met to justify scientific work, particularly if this standard is chosen because it prevails in other areas of science. It is true that psychology was first accepted as a science on the basis of demonstrations that certain psychological questions could be attacked by methods comparable in precision to those of the more established sciences. This precedent should, however, not guide current decisions regarding research strategies appropriate to advance the field. Progress is made in science when we improve the current state of knowledge, not simply when we achieve arbitrary standards of precision typical of research in other areas. Optimum research strategies of psychologists must be determined by the nature of psychological phenomena, not by the models available from other areas of science.

The key to developing a more complete psychological science is found in improvising methods for investigating currently inaccessible phenomena that interest us, not in continuing to apply existing methods to those phenomena amenable to the existing methods while we ignore the rest.

The how of naturalistic memory research

We can now turn our attention to the nature of alternative strategies. The alternative strategies must be able to deal with acquisition periods and with retention intervals of long duration. With a naturalistic approach, retention tests generally are still administered under standard laboratory conditions, but the acquisition of content occurs in a nonlaboratory environment (e.g., school, home, office, playground); the acquisition period as well as the retention interval may be very long, and the conditions prevailing during acquisition and during the retention interval are not controlled by the investigator.

Strategies capable of meeting these conditions have been available for more than half a century in the form of multiple-regression techniques, but they have been largely ignored by experimental psychologists. Cronbach (1957) called attention to this major problem in this field in his presidential address to the APA more than a quarter of a century ago. He pointed out that correlational psychology and experimental psychology have developed independent of each other, and he deplored the fact that psychologists seem to be limiting their investigations to one or the other method of inquiry, rather than to an attempt at integration. Unfortunately, what he said more than 25 years ago is still true and, in my opinion, is largely responsible for our slow progress in extending memory research to most naturalistic situations. Cronbach (1957) pointed out that the correlational method can be used to study what humans have not learned to control or can never hope to control: "Nature has been experimenting since the beginning of time, with a boldness and complexity far beyond the resources of science. The correlator's mission is to observe and organize the data from nature's experiments" (p. 672). He further discussed the fact that social psychologists, child psychologists, and others continuously avail themselves of this resource, but perception and learning psychologists do not. They have given scant attention to individual differences, using them primarily as a basis for estimating experimental error. This has been largely true of traditional memory research, which has followed the direction taken by Ebbinghaus. Although regression is now frequently used in the analysis of experimental results, the technique has not been used to explore individual differences or long-term relations among variables in naturalistic settings.

Cronbach criticized the use of single-variable designs by experimental psychologists as manifestly in conflict with their awareness of the multifaceted nature of tasks and responses: "The correlational psychologist discovered long ago that no observed criterion is truly valid and that simultaneous consideration of many criteria is needed for a satisfactory evaluation of performance" (p. 676). He quoted Miller (1957) to the effect that theoretical progress is obstructed when one restricts oneself to a single measure of response, and he concluded that experimenters have much to gain by treating their dependent variables as a continuous multivariate system.

We can add to Cronbach's observations that the multiple-correlation technique is perfectly suited to cope with the long acquisition and retention intervals that constitute an insurmountable problem to the memory experiment. Industrial and educational psychologists have used multiple-correlation techniques for more than half a century in situations that require relating criterion measures to test scores obtained years earlier. The classic problem of predicting college grades on the basis of SAT scores or high school records illustrates this type of application. The correlational approach not only allows us to bridge the time intervals but also can be used to treat time as an independent variable and determine the effect of time on the relations between other independent and dependent variables.

During the past decade, I have used a correlational approach in three major investigations of memory, each based on a large number of subjects, and a cross-sectional design in which some subgroups had acquired the relevant knowledge quite recently, whereas others had acquired the knowledge at intervals of up to 50 years earlier (Bahrick, 1983a, 1984; Bahrick, Bahrick, & Wittlinger, 1975). In each of these investigations it was possible to obtain retention functions that covered a 50-year time span and to use memory content acquired over a period of several years. The functions, when adjusted by multiple-regression techniques, show as much stability as functions obtained in the laboratory for short intervals. Furthermore, each of these investigations assessed the effects of many different independent variables operating during the acquisition period and during the retention interval. The effect of each variable can be statistically removed, or it can be projected over a 50-year period. This is done simply by substituting the appropriate value of the variable (including the value of zero) in the regression equation and reevaluating the equation. Thus, one can determine how well the scores in Spanish reading comprehension are predicted by grades received in Spanish courses 50 years earlier and compare this to the effect due to the number of courses taken or to the number of days the individual spent in Spanish-speaking countries during the 50-year interval. Even if experiments dealing with such long time periods were possible, it would take a great many of them to yield the information available from a single correlational study. In addition, each of these investigations involved the use of many dependent variables, not just one or two, as is typically the case in the experimental approach. Thus, we can determine the differential effects of travel in Spanish-speaking countries on Spanish reading comprehension, Spanish recall vocabulary, or Spanish idiom recognition simply by evaluating the respective regression equations for each of these dependent variables. This approach demonstrates that no individual criterion can validly reflect retained knowledge and that simultaneous consideration of many criteria is essential to understand complex cognitive phenomena (Cronbach, 1957).

It is now appropriate to consider the limitations and problems of this method of investigating memory, lest we fall into the trap of treating our methodological advances as panaceas. One obvious shortcoming of the approach is that it confounds the age of the memory trace with the age of the individual, and this confounding makes it difficult to interpret the decline of retention. An additional investigation (Bahrick, 1983b) comparing retention among groups who learned the same material at different ages is needed to sort out these two interpretations. It may, however, be impossible to obtain the additional observations necessary to distinguish between explanations (e.g., because a particular content is always acquired by subjects at a certain age). In naturalistic memory research, the correlational approach is rarely designed to test hypotheses; it is therefore unlikely to yield unequivocal statements about causation, and often it must be supplemented with an experimental or quasi-experimental study (Bahrick, 1983b).

Another problem in interpreting retention functions based on multiple-regression equations is related to the weights representing the various independent variables in the equation. The stepwise method, most commonly used, adds variables to the program in accordance with the order of magnitude of their correlations with the residual variance of the dependent variable. If, instead of stepwise regression, some other, more arbitrary method of entering variables is followed, the weights of the independent variables will not be the same. Statements regarding the relative importances of the individual variables over the course of the retention interval are therefore contingent on the assumptions underlying the stepwise procedure.

Still other problems relate to the assumption of interval scaling inherent in the use of product-moment correlations and to the assumption of regression equations based on intercorrelation matrices. Although that assumption may be fulfilled for the individual indicants of the dependent and independent variables (e.g., number of Spanish words recalled versus the retention interval measured in years), the assumption may no longer hold if interpretations are extended to a theoretical construct such as "Spanish recall vocabulary" to be revealed by the dependent indicants. The indicant may reflect the construct only in an ordinal sense, not in an interval sense, because of floor effects or ceiling effects or other changes in sensitivity of measurement. As Nelson (1985) has pointed out, there may be no justification for assuming that the dependent variable is a linear indicant of the construct to be revealed, and if the function is nonlinear, then a product-moment correlation of the indicant may misrepresent the relationship in question. Cautious interpretation of results is therefore essential, and one must avoid the implication that the obtained functions can be generalized to theoretical constructs or to other indicants. Such generalizations may become more appropriate when several related indicants of a construct yield the same types of retention functions.

The most fundamental limitation on the usefulness of multiple-regression methods in life-span memory research is the difficulty of obtaining valid assessments of the important independent variables. These variables must reveal how much knowledge the individual subject originally had and to what extent he or she was exposed to relevant information during the retention interval. The events in question may have occurred many years earlier, and the original exposure and subsequent reexposure usually constitute multidimensional phenomena that may not be easily reflected in the form of simple scales. For these reasons, valid assessment of these phenomena constitutes a major challenge to the investigator. Clearly, the choice of knowledge systems that lend themselves to investigations of naturalistic memory research is restricted by these considerations. Fortunately, success and failure in overcoming this problem are easily diagnosed. The magnitudes of the multiple correlations of independent variables with each of the dependent variables will reveal to what extent the available indicants can account for variance in retention. Thus, in the study of retention of Spanish language learned in school (Bahrick, 1984), the reports of subjects regarding the number of courses taken, the grades received, and the time elapsed since the courses were taken account for approximately 50% of the variance on the various subtests for retention of Spanish. This alleviates concerns about the reliability of the reports, about problems regarding the comparability of grades, and about cohort effects and all other sources of error. Two other investigations of life-span memory yielded multiple correlations of approximately the same magnitude, indicating that there are various knowledge systems that permit this approach. Identification of suitable indicants of independent variables and development of appropriate scales of measurement constitute problems for the investigator that are unlike those encountered in most laboratory research and will differ for every investigation. In some cases we were able to obtain archival data (e.g., records from the college registrar or the city directory), and in other instances it was possible to obtain independent memory reports from two or more individuals to corroborate necessary information. The methodology of life-span memory research is only in its infancy, but the preliminary indications are that a cross-sectional approach, combined with the technology of multiple-regression analysis, is best suited to do justice to the complexity of changing knowledge systems maintained over long time periods.

Other methods of naturalistic memory research are being developed to deal with the great variety of naturalistic memory content. Linton (1975) effectively used a diary to establish the accuracy of individual episodic memory over a period of years, and Neisser (1982) took advantage of taped records to study the accuracy of John Dean's testimony regarding White House conversations. Warrington and Silberstein (1970) pioneered methods of assessing long-term memory for shared episodic memories by testing recall and recognition of significant public events. The events were originally selected from the *New York Times* review of the year, but the method has been extended to include memory for well-known faces (Warrington & Sanders, 1971), the names of television shows (Squire & Slater, 1975), the names of racehorses, and so forth. The method makes it possible to investigate event memory over very long time periods, but the assumption that the original exposures to all events were equal is troublesome, and it is difficult to assess the extent to which subsequent exposures during the retention interval augment retention scores. Control groups of teenagers too young to have experienced the events (Squire & Slater, 1975; Warrington & Sanders, 1971) or adults who lived abroad during part of the period covered by the test are useful in assessing the degree of such confounding. Perhaps the method will ultimately be combined with a multiple-regression technique capable of correcting for these effects and at the same time take into account individual-difference variables, such as educational level, intelligence, gender, and so forth. The neglect of individual-difference variables in the study of memory has been a consequence of the predominant experimental emphasis and has been deplored by Linton (1975) and Bruce (Chapter 4, this volume) in recent papers. They advocate a Darwinian, ecological orientation that would continue to emphasize the search for general principles. It is a safe prediction that ecological memory research will lead to the development of a plethora of new methods suitable for investigating diverse memory content not now subject to exploration.

What are the implications for future laboratory research?

Scientific knowledge is cumulative, and memory research will be no exception. We must continue to build on the legacy of 100 years of experience, and the evolution of laboratory methodology is the most significant portion of that legacy. New methods will supplement rather than replace the methods now available, and laboratory manipulation will remain preferable to naturalistic observations whenever the phenomena of interest permit it. The work on the accuracy of eyewitness testimony (Loftus, 1979) illustrates that some memory problems of obvious ecological importance can be examined with traditional methods without sacrificing validity. For other areas of ecologically important research, the laboratory will serve as an adjunct to aid in the resolution of questions left unanswered by naturalistic observations.

I see the future of memory research as pluralistic and pragmatic, with few constraints based on assumptions regarding content, process, or method. Such an eclectic approach lacks theoretical elegance, but I see it as an appropriate sequel to the sterility of a long period of overly restricted research.

References

Bahrick, H. P. (1983a). The cognitive map of a city – 50 years of learning and memory. In G. H. Bower (Ed.), *The psychology of learning and motivation. Advances in research and theory 17* (pp. 125–163). New York: Academic Press.

Bahrick, H. P. (1983b). Memory and people. In J. Harris & P. Morris (Eds.), *Everyday memory, actions, and absentmindedness* (pp. 19–34). New York: Academic Press.

Bahrick, H. P. (1984). Semantic memory content in permastore: Fifty years of memory for Spanish learned in school. *Journal of Experimental Psychology: General, 113,* 1–29.

Bahrick, H. P., Bahrick, P. O., & Wittlinger, R. P. (1975). Fifty years of memories for names and faces: A cross-sectional approach. *Journal of Experimental Psychology: General, 104,* 54–75.

Bahrick, H. P., & Karis, D. (1982). Long-term ecological memory. In C. R. Puff (Ed.), *Handbook of research methods in human memory and cognition.* New York: Academic Press.

Boring, E. G. (1950). *A history of experimental psychology* (2nd ed.), New York: Appleton-Century-Crofts.

Bruce, D. (1985). The how and why of ecological memory. *Journal of Experimental Psychology: General, 114,* 78–90.

Bryan, W. L., & Harter, N. (1897). Studies in the physiology and psychology of telegraphic language. *Psychological Review, 4,* 27–53.

Cronbach, L. J. (1957). The two disciplines of scientific psychology. *American Psychologist, 12,* 671–684.

Danziger, K. (1985). The origins of the psychological experiment as a social institution. *American Psychologist, 40,* 133–140.

Elmes, D. G., Kantowitz, B. H., & Roediger, H. L., III (1985). *Research methods in psychology* (2nd ed.). St. Paul: West.

Festinger, L., & Katz, D. (Eds.). (1953). *Research methods in the behavioral sciences.* New York: Dryden Press.

Galton, F. (1883). *Inquiries into human faculty and its development.* London: Macmillan.

Kintsch, W. (1974). *The representation of meaning in memory.* Hillsdale, N.J.: Lawrence Erlbaum.

Linton, M. (1975). Memory for real world events. In D. A. Norman & D. E. Rumelhart (Eds.), *Explorations in cognition.* San Francisco: Freeman.

Linton, M. (1978). Real world memory after six years: An in vivo study of very long-term memory. In M. M. Gruneberg, P. E. Morris, & R. N. Sykes (Eds.), *Practical aspects of memory* (pp. 69–76). New York: Academic Press.

Loftus, E. F. (1979). *Eyewitness testimony.* Cambridge, MA: Harvard University Press.

Miller, N. E. (1957). Objective techniques for studying motivational effects of drugs on animals. In E. Trabucchi (Ed.), *Proceedings of the international symposium on psychotropic drugs.* Amsterdam: Elsevier.

Nelson, T. O. (1985). Ebbinghaus' contribution to the measurement of retention: Savings during relearning. *Journal of Experimental Psychology: General,*

Neisser, U. (1978). Memory: What are the important questions? In M. M. Gruneberg, P. E. Morris, & H. N. Sykes (Eds.), *Practical aspects of memory* (pp. 3–24). London: Academic Press.

Neisser, U. (Ed.). (1982). *Memory observed: Remembering in natural contexts.* San Francisco: Freeman.

Parkman, J. M. (1972). Temporal aspects of simple multiplication and comparison. *Journal of Experimental Psychology, 95,* 437–444.

Squire, L. R., & Slater, P. C. (1975). Forgetting in very long-term memory as assessed by an improved questionnaire technique. *Journal of Experimental Psychology: Human Learning and Memory. 104,* 50–54.

Warrington, E. K., & Sanders, H. I. (1971. The fate of old memories. *Quarterly Journal of Experimental Psychology, 23,* 432–442.

Warrington, E. K., & Silberstein, M. (1970). A questionnaire technique for investigating very long term memory. *Quarterly Journal of Experimental Psychology, 22,* 508–512.

7 Issues of regularity and control: Confessions of a regularity freak

David C. Rubin

The laboratory offers a high degree of experimental control. That is why laboratories were devised in the first place, and that is why scientists often forsake real-world problems to enter them. This chapter is an argument that, given our present state of knowledge, control is more often a vice than a virtue. It is not experimental control that is now desirable, but rather regularity of results. The time for control will come, but psychology entered the laboratory too quickly. Psychology must first spend time observing and quantifying behavior in its fuller state of complexity. This chapter describes the rationale for this approach, followed by examples of research that has applied it to the topic of human memory.

The best way to start arguing for a flight from the laboratory in the area of memory research is to examine how we entered the laboratory in the first place. Ebbinghaus (1885/1964), in arguing that human memory could be studied in a scientific fashion, provided as clear a definition of the experimental method as exists in the psychological literature. In a section titled "The Method of Natural Science," he writes as follows:

> We all know of what this method consists: an attempt is made to keep constant the mass of conditions which have proven themselves causally connected with a certain result; one of these conditions is isolated from the rest and varied in a way that can be numerically described; then the accompanying change on the side of the effect is ascertained by measurement or computation. (Ebbinghaus, 1885/1964, p. 7)

> When, however, we have actually obtained in such manner the greatest possible constancy of conditions attainable by us, how are we to know whether this is sufficient for our purpose? When are the circumstances, which will certainly offer differences enough to keen observation, sufficiently constant? The answer may be made: When upon repetition of the experiment the results remain constant. (p. 12)

Notice that Ebbinghaus insisted that quantification and control are necessary for science. But how did he know if sufficient control had been obtained? Not by

Support for the preparation of this chapter was provided by NIA grant AG04278 and NSF grant BNS-8410124.

measuring how accurate the controls were, but by measuring their effects on the regularity of the observed behavior. Ebbinghaus looked for evidence of sufficient control in the results, not in the environment. I shall not argue with any of what Ebbinghaus said, except to note that he made one assumption that is almost always correct in the physical sciences and almost always incorrect in studying human behavior. He assumed that increasing control over the external environment increases the regularity of the behavior observed. It is much more common that the opposite is true – a counterintuitive claim that will soon be supported. This one minor flaw in a brilliant work has slowed progress in memory research and in psychology in general. Ebbinghaus did exactly what was needed to demonstrate to a skeptical world that a scientific study of memory was possible. The problem is that his success hid his erroneous assumption for so long.

Less control provides more regularity

The real world, not the laboratory, offers the best chance of observing regularity. For some behaviors and some initial levels of control, my counterintuitive claim must be wrong. However, when the average degree of control that has existed in the laboratory is considered, the claim is basically correct. When the environment is controlled in the laboratory, it tends to become simpler than the environment in which people normally operate. It tends to lack the kind of stimuli to which people normally respond. The simpler, or impoverished, environment of the laboratory is a stimulus that fails to exert stimulus control over behavior. The result is an increase in nonrepeated, seemingly random, behavior. This argument could be made in terms of using stimuli with evolved salience, but it can be made equally well on the basis of past learning. This argument asks for representative stimuli, as Brunswik (1955) or Petrinovich (Chapter 2, this volume) might, but not for reasons of representative sampling.

As a concrete example of the claim that more control yields less regularity, let us return to Ebbinghaus and the domain of verbal material. Consider a thought experiment in which two subjects randomly selected from a large introductory psychology course are both asked to learn and later to recall many lists, each 100 syllables long. Some of the lists are randomized nonsense syllables translated from German and are of known meaningfulness and pronunciability. Some of the lists contain 100 syllables of randomized nouns normed on dozens of different properties by a dull verbal-learning researcher (Rubin, 1980). The stimuli in the first two kinds of lists are presented at a rate of one every 3 sec. Some of the lists contain 100 syllables arranged in simple sentences, with the order of the sentences randomized. Each sentence is presented as a whole, and each subject signals, within set limits, when the next sentence should be presented. Some of the lists are stories 100 syllables long, and, finally, some of the lists are poems 100 syllables long. For the last two kinds of lists, the entire 100 syllables are presented at once, and thus the experimenter has no control over and no knowledge of the encoding time spent on each individual syllable. Presentation times are chosen for the different kinds of lists so that, on the average, each subject recalls 50 syllables from each kind of list.

Our task as psychologists is to predict the degree of agreement between the two subjects. In particular, we are to predict the type of list on which the two subjects will most often recall the same syllables. If we choose, we may also predict the type of list on which the two subjects will most often agree on the order of recall of those 50 syllables, the latency between the recall of particular syllables, or almost any other dependent measure. Agreement between the two subjects is a measure of regularity, of how well the situation controls behavior. In a thought experiment with more than two subjects, the larger the agreement between randomly selected pairs of subjects, the lower the error variance. The lists that are the simplest, most controlled, and least affected by the idiosyncrasies of the past experiences of the individual subjects are the nonsense syllables. The lists that are the most complex, least controlled, and most affected by the idiosyncrasies of the past experiences of the individual subjects are the poems. Would anyone choose the nonsense syllables?

As the lists become more complex, they become more structured, but it probably is not the degree of the structure alone that determines the ability of the stimuli to control behavior. Rich past histories, genetic or environmental, tend to increase a stimulus's control of behavior and make responses more similar among individuals, even when the degrees of formal structure among classes of stimuli do not clearly differ.

The thought experiment just described was intended to put in concrete terms the argument that more experimental control often leads to less regularity. Later we shall consider actual research in human memory in which minimal control produced exceedingly regular behavior.

More control provides less knowledge

Regularity is all we really need at our present state of theoretical advancement in most memory research. Control added beyond that necessary to gain repeatable results is undesirable. In addition to yielding decreased regularity, an increase in control has the effects of hiding unexpected results from the researcher and of decreasing the extent to which the results can be generalized. A well-controlled experiment allows the effects of only the independent variables in the design to be observed. Important but unexpected factors have little chance of being discovered if a controlled experiment is designed properly; they simply enter into the error variance. In addition, the predictions about the dependent variable typically are about changes in magnitude across conditions, and so the dependent variable usually is too simple to provide a sufficiently complete description of behavior to facilitate the formation of post hoc hypotheses (Rubin, 1985). "Sloppier" experiments, with less control of the experimental conditions and less control of the responses the subjects are allowed to make, provide greater chances for unexpected factors to be noticed. Moreover, if unexpected factors are not observed, we can have greater confidence that, if present at all, they will have only small effects; see Mook (Chapter 3, this volume) for a counterargument. Similarly, if regularity is sought, but controls are kept to a minimum, then the results of the observation can be generalized at least to the extent to which the conditions of observation varied. For example, in a sloppy study of memory, if the retention interval and the degree of initial learning are allowed to vary across subjects, and if subjects all produce similar behaviors, then we can generalize over variations in retention interval and degree of initial learning. In short, given two studies, if extraneous factors affect the result of interest, then we are more likely to be able to document those factors with the more open-ended, sloppier study, and if the two studies turn out to have equally regular results, then the results of the sloppier study can be generalized to a wider range of situations.

More control requires more knowledge

It has been claimed that regularity, not control, is what is needed at our current state of advancement. But certainly there must be some conditions under which control is the main objective and different conditions under which regularity is the main objective. Regularity should be the goal in a science that does not have theories to predict specific outcomes from experiments. Of course, all scientific inquiry must have some guiding hypotheses, but unless those hypotheses are sufficiently well developed to make predictions that other competing assumptions will not, there is little reason to test them. Rather, what we need are repeatable phenomena at a level of complexity that provides constraints for the formulation of broad classes of theories. Control should be the goal in a science in which theories have been developed that warrant serious testing. For such theories, the proper controls offer elegant tests. In particular, in situations where little control is applied, different theories often make the same predictions, but with more control these same theories can be forced to make different predictions. Whenever we have enough knowledge to form and test such competing theories, control is to be preferred. Unfortunately, such theories are still rare in cognitive research.

An example from developmental psychology may be helpful. General hypotheses led Piaget to discover and document the phenomenon of conservation in the child. Once this phenomenon was shown to be robust, competing theories could be developed and tested. The first step was to demonstrate a repeatable phenomenon that constrained possible theories and that allowed for experimental manipulation. Only after that was accomplished could competing theories be formulated. Progress would have been much slower if complex theories had preceded observation. Numerous analysis-of-variance experiments could have been run, deciding among instances of a class of theories, all of which were flawed.

Some subtle and some obvious implications accompany the goal of finding regularity and the goal of maximizing experimental control. When control is sought, the actual results obtained often are not intended to be generalized. Very specific conditions are obtained for a test of a theory, and these conditions are the only ones for which the interpretation of the results is important (Mook, Chapter 3, this volume). Changing one of the conditions slightly might alter the results completely, but if this condition is not of interest to the theories being tested, or if the theories predict such a change, the change is not of consequence. Unless a strong theory exists to state which of many possible changes in conditions should have large effects, however, such large changes in results with minor changes in conditions will reduce the accumulation of knowledge to chaos, as Petrinovich (Chapter 2, this volume) points out.

The role of theories also changes as one goes from emphasizing control to emphasizing regularity. When control is the major goal, a single theory, or a set of theories, determines what factors to control and manipulate and what questions experiments should be designed to answer. When regularity is the major goal, theories take a more subservient role in relation to the data and are used mostly to guide research in general terms and to interpret the observed data.

Regularity is proving the null hypothesis

The emphasis on regularity, rather than control, changes the role of inferential statistics in experimental inquiry. Current inferential statistical methods in psychology bias against the search for regularity. Inferential statistics note differences, not regularities. Nonetheless, understanding behavior often involves noting regularities, not differences. To note regularities usually is to accept the null hypotheses.

The statistical issue whether or not empirical support can be gained from accepting the statistical null hypothesis is a classic issue that has received considerable attention. In the sixties, it was the subject of a lengthy series of exchanges in the *Psychological Review* and *Psychological Bulletin* (Binder, 1963; Edwards, 1965; Grant, 1962; Wilson, Miller, & Lower, 1967). More recently, Greenwald (1975) has developed a model of how prejudice against gaining support from accepting the null hypothesis produces detrimental effects on the advancement of science. Thus, the view that accepting the null hypothesis cannot provide evidence for an empirical hypothesis is not held by all schools of statistics or by all psychologists. Two issues will be given as examples.

Those who argue that accepting the statistical null hypothesis can offer no support for a theory point to the fact that it is easy to do an experiment with so little power that the null hypothesis will be accepted even though a real effect is present. Those on the other side of the issue argue that because the means of two groups will almost always differ by some small, perhaps infinitesimal amount, it is always possible to reject the null hypothesis by increasing the power of the experiment. "Putting it crudely, if you have enough cases and your measures are not totally unreliable, the null hypothesis will always be falsified, *regardless of the truth of the substantive theory*" (Meehl, 1978, p. 822). There is a parallel between the two approaches. The power of an experiment must be chosen appropriately no matter whether one is seeking to gain support by rejecting or accepting the null hypothesis. Accepting the null hypothesis does not indicate that two means are identical, only that they are equal within the power of the experiment to resolve them.

The second criticism against gaining support from accepting the null hypothesis is that the null hypothesis can be confirmed because a sloppy experiment was performed, introducing random error. The counter to this is that the null hypothesis can be rejected because a sloppy experiment was performed, introducing nonrandom error. Again, there is a parallel. The quality of an experiment must be checked no matter whether the null hypothesis is to be accepted or rejected. Experimenter error can lead to the null hypothesis being either falsely accepted or rejected.

The preceding arguments were not intended to overcome all the biases present in psychology today against gaining support from accepting the null hypothesis (Greenwald, 1975). It can be argued that there are some reasons to prefer rejecting the null hypothesis (Wilson et al., 1967). All that should be made clear is that gaining support from accepting the null hypothesis is not prohibited by most statistical theory and that it may be the proper way of couching certain questions. Conceptually, support for regularity can be gained most directly through inferential statistics by acceptance of the null hypothesis, because usually it is a claim of no noticeable difference, rather than a claim of greater similarity than would be expected by chance.

The resistance of some to gaining support for a theory by accepting the null hypothesis may just be an aspect of the near monopoly held by inferential statistics in the study of human memory, as well as in most other areas of psychology. Most papers published in psychology make use of inferential statistics. Most undergraduate and graduate students in psychology are required to take a course in inferential statistics. In fact, if all the courses required for a graduate or undergraduate psychology degree in all psychology departments were listed, statistics probably would be the mode. For some, it is hard to imagine how it could be otherwise; yet this is not the case for all other sciences.

Given the current state of the advancement of psychology, often it is necessary to demonstrate that results cannot be attributed to chance. As the field advances, or as more regular data are obtained, such demonstrations should no longer be necessary. Thus, in physics, for example, the use of inferential statistics is exceedingly rare (Binder, 1963; Meehl, 1978). The null-hypothesis question (Is the speed of light constant in a vacuum?) is asked, rather than the more primitive psychological form (Is the speed of light different from zero at the .05 level?). One knows that results could not have occurred by chance. The same is true in certain areas of psychology. In psychophysics and in animal learning, it is possible to publish papers without using inferential statistics. There are questions of interpretation of the results, but the interpretations do not include the possibility that the results occurred by chance. In general, it is likely that as psychology advances, the role of inferential statistics in psychology will decrease. I, for one, look forward to the day when psychologists studying cognition will be embarrassed by the period in which they repeatedly had to report in journal articles that their results did not occur by chance.

The differences between the approaches of seeking regularity and seeking control may have been exaggerated slightly in order to make them clearer. In actual practice, the two extremes always mix and always share some common properties. Both can be done well or poorly. Both can be done with or without intelligence and creativity. Both need results that are repeatable under their respective conditions of observation. Both are of little interest if such repeatable results have no implications for theory development. Neither approach can be done to the exclusion of the other. Nonetheless, seeking regularity and seeking control remain different approaches to psychology.

Searching for regularity

Arguments about the way science should be considered are pleasant diversions from research. It is the research itself, however, that is the real determinant of which arguments are best. If regularity, and not control, should be our current goal, then I should be able to demonstrate progress from this approach. If the research presented here convinces psychologists to alter their research behavior, then the arguments will have been superfluous. If the research fails to impress anyone, then the arguments, at best, will have been mere curiosities. In research, we put in our effort, and we take our chances.

Having wandered around the "real world" for some time now without a proper laboratory to protect me, I have stumbled across more than my fair share of regularity. By examining what works and what does not work, I have developed some heuristics that I believe increase the chances of finding interesting regularities.

Heuristic 1

Use as little control as possible in the beginning. Do not worry about the subjects' prior exposure to the material they will learn, or even where, when, or how well the subjects initially learned the material they will recall. No effort should be made to simplify or control the material being used or the context in which it is being presented and recalled.

Heuristic 2

Do not decide on a dependent measure until after looking at pilot data. Examine the data accumulated for possible regularities, and then adapt the dependent measure to what the data show. Psychologists tend to use "amount" measures as their default, such as amount recalled or amount of time taken. These usually do not show the greatest regularity in nonlaboratory situations. Such amount measures are very sensitive to the variables that are not controlled outside of the laboratory, such as motivation level (Weiner, 1966), retention interval (Wickelgren, 1972), and type of encoding used (Craik & Lockhart, 1972). This is one reason why amount measures are so popular in the laboratory. Of course, there are exceptions, but, usually, dependent measures based on relations among which items or which aspects of items are recalled are more stable in nonlaboratory settings. Such measures might include the order of recall, or which, rather than how many, parts of a stimulus are recalled.

Heuristic 3

Do not be tied too strongly to any one theory or hypothesis when starting to collect data. Rather, try to think of the greatest possible number of theories that could be used to explain possible findings (Broadbent, 1973). This heuristic is so obvious that I would leave it out if my reading the journals did not convince me it needed to be mentioned. No one but the author of an article knows what was the true course of events leading to published research, but research usually is written as if one specific hypothesis and, except for confounding factors that were controlled, only one hypothesis was considered. Broadbent (1973) argues for the folly in this approach. First, a researcher often tests a pet theory by predicting an observation that would also be predicted by a host of other theories (Meehl, 1978). Thus, rather than testing the theory of interest, a whole set of theories is tested, and little support is gained for the pet theory itself. Second, and more seriously, if the predicted observation fails to materialize, the researcher is in a difficult position. If an alternative theory does not exist, the researcher may be tempted to search for explanations for the failure, without discarding the pet theory itself (Petrinovich, Chapter 2, this volume). That is, the researcher may not find it easy to be as impartial a judge as would be possible if several alternative theories had been postulated. Efficient progress in science will be fostered by serious consideration of sets of alternative theories and by emotional detachment from any one particular theory.

I shall draw examples almost completely from my own work so that I can report the actual steps that went on in the research. For each example given, I shall show how the three heuristics functioned. Where possible, I shall include data not previously reported.

Example 1: The tip-of-the-tongue phenomenon

When a person can almost, but not quite, recall a word after being given its definition, many facts about the word often are known, such as how many syllables are in the word and the first letter of the word (Brown & McNeill, 1966). Heuristic 1 applies to the conditions of learning in this situation. The word that is being partially recalled was learned without laboratory control. The experimenter has no knowledge of the context or spacing of the learning, the amount of prac-

Table 7.1. *Number of correct letters*

	Target word										
Direction of scoring	p	h	i	l	a	t	e	l	i	s	t
Left	27	24	16	16	2	0	0	0	0	0	0
Right	0	0	0	0	0	0	0	0	18	18	18

tice, the potential interference from other words learned at approximately the same time, the retention interval measured from the word's last use, or a host of other factors known to affect memory. In this study, heuristic 1 also applied to the recall situation used (Rubin, 1975). Subjects were simply asked to recall the letters of the word, using blanks to indicate letters they could not recall. Brown and McNeill found that subjects tended to know the first letter of a word by asking subjects if they knew the first letter. In contrast, I asked subjects to record all they knew, hoping to find out whatever it was that they in fact did know. In sum, as little control as possible was applied to both the learning and the recall situations.

A response measure was needed to capture the regularity present in the recall. Subjects in pilot studies appeared to recall clusters at the beginnings and ends of words. That is, they not only knew the first letter that Brown and McNeill had asked them to report but also knew the first and last few letters. The subjects, however, were not especially accurate on how many letters they did not know in the middle of a word. A dependent measure was therefore chosen that scored letters as correct if they were in the correct positions counting from either the beginning or the end of the word. Starting at the beginning of a word, a letter was scored correct only if it and the letter before it were correct. Starting at the end of a word, a letter was scored as correct only if it and the letter after it were correct. This measure was an adaptation of the common transitional error probability; so it, like the rest of the measures to be introduced here, was far from novel. Only the contexts in which the measures were used were different. Table 7.1 shows the results of applying this transitional-probability type of measure to the recall of 37 subjects who were in the tip-of-the-tongue state when presented with the definition of the word *philatelist*.

The theory used to describe the results was not the idea that guided the research. Brown and McNeill reported that their subjects, when in the tip-of-the-tongue state, knew that the letter *p* began the word *philatelist*. It seemed likely that the subjects who knew *p* also knew at least the phoneme indicated by the first two letters, *ph*. My hunch was partly correct, but it also appears that subjects in the tip-of-the-tongue state actually know the entire first morpheme, *phil*. The hypothesis of morpheme-like recall was driven by the data. The hypothesis did not lead me to do the experiment. I tried to find out something about the tip-of-the-tongue phenomenon by applying as little control as possible and by fit-

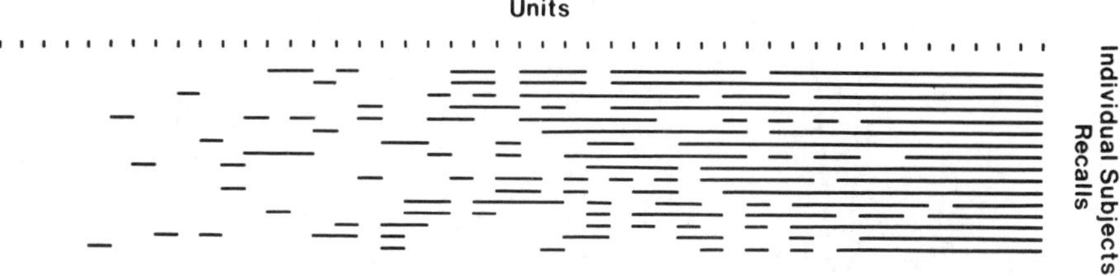

Figure 7.1. A scalagram analysis of the recalls of 16 older men for the 47 units of the Lincoln story. Both the subjects and the units are rank-ordered by probability of recall.

ting the dependent measure to the regularity observed. The particular hypothesis served only to describe the results. I had a whole set of possible hypotheses based on single-letter, phoneme, syllable, and morpheme clusters that I was ready to accept, given different possible outcomes. The interpretation was then checked using a different method and a different sample of subjects.

Example 2: Prose memory

When I started research on prose memory in 1970, such materials were considered by many as not controlled enough for laboratory study. Heuristic 1 was applied, in that I was working in the least controlled situation in which I thought that lawful results could be found. While scoring some pilot recalls, I noticed that subjects tended to recall different amounts of material, but tended to recall, or not recall, the same units. It was almost as if some parts of the passage were always recalled, some parts were never recalled, and some parts were recalled only by those subjects who recalled most of the passage. Applying heuristic 2, dependent measures were chosen to capture this regularity. Scalagram analysis (Guttman, 1947; Kenny & Rubin, 1977) was the first measure to be adapted to describing the regularity observed. In scalagram analysis, the complete data matrix of individual subjects recalling or failing to recall individual units is displayed. Both the subject axis, which runs horizontally, and the units axis, which runs vertically, are rank-ordered by amount recalled. Figure 7.1 displays the data for 16 subjects in a normative aging study (mean age = 68 years) who recalled the Lincoln story after a 10-min retention interval (Rubin, 1978). Perfect scalability would result in solid lines for those in the upper part of the figure, followed by uninterrupted blanks, and would imply that for all subjects there exists a single rank order of units from most to least likely to be recalled. Violations of this ideal are counted, and a normalized index is reported. The coefficient of reproducibility for Figure 7.1 is .84, indicating that if I were told exactly how many units each subject recalled and if I were given the group's overall rank order, then I could predict exactly which units each subject would recall and be correct an average of 84% of the time.

A second, even simpler dependent measure was formed for the same data: the number of subjects recalling each unit (Rubin, 1978, 1985). This measure, which

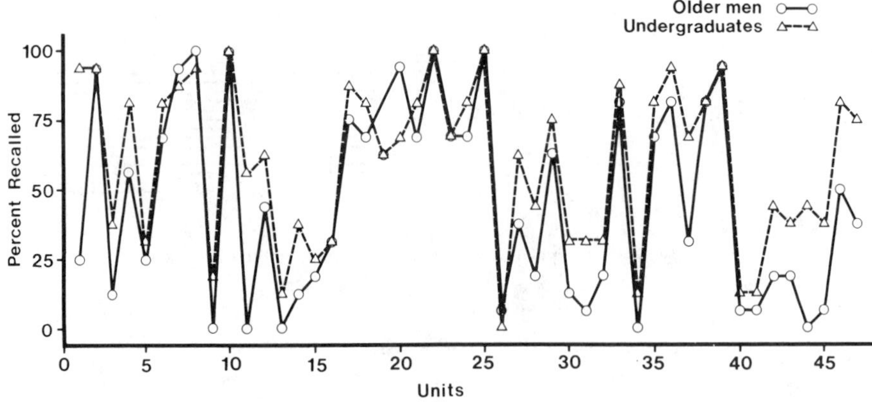

Figure 7.2. The probability of each of the 47 units of the story shown in Figure 7.1 being recalled by the subjects whose data are shown in Figure 7.1 and by 16 undergraduates.

is equivalent to adding across scalability figures such as Figure 7.1 to obtain one value for each unit of the story, was used to describe another regularity noticed in the data. Figure 7.2 displays the same data as Figure 7.1, as well as recalls from 16 undergraduates. The horizontal axis displays the units of the Lincoln story in the order in which they occur in the story. The vertical axis displays the percentage of the 16 subjects in each group who recalled each unit. The older subjects recalled only three-quarters as much as the undergraduates (45% versus 60%), but they tended to recall the same units. The correlation between the two groups on which units they recalled, calculated over the 47 units of the Lincoln story, is .85, compared with an average reliability (Cronbach's alpha) of .90 (Cronbach, 1951). This indicates that the recalls of the two groups correlate with each other almost as well as the recall of each group would be expected to correlate with those for new groups of subjects drawn from the same population.

Heuristic 3 suggests that one should not be strongly tied to any one theory, but rather should think of as many theories as possible. A dozen theories for why specific units would be recalled were considered. The factors in these theories varied from serial position to the contribution of each unit to the overall image produced by the story. If reliable differences had been observed between the two age groups, they could have been probed using all of the dozen theories.

Example 3: Very long term memory

The same techniques that were applied to prose learned in the laboratory can be used to study material learned without the benefit of laboratory control. As might be expected from the arguments made earlier, such material often can

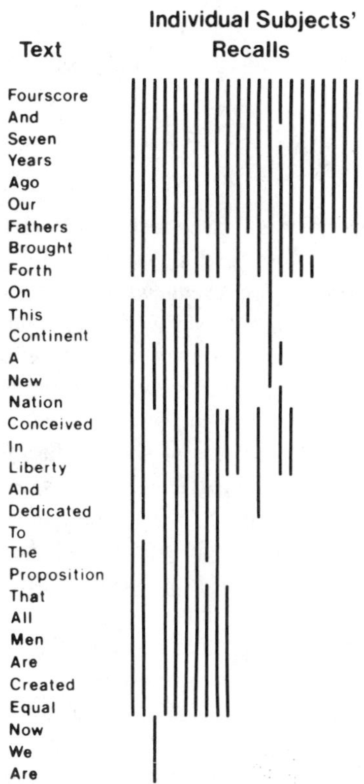

Figure 7.3. Recalls of the Gettysburg Address. The subjects are rank-ordered by the amount they recalled.

demonstrate greater regularity than that learned under more controlled conditions. Figure 7.3 is a scalagram like that of Figure 7.1, except that the units have been left in their original sequential order instead of being rank-ordered by amount recalled. Figure 7.3 displays the recalls of 26 subjects for the exact words of the Gettysburg Address (Rubin, 1977). The only errors that were scored as correct were spelling errors and the substitution of *forefathers* for *fathers,* a substitution made by 12 of the 22 subjects who recalled the word. The units in Figure 7.3 were not reordered by amount recalled because the actual order of the words in the passage is such a good predictor. Using the rank order of units of the group as a whole and the number of units each individual recalled, exactly which word each individual recalled can be predicted 97.6% of the time. Using primacy, instead of the empirical rank order, results in only a slight drop to 97.0%. Thus, not only do all subjects tend to recall the same words, they also tend to start at the beginning, recalling as much as they can until they stop. For this example, competing hypotheses were not considered. The regularity observed was strong enough to rule out most reasonable alternatives before they could even be considered. It should be noted that these data, collected without any laboratory control of learning or retention interval, are considerably more regular than the laboratory data of Figure 7.1.

Example 4: Semantic domains

The organization of semantic memory and its effect on the retrieval of information learned in and out of the laboratory have a long history in experimental psychology (Bousfield, 1953; Bousfield & Sedgewick, 1944; Kausler, 1974). Following heuristic 1, no control was exerted over when, how, and where the instances recalled were learned. For a semantic domain such as *animals,* the learning began very early and probably progressed at a slower rate through high school to college. For a semantic domain such as *all the faculty members at the university,* the learning had a much later onset and was of shorter duration. The recall situation was also as uncontrolled as possible, given that the subjects had to be informed to recall a specific semantic domain. Subjects were simply asked to recall as many instances of a semantic domain (e.g., animals) as they could. The open-ended nature of the recall situation allowed the subjects rather than the experimenter to define the instances of the semantic domain.

Following heuristic 2, the dependent measure was adapted to fit the regularity observed. Certain words tend to be recalled together in clusters. Because these clusters usually are small (Gruenewald & Lockhead, 1980), a measure based on local ordering was adopted. The similarity between any two items was defined as the number of subjects recalling the two items next to each other. This measure had the added advantages of a clear theoretical interpretation under most associative and search models of memory and a historical tie to the measure of clustering introduced by Bousfield (1953). Similarity matrices of the most commonly recalled instances of a domain were then constructed. The subjects thus determined which items would be considered as the central members of a domain and how the items would be related. The results are exceptionally stable and provide similarity spaces that are in good agreement with those obtained from other techniques such as similarity ratings (Rubin & Olson, 1980). Figure 7.4 shows an example of the similarity space that resulted from 20 recalls of the *animal* domain by a single subject. The figure shows clear clusters for American wild animals, African wild animals, farm animals, and small animals, including *mouse* and the pets *cat* and *dog*.

Of course, what is being studied both here and in the more traditional laboratory list-learning studies of clustering is the preexperimental, unobserved, and uncontrolled processing that led to the memory of the semantic domain being organized in the first place. Thus, the acquisition and retention of the material that is recalled in the method just described or that leads to the clustering of lists learned under experimental control are equally uncontrolled in both methods. In one case, however, a veneer of experimental control is applied to the experiment

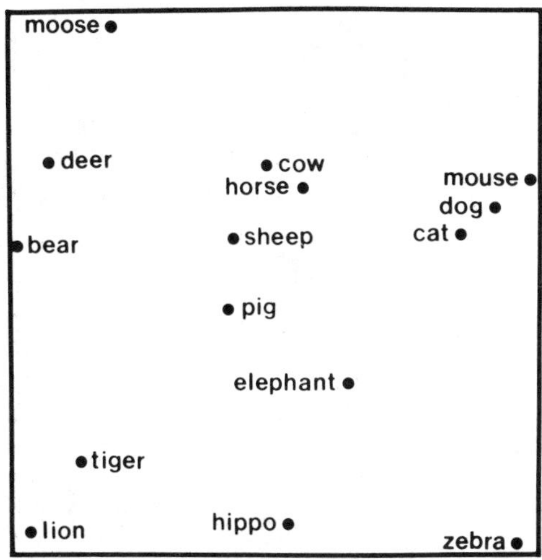

Figure 7.4. Similarity space produced from 20 repeated recalls of one subject. (From Rubin & Olson, 1980)

reported, at the cost of producing "noisier" data and less opportunity for uncovering unexpected results. This point is most obvious for this example, but it also holds for the other examples presented here.

Example 5: Recall of coins

At this point, the application of the heuristics should be predictable. For the recall of coins, little control was exerted over the conditions of encoding. Information about coins is learned over a long period of time, with repeated exposures occurring daily for most subjects. The exact amount and spacing of each subject's exposures and the amount of attention given to coins at each exposure were uncontrolled and unknown. Some subjects probably collected coins, studying in great detail their dates, mint marks, and other characteristics that affect their numismatic value. Other subjects did not. Minimal control was exerted over the conditions of recall. Subjects were simply asked to draw, in empty circles, the two sides of common coins. This was the most open-ended question that could be devised that would elicit information about the recall of coins. Recognition could have been used to assess memory for coins, but the foils and the target presented to the subject provided considerable information, and in our experience the particular foils used greatly affected the results (Kontis, 1982).

Following heuristic 2, a dependent measure was chosen to capture the regularity noted. Subjects' recalls were partial, but they tended to recall the same items in the same locations. As with the earlier examples, the amount recalled for a particular unit, rather than simply the total amount recalled, was chosen as a measure. In particular, the number of subjects who recalled each inscription in

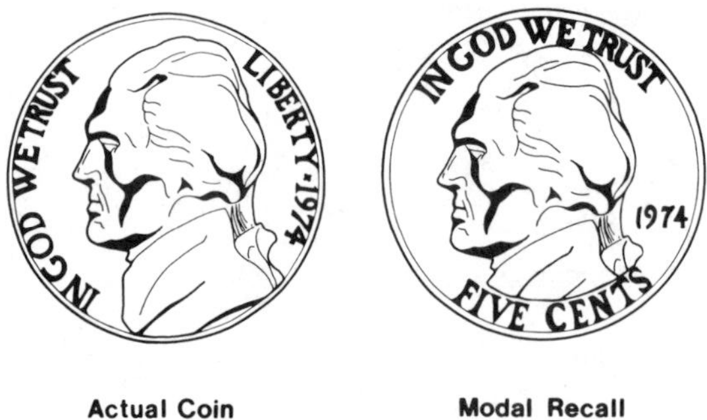

Figure 7.5. An actual nickel and the nickel recalled by averaging over subjects' recalls. (From Rubin & Coutis, 1983).

each possible location on a coin was scored (Rubin & Kontis, 1983). Tables of such item–location pairings were reported, and modal coins were constructed by filling in the coin sequentially with the most frequently recalled item–location pair that did not already have its item or location used. Figure 7.5 shows the actual nickel and the modal nickel.

Following heuristic 3, theoretical preconceptions were kept to a minimum. The modal nickel shown in Figure 7.5 was identical with the modal penny, dime, and quarter drawn by subjects, except for the particular value and the particular profile drawn. The discussion centered on the role of schematic knowledge and the conditions necessary to have people store and recall detailed information not covered by a schema. The discussion was a way to describe the regularity observed and to suggest further experiments; it was not used to guide the initial formulation of the research. Once the regularity was observed, competing explanations were considered in an attempt to understand what had been found.

Example 6: The autobiographical memory of college students

For this example, the regularity to be discussed was described in an article by Crovitz and Schiffman (1974). The regularity was so impressive that it begged for further understanding. Crovitz and Schiffman presented 98 subjects with 20 common nouns and asked each to record the event from his or her life that each word evoked. The subjects were then asked to date their memories in terms of how long ago the incidents had occurred. Figure 7.6 shows the number of memories per hour that were reported as a function of hours since the incidents. Both axes are logarithmic; so the straight line is a power function. The points plotted are the common time markers of English ranging from 1 to 23 hours earlier to 1 to 17 years earlier. The straight line is of the same form as would be expected from laboratory studies of retention, and it supports the interpretation that the line represents the retention function for autobiographical memory (Rubin, 1982).

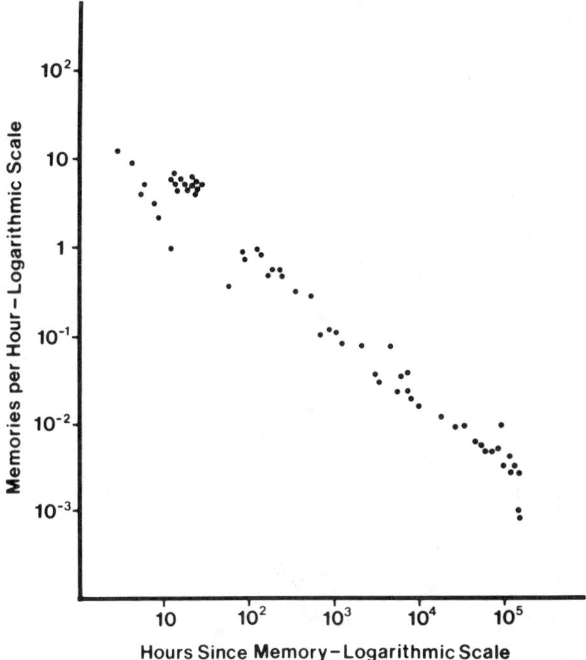

Figure 7.6. The distribution of autobiographical memories over time. (Adapted from Crovitz & Schiffman, 1974).

Crovitz and Schiffman had no control or knowledge of the learning, rehearsal, or other aspects of the encoding of the memories. They provided only the barest of constraint during recall. Moreover, the same results are obtained if even less constraint is applied by asking subjects to recall autobiographical memories in the absence of any cue words (Rubin, 1982). Thus, heuristic 1 was followed. Heuristic 2 was applied in that the plot shown in Figure 7.6 was formed to capture the regularity present in the data. In my work, I have attempted to follow heuristic 3 by formulating several possible theoretical explanations for the phenomenon and then attempting either to rule them out or to provide support for them.

Example 7: Autobiographical memory in older subjects

One extension of the Crovitz and Schiffman study involves the use of older subjects. Older subjects have had more years to build an autobiography to report than have younger subjects and therefore can provide information about changes over long time periods that undergraduates cannot. The same uses of heuristics 1, 2, and 3 apply here as in the younger subjects, and the results are the same for the most recent 20 years of both groups' lives. For periods further back than 20 years, the older subjects' data do not continue to decrease, but

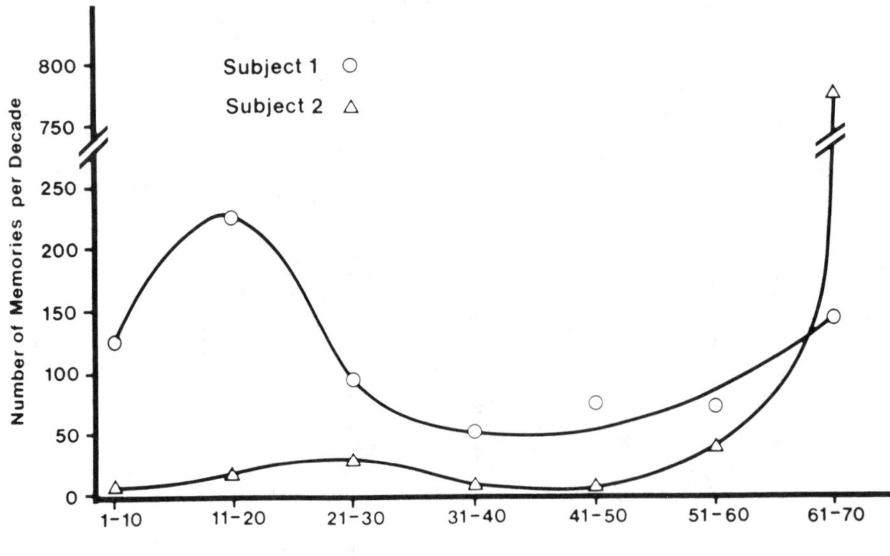

Figure 7.7. The distribution of autobiographical memories from two 70-year-old subjects.

rather show an increase for some periods in their youth. These findings hold for the reanalysis of data from several laboratories (Rubin, Wetzler, & Nebes, 1986). To describe these results, a simple histogram, rather than the more complex log-log transformation, is best. Figure 7.7 shows the histograms for two 70-year-old subjects who each provided dated memories to 921 cue words. The data are grouped into decades of life. It should be noted that it was the search for an understanding of an observed regularity that led to the reanalysis of existing data from other laboratories and that in turn led to the search for theoretical explanations.

Some lessons from the examples

Heuristic 1 suggests that experimenters should use as little control as possible. This was clearly followed in the examples presented here. In most cases, no control over or even knowledge of the host of parameters used to describe learning in the laboratory was used. This not only allowed a wide range of conditions of learning to be sampled in one experiment but also indicated that such a variety in conditions would not lead to a corresponding variety in results. Thus, whatever results were obtained could be generalized to a wide range of learning situations. The procedures used to obtain recalls also exerted as little control as possible, allowing the subjects to reveal what memories they had in a way that was as unbiased by the experimenter as was possible. In this way, subjects were free to present organization that the experimenter did not know to be present when the investigation was begun. For example, subjects demonstrated morpheme-like clustering in the tip-of-the-tongue phenomenon, marked primacy in very long term memory for sacred material, specific kinds of clustering in semantic domains, location-specific recall of items on coins, and interpretable distributions of memories over retention intervals in autobiographical memory. Nonetheless, the data observed were more regular than those usually obtained under strict laboratory control. That is, the variability among subjects on the dependent measures used usually was smaller than would be expected in the laboratory using standard measures. In fact, in many examples, the data were so regular that the results from individual subjects could be displayed (Figures 7.1, 7.3, 7.4, and 7.7), allowing for the form and degree of individual differences among subjects to be specified in detail (Bruce, Chapter 4, this volume).

Heuristic 2 suggested that the dependent measure to be used be tied to the regularity observed in the data. The dependent measures varied from example to example. In all cases they were more complex than the total amount recalled, but not much more complex. The measures were always the recall of a particular unit relative to other units of recall. The measures used may, at times, have been novel in the domain in which they were applied, but they were not novel measures. All the measures presented here have been used before, and most have known statistical properties. The main difference between the work presented here and more hypothesis-driven experimental work using the same measures is that here the measures were chosen to describe regularities noticed in the data, rather than being chosen a priori to test a hypothesis. Once the regularities were described in a quantitative fashion, they could be used to constrain and, through experimental manipulation, to test theories. In fact, the slightly more complex measures used here offer more of a challenge to theories than does the simpler amount-recalled measure. For instance, predicting the relative frequency of recall of units from a prose passage read or recalled under various conditions allows for a more efficient test of a complex theory than does predicting the amount of recall from those conditions (Rubin, 1985).

Heuristic 3 suggests that researchers should not be tied to one theory to try to explain the regularity they observe. As the examples demonstrate, this often leads to research that appears more data-driven than theory-driven. Theory, especially the kind of theory that has motivated laboratory research, however, is not ignored. It determines the general areas in which regularity is sought and what kinds of regularity are worth pursuing, and once theoretically interesting regularities are found, it shapes the experiments that are performed. If one were to criticize the collection of examples used to argue my points, one could say that as a collection they fail to cumulate into a body of knowledge in the way that a series of theory-driven experiments would. However, each example was an attempt to add to the cumulative knowledge base of an area of research at a very basic level. Rather than explicitly questioning the existing assumptions of these areas, an attempt was made to avoid as many of the assumptions as possible. The attempt was made by providing little control or constraint over the subject and the data analysis, thereby allowing the structure present in memory to become apparent.

How, when, and *why* should memory be studied outside of laboratory controls? *How?* By using the three heuristics discussed in the second half of this chapter. *When?* When a theory does not yet exist in an area of research that makes predictions worth the effort of testing. *Why?* Because there is more regularity and more chance of finding theoretically interesting results in data collected using the naturally occurring learning, the wide range of conditions, and the minimal control that are more common outside of the laboratory.

References

Binder, A. (1963). Further considerations on testing the null hypothesis and the strategy and tactics of investigating theoretical models. *Psychological Review, 70,* 107–115.

Bousfield, W. A. (1953). The occurrence of clustering in the recall of randomly arranged associates. *Journal of General Psychology, 49,* 229–240.

Bousfield, W. A., & Sedgewick, C. H. W. (1944). An analysis of sequences of restricted associative responses. *Journal of General Psychology, 30,* 149–165.

Broadbent, D. E. (1973). *In defense of empirical psychology.* London: Methuen.

Brown, R., & McNeill, D. (1966). The "tip-of-the-tongue" phenomenon. *Journal of Verbal Learning and Verbal Behavior, 5,* 325–337.

Brunswik, E. (1955). Representative design and probabilistic theory in a functional psychology. *Psychological Review, 62,* 193–217.

Craik, F. I. M., & Lockhart, R. S. (1972). Levels of processing: A framework for memory research. *Journal of Verbal Learning and Verbal Behavior, 11,* 671–684.

Cronbach, L. J. (1951). Coefficient alpha and the internal structure of tests. *Psychometrika, 16,* 297–334.

Crovitz, H. F., & Schiffman, H. (1974). Frequency of episodic memories as a function of their age. *Bulletin of the Psychonomic Society, 4,* 517–518.

Ebbinghaus, H. (1964). *Memory: A contribution to experimental psychology.* (H. A. Ruger & C. E. Bussenius, Trans.). New York: Dover. (Original work published 1885)

Edwards, W. (1965). Tactical note on the relation between scientific and statistical hypotheses. *Psychological Bulletin, 63,* 400–402.

Grant, D. A. (1962). Testing the null hypothesis and the strategy and tactics of investigating theoretical models. *Psychological Review, 69,* 54–61.

Greenwald, A. G. (1975). Consequences of prejudice against the null hypothesis. *Psychological Bulletin, 82,* 1–20.

Gruenewald, P. J., & Lockhead, G. R. (1980). The free recall of category examples. *Journal of Experimental Psychology: Human Learning and Memory, 6,* 225–240.

Guttman, L. (1947). The Cornell technique for scale and intensity analysis. *Educational and Psychological Measurement, 7,* 274–279.

Kausler, D. H. (1974). *Psychology of verbal learning and behavior.* New York: Academic Press.

Kenny, D. A., & Rubin, D. C. (1977). Estimating change reproducibility in Guttman scaling. *Social Science Research, 6,* 188–196.

Kontis, T. C. (1982). *In search of the schema for a common object.* Unpublished senior honors thesis, Duke University, Durham, NC.

Meehl, P. E. (1978). Theoretical risks and tabular asterisks: Sir Karl, Sir Ronald, and the slow progress of soft psychology. *Journal of Consulting and Clinical Psychology, 46,* 806–834.

Rubin, D. C. (1975). Within word structure in the tip-of-the-tongue phenomenon. *Journal of Verbal Learning and Verbal Behavior, 14,* 392–397.

Rubin, D. C. (1977). Very long-term memory for prose and verse. *Journal of Verbal Learning and Verbal Behavior, 16,* 611–621.

Rubin, D. C. (1978). A unit analysis of prose memory. *Journal of Verbal Learning and Verbal Behavior, 17,* 599–620.

Rubin, D. C. (1980). 51 properties of 125 words: A unit analysis of verbal behavior. *Journal of Verbal Learning and Verbal Behavior, 19,* 736–755.

Rubin, D. C. (1982). On the retention function for autobiographical memory. *Journal of Verbal Learning and Verbal Behavior, 21,* 21–38.

Rubin, D. C. (1985). Memorability as a measure of processing: A unit analysis of prose and list learning. *Journal of Experimental Psychology: General, 114,* 213–238.

Rubin, D. C., & Kontis, T. C. (1983). A schema for common cents. *Memory & Cognition, 11,* 335–341.

Rubin, D. C., & Olson, M. J. (1980). Recall of semantic domains. *Memory & Cognition, 8,* 354–366.

Rubin, D. C., Wetzler, S. E., & Nebes, R. D. (1986). Autobiographical memory across the lifespan. In D. C. Rubin (Ed.), *Autobiographical memory* (pp. 202–204). Cambridge University Press.

Weiner, B. (1966). Effects of motivation on the availability and retrieval of memory traces. *Psychological Bulletin, 65,* 24–37.

Wickelgren, W. A. (1972). Trace resistance and the decay of long-term memory. *Journal of Mathematical Psychology, 9,* 418–455.

Wilson, W., Miller, H. L., & Lower, J. S. (1967). Much ado about the null hypothesis. *Psychological Bulletin, 67,* 188–196.

8 Finding the bloody horse

Alan Baddeley

> You praise the firm restraint with which they write –
> I'm with you there, of course:
> They used the snaffle and the curb alright,
> But where's the bloody horse?

The quotation comes from the South African poet Roy Campbell and refers to the work of South African novelists of the earlier years of this century. The sentiment is, however, much more widely applicable, and it could, without too much distortion, be applied to the work over the last 50 years of students of memory such as myself. Science needs controlled observation and hence is always open to the risk that excessive control, "the snaffle and the curb," may stifle the phenomenon that is being observed, "the bloody horse." Such a criticism is not, of course, novel: "If *X* is an interesting or socially significant aspect of memory, then psychologists have hardly ever studied *X*" (Neisser, 1978, p. 4).

The tension between the need for control and the need to preserve the essence of the phenomenon under investigation has been present since the scientific study of memory began 100 years ago, with two investigators both beginning to tackle the question of how human memory could best be studied. In Germany, Ebbinghaus opted for a highly constrained experimental approach in which the phenomena of memory were stripped down to the minimum, with everything rigidly controlled. If it proved difficult to hold something constant, as was the case with meaning, then every effort was made to exclude it from the study. Ebbinghaus was brilliantly successful in demonstrating that lawful relationships could be revealed in this way, but he did so at the cost of turning the psychology of memory away from some of its central questions and laying the foundations for what many would now regard as 80 years of sterility. It would be wrong to blame Ebbinghaus for this, because there is no doubt that his achievements were substantial. His successors, alas, tended to lack his originality, with the result that the more easily imitated feature of his work, its preoccupation with rigid control, increasingly came to dominate the study of memory. The snaffle and the bit proved much easier to pass on than the horse.

At the same time as Ebbinghaus was struggling with the problem of experimental control in the study of memory, Sir Francis Galton was writing his *Inquiries into Human Faculty,* an intriguing mélange of anecdote and careful measurement, of introspection and sophisticated statistical analysis (Galton, 1883). In the intervening century, Galton has been remembered for his contributions to statistics, to the question of the inheritance of intelligence, and to subjective ratings of visual imagery, but his contribution to memory had been largely neglected until the recent rediscovery of the importance of autobiographical memory (Rubin, 1986).

The Galton tradition could be said to represent a concern with the richness and complexity of memory in the world, in contrast to the much more limited and constrained reflection of memory through laboratory-based tasks. This tradition was continued by Bartlett, although Bartlett himself was at pains to distinguish his own view from that of Galton. He did so, however, not by turning his back on everyday memory but by questioning Galton's reliance on statistical procedures, an aspect of his work that is quite separate from Galton's contribution to the natural history of memory. Indeed, although it has not been a major theme in British psychology, there has been a trickle of research on naturalistic aspects of human memory and learning that has continued since Bartlett's day. Examples include work in the Bartlett tradition on prose recall by Gomulicki (1956) and Kay (1955), Hunter's work on the mnemonist and calculator Aitken (Hunter, 1977), and Morton's research on incidental memory for the layout of a telephone dial, or rather lack of it (Morton, 1967). A considerable expansion of research in this area began in the 1970s and was first reflected in the symposium organized by the Welsh section of the British Psychology Society in 1978, published as *Practical Aspects of Memory* (Gruneberg, Morris, & Sykes, 1978). It was at that meeting that Neisser made his oft-quoted comment on the irrelevance of much memory research. Although it was a fair comment on the previous 20 years of research, the conference itself was a striking refutation of the generality of the comment. [The continuing interest in naturalistic memory in Britain is well reflected in Wilson and Moffat's *Clinical Management of Memory Problems* (1984) and *Everyday Memory,* by Harris and Morris (1984).]

And so the Galton tradition, with its interest in the richness and complexity of memory in the real world, survived and probably is healthier now than at any time in the last 50 years. Do we therefore need reminding of its importance? Unfortunately, I think we do. Any science needs to be concerned with standards, as well as with novelty and originality. It is, on the whole, very much easier to monitor the methodological rigor of a piece of work than to assess its originality. It is always easier to apply the snaffle and the curb than to find the horse. Psychology, in general, and its journals, in particular, are still very conscious of the need to be psychologically "respectable," and one route to such respectability is to require the "highest" standards of evidence, regardless of practical difficulties; on this view, the criteria are exactly the same whether one is carrying out the 57th manipulation on some highly constrained laboratory paradigm or exploring a totally new aspect of memory in the outside world. According to this approach, the aim of an experiment is to achieve certainty; to increase the amount of information by significantly narrowing down the alternatives is not enough.

Such constraints are by no means absolute. As Bertrand Russell observed many years ago, if one has written a highly respectable and preferably very boring book, then one is much more likely to be able to get away with producing something that is readable. In my own case, though I cannot claim to have written anything as eminent and impenetrable as *Principia Mathematica,* I have generated and indeed continue to generate my share of the boring and the respectable, which means that I probably am accorded more licence than would otherwise be the case. Nonetheless, it continues to be difficult to publish work that is essentially concerned with the natural history of memory, work that appears to be intrinsically interesting but that does not allow unequivocal theoretical conclusions. I am not yet sufficiently paranoid to believe that this is any easier for any of my colleagues interested in naturalistic memory. Hence, despite the fact that there is now a much more general sympathy for a study of naturalistic memory, I think it is still important to remind ourselves of the need to map our laboratory findings onto the real world and to be willing to accept and publish work that is still very much at the stage of natural history. At some point we shall reach a stage at which simple observations of memory in the real world will be insufficiently novel to merit publication. At present, however, I think we are still a long way from that point.

What is memory for?

The Ebbinghaus approach, with its concern for control and measurement, tends to bypass a central question about human memory, namely, its functional role. At a very general level, it is clear that unless a system can store information, then it cannot learn, and if it cannot learn, it will not acquire language or be able to perform more than a fraction of the cognitive skills that are necessary for coping in a technological society. Hence, the use of memory is obvious if one treats memory as a general capacity for storing information. There is, of course, abundant evidence that memory is not a unitary function, and this in turn raises the question of the functions of the various subcomponents of human memory. Much of my own research over the last decade has been concerned with this question – in the case of short-term memory, leading to an extensive series of experiments on working memory, and in the case of long-term memory, leading to questions about the ecological relevance of standard measures of human memory.

The traditional view of short-term memory was that it formed an essential bridge between the long-term memory store and sensory input, being responsible for the setting up of control processes, for rehearsal and learning, and for establishing and maintaining retrieval plans (Atkinson & Shiffrin, 1968). Set against this general conclusion was the observation by Shallice and Warrington (1970) that patients who appeared to have grossly defective short-term memory nonetheless appeared capable of normal learning and relatively normal cognitive processing.

In an attempt to explore this apparent paradox, Graham Hitch and I carried out a series of experiments in which we studied the effects on learning, comprehension, and reasoning of a concurrent secondary digit-span task that was assumed to absorb most of the available short-term-memory capacity. The effect of this manipulation was much less dramatic than the modal model would have predicted, and that encouraged us to reconceptualize short-term memory as a multicomponent system (Baddeley & Hitch, 1974). Subsequent work has extended the working memory model to a wide range of tasks (Baddeley, 1986), including the understanding of fluent reading (Baddeley & Lewis, 1981), the development of working memory (Hitch & Halliday, 1983), developmental dyslexia (Baddeley, 1986), and, currently, the understanding of complex psychomotor tasks. Neuropsychological applications of the concept have also proved fruitful, not only in explaining specific short-term-memory deficits but also in attempting to understand the breakdown in function that occurs with subjects suffering from frontal-lobe damage or dementia (Baddeley, 1986).

Our interest in the functional aspects of long-term memory has had a rather more immediate practical aim in view. One of the most sensitive indicators of brain damage resulting from head injury, normal aging, or senile dementia is by the performance of patients on standard laboratory memory tests such as paired-associate learning. One of the most frequent complaints of patients suffering from such afflictions is that their memory is impaired. It is unlikely that patients are inconvenienced by the need to learn pairs of unrelated words; it is much more likely to be the case that problems occur because of an incapacity to cope with the daily routine, particularly such prospective memory tasks as remembering appointments, a capacity that may well be quite unrelated to verbal learning ability. For example, in one study we selected two groups of subjects, one good at verbal free recall and the other rather poor at this task (Wilkins & Baddeley, 1978). We then required them to perform a prospective memory task, analogous to remembering to take pills, in which the subject had to press a button at regular intervals four times per day. Those with good verbal memories were significantly *less* accurate in their prospective memory performance than were those with poor verbal recall.

Alan Sunderland, John Harris, and I explored the memory deficits associated with closed-head injury, studying the performances of our subjects on standardized memory tests and also attempting to obtain some indication of their everyday-memory problems by means of interviews with the patient and a relative, as well as through diaries (Sunderland, Harris, & Baddeley, 1983). We obtained an interesting but complex pattern of results suggesting the following conclusions: First, subjects were not reliable sources of evidence on their own memory problems; in particular, patients who had suffered their head injuries relatively recently gave estimates of their memory that did not relate either to their objective performances or to assessments of their performances by relatives. A somewhat more consistent pattern emerged in the case of diaries and relatives' assessments. These tended to give a more coherent picture and also to correlate with some objective memory tests, but not with others. The test that correlated most closely with observations of everyday memory was the logical memory test taken from the Wechsler Memory scale. This requires the subject to remember a paragraph that tells a simple story, recalling it both immediately and after a delay. Both immediate recall and delayed recall showed impressively high correlations with relatives' questionnaires ($r = .72$ and $r = .63$, respectively). Another measure of the sensitivity of a memory test is its ability to discriminate between those patients who had and those who had not suffered head injury. On this criterion, prose recall was a significant but much less impressive measure than were other tasks such as one involving the recognition of recurring nonsense figures, or a task measuring speed of retrieval from semantic memory, neither of which was significantly related to complaints of everyday-memory problems.

The pattern therefore suggested that the optimal test to be used when studying the memory deficits of patients will depend crucially on the question being asked. Certain measures are sensitive indicators of the presence of brain damage, but do not give a clear indication whether or not the patient is likely to suffer memory problems that will interfere with the ability to carry on a normal life. In contrast, other measures are less sensitive to the presence or absence of brain damage, but provide a better indication whether or not the patient is likely to encounter memory problems in coping with everyday living.

One weakness of this study is its reliance for validation on subjects' and relatives' abilities to recall instances of lapses of memory. In the case of the patient, this is obviously open to a range of difficulties. A patient who has a memory problem is likely to forget that lapses have occurred, and indeed patients with substantial memory problems often lack insight. One of the most amnesic patients I have ever tested interrupted the experiment every few minutes with the expression "I pride myself on my memory," completely forgetting that she had made this remark many times previously in the same session. Although this problem can be avoided to some extent by relying on a relative's assessment, in a later study in which we were examining the memory problems of the elderly, this advantage was lost, probably because the relative also was elderly and hence tended to forget occurrences of memory lapses in the patient (Sunderland, Watts, Baddeley, & Harris, 1986).

Another problem stems from the different life-styles pursued by different subjects, particularly when their ages are grossly different. For example, studies of normal elderly people carried out by Harris and Sunderland indicated that they reported substantially *fewer* memory lapses than did young subjects (Sunderland, Harris, & Baddeley, 1984). Although some of that difference could have stemmed from the greater tendency of the elderly to forget their lapses, that probably was not the whole explanation. Moscovich and Minde carried out a study, described by Harris (1984, p. 77), in which elderly and young subjects were asked to give subjective estimates of their memory capacities and then were required to remember to telephone the experimenter at a specific time in the future. The elderly reported fewer lapses and were more reliable in the subsequent prospective memory test. It seems likely that older subjects live more ordered lives and also make better use of external reminders, such as calendars and diaries. For whatever reason, however, as others have pointed out (Herrmann, 1984; Morris, 1984), diaries and subjective estimates do involve many methodological problems. I would suggest that they do not offer a satisfactory measure of everyday memory and thus cannot be regarded as adequate forms of quantitative validation.

If laboratory tests lack ecological validity, and if subjective estimates are unreliable, then how can everyday-memory problems be estimated? An ongoing project by Barbara Wilson, Janet Cockburn, and myself is attempting to tackle this thorny question as follows. Although questionnaire-and-diary studies probably are unreliable as sources of quantitative information about memory problems, they probably do provide reasonable qualitative indications of those aspects of everyday life that are most disrupted by memory lapses. Barbara Wilson, at the Rivermead Rehabilitation Centre in Oxford, attempted to combine qualitative information from questionnaires with quantitative evidence from laboratory tasks by devising a range of subtests, each of which aimed to give an objective measure of the subject's susceptibility to memory errors of a particular type.

The resulting Rivermead Behavioural Memory Test has 11 subcomponents; one requires the subject to remember the name of a person shown in a photograph, a second involves remembering to perform an act at a prespecified time, a third involves recognizing a small set of previously presented pictures, a fourth requires the learning of a simple route, and so forth (Wilson, Cockburn, & Baddeley, 1985). In a pilot study, a sample of 25 patients at the Rivermead Rehabilitation Centre, who were described by their therapists as having memory problems sufficient to interfere with their therapy, passed a mean of only 3.8 of the subtests, whereas other patients who were categorized by their therapists as without serious memory problems passed a mean of 10, and normal controls passed all of the subtests (Wilson, Baddeley, & Hutchins, 1984).

We are currently carrying out a more extensive validation study involving a larger sample of subjects and using as our validating score therapists' observations of memory lapses in the patients over a 2-week period. The results thus far are very promising, yielding a correlation between overall score and number of lapses reported of 0.75. We hope that the test not only will be useful in pinpointing areas of potential memory problems, hence helping the therapists, but also may provide a measure of memory performance that has sufficient face validity to be acceptable and unthreatening to the patient, while being sufficiently sensitive to indicate any clinically significant deterioration in memory performance.

Naturalistic memory and theory

I have thus far spoken as though everyday-memory studies simply provide a richer and more profitable way of revealing important facts about human memory. If that were the case, then the journals would be full of such studies, and one would not need to have essays such as this. In practice, of course, carrying out good studies under everyday conditions is extremely difficult. This is particularly so if one wishes to ask theoretically cogent questions about the phenomena observed. In the absence of such theoretical development, everyday-memory studies are likely to end up as a branch of psychology that resembles the traditional Victorian museum: full of curios and quaint artifacts, but lacking in any coherent pattern or structure.

In order to ask theoretical questions, it is almost always necessary to manipulate the phenomenon in some way, and often this requires a study that is halfway between a naturalistic approach and an experimental approach. I would like to illustrate this using a series of three experiments carried out by Amancio da Costa Pinto of the University of Porto and myself.

We were interested in the long-term recency phenomenon and its relevance, if any, to everyday memory. In an earlier study, Hitch and I had shown that a clear long-term recency effect could be obtained if rugby football players were required to try to recall the teams they had played against earlier in the season. There was a marked recency effect, with the probability of recall being a function of the number of interpolated games, rather than elapsed time (Baddeley & Hitch, 1977). Unfortunately, although the phenomenon of long-term recency may be very common (showing up in questions such as when one last visited London, or the last party one attended), exploring the phenomenon empirically is far from simple, largely because of the difficulty of finding suitable tasks. We decided to look at recollection of parking location in the hope that this might be a suitable test, and over a 2-week period we noted the locations in which cars were parked outside our Applied Psychology Unit (APU). We then surprised our colleagues by asking them to attempt to recall where they had parked each morning and afternoon over the last 2 weeks. Their recall performances are shown in Figure 8.1, from which it is clear that recency was obtained.

In contrast to the previous study, in which our rugby players often had missed several opponents' names, attendance at the APU was relatively consistent, with the result that elapsed time and number of interpolated visits were too highly correlated to be statistically separated as determinants of forgetting. We therefore decided to move to a semiexperimental design in which members of our subject panel were invited to attend a test session and subsequently were asked to recall their parking locations after a delay of 2 hours, 1 week, or 1 month. If our previously observed recency effect was due to the fading of the memory trace over a 2-week period, then we would expect to see substantial differences in levels of retention across the three groups. In fact, no such differences occurred, with the three groups making correct recalls on 72%, 73%, and 72% of the oc-

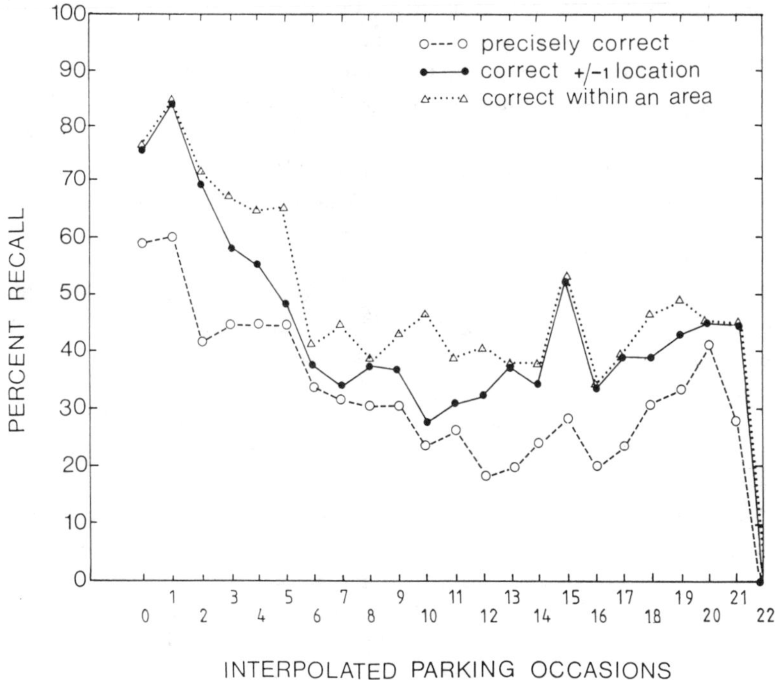

Figure 8.1. Recall of parking location as a function of number of interpolated parking occasions.

casions, respectively. Note that such a result also rules out a general-interference interpretation, because our subjects clearly were likely to have parked many times in the intervening period. That leaves either a specific strong-interference interpretation, which says that only highly similar parking locations will cause forgetting, or some more complex interpretation in terms of trace discrimination (Glenberg et al., 1980).

We decided to test these possible interpretations further by requiring our subjects to come for two test sessions, separated by a week. We then tested the retention of one group at 4 weeks after their initial visit, at which time the second visit should provide a source of retroactive interference (the RI group). We tested the second group 4 weeks after their second occurrence, in which case the first visit should form a source of proactive interference (the PI group). Overall recall was significantly lower than that shown in the previous study, and in the conditions recalled after 4 weeks, recalls were not significantly different between the PI group (47%) and the RI group (39%). On the other hand, the first visit of the PI group, some 6 weeks earlier, was very poorly recalled (20%), whereas the second visit of the RI group, some 2 weeks earlier, was relatively well recalled (61%). This pattern of results appears to fit most neatly into a discrimination hypothesis such as that proposed by Glenberg and associates and Hitch and Halliday, in which the subject attempts to discriminate one of two competing traces; for a given temporal separation between the two traces, the discrimination becomes progressively more difficult as the delay increases.

We are, then, in this naturalistic study, able to reject both a decay interpretation and a simple interference-theory interpretation. Furthermore, our results broadly fit a discrimination model that was developed to explain laboratory-based long- and short-term recency effects. However, further development and testing of such a model will require many more observations than it is feasible to make under the constraints of studying parking location. Consequently, if we are to make further theoretical progress, then we shall be forced back to the laboratory, where it is possible to obtain many more data under far more closely specified conditons.

I would like to conclude with a cautionary tale. Although the richness of the real world often will yield interesting new insights, it is sometimes the case that the opposite occurs, when a clear and apparently highly relevant phenomenon discovered in the laboratory fails to survive the rigors of everyday life. One such case occurred in studies carried out by Bob Logie, Muriel Woodhead, and myself regarding face recognition (Logie, Baddeley, & Woodhead, in press).

Our main concern over a whole series of experiments was to explore ways in which subjects could be taught to improve their capacities for recognizing unfamiliar faces. We explored a range of strategies for enhancing face learning, both ancient and modern, and came up with depressingly meager results (Baddeley, 1986; Baddeley & Woodhead, 1983). We did, however, come up with one apparently serendipitous finding, namely, that the particular pose that was featured in the picture of the face to be recognized was a rather important variable, with a three-quarter view being better than a frontal or profile pose. If this could be determined to be reliable, then it would have practical implications for the standard procedures of taking photographs for passports, driving licences, and so forth. We were, however, reluctant to issue advice without first checking our findings under more realistic conditions than those of the laboratory, where subjects had been shown one photograph and required to recognize another. We therefore decided to set up a grand field study in which the elegant design of the laboratory would be combined with the richness and relevance of the outside world.

We sought the help of a local newspaper in a study in which the citizens were invited to search for a number of targeted persons within their town. Three local towns were used, with an elaborately counterbalanced design such that each target appeared in one of the three poses in the edition distributed in one of the three towns. Our targets were then required to walk through the three towns in the morning and in the afternoon. We were assured by our local newspaper that there would, at the very least, be several hundred respondents, and we duly sat by the telephone at 9 o'clock on Saturday morning and waited for the information to flow in. At 5 p.m. we received our only response, a correct identification of one target in the profile view!

What could we learn from this fiasco? The lack of response could mean that the task we set our subjects was very difficult, or it could simply be that we needed to motivate the populations of the three towns we studied rather more strongly. Our second experiment was therefore somewhat more cautious. We knew that our subject panel tended to be highly motivated and highly cooperative; so we decided to recruit them to look for our targets during their Saturday morning shopping. We offered all the subjects who came to be tested at the APU over a period of time the opportunity of participating, giving a small sum to those who agreed to take part. On the eve of the crucial day, they were instructed to examine a set of six photographs and spend 15 min trying to memorize them. They comprised two targets in each of the three poses. Next morning, our subjects were instructed to refresh their memory and then set out shopping, keeping an eagle eye open for the targets, who would be in clearly specified areas. Subjects were to indicate the detection of a target by noting the location and time of detection and the clothing that the target was wearing, recording their responses on a form provided. Between them, the 33 subjects made a total of 30 responses, of which 28 were false alarms. It is clear from this that the task of searching for a set of relatively unfamiliar faces in a crowd is extremely difficult. Although this may have some general implications for the likelihood of newspaper photographs leading to the detection and apprehension of persons wanted by the police, it did not tell us very much about our original question concerning the optimal pose. Experiment 1 had yielded one detection in a profile view, and experiment 2 yielded one detection each for a frontal target and three-quarter target.

Undeterred, we decided to try again, this time attempting to make the task much easier by using a single target and specifying the route that he would follow and the direction in which he would walk. Our subjects were instructed to make at least one circuit of the route, going in the opposite direction to the target. Hence, we assumed that we could be certain that the target and the searchers would meet face to face. At last, we managed to achieve a reasonable detection rate, together with some indication that angle of pose does influence performance. Subjects searching for a target they had seen photographed in profile had a 66% hit rate and a 34% false-alarm rate, significantly poorer than for a frontal or three-quarter view, both of which gave a detection rate of 75% and a false-alarm rate of 15%. There was, however, no suggestion that the three-quarter view was superior to the more traditional frontal pose.

We ran one final experiment in which we moved back into the laboratory, this time having our target enter a room in which group testing was proceeding, make an announcement, and then leave. At the end of the session, subjects were unexpectedly asked to select the announcer from a set of photographs, with some subjects having the target in frontal view, some in profile, and some in three-quarter view. Under these circumstances, we got our predicted order of difficulty, with a 48% detection of profile, a 54% detection of frontal view, and a 68% detection of three-quarter view. It appears, then, that we do have a genuine phenomenon, but one that is not sufficiently robust to survive the rigors of life outside the laboratory.

As our study suggests, moving out of the laboratory is not without its problems, but it is necessary if we wish to generalize our results to the world outside the psychology department. And if the result is sometimes to suggest that our laboratory phenomena are less robust than we had hoped, on other occasions naturalistic observation and the exploration of everyday cognition can reveal important and interesting new phenomena that extend and challenge our existing theories.

References

Atkinson, R. C., & Shiffrin, R. M. (1968). Human memory: A proposed system and its control processes. In K. W. Spence (Ed.), *The psychology of learning and motivation: Advances in research and theory* (Vol. 2, pp. 89–195). New York: Academic Press.

Baddeley, A. D. (1979). Working memory and reading. In P. A. Kolers, M. E. Wrolstad, & H. Bouma (Eds.), *Processing of visible language* (pp. 355–370). New York: Plenum.

Baddeley, A. D. (1986). *Working memory.* Oxford: Oxford University Press.

Baddeley, A. D., & Hitch, G. J. (1974). Working memory. In G. Bower (Ed.), *Recent advances in learning and motivation* (Vol. VIII, pp. 47–90). New York: Academic Press.

Baddeley, A. D., & Hitch, G. J. (1977). Recency re-examined. In S. Dornic (Ed.), *Attention and performance* (Vol. VI, pp. 647–667). Hillsdale, NJ: Lawrence Erlbaum.

Baddeley, A. D., & Lewis, V. J. (1981). Inner active processes in reading: The inner voice, the inner ear and the inner eye. In A. M. Lesgold & C. A. Perfetti (Eds.), *Interactive processes in reading* (pp. 107–129). Hillsdale, NJ: Lawrence Erlbaum.

Baddeley, A. D., & Woodhead, M. M. (1983). Improving face recognition ability. In S. Lloyd-Bostock & B. Clifford (Eds.), *Evaluating witness evidence* (pp. 125–136). London: Wiley.

Galton, F. (1883). *Inquiries into human faculty and its development* (Everyman edition). London: Dent.

Glenberg, A. M., Bradley, M. M., Stevenson, J. A., Kraus, T. A., Tkachuk, M. J., Gretz, A. L., Fish, J. H., & Turpin, B. M. (1980). A two-process account of long-term serial position effects. *Journal of Experimental Psychology: Human Learning and Memory, 6,* 355–369.

Gomulicki, B. R. (1956). Recall as an abstractive process. *Acta Psychologica, 12,* 77–94.

Gruneberg, M. M., Morris, P. E., & Sykes, R. N. (Eds.). (1978). *Practical aspects of memory.* London: Academic Press.

Harris, J. E. (1984). Remembering to do things: A forgotten topic. In J. E. Harris & P. E. Morris (Eds.), *Everyday memory, actions and absentmindedness* (pp. 71–92). London: Academic Press.

Harris, J. E., & Morris, P. E. (Eds.). (1984). *Everyday memory, actions and absentmindedness.* London: Academic Press.

Herrmann, D. J. (1984). Questionnaires about memory. In J. E. Harris & P. E. Morris (Eds.), *Everyday memory, actions and absentmindedness* (pp. 133–172). London: Academic Press.

Hitch, G. J., & Halliday, M. S. (1983). Working memory in children. *Philosophical Transactions of the Royal Society of London B, 302,* 325–340.

Hunter, I. M. L. (1977). An exceptional memory. *British Journal of Psychology, 68,* 155–164.

Kay, H. (1955). Learning and retaining verbal material. *British Journal of Psychology, 46,* 81–100.

Logie, R. H., Baddeley, A. D., & Woodhead, M. M. (in press). Face recognition, pose and ecological validity. *Applied Cognitive Psychology.*

Morris, P. E. (1984). Validity of subjective reports on memory. In J. E. Harris & P. E. Morris (Eds.), *Everyday memory, actions and absentmindedness* (pp. 173–190). London: Academic Press.

Morton, J. (1967). A singular lack of incidental learning. *Nature, 215,* 203–204.

Neisser, U. (1978). Memory: What are the important questions? In M. M. Gruneberg, P. E. Morris, & R. N. Sykes (Eds.), *Practical aspects of memory* (pp. 3–24). London: Academic Press.

Neisser, U. (1982). *Memory observed: Remembering in natural contexts.* San Francisco: W. H. Freeman.

Rubin, D. (1986). *Autobiographical memory.* Cambridge University Press.

Shallice, T., & Warrington, E. K. (1970). Independent functioning of verbal memory stores: A neuropsychological study. *Quarterly Journal of Experimental Psychology, 22,* 261–273.

Sunderland, A., Harris, J. E., & Baddeley, A. D. (1983). Do laboratory tests predict everyday memory? A neuropsychological study. *Journal of Verbal Learning and Verbal Behavior, 22,* 341–357.

Sunderland, A., Harris, J. E., & Baddeley, A. D. (1984). Assessing everyday memory after head injury. In J. E. Harris & P. E. Morris (Eds.), *Everyday memory, actions and absentmindedness* (pp. 191–206). London: Academic Press.

Sunderland, A., Watts, K., Baddeley, A. D., & Harris, J. E. (1986). Subjective memory assessment and test performance in the elderly. *Journal of Gerontology, 41,* 376–385.

Wilkins, A. J., & Baddeley, A. D. (1978). Remembering to recall in everyday life: An approach to absentmindedness. In M. M. Gruneberg, P. E. Morris, & R. N. Sykes (Eds.), *Practical aspects of memory* (pp. 27–34). London: Academic Press.

Wilson, B., Baddeley, A., & Hutchins, H. (1984). *The Rivermead Behavioural Memory Test: A preliminary report* (Technical Report 84/1). Rivermead Rehabilitation Centre, Oxford.

Wilson, B. A., Cockburn, J., & Baddeley, A. D. (1985). *The Rivermead Behavioural Memory Test.* Reading, England: Thames Valley Test Co. (22 Bulmershe Road).

Wilson, B. A., & Moffat, N. (1984). *Clinical management of memory problems.* London: Croom Helm.

9 Some bad and some good reasons for studying memory and cognition in the wild

Thomas K. Landauer

Why should we take research on cognition out of the laboratory into the real world? First, let me mention some reasons that I do not find compelling.

Some bad reasons

Laboratory studies produce erroneous results

"We do not need to move to the real world, because principles and facts that have been discovered in laboratory research on cognition do not apply to real life." Although one hears assertions to this effect, I know of almost no instances in which real-life tests of well-established principles have been carried out in a sensible way and have failed. On the other hand, there have been many examples of tests and real-world applications of principles regarding human learning and cognition that were discovered in the laboratory and have proved entirely satisfactory. Moreover, Neisser's pessimism (1978) notwithstanding, some of the principles are highly nonobvious. My own favorite example concerns the spacing of practice. This demonstrably counterintuitive finding (Melton, 1970; Rothkopf, 1963; Rothkopf & Coke, 1963) initially emerged from a long and tortuous set of experiments in the most classic and abstract verbal learning tradition. By now, literally dozens of applications to instruction, the teaching of classroom materials, and the practice of motor skills have been reported in the literature. I estimate the success-to-failure ratio as at least 10:1. Often the benefits are quite dramatic. For example, Ross and I showed that merely telling students how to use spaced practice greatly increased their ability to memorize a telephone number (Landauer & Ross, 1977), and Ainslie and I demonstrated that a very long delay for a review examination on a full course of technical information resulted in much better retention over a year (Landauer & Ainslie, 1975).

There have, of course, been many instances in which variables with significant effects in the laboratory have been found to have little influence in practical situations. However, this is almost always a matter of sufficiency or importance,

rather than correctness. A recent example from my own work concerns the effects of prior associations on the values of name assignments for commands in a computer text-editing environment (Landauer, Galotti, & Hartwell, 1983). Prior association, of course, has a strong effect in list learning, where associative pairing is the subject's only task. But in learning to use a text editor, these effects apparently were hidden by more important learning difficulties. It took people so long to master other conceptual problems that there was plenty of time to learn either easy names or more difficult names for a small number of commands without affecting overall training time.

What sometimes has led people to believe that laboratory studies of cognition are not applicable is the mere fact that they have not yet been applied. This is partly because experimental psychology has made but few and feeble attempts to make itself useful. But to make matters worse, the reason that some principles have not been applied is simply that some people have thought that they were not applicable. The repetition-spacing principle mentioned earlier is a good example. A common intuition of both learners and educators is that it is better to mass repetitions than to distribute them. Even psychologists who write treatises on how to memorize or study seldom mention repetition spacing, despite the fact that it is very easy to apply and gives extremely robust results, improving learning rates by factors of two or more in many cases. This volume contains three chapters reporting promising results from using practice spacing regimens in rehabilitation for dementia patients (Chapters 32–34, this volume). Exciting as this development is, it illustrates a depressing moral. Why was this powerful, well-proven technique from our laboratories so long in being put to work in the clinic, whereas mnemonic techniques from the nonscientific (huckster?) memory-training tradition were doggedly pursued despite daunting practical problems (amnesics have trouble learning "one's a bun, two's a shoe . . . ")?

Laboratories do not generate enough ideas or hypothesis tests

I do not think we need to move from the laboratory to the wild simply to have a way to test theories formed on the basis of work in the laboratory. This remark needs qualification. Certainly it would be good to have broader tests and broader sources of ideas, and I shall argue later that phenomena and problems encountered in realistic environments have special status. But this is not merely because they feed the mill. There is no dearth of theories, theory tests, or idea sources within the laboratory context itself. The set of theories of cognition that have stood up to all tests imagined for them in the laboratory is null. Simply finding tests, any tests, is therefore not a good reason to go elsewhere. Indeed, because theories often are about the effects of pure or isolable factors, controlled experiment often provides the only possible test. When it comes to testing theories, the laboratory almost always holds the advantage over the real world. Hypothesis tests require clear control in order to know what went right or wrong, what caused what, and often that is precisely what is lacking in the real world. It

seems much more logical to derive hypotheses on the basis of work on everyday function and then test them against careful experiment, rather than doing the opposite. What does need to be tested in the real world is the completeness of theories as descriptions of the things in which we are interested. It is not correctness that real-world studies must tell us about, but completeness.

Some good reasons

Test of adequacy

My last remark implies that the laboratory may not always provide a good test of adequacy. Why not? The main reasons have to do with the nature of the mind and the nature of the nature in which mind operates. The human mind is an enormously complex, powerful, and adaptive information-processing instrument. If one considers it merely a match for present-day general computers (a sort of inverse Turing machine), it is capable of performing a huge, possibly infinite variety of tasks in a possibly infinite number of ways. That is, it can reprogram itself to use a vast array of different algorithms, data, and methods to try to do almost anything it is asked to do. In the case of the mind, programming probably is accomplished by experience, education, learning, and strategic intent. Flexible programming, both intrinsic and extrinsic, makes the mind what it is, not a fixed set of structures. This makes it extremely difficult to choose what functions of the mind to study in the laboratory. Whatever tasks it faces, the mind will attempt them somehow, and the way it does so likely will depend on just how a task is set, what experiences it has had before, and so forth. This makes it easy to end up doing experiments about experiments and evolving a discipline that is at best pure intellectual play, and at worst scholastic and solipsistic.

The human mind evolved to function in a complex world, where it operates on large masses of previous experience and instruction, where it learns, makes decisions, retrieves information, and forgets in a matrix of multiple, probabilistically distributed demands. If the mind is studied only in the laboratory, it will be very easy to miss some of the functions for which it is designed, some of the environmental and experiential support on which its function depends, and some of the obstacles with which it needs to contend. In the laboratory, phenomena and factors to be examined will necessarily be chosen in the first instance by intuitive hunch, based only on informal observation. Critical processes are bound to be taken for granted, and important variables will go unstudied. Strong interactions in the way the system functions under various circumstances and in the presence of various factor levels will go unnoticed. Particularly important, the control processes by which the mind switches among different tasks or shares capacity between them (by analogy to computers, its scheduler algorithms) will almost certainly be neglected. Such resource allocations can have extremely important effects on the characteristics of the functions involved. Others have noted that the weak correlations between reported cognitive failures and performances on labo-

ratory assessments of cognitive abilities may well be due to the fact that the way in which life is arranged and its demands are traded often is responsible for success or failure, rather than the sheer ability of component processes (Rabbitt, Chapter 17, this volume).

When Landauer and associates (1983) tried to find a benefit in naming computer commands with words like those that a naive user would employ, they found no appreciable benefit. They concluded that the reason was because the learning of the new and peculiar set of functions entailed a relatively minor learning problem that the users could accomplish in the interstices of other task components. By contrast, the results suggested that the mapping of differing command names to functions that required differing syntax had a strong effect. This issue of the mapping of differences in a response set to the structure of a set of concepts was something that had rarely found its way into the laboratory (there were some precedents, but they were distant and not highly developed).

Variables missing from laboratory tasks may contribute to superior performance as well. Chess masters, for example, can remember more board positions than ordinary players or nonplayers by a wide margin (Chase & Simon, 1973). Analysis of the basis of these expert skills has gone far towards improving the sophistication and completeness of our views of cognitive processes. Note that in this instance the degree to which the study of natural skills required working in the real-life environment was minimal. Instead, what turned the trick was to bring a natural task and its natural adepts into the laboratory for systematic observation.

A still unpursued example of a similar sort is the learning of words. Recognition vocabulary for words grows at a rate that must approach 30 or 40 words per day during the most active learning years. Recent attempts to mimic the processes by which word meanings might be acquired from reading fell short of accomplishing any such rate (Jenkins, Stein, & Wysocki, 1984). It seems likely that the reason for such findings is that the words experimenters attempt to teach children in the laboratory are not the words the children will learn in nature. What is the difference? Is there some sort of detailed readiness afforded by the current knowledge structure in each child's head that complements the raw materials of language exposure available in the same child's environment? To pursue such speculation would require detailed in situ description and analysis of the relevant experiences of individuals. It seems most unlikely that the answer will come from isolated laboratory experiments, although bringing the phenomenon back into the laboratory when we have a better idea of how to mimic it may be required for a final evaluation of whatever theory emerges.

Setting the problems for research

Why should we be more interested in the mind in its wild state than in its tame state? I began by pointing out that there are more than enough problems to be pursued that arise and can be answered in the laboratory without recourse to nature. Why, then, should the questions found in the real world be any more attractive? There are several answers. A good enough answer is that most of us are especially curious about how we humans behave. Because human behavior can vary widely in different contexts, the only true sense in which humans can be said to have characteristic behavior is when they act in their natural environment.

Much of the work to date on everyday memory can be seen as motivated by curiosity about the interesting phenomena and quirks of human cognition. Indeed, there seems to be an overabundance of studies of what might be called oddities, curios, wonders, and freaks of cognition. People have studied memory for patterns on pennies and phone dials, memory for the Lord's Prayer, people's recognition of famous faces or old friends, and the performances of mnemonists, idiot-savants, and brain-damaged patients. What we are mostly lacking so far are studies of normal and truly everyday functions. Of course, extremes of function, failures and remarkable successes, can be quite revealing. They often tell as much about what a process must be like as does its typical performance. But such pieces of exceptional data are much more useful in the company of detailed and systematic knowledge of the normal, of which we are currently seriously deprived.

Thus, what we need is knowledge of the normal functions of the human mind in its natural habitat, a characterization of the host of cognitive successes, as well as the minority of cognitive failures. The tip-of-the-tongue phenomenon is interesting (Brown & McNeil, 1984; Freedman & Landauer, 1966), but against an all but unexamined baseline of expected performance, it is merely a curious phenomenon unto itself, rather than a description of what the human mind does for a living. We should be looking for the kinds of things that Agatha Christie seemed to know about memory and cognition, as well as those about which William James pondered. In *Cards on the Table* (Christie, 1984), Hercule Poirot describes the solution of a mystery thus:

> I got everyone in turn to tell me just what they remembered of the room. From that I got some very valuable information. First of all, by far the most likely person to have noticed the dagger was Dr. Roberts. He was a natural observer of trifles of all kinds – what's called an observant man. Of the bridge hands, however, he remembered practically nothing at all (despite the fact that a grand slam was in progress while the murder was committed). I did not expect him to remember much, but his complete forgetfulness looked as though he had something else on his mind all the evening. . . . Mrs. Lorimer I found to have a marvelous card memory, and I could well imagine that with any one of her powers of concentration a murder could easily be committed close at hand and she would never notice anything.

Note her appreciation of the role of attention and her intuition that a good card memory does not imply a good memory for anything else. Agatha Christie's mysteries are replete with such inferences based on what people would or would not have remembered at various times. It is hard to vouch for the accuracy of Christie's intuitions, but they point to a kind of knowledge that is not well articulated in our science. It is worth noting, as in the example just given, that the factors that often figure in her deductions are control processes that determine what information someone would or would not have noticed and used, individual differences in ability or in what the person cares about and pays attention to, and what the normal expectations are for what things people would or would not have remembered.

Among the new kinds of knowledge needed are the following: First, we need much more in the way of qualitative naturalistic descriptions of the kinds of problem solving, memory use, learning, retrieval, calculation, and so forth, that go on in everyday life. How much of human problem solving is complex pattern recognition, and how much Aristotelian logic? How much of the information people use is new, how much is old, and how much is inferred from the old? Second, we need quantification of what kinds of information are required and used, as well as the corresponding distribution of contexts in which the information content of memory is encountered and employed. Work such as that of Ross (1984) shows that people's success in solving logical problems depends heavily on their having been reminded, by apparently irrelevant details, of earlier solved problems. This suggests that to understand how people think requires knowledge of the ecology in which they function. To merely know what to explain, we need much more information on what people actually do with their minds.

Third, we need to know what proportion of what is learned in everyday life (in reading, in school classes, in conversations, at work, from manuals, on television) is used, when it is used, how likely it is to be forgotten before it is used, what sorts of things typically are remembered, what are distorted and how, and so forth. There has been a tiny handful of studies in the literature that have traced the retention of material learned in classes over the kinds of time periods in which it might actually be used (Bahrick, Chapter 6, this volume; Landauer & Ainslie, 1975). But even here, the methods used for measurement reflect the kinds of things assessed at the end of school classes or on common selection tests. These kinds of tests are aimed at telling which students did best, so that the better ones can be given higher-paid jobs, or so that their future education or career paths can be guided. Methods simply have not been developed by which to assess the totality of the information gained, or its relevance to later performance, or later recollection in some way during the natural course of life. The work of Ley (1978) on patients' memory for medical instructions is a notable start in the right direction. In this work, the questions asked and the goal toward which the instruction was aimed were clearly related to what the patient needed to carry away from the medical appointment. We need similar kinds of information about all the sources of knowledge that people are exposed to in order to better engineer, schedule, and time their educational and instructive events, but we also need this kind of information merely to be able to describe, investigate, and understand normal function.

A quantitative approach is represented by a small exploratory sally we recently made into the acquisition of knowledge from reading. We were interested in how much new information people actually gain from normal reading, and we measured it by having people try to fill in words randomly deleted from passages. The preliminary results show that people initially remember about one-third to one-half a bit of new information for every word as they read, and they lose about half of this in the following 2 weeks. Similar work to discover the rates of gain and loss of information from other sources could eventually paint a picture of the everyday dynamics of the human knowledge store – how and what it adds, loses, and "contains" as the individual moves through daily life.

Fourth, we need descriptions of the nature and quality of everyday memory and problem-solving activities in a representative way that will tell us their place in ongoing life. We need some methodology such as having keen observers spend the entire day, everyday, for months, with particular individuals, seeing what it is like. The kind of attention that has been lavished on the social life of children and apes also needs to be applied to the intellectual life of adults. I have often been curious how it happens that my wife and I can have conflicting but very clear recollections of the content of a recent event, of who did what at what time and who did not, or who said what to whom. Important aspects of human social relations (and psychotherapy) hinge on these kinds of memories. It would be nice to know something about how likely these memories are to be correct, as well as what determines when they are correct and what form errors take when they are not. What kinds of happenings do we remember how well for how long? What is the comparative quality of recollection for prices, dates, names, happenings, feelings, and actions? How large are individual differences in such matters? How much do individual differences interact with context effects and differences in material?

Ulric Neisser (1978) analyzed the striking differences and correspondences between John Dean's testimony to a congressional committee about what had been said in White House conversations about Watergate and the tape transcripts of the same conversations. Neisser's method was informal and intuitive, but it produced surprising observations and interesting interpretations. It would be quite valuable to develop and extend this approach. For example, the conversations of normal people, perhaps spouses, could be unobtrusively recorded over extended periods. Later, both parties could be queried about what had been said by whom. Confidence ratings could be obtained, retention intervals controlled, and so forth. With larger numbers of participants and other measures of their abilities and motivations, or with diaries or questionnaires about surrounding life events, much richer and more rigorous investigations of the determinants of everyday-memory preservation and transformation might be possible. I would dearly like to know how accurate my average real-life memory is. Judges and lawyers should want to know too, and so should we memory theorists.

Support of invention

A final and important reason for interest in the function of cognition in its natural habitat, and a promising venue for its study as well, lies in the application of psychology to design and invention. This happens in several contexts.

The learnability and usability of machines and other useful objects are greatly determined, of course, by the capabilities and limitations of users. The previously mentioned experiments on text editing were aimed at finding principles to guide designers in the production of computer systems that would be easier to learn to operate. One lesson learned was that many of the important factors in what makes such systems easy could not be discovered without bringing a full-scale system into the laboratory as an object of study. The other side of the coin is that serious attempts to understand ease of learning in the use of "cognitive tools" like computer systems are certain to expose gaps in our knowledge and set us new research problems of guaranteed human relevance. Recall that Pasteur's discoveries about bacteria were driven by a need to understand practical problems of fermentation. Applied problems frequently offer splendid cases of "everyday function." They force us to make our theories complete by reminding us saliently of their inadequacies.

To me, one of the most exciting possible applications for natural-cognition research is as an underpinning for the invention of new aids and prosthetics for mental performance. Modern computing technology, both its amazing hardware and the clever things that software can now do, opens up enormous opportunities for psychologists. Psychology was not, in the past, a fecund mother of invention. This was largely because there were no appropriate raw materials or technology to be fashioned into inventions that would help people with complex information-processing tasks. Computers have changed all that. It is time for us to start trying to understand what people do not do as well as they might, and why, and then go out and invent cognitive aids.

Here is a modest starting example of cognitive-tool invention from our laboratory. Furnas, Gomez, Dumais, and I have been worrying about why people, as often as not, fail to find information in a data base, even though it is there. Some fairly extensive data collection and analysis made it clear that the main reason is that things are stored under names different from those people use to look them up (Furnas, Landauer, Gomez, & Dumais, 1983). Further simulation and experimental studies indicated that simply providing many more key-word names (typically 30 instead of the customary 1 to 5) for a piece of data could improve by a factor of four to eight the likelihood that people would find what they wanted. Apparently this had never been tried before, partly because of a faulty intuition of indexers. Each indexer can think of only a few words and therefore judges these to be the only important ones; but in fact, each person thinks of a different few words than did the last person. Old systems also limited the number of index entries because of the constraints of paper-and-ink technology. Based on our "naturalistic" findings and high-powered but straightforward computer techniques, we have already invented some new systems that can increase human information-retrieval success by factors of as much as five (Furnas, 1985; Gomez & Lochbaum, 1984).

Redesign and invention based on knowledge of human cognitive performance are also needed in education, in job training, in the reorganization of social institutions to make them run more smoothly, and, of course, in therapy for cognitive disorders. In all of these cases, we need much better descriptions and much deeper analysis of the normal functions, processes, capabilities, and, especially, the limiting factors in the way people perform tasks. We need this kind of knowledge in order to be able to exploit information technology to amplify and complement human cognitive abilities. The new technologies will give us tools by which we can provide ways to overcome limitations and devise new ways to do things unimagined before. Mathematics and most other fields of knowledge have depended on the tools of making marks on paper. How the human cognitive performances of the future will depend on the use of electronic records and manipulation is impossible to know. But surely it would be nice if their evolution were guided by systematic psychological knowledge of the characteristics of the humans who use them. And just as surely, active participation in the research and development that bring these new tools into being will be beneficial to the development of psychological science.

Conclusion

In conclusion, it seems to me that a focus on real-life functions will serve to keep the object of study steady. The beast will not change its shape as it lies on the microscope table. Studying cognition in the wild will make us look at all of the variables and at all of the complexity, which will make our job much harder. But steadfastly studying those processes that have important places in the cognitive life of humans, and only those processes, will at least give us a finite goal to pursue.

Finally, lest I have not mentioned it often enough, the real test of whether or not something is being studied in the right context is not whether the place of study is the laboratory or the field, but whether or not the phenomenon being studied is a naturally important one. Face validity of the task, merely that it is one that people sometimes actually perform, is a poor guide. Some "real" tasks may be trivial and unrevealing. On the other hand, some abstract and artificial tasks may be necessary to understand what is going on in a real process. Laboratory experiments often are best even for the study of natural phenomena. Only by control of the introduction of variables and the random assignment of factor levels and conditions can cause be inferred. Once one knows what one wants to study, and I am urging knowing that by observing performance in its real context, then analyzing it into its essential components often will require controlled experiments. There is no reason why these cannot be done in the laboratory.

Moreover, there certainly may be fundamental processes, such as "learning," whose study in the purely laboratory setting will be extremely important for an understanding of function in vivo. Such studies should not be ridiculed for the wrong reasons – a wrong reason being merely that they are abstract or done in the laboratory. They should be open to question, however, if the motive for studying them was not derived from observation and analysis of phenomena at work in the actual functioning of the organism in the system of life in which it is usually embedded.

References

Brown, R., & McNeil, D. (1984). The "tip of the tongue phenomenon." *Journal of Verbal Learning and Verbal Behavior, 5,* 325–337.

Chase, W. G., & Simon, H. A. (1973). The mind's eye in chess. In W. G. Chase (Ed.), *Visual information processing* (pp. 215–282). New York: Academic Press.

Christie, A. (1984). *Cards on the table.* New York: Berkley Publications.

Freedman, J., & Landauer, T. K. (1966). Retrieval of long-term memory: "Tip-of-the-tongue" phenomenon. *Psychonomic Science, 4,* 309–310.

Furnas, G. W. (1985). Experience with an adaptive indexing scheme. In L. Borman & B. Curtis (Eds.), *Proceedings of Human Factors in Computing Systems* (CHI '85). New York: Association for Computing Machinery.

Furnas, G. W., Landauer, T. K., Gomez, L. M., & Dumais, S. T. (1983). Statistical semantics; analysis of the potential performance of keyword systems. *Bell System Technical Journal, 62,* 1753–1806.

Gomez, L. M., & Lochbaum, C. C. (1984). People can retrieve more objects with enriched key-word vocabularies. But is there a human performance cost? In B. Shackel (Ed.), *Human–Computer Interaction* (Interact '84) (pp. 257–262). Amsterdam: North Holland.

Jenkins, J. R., Stein, M. L., & Wysocki, K. (1984). Learning vocabulary through reading. *American Educational Research Journal, 21,* 767–787.

Landauer, T. K., & Ainslie, K. I. (1975). Exams and use as preservatives of course-acquired knowledge. *Journal of Educational Research, 69,* 91–104.

Landauer, T. K., Galotti, K. M., & Hartwell, S. (1983). Natural command names and initial learning: A study of text editing terms. *Communications of the ACM, 26,* 495–503.

Landauer, T. K., & Ross, B. H. (1977). Can simple instructions to space practice improve ability to remember a fact? An experimental test using telephone numbers. *Bulletin of the Psychonomic Society, 10,* 215–218.

Ley, P. (1978). Memory for medical information. In M. M. Gruneberg, P. E. Morris, & R. N. Sykes (Eds.), *Practical aspects of memory* (pp. 120–127). London: Academic Press.

Melton, A. (1970). The situation with respect to the spacing of repetitions and memory. *Journal of Verbal Learning and Verbal Behavior, 9,* 596–606.

Neisser, U. (1978). What are the important questions? In M. M. Gruneberg, P. E. Morris, and R. N. Sykes (Eds.), *Practical aspects of memory* (pp. 3–24). London: Academic Press.

Neisser, U. (1981). John Dean's memory: A case study. *Cognition, 9,* 1–22.

Ross, B. H. (1984). The effects of remindings on learning a cognitive skill. *Cognitive Psychology, 16,* 371–416.

Rothkopf, E. Z. (1963). Some observations on predicting instructional effectiveness by simple inspection. *Journal of Programmed Instruction, 2,* 19–20.

Rothkopf, E. Z., & Coke, E. (1963). Repetition interval and rehearsal method in learning equivalences from written sentences. *Journal of Verbal Learning and Verbal Behavior, 2,* 406–416.

Part II

Cognition in adulthood and late life: Findings in real-life settings

10 Introduction to Part II: What do we know about the aging of cognitive abilities in everyday life?

Leonard W. Poon

Neisser's critique (1978) of the functional significance of modern theories of memory played an important part in energizing both laboratory and real-world research. His paper renewed interest in and fueled discussions of the issues of generalizability, predictability, and validity of laboratory methods and findings.

The chapters in Part I of this book have outlined the rationale and arguments underlying the debate concerned with carrying out cognitive research in the laboratory and in the real world. These chapters have clarified the how, when, and why of studying real-world or everyday cognition. This clarification of the conceptual utility of representativeness, generalizations, ecological and external validity, and functional explanations paves the way for reviews of findings on everyday cognition in Part II of this book.

What do we know about cognitive abilities in everyday life along the adult life span? I believe that there is a two-part answer to the question. On the one hand, researchers have gained substantial knowledge about everyday cognition since the 1970s. The 1978 and 1987 conferences on *practical aspects of memory* (Gruneberg, Morris, & Sykes, 1978) testify to the depth of interest and research. From the perspective of the adult life span, researchers have begun to examine cognitive phenomena with greater precision (Smith, 1980). Although it has not been demonstrated empirically, it has been said that the magnitudes of age differences reported in the research literature over the last three decades have shrunk. This could be due to the sytematic exploration of the influences of other concomitant variables that could account for meaningful amounts of variance that previously were attributed to chronological age. Age is one of many variables that account for individual differences. Other concomitant factors include cognitive strategies, nature of the stimuli, criterial tasks, environmental influences, and so forth (Poon, 1985; Smith, 1980).

On the other hand, the literature available on everyday cognition along the adult age span is descriptive, cross-sectional, and atheoretical. This is not a bad state of affairs, given the preliminary nature of most of these investigations. Theoretical concepts must be derived from robust phenomena, and meaningful hypotheses about human behaviors will be postulated in due time. The need for information about the influence of the cohort on different types of everyday cognition is more pressing. Conclusions about changes in behaviors along the life span based on cross-sectional studies alone would be tenuous.

The 16 chapters in Part II are organized into two sections. The first section (Chapters 11–20) reviews the literature on a number of common, daily memory activities along the adult life span: reading, speech comprehension, imagined and perceived memory, word finding, finding one's way, problem solving, and remembering upcoming events. The second section (Chapters 21–25) reviews the influences of common individual-difference factors on the observed behavior: motivation, memory awareness, expertise, and individual world-knowledge systems. Chapter 26 provides the synthesis bridging laboratory and everyday-cognition research.

Over the course of a day, we spend a significant part of our time absorbing information visually and auditorially. Changes in reading and speech comprehension over the adult life span are reviewed in Chapters 11–13. J. Hartley (Chapter 11) focuses on the effects of individual differences in readers on prose memory performance. Hartley finds that prior knowledge and reading comprehension skills are important for prose memory at each stage of adulthood. Aside from these two exceptions, there are no uniform relationships between prose memory and a wide range of reader variables for the adult age ranges measured in her studies. Meyer and Rice (Chapter 12) report a comprehensive review of the effects of the text, the reader, and the task on prose memory. Their review shows that there are some discrepancies in the literature regarding the locus of adult age differences in reading comprehension and memory. However, the discrepancies can be explained by examining learner, task, and text variables.

Unlike reading, a process in which a person can scan the material forward and backward, speech processing is a linear, sequential process. That is, speech is received one word at a time, and at varying speech rates. Stine, Wingfield, and Poon (Chapter 13) systematically examine how young and elderly adults select segments of normal and unstructured speech passages and evaluate how speech rate and speech structure affect age-related differences in the memory and recall of a passage.

Whereas Chapters 11–13 focus on age differences in memory for written and spoken information, Chapter 14 (Cohen and Faulkner) is concerned with the nature of memory representation and the distinction between perceived and generated memories. Many memories are for things that are imagined or never happened. Do older adults have more difficulty in differentiating perceived and generated memory? Cohen and Faulkner's research shows that older adults are particularly prone to make reifying errors, believing that what is only imagined or never occurred is actually perceived. These results have important implications for adult age differences in eyewitness testimony and autobiographical memories.

Bowles, Obler, and Poon (Chapter 15) review the adult life span and clinical literature on the common naming and word-retrieval complaints of older persons, the so-called tip-of-the-tongue phenomenon. This phenomenon is particularly interesting to everyday-cognition investigators because it has been studied in the naturalistic setting, in the clinical setting, and in the laboratory. This chapter reviews findings from all three settings with young and elderly adults and aphasic and demented patients.

Two chapters are devoted to changes in spatial abilities over the adult life span. Examples of these abilities are locating a misplaced object or finding one's way in an unfamiliar part of town. Kirasic (Chapter 16) reviews the literature on isolating individual characteristics, adaptive processes, and performances in different spatial situations. Rabbitt (Chapter 17) examines adult age differences in finding one's way in a familiar locale and finds that a measurement of fluid intelligence can account for a significant amount of the performance variance.

Two complementary chapters are presented on adult age differences in everyday problem solving. Chapter 18 (A. Hartley) assists the reader in defining and understanding problems and hassles people face in everyday situations. Chapter 19 (Denney) examines the accuracy of predicting problem-solving performances in terms of task validity and performance stability. A developmental model for problem-solving performance is presented.

Chapter 20 (Sinnott) describes the differences in prospective and intentional memory performances in everyday situations. The study of prospective memory is very much in its infancy, and Sinnott points out a number of substantive and methodological issues that should be explored.

Chapters 21–25 describe four different sources of confounding that are frequently overlooked in the study of cognition in real-world or laboratory situations. Perlmuter and Monty (Chapter 21) demonstrate how motivation in choice and perceived control by the subject can facilitate performance significantly. Dixon (Chapter 22), Cavanaugh (Chapter 23), and Camp (Chapter 25) address the issue of awareness and its relationship to performance. Dixon's chapter focuses on questionnaire research on metamemory over the adult life span. Cavanaugh's chapter examines the conceptual bond between awareness and performance, and Camp's chapter examines awareness in a broader world-knowledge-system context. Charness (Chapter 24) reviews the interactive influences of expertise and chronological age on performances.

Finally, Kausler (Chapter 26) synthesizes laboratory and real-world cognitive research and notes that research on adult age differences in everyday memory performances need not abandon the traditional laboratory approach. The focus of that research, Kausler recommends, should be on the analysis of conditions likely to affect the proficiency of everyday-memory processes, rather than on tests of either the validities of theories accounting for general decrements in memory with aging or the generalizability to late adulthood of the minor memory phenomena discovered by basic researchers.

These 16 chapters in Part II of this book provide the necessary context in which to evaluate what we know about cognition in everyday situations. It is hoped that the data and reviews will inspire the readers to advance our knowledge of adult age differences in cognitive abilities in and out of the laboratory.

References

Gruneberg, M. M., Morris, P. E., & Sykes, R. N. (Eds.). (1978). *Practical aspects of memory.* London: Academic Press

Poon, L. W. (1985). Differences in human memory with aging: Nature, causes, and clinical implications. In J. Birren & K. W. Schaie (Eds.), *Handbook of the psychology of aging* (pp. 427–462). New York: Van Nostrand Reinhold.

Smith, A. D. (1980). Advances in the cognitive psychology of aging. In L. W. Poon (Ed.), *Aging in the 1980s: Psychological issues* (pp. 223–225). Washington, DC: American Psychological Association.

Neisser, U. (1978). What are the important questions? In M. M. Gruneberg, P. E. Morris, & R. N. Sykes (Eds.), *Practical aspects of memory* (pp. 3–24). London: Academic Press.

Part IIA

Everyday cognitive abilities

11 Memory for prose: Perspectives on the reader

Joellen T. Hartley

Memory serves many functions in the everyday transactions between the individual and the world. For example, we remember to stop at the grocery store, we remember where the grocery store is located, we remember how to drive an automobile in order to get to the grocery store, and, once there, we remember that we need to acquire the makings of a company meal scheduled for 2 days hence. These pieces of remembered information could be acquired in a number of ways, but in many everyday examples the remembered information is acquired through the processing of spoken or written language. We might, for example, hear or read instructions on how to drive a stick-shift automobile. The sequence of operations described in the verbal instructions would be stored and translated into a sequence of motor actions. Of course, the activity would not progress smoothly until such time as the motor actions became relatively automatic, but the initial representation of the activity could be acquired through spoken or written language. This chapter is concerned with the acquisition of information from written language (referred to as "prose" or "discourse"). The acquisition of information from spoken language is taken up in Chapter 13 by Stine, Wingfield, and Poon.

This chapter begins with a brief natural history of research in the area in which various kinds of studies intersect: discourse-processing, memory, and aging studies. Next, the current status in this research area is described, and the interpretation of current findings within existing models is outlined. Attention is then directed to describing an example of research concerned with the characteristics of the prose processor (the reader) and how these characteristics influence performance on prose memory tasks. Finally, a brief consideration of "the reader in the real world" highlights some issues that have not been addressed, particularly as they relate to discourse memory in older adults.

Support for research reported here was provided by grant AGO3362 from the National Institute on Aging. The author extends appreciation to P. A. Bellucci, J. J. Cassidy, T. A. Graves, D. W. Lee, and T. J. Mushaney for valuable assistance in the process of data collection and analysis.

A brief natural history of research on prose memory and aging

The study of memory for written and spoken discourse in adulthood was motivated by a general concern that the traditional methods of verbal learning (serial list learning, paired-associate list learning, free-recall list learning) failed to capture either the breadth or the complexity of memory functioning in adults in the real world; see Hartley, Harker, and Walsh (1980), Hultsch and Pentz (1980), and Walsh and Baldwin (1977) for elaboration. Outside of the formal classroom, there is little reason to believe that people memorize lists of words or unrelated concepts; yet scientific knowledge about developmental changes in memory has been based on these tasks. The findings from cross-sectional studies of list learning comparing older adults with younger adults offer little hope to those of us who plan to grow old: We can expect to remember about one-third to one-half less from our new experiences than will younger adults. Cognitive geropsychologists have invested many hours exploring the causes of these age-related deficiencies in memory, as reviewed by Craik (1977) and Hartley and associates (1980). In general, all hypotheses are based on mechanisms of age-related decrements in memory function. But if decrement is the model, then clear evidence of decrement must be demonstrated in all forms of memory. Alternatively, if decrement is not consistent across memory tasks, theories must be elaborated that will specify qualitatively different kinds of memory, some that do and some that do not undergo change during late adulthood. This second alternative is not parsimonious, and it would be preferable to show that there is reasonable uniformity in age-related memory changes that are independent of the particular task or type of material. The study of memory for prose is one of the new directions that aging research has taken in response to the challenge of assessing memory change with tasks that are ecologically valid and that expand the data base for theory building (Rubin, Chapter 1, this volume).

The earliest studies of prose memory in older adults were hampered by lack of a measurement system that was reliable and was accepted as valid by a broad group of researchers. When Gordon and Clark (1974) explored prose memory in older adults, they measured memory by scoring the number of intuitive "idea units" that were produced during written recall. An idea unit is difficult to define so that it can be reproduced in another laboratory. The methodological breakthrough in this area of research was the development of systems for representing the semantic contents of a discourse (Frederiksen, 1975; Kintsch, 1974; Meyer, 1975). These systems provided a tool for quantifying the recall of prose in a way that was replicable from laboratory to laboratory. All of the systems assume that the proposition (a relationship between a set of concepts) is the elementary unit of meaning in a discourse. None of the systems requires that the original proposition be recalled verbatim; rather, any proposition that reproduces the meaning of the original proposition is accepted as correct. Thus, emphasis is directed away from rigid reproduction and toward reconstruction of meaning. As the representation systems became generally available to the scientific community, there was a burst of energy directed into new lines of research on developmental changes in memory for discourse in adulthood.

The first generation of research on memory for prose in adulthood included studies that used intuitive idea-unit measurements as well as the newly available discourse-representation systems. The goal of much of the early research was to determine whether or not there were age differences in memory performance when prose materials were used instead of traditional word lists. Gordon and Clark (1974) found clear age differences for both recall of idea units and recognition of a well-structured story. A series of studies by Taub (1976, 1979) reported overall age differences in both recall and recognition of prose passages, but a complication was introduced: If the older adults were highly verbal (measured by WAIS vocabulary performance), age differences were not observed. Subsequently, other research groups also reported that older and younger adults did not differ on prose memory tasks (Harker, Hartley, & Walsh, 1982; Meyer & Rice, 1981). Still other research groups reported that there were reliable age differences in memory for prose (Cohen, 1979; Zelinski, Gilewski, & Thompson, 1980). The picture was by no means clear.

Despite inconsistencies in the early findings, a second generation of research was undertaken to test predictions about aging and memory for prose based on existing theories of memory and discourse processing. For example, there has been a long-standing hypothesis that older adults do not organize information when learning word lists (Hultsch, 1969). If that is true, and if their failure to organize extends to prose materials, then the higher-level organization that is inherent in a well-formed text may be ignored by older subjects. It is known that readers are generally sensitive to text structure, and propositions that are at a "higher" level in the structure (more central to the gist of the text) are more likely to be recalled (Meyer, 1975). This "levels effect," which is based on relative recall of information types rather than on the absolute amount of information recalled, provides an index of the reader's ability to organize the textual information in memory. As with earlier studies, there is inconsistency in the literature about the levels effect when older adults are compared with younger adults. Interestingly, almost every combination of results has been reported with respect to age differences in the levels effect: (1) Some researchers found no evidence that the levels effect was different in older adults (Petros, Tabor, Cooney, & Chabot, 1983; Zelinski, Light, & Gilewski, 1984). (2) Some researchers found evidence that older adults recalled as many of the high-level propositions, but fewer of the low-level propositions (Zelinski et al., 1980). (3) Still other researchers found evidence that older adults recalled fewer of the high-level propositions and the same number of lower-level propositions (Dixon, Simon, Nowak, & Hultsch, 1982). To complicate the issue even more, Dixon, Hultsch, Simon, and von Eye (1984) reported that the nature of age differences in the levels effect depended on the verbal ability of the research participants: When low-ability subjects were compared, older adults recalled relatively fewer of the high-level propositions; when high-ability subjects were compared, older adults recalled the same number of high-level propositions as younger adults, but relatively fewer of the low-level propositions. (See Chapter 12, this volume, for an attempt to resolve the conflicting levels-effect findings.) In summary, it is fair to say that the predictions of an organizational-deficiency hypothesis have not provided a satisfactory explanation of the nature of age differences in memory for prose. Perhaps this is not surprising, given the differences in the nature of organization in typical word lists and in typical prose.

Several investigators have tested hypotheses based on a levels-of-processing approach to memory (Craik & Lockhart, 1972). As extended to age differences in memory, these hypotheses propose that older adults experience difficulty (for various proposed reasons) when processing information at deeper, semantic levels of processing, as reviewed by Craik (1977) and Hartley and associates (1980). Although it seems counterintuitive that prose could be processed at other than a semantic level, the hypothesis was tested in an experiment by Simon, Dixon, Nowak, and Hultsch (1982) that manipulated the orienting task during reading. Young adults recalled more information in the "deeper" processing condition than did older adults. However, when the groups were compared for intentional learning, age differences were not found, compromising an interpretation based on levels-of-processing notions. The one clear message from the studies conducted within the memory-theory domain is that existing theoretical accounts of memory and its aging generally are unable to account for the findings in the prose studies.

When an analysis of age differences in prose memory is based on discourse theory (in which characteristics of a text are important explanatory concepts), rather than memory theory (in which the information-processing characteristics of the reader are important explanatory concepts), the discrepancies among the existing studies still are not resolved. For example, Meyer and Rice (1983a) reported that different discourse structures (descriptive versus comparative) were recalled differently, but age differences were not modulated by structure. (In Chapter 12 of this volume, Meyer and Rice elaborate further on this research.) Harker and associates (1982) found that the different types of propositions (predicate, modifier, connective) that result from application of the Kintsch (1974) representation system are recalled in the same pattern by older and younger persons. In the study of Harker and associates, the absence of overall age differences may have accounted for the results. However, in two recent studies in my own laboratory that have found reliable age differences, there was no evidence that older adults recalled fewer of any one type of proposition (Hartley 1986). Finally, a study by Spilich (1983) estimated the parameters of the text-comprehension model proposed by Kintsch and van Dijk (1978) for older and younger adults. Overall recall differences were found, and Spilich attributed these to age-related differences in working memory capacity and contents. The results reported by Spilich (1983) stand alone at present, and the history of research in this area suggests that evaluation of the working memory hypothesis must await reports of replication studies.

This review has neglected, to this point, to elaborate on a potentially important set of complications that overlies the work in this research area. Specifically, the studies have rarely been comparable with respect to characteristics of the subjects (e.g., verbal ability, education), characteristics of the texts (e.g., structure, length), and characteristics of the task (e.g., how material is presented, how memory is tested). It has been suggested (Hultsch & Dixon, 1984; Meyer & Rice, 1983b) that subject differences, text differences, and task differences could well be the important dimensions underlying variability in the existing data. Meyer and Rice (1983b) proposed a three-sided model of the prose-processing situation. The three vertices are learner, text, and task characteristics. Hultsch and Dixon (1984) suggested that the tetrahedral model elaborated by Jenkins (1979) to organize the results of memory research in general could be usefully extended to discourse studies in order to resolve some of the discrepancies in the findings with respect to age differences. The four points in this tetrahedral model are the subject, the orienting task, the criterial task, and the materials. In addition, the interactions among all components of the model allow for wide-ranging variation in performance. Each of these models recognizes the importance of individual and cohort-related differences in abilities and experience. Thus, these models provide a source of new and interesting hypotheses for exploring age-related differences in memory for discourse.

Meyer and Rice (Chapter 12, this volume) elaborate on Meyer's three-sided model, concentrating especially on the text and task variables and their interactions with each other and with the prose learner. The remainder of this chapter focuses on the prose learner, including his or her verbal abilities and education, knowledge, goals and strategies, chronological age, verbal experience, and personality factors.

Current status of research on the reader

In this section, the characteristics of the reader (learner) are considered as potential sources of variability in prose memory performance. Six groups of variables are considered in detail, drawing on evidence from a number of studies, including data from my own laboratory (Hartley, 1986). The plan is (1) to define the variables, (2) to note their relationships to discourse memory, and (3) to discuss their relevance in aging studies. For some of these variables, a great deal of information is available; for others, the information is minimal and speculative.

Verbal ability and education

Verbal ability and education are considered simultaneously because they tend to be positively correlated. Verbal ability also tends to covary with age: All other things being equal, older individuals score higher on tests of verbal ability until quite late in life. In fact, this pattern of confounded relationships among verbal ability, education, and age poses a dilemma for the researcher who would like to equate older and younger groups on the verbal-ability and education variables. It probably is not possible to do this in a meaningful way. For example, to equate for verbal ability on the basis of vocabulary is a problem because vocabulary continues to increase over the life span. To equate for education poses a somewhat different problem because of cohort differences in the availability, rigor, and purposes of education; see Hultsch and Dixon (1984), Krauss (1980), and Meyer and Rice (Chapter 12, this volume) for more discussion of this issue.

The term "verbal ability" has been narrowly defined in the literature on aging and prose memory. Almost universally, researchers in this area have used a vocabulary score as the single index of verbal ability, primarily because of the relative ease of obtaining the measure and also because of an attempt to maintain consistency with the existing literature. A complication is that different research groups have used different vocabulary measures, a practice that has made direct comparisons from study to study somewhat difficult. The most widely used measure is the vocabulary subtest of the WAIS (Wechsler, 1955). Other measures that have been used are the Shipley Institute of Living Vocabulary Test (Shipley, 1940), the Verbal Meaning subtest of the Primary Mental Abilities Test (Thurstone & Thurstone, 1949), and the Advanced Vocabulary Test from the Kit of Factor-Referenced Cognitive Tests (Ekstrom, French, Harman, & Dermen, 1976). These tests will be referred to as the WAIS, the Shipley, the PMA, and the ETS vocabulary tests, respectively. The main difficulty in comparing these tests is that they vary in level of difficulty and may not discriminate equally well across the whole range of abilities and ages for which they have been used.

A summary of the results of 12 representative prose memory studies is presented in Table 11.1. Several of these studies included middle-aged groups as well as the standard younger and older age groups, but the two extreme age groups are the only ones included here. It should also be recognized that the definitions of "younger" and "older" varied in these studies, but generally the ranges for young subjects were from 16 to 40 years, and for old subjects from 60 to 80 years. For each study, the specific vocabulary test, vocabulary scores, and average years of education are given. In addition, the length of the text and its general type are noted. A notation is included to indicate when text presentation was not written. Finally, the directions of the age comparison and criterion memory task are given. In some investigations, multiple experiments were included and are given here for purposes of comparison.

The most striking feature of Table 11.1 is that in all but three of the studies there were significant memory differences favoring the younger adults. The second feature is that when all studies are considered together, the recall advantage of the younger adults seems to be independent of the level of vocabulary ability or education. This conclusion contradicts the generally held belief that age differences in prose memory are absent when highly verbal older adults are included (but see Chapter 12, this volume, for a different conclusion). The importance of verbal ability (narrowly defined) has been suggested as an explanation for two reported failures to find age differences in prose memory (Harker et al., 1982;

Table 11.1. *Summary of results from representative studies describing verbal ability/recall relationships*

Source	Vocabulary measure[a]	Vocabulary score		Education (years)		Text (words/type)	Age comparison	Criterion task
		Young	Old	Young	Old			
Taub (1979)	WAIS	57	58	14	13.4		Y = O	Recognition
		51	50	12.4	13.1		Y > O	Recognition
		30	40	12.1	12.4		Y > O	Recognition
Gordon & Clark (1974)	WAIS	74	73	16.6	16.7		Y > O	Recall, Recognition
Cohen (1979), Exp. 2	WAIS	69	69	Y = students & grad. students; O = professional training		300/story[b]	Y > O	Recall
Meyer & Rice (1981)	WAIS	56	58	15.3	15.4	641/essay	Y = O	Recall
Light & Anderson (1985)								
Exp. 1	WAIS	74.4	75.2	Students & alumni		161/essay	Y > O	Question/answer
Exp. 2	WAIS	71.0	75.1	16.4	17.2	161/essay	Y > O	Forced recognition
Zelinski et al. (1984)								
Exp. 1	PMA	39.2	34.6	11.2	12.4	290/story	Y > O	Recall
Exp. 2	PMA	46.7	47.2	17.1	16.3	230/story	Y > O	Recall
Exp. 3	Shipley	32	36	15.6	16.7	>600/essay	Y > O	Recall
Harker et al. (1982)	Shipley	31 (Y1) 35 (Y2)	37	Y1 = students; Y2 = grad. students; O = alumni		400/essay	Y = O	Recall
Hartley (1986)	Shipley	31.3	36.6	13.9	15.8	400/essay & story	Y > O	Recall
Hartley (unpublished)	Shipley	32	36	14.0	15.5	200/essay	Y > O	Recall
Simon et al. (1982)	ETS	7.6	10.3	13.8	12.7	500/essay	Y > O	Recall
Hultsch & Dixon (1983)	ETS	6.7	10.0	12.9	11.9	115/biography	Y > O	Recall
Dixon et al. (1982)	ETS	14.1	14.0	13.0	12.9	180/news[c]	Y > O	Recall

[a]Maximum scores: WAIS = 80;
PMA = 50;
Shipley = 40;
ETS = 18.

[b]Spoken presentation, oral recall.

[c]Both written and spoken presentation.

Meyer & Rice, 1981). Each of these investigations used groups of older adults who were college graduates and who achieved high vocabulary scores. However, Table 11.1 shows other studies that included older adults who were equally well educated and had equally high vocabulary scores on the same vocabulary tests, and yet recalled less from prose passages than did younger adults.

The data shown in Table 11.1 from Hartley (1986) are particularly instructive for considering the effects of vocabulary and education. There were, in fact, two older groups included in the investigation. These older groups differed in characteristics only in that one group was composed of currently enrolled university students, whereas the other group was not. Despite their current involvement with the educational process (making them similar to the younger students who formed the young group), these older students did not differ on any measure of performance from the older nonstudents. Recalls of text were identical for the two old groups and were significantly lower than that for the young group. This study can be compared rather directly with the study reported by Harker and associates (1982), because the same vocabulary measure was used, two of the texts were the same, and the absolute levels of vocabulary and education were virtually equivalent. One study found reliable age differences (Hartley, 1986); the other did not (Harker et al., 1982). The reason for the discrepancy between the two studies is not clear, but it may be related to the fact that recall was noticeably lower for all groups in the study of Harker and associates, suggesting that scoring criteria may have differed. In summary, the overwhelming majority of the evidence shown here fails to support the claim that well-educated older adults with high vocabulary scores will remember the contents of prose as well as younger adults.

The data presented here do not preclude the possibility that age differences are smaller in magnitude when high-verbal older adults are included in the study. There is some evidence that this occurs. In a series of analyses to examine the relationship between vocabulary and prose memory, Meyer and Rice (1983a) partitioned a larger data set for older and younger adults into comparison groups on the basis of vocabulary scores. Pairwise comparisons were made for high-verbal old versus randomly selected young, high-verbal old versus high-verbal young, low-verbal old versus low-verbal young, and low-verbal old versus matching low-verbal young. Age differences were reliable for all comparisons, except for the high-verbal old versus randomly selected young. Taken as a whole, however, these data generally coincide with the conclusion that high verbal ability in the older sample does not guarantee a lack of age difference in prose memory.

Although verbal ability has been defined in terms of vocabulary measures, knowledge of the meanings of words is only one dimension of verbal ability. In their study of the cognitive correlates of verbal ability, Hunt, Lunneborg, and Lewis (1975) defined verbal ability as a composite score on four subtests of a standardized precollege test: English usage, spelling, reading comprehension, and vocabulary. This measure, as noted by Hunt and associates, defines verbal ability in terms of knowledge about words and their usage. It is assumed, of course, that this is a set of highly correlated skills. Perfetti (1983, 1985) has argued that the components of verbal ability should include more basic cognitive skills and has proposed that an adequate definition of verbal ability includes simple verbal processes (e.g., letter recognition, word decoding), complex verbal processes (e.g., any process that accesses more than one verbal code), and verbal knowledge (e.g., vocabulary, schema knowledge).

Very little information has been published concerning adult age differences in components of verbal ability beyond vocabulary measures. The most extensive investigation of the relationship between components of verbal ability and prose memory was reported by Hultsch, Hertzog, and Dixon (1984). These investigators obtained scores for young, middle-aged, and old adults on a series of standardized intellectual-ability measures, as well as prose memory. Although not specifically selected to index verbal ability, the battery included measures of verbal association, memory for words, vocabulary, and various fluencies. Factor analysis of the set of measures produced three specific ability factors and a general intelligence factor. The interesting finding was that prose memory was predicted by more than one of the factors. Age differences in the ability measures were correlated with age differences in prose recall, but age differences remained even after ability differences were taken into account. Taking a somewhat different approach, in a preliminary attempt to extend the Perfetti (1983, 1985) model to aging studies, it was shown that some simple verbal processes, such as word-naming latency, may account for a portion of the age-related variance in prose memory (Hartley, 1986). These results suggest that a broader definition of verbal ability and/or related abilities would provide an important insight into characteristics of the prose reader that could mitigate or exacerbate the effects of age on prose memory.

Prior knowledge

As used here, the term "prior knowledge" refers to the amount of information that a reader possesses about a specific topic that is currently being studied for retention. (It is, of course, possible that general knowledge plays a role in prose memory for any specific topic, but that relationship will not be explored here.) The facilitating effect of prior knowledge on acquisition of new information about the relevant topic has been well documented in a series of experiments by Voss and his colleagues (Spilich, Vesonder, Chiesi, & Voss, 1979; Voss, Vesonder, & Spilich, 1980). Prior knowledge is thought to allow for easier and better integration of new information about the topic. If the topic already has a representation in memory, then new information will simply fill into existing slots or create new slots within the existing representation. If the topic is completely new, then a representation must be constructed during prose processing, and the content slots filled in at the same time. In contrast to information about verbal ability and prose memory, there is little information about prior knowledge and prose memory in older adults.

Hultsch and Dixon (1983) manipulated prior knowledge by selecting age-specific topics for short texts. The texts were brief biographical sketches of entertainers. The results of the study suggested that prior knowledge affected the magnitude of age differences in memory for the texts. Specifically, age differences were eliminated when the text was about the old-specific entertainer, but were present when the text was about the young-specific entertainer. The elimination of age effect in this study resulted from a relative increase in recall for the older subjects, coupled with a relative decrease in recall for the younger subjects. Because older and younger adults may possess differing amounts of prior knowledge about the topics used in a prose memory study, it will be important to study the effects of this variable further. The approach taken by Hultsch and Dixon (1983) would be a fruitful way to proceed; however, those authors noted that it may be difficult to select topics that are sufficiently age-specific to allow for clear separation of the age groups on recall measures. At first glance, this problem suggests that the effects of prior knowledge may simply not be important; but consistent small effects on recall may be as important to know about as large effects.

Goals and strategies of the reader

It seems reasonable to assume that when adults approach a prose memory task, they bring to the situation a variety of strategies to guide performance during reading and recall periods. As used here, "strategies" are metacognitive behaviors similar to the "executive routines" proposed by Brown (1977) in her model of the thinking process. Strategies serve to guide and to monitor interaction with a task and probably are related to the learning goals that the reader brings to the text-processing task. For example, if the goal is to memorize the text, then one set of strategies might be activated. If the goal is to derive some overall summary of the information in the text, the strategies might be different (Fischer & Mandl, 1984). Strategies probably take up space in one's cognitive awareness (working memory) and may actually impede information acquisition unless they are highly automatic. In light of the proposition that working memory capacity may be reduced in older adults and that this may partially account for age differences in recall (Spilich, 1983), it is important to understand the use of strategies in older adults.

Goals. In a study concerned with orienting-task effects during text reading, Simon and associates (1982) manipulated the goals of the reader. The interesting comparison was between the two "deep" semantic conditions: reading to give advice and reading to remember. The text was about a family in financial difficulty. There were no age differences in recall for the intentional-learning condition (a surprising result), but substantial age differences for the advice condition. Both the overall recall level and the recall of higher-level propositions were reduced in the older adults in the advice condition. Perhaps the goal of formulating sound advice about a very serious situation activated strategies in the older readers that directed their attention to specific details of the situation rather than to the overall organization of the information in the text. The activation of different strategies may have reflected experience with the kind of financial situation described. The point is, the orienting task may have had an effect separate from forcing semantic processing as proposed by the authors.

Further evidence that the learner's goals may affect recall of prose information has been found in two studies conducted by Hartley and Hartley (Hartley, Hartley, & Johnson, 1984; Johnson, Hartley, & Hartley, 1984). In a series of training sessions, older and younger novice computer users were taught to use a computer text editor. Lessons were presented as brief texts about the operation of editing functions. At the beginning and end of each lesson, the learners provided a written summary of the information that had been accumulated to date. In each of the two experiments, younger adults tended to produce more of the information than older adults, but the differences were not significant. Only when the data from both of the experiments were pooled (yielding 48 subjects in each age group) did the recall difference become statistically significant. Contrary to the findings of Simon and associates (1982), these results suggest that the magnitudes of age differences in prose recall may be minimal if the learner's goal is other than memorization.

Strategies. Two investigations have directly measured aspects of the prose learner's strategies for dealing with the reading and recalling of a text. In each of these studies, the reader's assigned goal was to be able to recall as much of the text as possible. The results of the first investigation were reported by Rice and Meyer (1983). These investigators developed a questionnaire that was given to a large number of participants in two different prose memory studies involving young, middle-aged, and older subjects. The questionnaire asked the learners about the strategies they used while reading the text and while recalling the text. In addition, information was gathered about reading frequency, reading enjoyment and skill, number of hours spent reading during a typical week, and types of materials routinely read. Factor analyses were performed on the questionnaire, and the factor scores were used in a regression equation to predict prose recall scores. The best predictor of recall turned out to be a recall-strategy factor: specifically, a strategy in which the learner wrote the text down according to the original paragraph structure, using the currently written segment to cue recall of the next segment (Rice and Meyer called this the paragraph strategy). The only reading-strategy factor that was related to recall efficiency was one that included a main-point identification strategy. These results are interesting in several respects. First, the fact that strategic factors predicted recall is important. Second, the fact that the recall strategy was the most important factor seems counterintuitive, especially because that strategy did not correlate with any of the reading-strategy factors. Rice and Meyer (1983) suggested that the paragraph strategy reflected the reader's sensitivity to the structure of the text. However, because the strategy was not consistently correlated with other measures of sensitivity to structure, it is difficult to accept this interpretation.

In a recent study, the Rice and Meyer strategy questionnaire was administered to subjects in three age groups who participated in a prose learning experiment in my laboratory (J. Hartley, unpublished data). Because the number of subjects was small relative to the number of items on the questionnaire, the factor-analysis procedures were somewhat different. Whereas Rice and Meyer (1983) included all reading and recall questions in a single factor analysis, I performed two separate analyses: one for the reading strategies and one for the recall strategies. The factors nevertheless were very similar to those obtained by Rice and Meyer. In agreement with Rice and Meyer, the paragraph strategy was a significant predictor of recall. None of the reading-strategy factors was, by itself, a significant predictor. In addition, there were age differences in the tendency to use the paragraph strategy for recall, with younger adults reporting greater use of the strategy than older adults.

Taken together, these studies suggest that the goals and strategies of the reader may be important factors in understanding the nature and extent of age differences in prose memory.

Age

The usual research strategy for studying the relationship between age and prose memory uses chronological age as a variable for forming independent experimental groups. When group differences are found, it is generally assumed that age is the relevant variable. The possibility that cohort (year of birth) factors may play a role has been virtually ignored in prose memory studies; yet the problem may be as serious in prose memory studies as it is in list-learning studies. Because age and cohort factors cannot be separated experimentally, a different approach is needed to evaluate the two effects: If age is the relevant factor, then we might expect that prose memory will be negatively correlated with age within the older cohort itself, especially if the older cohort is composed of individuals beyond the age of 65 years. The logic for this expectation rests on the assumption that cognitive deterioration related to age should accelerate in the last decade of the expected life span. If the cohort is the relevant factor, then we might expect relative stability within, let us say, a 10-year cohort group. Surprisingly, within-group correlations are seldom reported, but when they are, the results are instructive. In a large-scale study of the relationship between reader variables and text variables, Rice and Meyer (1983) found no relationship between total recall and age in an older group that included 159 individuals between the ages of 61 and 80 years. Clearly, the 19-year age span represented in that study was sufficiently long for measurable age-related cognitive changes to occur; yet prose recall did not very across the span. In two studies in my laboratory, the correlation between age and prose memory within the older groups has been in the expected direction. In one study that included 48 older adults between the ages of 63 and 76 years, the correlation between the prose memory measure and chronological age was –.19, $p < .10$. In a second study that included 24 older adults aged 61–75 years, the correlation was –.29, $p < .10$. In the second study, when the older group was expanded to 44 subjects and the age range was increased to 61–90 years, the correlation was –.36, $p < .01$. Thus, although a single-cohort analysis was suggestive of the expected age relationship, an expansion of the older age range to include more than one cohort was needed before a statistically significant relationship was observed.

These data, taken as a whole, do not rule out the possibility that cohort factors may be the important differences, rather than age factors. It does seem clear that prose memory remains reasonably stable over a fairly long period of time in older adulthood. It is difficult to reconcile this conclusion with the fact that substantial differences in prose recall are seen when the extreme age groups (old and young groups) are compared. Perhaps the extreme age-group differences reflect both cohort differences and age-related changes in discourse memory processes. At present, there is not sufficient evidence to determine the unique contribution of age itself to prose memory differences.

Personality factors

The relationships between memory functioning and personality variables have received little attention in studies of aging. There is frequent casual mention of the possibility that dispositions and motives may play roles in memory, but there is, to my knowledge, no empirical evidence that personality characteristics are related to memory performance in older adults. In a recently completed thesis, Patricia Bellucci (1984) measured the need for cognition (Cacioppo & Petty, 1982) and the locus of control (Levenson, 1972), as well as single-trial free recall and prose recall, in groups of younger and older adults from the Long Beach, California, area. ''Need for cognition'' is defined by Cacioppo and Petty (1982) as the tendency to engage in and enjoy thinking. People scoring high in the need-for-cognition measure generally enjoy more complex cognitive tasks and tend to organize information into a meaningful structure (Cacioppo & Petty, 1982). It was hypothesized that this variable would be positively correlated with performance on memory tasks that required cognitive effort, such as prose memory and free recall of a list of words. Because cognitive effort might be more ''effortful'' for older adults, it was expected that older adults would show a stronger relationship between the personality variables and memory than would younger adults. The internality scale (the degree to which one believes that one controls personal outcomes) of the locus-of-control measure (Levenson, 1972) was also expected to be related to the memory measures. In a sample of 24 young adults, neither locus of control nor need for cognition was correlated with memory performance, although the personality measures were reliably correlated with each other and showed a typical distribution for college students. In a sample of 48 old adults, the only correlation that approached significance was between need for cognition and free-recall performance ($r = .20$, $p = .08$). Again, the two personality variables were correlated with each other and showed a reasonable distribution of scores across the sample. Thus, whereas prose memory was dependent on age group, it was independent of the personality measures within each age group. Prior to reaching a strong conclusion concerning the lack of impact of personality variables on memory, other dimensions of personality should be investigated. However, in a sample of subjects who were typical for experimental investigations of prose memory and aging, two personality variables that might be expected to correlate with cognitive performance were of no importance for two different measures of memory.

Reading habits and history

There is some evidence that the reading habits and reading history of the individual are related to performance in a prose memory task. The work reported by Rice and Meyer (1983) and discussed by Meyer and Rice (Chapter 12, this volume) provides information across a wide age span and a large number of subjects. Specifically, Rice and Meyer (1983) found that total recall and several other measures of prose memory were superior for those persons who read extensively and enjoyed doing so. This was true for young, middle-aged, and old groups. Research in my laboratory (described in the next section) has produced similar relationships. it would be tempting to use this information to suggest that the ability to read and remember prose is a skill that benefits from continued practice across the life span. Because the evidence is correlational, however, it is equally likely that those persons who have good reading and remembering skills continue to read extensively across the life span. The fact that enjoyment of reading is related to prose memory ability suggests that the latter explanation is more appropriate.

A substantive research example

For the past few years, I have been interested in discovering which classes of reader characteristics correlate with prose memory performance in older and younger adults and which do not. Table 11.2 shows a subset of the information that was available from a recent study (J. Hartley, unpublished data). Many of these measures are ones that normally might not be reported, either for lack of page space in a manuscript or because they do not speak to the major theoretical thrust of the experiment itself. However, from the point of view of cognition in everyday life, they are interesting and potentially important. The variables in Table 11.2 are organized into several sets of reader variables and a

Table 11.2. *Reader characteristics for three age groups*

Variable	Young (18–29 years) (n = 24)	Middle-aged (44–58 years) (n = 26)	Old (61–90 years) (n = 44)
Age	22.3	51.5	73.8
Recall (% of total propositions)	37.8	32.2	27.4[a]
Standard-ability measures			
Reading comprehension	.65	.68	.55[a]
Word fluency	51.2	48.6	41.6[a]
Vocabulary	31.8	35.8	36.2[a]
Abstract reasoning	17.1	15.3	13.3[a]
Education (years)	13.9	16.0	14.8[a]
Health & habits			
Self-rated health (maximum = 10)	8.6	9.0	7.7[a]
Complaint-based health (maximum = 24)	22.8	22.1	19.9[a]
Number of medications	2.0	2.9	2.6
Weekly coffee/tea intake	6.0	20.3	13.3[a]
Weekly alcohol intake	3.8	3.8	3.0
Reading per week (hours)	16.7	18.9	14.6
Text factors (self-assessed)			
Prior knowledge[b]			
Interest[b]			

[a] $p < .05$.
[b] Groups did not differ on text-by-text comparison.

set of variables concerned with the reader's interaction with the text. With the exception of the prose-recall and standard-ability measures, all measures were based on self-report. The measures of standard abilities were as follows:

1. Reading comprehension – percentage correct for those questions attempted from the first half of the Davis Reading Test, Form 1B (Davis, 1944).
2. Word fluency – number of words produced in 5 min that start with the letter *s* (Primary Mental Abilities Test) (Thurstone & Thurstone, 1949).
3. Vocabulary – vocabulary subtest of the Shipley Institute of Living scale (Shipley, 1940) (maximum = 40).
4. Abstract reasoning – reasoning subtest of the Shipley Institute of Living scale (Shipley, 1940) (maximum = 20).

Table 11.3 shows the correlation coefficient between each of the measures and a measure of prose recall that was derived from performance on four different 200-word texts.

Standard-ability measures. The reading-comprehension, word-fluency, and vocabulary measures are all components of verbal ability, as defined by Perfetti

Table 11.3. *Correlations between text-recall measure (% correct) and reader characteristics*

Variable	Whole sample (n = 94)	Young (18–29 years) (n = 24)	Middle-aged (44–58 years) (n = 26)	Old (61–90 years) (n = 44)
Standard-ability measures				
Reading comprehension	.54[a]	.65[a]	.52[a]	.35[a]
Word fluency	.37[a]	−.17	.24	.60[a]
Vocabulary	.11	.50[a]	.24	.22
Abstract reasoning	.45[a]	.19	.37[a]	.40[a]
Education	.26[a]	−.14	.22	.57[a]
Health & habits				
Subjective health	.01	−.22	−.22	−.05
Complaint-based health	.12	−.24	.06	.00
Number of medications	−.09	−.22	−.10	.08
Weekly coffee/tea intake	−.18[a]	.08	−.21	−.20
Weekly alcohol intake	.05	−.08	.00	.15
Reading variables				
Typical hours per week	.26[a]	.00	.15	.36[a]
Reading enjoyment	.17[a]	.12	.24	.29[a]
Self-assessed reading skill	.20[a]	.17	−.10	.30[a]
Text factors (self-assessed)				
Prior knowledge	.34[a]	.43[a]	.33[a]	.32[a]
Interest in topic	.11	.14	.12	.09

[a]$p < .05$ for correlation coefficient.

(1983). Of these, reading comprehension was the only variable that was correlated consistently with prose memory across the three age groups. The vocabulary measure, usually the only index of verbal ability, was correlated with recall for the young group only. This was unexpected and may reflect the fact that the vocabulary scores for the two older groups were so uniformly high that variability was constrained for these groups. Nevertheless, despite their high level of vocabulary, the two older groups recalled significantly less information from the texts than did the young group.

Although not usually considered an index of verbal ability, the abstract-reasoning measure does index the ability to manipulate concepts mentally in order to extract an important principle. It is not, therefore, surprising that this measure would correlate with prose memory. This measure was less important for the young group than for the two older groups, reflecting either a ceiling problem on the measure in the young group or the increased importance of flexible thinking for prose memory in the older groups.

Education. The number of years of education was related to prose memory only for the oldest group, but this group did not differ from the youngest group in number of years of education. In these data, therefore, vocabulary and education seemed to exert independent influences on measures of prose memory at different points in the life span.

Health and habits. In general, the health and habits measures were not correlated with the measure of prose memory. Although some of the relationships appear to be in an expected direction, none was significant in the sample sizes included in the study. It is possible that these measures would assume more importance in a larger, more heterogeneous sample. The subjects included in the present study were typical volunteers who were reasonably healthy and prudent in their habits. The absence of significant correlations between these variables and prose memory could be interpreted by an optimist as indicating that when health is good and vices are minimal, memory for written discourse will not suffer. A scientist would prefer to see more evidence before accepting this interpretation.

Reading variables. The instrument used by Rice and Meyer (1983) for assessing reading variables was given to all participants in the present study. None of the variables was related to prose memory in the young and middle-aged groups, but three of the four variables were related to prose memory in the oldest group. It appears that older adults who read more, enjoy it, and see themselves as possessing good reading skills remember more from texts than do those older adults who do not. Rice and Meyer (1983) found these variables to be related to prose memory for all age groups included in their study. The differences in procedures between the two studies were sufficiently large, however, to preclude meaningful comparison and resolution of the discrepant results.

Text factors. Finally, prior knowledge of the topic was a significant correlate of memory for all age groups. Interest in the topic was unimportant for the texts included in the study. It should be noted that prior knowledge was the only variable, other than the reading-comprehension measure, that was a consistent correlate of prose memory in this study.

Conclusion. An overall assessment of these data suggests that prior knowledge and reading-comprehension skills are important for prose memory at each stage of adulthood. With these two exceptions, there were no uniform relationships between prose memory and a wide range of reader variables for the age ranges included in this study. There was, however, an interesting pattern in which more and more variables became significant correlates of the prose memory measure as age increased: There were three significant correlates in the young and middle-aged groups and eight significant correlates in the old group. The magnitudes of the correlation coefficients suggest that this pattern is real, rather than being merely a statistical power problem related to different sample sizes.

These data are particularly interesting when considered along with the Hultsch and associates (1984) study of the roles of intellectual factors in prose memory across adulthood. Those investigators found that increasing numbers of specific intellectual factors were related to prose memory in their older subjects. In the present study, intellectual factors as well as other factors showed a similar pattern.

The reader in the real world

Laboratory versus real-world tasks

Remembering the meaning of what has been read from a discourse is certainly an everyday activity in a literate culture. As suggested from information presented here, most adults seem to read on a daily basis, and the Long Beach sample discussed in the preceding section estimated that they devoted an average of 16–17 hours per week to reading. The ordinary person reads the newspaper at the breakfast table to find out about the fate of a favorite sports team or an interesting political figure. The ordinary person reads a novel at the beach or on the bus for the pure enjoyment or suspense it provides. The ordinary person attempts to read (usually on April 14) the latest publication from the Internal Revenue Service concerning the preparation of tax returns. Discourse memory, however, has been studied exclusively in the laboratory. What is the justification for assuming that this everyday cognitive behavior is the same in the laboratory as it is outside of the laboratory?

If we consider the general nature of the materials that are used in our laboratory tasks, we can be reasonably confident that we are asking our subjects to read the kinds of information to which they are routinely exposed: for example, news articles (Dixon et al., 1984), biographies (Hultsch & Dixon, 1983), stories (Cohen, 1979), and essays (Meyer & Rice, 1981). For the most part, the experimental manipulations with texts correspond to variations in texts that are present in everyday situations: for example, differing organizational structures (Meyer & Rice, 1983a) or different levels of familiarity (Hultsch & Dixon, 1983).

Where we fail to capture everyday behavior is with the criterion tasks. The majority of studies use a criterion task of complete written recall to assess memory. The everyday reader is seldom required to reproduce what has just been read. Although investigators are careful to assure the reader that verbatim recall is not required and that paraphrase is perfectly acceptable, the reader in the laboratory usually is sensitive to the fact that his or her memory is being evaluated. Interaction of the reader with the text is undoubtedly affected by this accurate perception of the experimental situation. My own experience has been that subjects of all ages spend a considerable amount of time studying a text in preparation for recall. It is not unusual for a reader to spend 10 sec studying an average sentence. Examinations of recall protocols frequently reveal that the phrasing of a text has been quite accurately reproduced. It is clear that, in many cases, the goal of the reader in a text-reading task is to memorize the text. I am not certain that we are really interested in discovering whether or not there are age differences in memorizing a text. Rather, we are more interested in how much and what readers at different developmental stages retain from encounters with written discourse that are as brief as a glance at the morning paper or as extensive as reading a manual on how to operate a newly acquired personal computer. There have been only a few studies that have been specifically designed to look at these more natural criterion tasks, such as preparing to give advice to people (Simon et al., 1982), or reading with a brief summary as the goal (Zelinski et al., 1984, Exp. 3), or reading with the goal of learning a new skill (Hartley et al., 1984). Our understanding of everyday prose memory would benefit from more investigations of this type.

Models of the reader

The fact that most experimental investigations of prose memory have manipulated text and task variables suggests that the reader is viewed as a "nuisance" variable, that is, something that adds unwanted variance that is of little interest. The characteristics of the reader often are measured so that we can use them as an excuse of last resort for unpredicted and unexplained oddities in our data. The implicit model of the "ideal reader" conforms to the mechanistic model of humans – that is, a passive information processor who reflexively responds to experimental manipulations. The "real reader" can be viewed more accurately as an active information seeker who brings a variety of skills, strategies, and self-generated performance criteria to the laboratory learning task. Two developmentally important questions arise: (1) To what extent are there age differences/changes in the component skills of prose memory? (2) Are there age-related differences/changes in the reader's strategies and performance criteria? The recent investigation of Hultsch and associates (1984) begins to answer the first question. There do seem to be age differences in some of the intellectual abilities that are related to discourse memory. There seems to be no published information concerning the second question.

The older adult as a reader in the real world

To the extent that strategies for reading and encoding information from prose develop with experience, the older adult may be a qualitatively different reader than the younger adult. For example, some investigators have found that the older adult tends to retain the ability to recall higher-level information in the discourse structure, but recalls less of the lower-level information (Dixon et al., 1984; Zelinski et al., 1980). This could be interpreted as a deficiency in the ability to process details, but it also could be interpreted as a shift in strategy that has resulted from experience. Little is known about the development of reading strategy in adults. Less is known about the interaction of strategy with changing cognitive capabilities. Do discourse-processing strategies evolve to enable the older adult to cope with age-related changes in sensory functions or cognitive speed? Do changes in very basic cognitive processes have an irreversible negative impact on more complex cognitive processes, such as memory for discourse? Most important, do any of these changes seriously limit the individual's overall ability to function as a cognitive entity in the world? The everyday cognitive entity – including some who have contributed to this volume – would like to know the answers to at least a few of these questions.

References

Bellucci, P. A. (1984). *Personality variables in memory for discourse.* Unpublished master's thesis, California State University, Long Beach.

Brown, A. L. (1977). Development, schooling, and the acquisition of knowledge about knowledge. In R. C. Anderson, R. J. Spiro, & W. E. Montague (Eds.), *Schooling and the acquisition of knowledge.* Hillsdale, NJ: Lawrence Erlbaum.

Cacioppo, J. T., & Petty, R. E. (1982). The need for cognition. *Journal of Personality and Social Psychology, 42,* 116–131.

Cohen, G. (1979). Language comprehension in old age. *Cognitive Psychology, 11,* 412–429.

Craik, F. I. M. (1977). Age differences in human memory. In J. E. Birren & K. W. Schaie (Eds.), *Handbook of the psychology of aging* (pp. 384–420). New York: Van Nostrand Reinhold.

Craik, F. I. M., & Lockhart, R. S. (1972). Levels of processing: A framework for memory research. *Journal of Verbal Learning and Verbal Behavior, 11,* 671–684.

Davis, F. B. (1944). Fundamental factors in reading. *Psychometrica, 9,* 185–197.

Dixon, R. A., Hultsch, D. F., Simon, E. W., & von Eye, A. (1984). Verbal ability and text structure effects on adult age differences in text recall. *Journal of Verbal Learning and Verbal Behavior, 23,* 569–578.

Dixon, R. A., Simon, E. W., Nowak, C. A., & Hultsch, D. F. (1982). Text recall in adulthood as a function of level of information, input modality, and delay interval. *Journal of Gerontology, 37,* 358–364.

Ekstrom, R. B., French, J. W., Harman, H. H., & Dermen, D. (1976). *Manual for kit of factor referenced cognitive tests.* Princeton, NJ: Educational Testing Service.

Fischer, P. M., & Mandl, H. (1984). Learner, text variables, and the control of text comprehension and recall. In H. Mandl, R. L. Stein, & T. Trabasso (Eds.), *Learning and comprehension of text* (pp. 213–254). Hillsdale, NJ: Lawrence Erlbaum.

Frederiksen, C. H. (1975). Representing logical and semantic structure of knowledge acquired from discourse. *Cognitive Psychology, 7,* 371–458.

Gordon, S. K., & Clark, W. C. (1974). Application of signal detection theory to prose recall and recognition in elderly and young adults. *Journal of Gerontology, 29,* 64–72.

Harker, J. O., Hartley, J. T., & Walsh, D. A. (1982). Understanding discourse: A lifespan approach. In B. A. Hutson (Ed.), *Advances in reading/language research* (pp. 155–202). Greenwich, CT: JAI Press.

Hartley, A. A., Hartley, J. T., & Johnson, S. J. (1984). The older adult as computer user. In P. K. Robinson, J. Livingston, & J. E. Birren (Eds.), *Aging and technological advances* (pp. 347–348). New York: Plenum.

Hartley, J. T. (1986). Reader and text variables as determinants of discourse memory in adulthood. *Psychology and Aging, 1,* 150–158.

Hartley, J. T., Harker, J. O., & Walsh, D. A. (1980). Contemporary issues and new directions in adult development of learning and memory. In L. W. Poon (Ed.), *Aging in the 1980s: Psychological issues* (pp. 239–254). Washington, DC: American Psychological Association.

Hultsch, D. F. (1969). Adult age differences in the organization of free-recall. *Developmental Psychology, 1,* 673–678.

Hultsch, D. F., & Dixon, R. A. (1983). The role of pre-experimental knowledge in text processing in adulthood. *Experimental Aging Research, 9,* 17–22.

Hultsch, D. F., & Dixon, R. A. (1984). Memory for text materials in adulthood. In P. B. Baltes & O. G. Brim, Jr. (Eds.), *Life-span development and behavior* (Vol. 6). New York: Academic Press.

Hultsch, D. F., Hertzog, C., & Dixon, R. A. (1984). Text processing in adulthood: The role of intellectual abilities. *Developmental Psychology, 20,* 1193–1209.

Hultsch, D. F., & Pentz, C. A. (1980). Encoding, storage, and retrieval in adult memory: The role of model assumptions. In L. W. Poon, J. L. Fozard, L. S. Cermak, D. Arenberg, & L. W. Thompson (Eds.), *New directions in memory and aging: Proceedings of the George A. Talland memorial conference* (pp. 73–94). Hillsdale, NJ: Lawrence Erlbaum.

Hunt, E., Lunneborg, C., & Lewis, J. (1975). What does it mean to be high verbal? *Cognitive Psychology, 7,* 194–227.

Jenkins, J. J. (1979). Four points to remember: A tetrahedral model of memory experiments. In L. S. Cermak & F. I. M. Craik (Eds.), *Levels of processing in human memory.* Hillsdale, NJ: Lawrence Erlbaum.

Johnson, S. J., Hartley, J. T., & Hartley, A. A. (1984, May). *Aging: Memory and performance of a newly-learned cognitive skill.* Paper presented at the annual meeting of the Western Psychological Association, Los Angeles.

Kintsch, W. (1974). *The representation of meaning in memory.* Hillsdale, NJ: Lawrence Erlbaum.

Kintsch, W., & van Dijk, T. A. (1978). Toward a model of text comprehension and production. *Psychological Review, 85,* 363–394.

Krauss, I. K. (1980). Between- and within-group comparisons in aging research. In L. W. Poon (Ed.), *Aging in the 1980s: Psychological issues* (pp. 542–551). Washington, DC: American Psychological Association.

Levenson, H. (1972). *Distinctions within the concept of internal-external locus of control: Development of a new scale.* Presented at the 80th annual convention of the American Psychological Association, 261–262.

Light, L. L., & Anderson, P. A. (1985). Working-memory capacity, age, and memory for discourse. *Journal of Gerontology, 40,* 737–747.

Meyer, B. J. F. (1975). *The organization of prose and its effect on memory.* Amsterdam: North Holland.

Meyer, B. J. F., & Rice, G. E. (1981). Information recalled from prose by young, middle and old adult readers. *Experimental Aging Research, 7,* 253–268.

Meyer, B. J. F., & Rice, G. E. (1983a, December). *Effects of discourse type on recall by young, middle, and old adults with high and average vocabulary scores.* Paper presented at the meeting of the National Reading Conference, Austin, TX.

Meyer, B. J. F., & Rice, G. E. (1983b). Learning and memory from text across the adult life span. In J. Fine & R. O. Freedle (Eds.), *Developmental studies in discourse.* Norwood, NJ: Ablex.

Perfetti, C. A. (1983). Individual differences in verbal processes. In R. F. Dillon & R. R. Schmeck (Eds.), *Individual differences in cognition* (Vol. 1). New York: Academic Press.

Perfetti, C. A. (1985). *Reading ability.* New York: Oxford University Press.

Petros, T., Tabor, L., Cooney, T., & Chabot, R. J. (1983). Adult age differences in sensitivity to semantic structure of prose. *Developmental Psychology, 19,* 907–914.

Rice, G. E., & Meyer, B. J. F. (1983). *Prose recall: Effects of aging, verbal ability, and reading behavior* (Research Report No. 13, Prose Learning Series). Tempe: Arizona State University, Department of Educational Psychology, College of Education.

Shipley, W. C. (1940). A self-administering scale for measuring intellectual impairment and deterioration. *Journal of Psychology, 9,* 371–377.

Simon, E. W., Dixon, R. A., Nowak, C. A., & Hultsch, D. F. (1982). Orienting task effects on text recall in adulthood. *Journal of Gerontology, 31,* 575–580.

Spilich, G. J. (1983). Life-span components of text processing: Structural and procedural changes. *Journal of Verbal Learning and Verbal Behavior, 22*, 231–244.

Spilich, G. J., Vesonder, G. T., Chiesi, H. L., & Voss, J. F. (1979). Text processing of domain-related information for individuals with high and low domain knowledge. *Journal of Verbal Learning and Verbal Behavior, 18*, 275–290.

Taub, H. A. (1976). Method of presentation of meaningful prose to young and old adults. *Experimental Aging Research, 2*, 469–474.

Taub, H. A. (1979). Comprehension and memory of prose by young and old adults. *Experimental Aging Research, 5*, 3–13.

Thurstone, L. L., & Thurstone, T. G. (1949). *SRA Primary Mental Abilities Test*. Chicago: Science Research Associates.

Voss, J. F., Vesonder, G. T., & Spilich, G. J. (1980). Text generation and recall by high-knowledge and low-knowledge individuals. *Journal of Verbal Learning and Verbal Behavior, 19*, 651–667.

Walsh, D. A., & Baldwin, M. (1977). Age differences in integrated semantic memory. *Developmental Psychology, 13*, 509–514.

Wechsler, D. (1955). *Manual for the Wechsler Adult Intelligence Scale*. New York: Psychological Corporation.

Zelinski, E. M., Gilewski, M. J., & Thompson, L. W. (1980). Do laboratory memory tasks relate to everyday remembering and forgetting? In L. W. Poon, J. L. Fozard, L. S. Cermak, D. Arenberg, & L. W. Thompson (Eds.), *New directions in memory and aging: Proceedings of the George A. Talland memorial conference* (pp. 519–550). Hillsdale, NJ: Lawrence Erlbaum.

Zelinski, E. M., Light, L. L., & Gilewski, M. J. (1984). Adult age differences in memory for prose: The question of sensitivity to passage structure. *Developmental Psychology, 20*, 1181–1192.

12 Prose processing in adulthood: The text, the reader, and the task

Bonnie J. F. Meyer and G. Elizabeth Rice

During the last five years, a substantial increase has occurred in the number of studies investigating aging effects in processing prose. As noted by Hartley in Chapter 11, many recent studies have reported age-related differences in quantity and quality of recall, whereas others have found no differences. In attempts to understand these discrepancies, analyses of this literature (Hultsch & Dixon, 1984; Meyer & Rice, 1983a) have been cast in terms of an interactional scheme among text, learner, and task variables (Figure 12.1). Because these variables interact in the comprehension process, it is impossible to discuss them adequately in isolation. However, this chapter emphasizes text variables, whereas Chapter 11 emphasized learner variables. Before examining text variables, we shall discuss learner and task variables, because their consideration is critical in understanding discrepancies in the literature on aging and prose learning.

Learner variables

Education and vocabulary

In considering the learner variables of education and vocabulary as partially responsible for the contradictory aging effects in prose learning, we are considering the long-standing problem in aging research of how to make old and younger age groups equivalent on cultural variables in cross-sectional studies (Birren & Morrison, 1961; Botwinick, 1978; Krauss, 1980). If studies examine only old adults with college degrees, their findings may not hold for the majority of old adults, who lack these degrees. In addition, degrees from various institutions and generations differ in educational value. Also, the fact that fewer older adults are highly educated reflects economic differences and changes in the ac-

Preparation of this chapter was supported in part by grant MH #31520 from the National Institute of Mental Health to Bonnie J. F. Meyer and by grant 03438 from the National Institute on Aging to Bonnie J. F. Meyer and G. Elizabeth Rice.

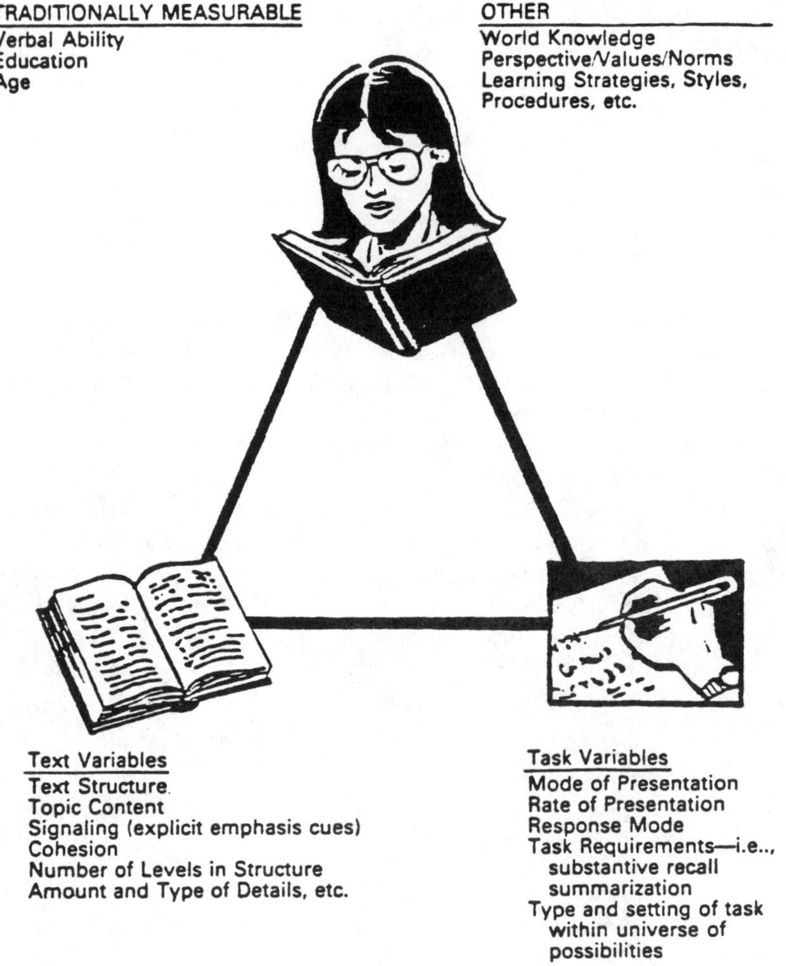

Figure 12.1. Learner, text, and task variables involved in reading comprehension by adults across the adult life span. (From Meyer & Rice, 1983a.)

cessibility of education over the last half-century, rather than differences in aptitude for academic achievement.

Meyer and Rice (1983a) showed that age differences in memory performance with prose materials may be present or absent depending on how the investigator equates the age groups on education and verbal ability. Most recent investigations with prose have reported education level and verbal ability of subjects, but a few have not reported vocabulary scores (Petros, Tabor, Cooney, & Chabot, 1983; Smith, Rebok, Smith, Hall, & Alvin, 1983; Zelinski, Gilewski, & Thompson, 1980). The study of Smith and associates showed no main effect for age, whereas the study of Petros and associates and that of Zelinski and associates showed age effects. Meyer and Rice showed that samples of young and old adults equivalent in education (16 years) could be mismatched in terms of verbal ability. Samples equivalent in education and verbal ability showed age deficits on some measures of prose recall, whereas no age deficits were found for samples in which old adults scored considerably higher on vocabulary tests than did young adults with the same amount of education. Thus, both education and verbal ability should be routinely reported.

The issue of getting equivalent cross-sectional samples on verbal ability is quite complex. First, vocabulary test scores improve with age, particularly from the age of 18 years to 25 years but also in the fifties and sixties, with some decline in the eighties (Botwinick, 1978; Wechsler, 1955). Thus, if we select a young group of college freshmen to match the vocabulary performance of an older group, we may be comparing our old group to a group of young adults with superior verbal aptitude, although current performances are equivalent. Another problem concerns the declining scores on standardized tests among the young. A common difficulty in conducting aging research is being able to locate young adults in university programs with vocabulary scores as high as those of alumni from the same school who are in the older age groups (Harker, Hartley, & Walsh, 1982). It is possible that verbal aptitudes, particularly those traits necessary for reading comprehension, will be equivalent for an undergraduate young group and an alumni old group with unequal vocabulary scores. The final problem relates to what test the experimenter elects to employ. Various vocabulary tests have been employed; little is known about how they compare for samples of young and older adults. See Meyer and Rice (1983a) for regression lines between two commonly used vocabulary tests: the vocabulary subtest of the WAIS and the Quick Word Test (Borgatta & Corsini, 1964).

A number of investigations (Meyer & Rice, 1983a; Poon, Krauss, & Bowles, 1984; Taub, 1979) have suggested that age differences in text recall interact with the level of verbal ability. Meyer and Rice (1983a) presented an analysis of four subsamples selected from a group of 314 younger and older adults, all of whom had read and recalled two expository texts. The subsamples were formed on the basis of their vocabulary scores on the Quick Word Test. The comparison groups were formed as follows: (1) random young versus high-verbal old (young adults selected at random from a pool of primarily college students versus the 50 highest-scoring old adults); (2) high-verbal young versus high-verbal old (the 50 highest-scoring young versus the 50 highest-scoring old); (3) low-verbal young versus low-verbal old (the 50 lowest-scoring young versus the 50 lowest-scoring old); (4) low-verbal old versus matching young (the 50 lowest-scoring old versus 50 young with comparable scores). Table 12.1 shows these four comparisons and their education, vocabulary, and performance data. These data suggest rather

Table 12.1. *Four comparisons of different young (Y) and old (O) age groups: learner variables and recall outcomes*

Four comparison groups	Learner variables		Age deficits?	
	Education	Vocabulary (Quick)	Total recall	Logical relations
Random young vs. high-verbal old	Y = 15.4, O = 16.1 [$F_{(1, 98)} = 2.2$, n.s.]	Y = 52, O = 82 [$F_{(1, 98)} = 121.03$, $p < .0001$] Predicted WAIS: Y = 62, O = 73	No Y = .35, O = .37[a] [$F_{(1, 98)} = .62$]	No Y = .40, O = .45 [$F_{(1, 98)} = 1.91$]
High-verbal young vs. high-verbal old	Y = 16.5, O = 16.1 [$F_{(1, 98)} = .83$, n.s.]	Y = 67, O = 82 [$F_{(1, 98)} = 60.03$, $p < .0001$] Predicted WAIS: Y = 71, O = 73	Yes Y = .42, O = .37 [$F_{(1, 98)} = 4.9$, $p < .03$]	No Y = .48, O = .45 [$F_{(1, 98)} = 2.14$]
Low-verbal young vs. low-verbal old	Y = 13.3, O = 12.5 [$F_{(1, 98)} = 2.61$, n.s.]	Y = 32, O = 46 [$F_{(1, 98)} = 59.71$, $p < .0001$] Predicted WAIS: Y = 51, O = 55	Yes Y = .31, O = .25 [$F_{(1, 98)} = 9.97$, $p < .002$]	Yes Y = .36, O = .31 [$F_{(1, 98)} = 5.90$, $p < .02$]
Low-verbal old vs. matching young	Y = 15.0, O = 12.5 [$F_{(1, 98)} = 21.91$, $p < .0001$]	Y = 46, O = 46 Predicted WAIS: Y = 59, O = 55	Yes Y = .38, O = .25 [$F_{(1, 98)} = 42.5$, $p < .0001$]	Yes Y = .41, O = .31 [$F_{(1, 98)} = 22.90$, $p < .001$]

[a]Mean proportion of ideas recalled.

Source: Meyer and Rice (1983a).

Table 12.2. *Characteristics of adults in prose learning studies that show no age deficits*

	Education		Vocabulary	
Study	Young	Old	Young	Old
Taub (1979)	14	13.4	57 (WAIS)	58
Meyer & Rice (1981a)	15.3	15.4	56 (WAIS)	58
Harker et al. (1982)	USC undergrads. USC graduate students	USC alumni	31 (Shipley Hartford)	37 35
Simon et al. (1982) (intentional)	14	13	7.6 (ETS Advanced)	10.3
Smith et al. (1983)	15.7	14.8	None reported	
Young (1983)	14.3	16.3	47 (Quick)	72
Mandel & Johnson (1984)	12.7	13.8	21.6 (30 items from WAIS)	24.7

clearly that there are age-related deficits in memory performance for adults with average or below-average abilities and little post-high-school education. The situation is not as clear for individuals with above-average verbal ability and college education. As mentioned earlier with regard to education, the age groups in comparisons 1 and 2 were equivalent in education. However, the vocabulary differences were greater for comparison 1, where no age differences in recall were found, than for comparison 2, where moderate age differences in recall were observed. Thus, with these groups, age differences in memory performance may be present or absent depending on how the investigator equates the age groups on education and verbal ability.

Table 12.2 lists the studies on prose learning and aging in which aging deficits were not found. As seen in Table 12.2, these studies examined subjects with some college education; all but the study of Smith and associates (1983), where vocabulary is not reported, indicate at least a slight superiority by the old adults for either years of education or vocabulary scores. Thus, the studies not finding age deficits may correspond best with sample 1 in Table 12.1.

In a study using samples of young and old adults corresponding to samples 2 and 3 listed in Table 12.1, Meyer and Rice (unpublished data) looked for an interaction between age and verbal ability; however, this interaction would be much easier to obtain by comparing samples similar to 1 and 4 in Table 12.1. There was an overall age effect and no age-by-verbal-ability interaction, although preplanned comparisons for age effects with high-verbal adults were not statistically significant (but approached significance, $p < .08$), whereas age effects were highly significant for lower-verbal adults.

Hultsch, Hertzog, and Dixon (1984) investigated this interaction by relating text performances by young, middle-aged, and old adults to a set of intellectual-ability factors: general intelligence (*g*), verbal comprehension, verbal productive thinking, and associative memory (Ekstrom, French, Harman, & Derman, 1976). The factor with the greatest overall relationship to text memory was *g*. Regression analyses indicated that age differences in text-recall performance were reduced drastically, but not eliminated, when partialled for intellectual ability. An age-by-verbal-comprehension interaction was not found, but an interaction was found between age and verbal productive thinking (as well as for associative memory). However, the lack of age deficits for older adults scoring high on these two measures held only for the immediate free-recall condition. At 1 to 4 weeks later, age effects were found for all groups.

In an attempt to reconcile the findings of Hultsch and associates and our work, we need to consider two issues: sample selection and vocabulary test. The sample of 150 young, middle, and old adults in the study of Hultsch and associates varied significantly on education (young, 14 years; middle-aged, 13 years; old, 11 years). However, Hultsch and associates pointed out that these differences matched the average years of education for these age groups reported by the 1977 U.S. Census. The subjects in their study were white female adults from a small city in central Pennsylvania. In contrast, Meyer and Rice (1983a) worked with volunteers from the Phoenix, Arizona, area, an area that attracts healthy, mobile, and relatively wealthy older adults. Their low-verbal old adults had an average of 12.5 years of education, and their high-verbal old adults had an average of 16.1 years of education.

In addition, Meyer and Rice used the Quick Word Test to measure vocabulary. Adults who score at the 25th percentile on the Quick test score at the 75th percentile on the vocabulary subtest of the WAIS. The high-verbal old adults scored at the 93rd percentile on the Quick test and hit the ceiling of the WAIS. The Quick is a tricky 100-item multiple-choice test (i.e., heart = beat, draw, core, or vein; shoot = bang, push, twig, or jump; algid = damp, weed, cold, or moss) that appears to require considerable associative memory and verbal productive thinking. Thus, the findings of Hultsch and associates that these factors relate to prose recall more than does verbal comprehension may not be contrary to the findings of Meyer and Rice, but may only reflect differences in tests used.

Thus, Hultsch and associates may have failed to replicate the findings of Meyer and Rice because their sample did not include extremely verbal and well-educated old adults, and their measures of verbal comprehension varied. It is interesting to note that the group of Hultsch and associates who scored high on verbal productive thinking showed larger deficits a week after exposure to the passages than initially. Meyer and Rice (unpublished data) reported that although the amounts, types, and organizations of recall between high-verbal young, middle, and old adults were equivalent immediately after reading passages, 1 week later the older adults' performances showed greater deficits on all measures in comparison with the two younger groups.

In summary, some of the differences among the various studies on prose learning and aging can be explained by differences in education and ability of subjects. Age deficits in prose recall appear to be found consistently for average and low-verbal adults with mainly high school education (Cohen, 1979; Dixon, Hultsch, Simon, & von Eye, 1984; Dixon, Simon, Nowak, & Hultsch, 1982; Glynn, Okun, Muth, & Britton, 1983; Meyer & Rice, 1983a, 1983b; Spilich, 1983; Spilich & Voss, 1982; Surber, Kowalski, & Pena-Paez, 1984; Taub, 1975, 1979; Zelinski et al., 1984). However, all of the discrepancy cannot be explained, because some studies with highly educated, high-ability old adults reported aging deficits (Cohen, 1979; Gordon & Clark, 1974; Meyer & Rice, 1983b; Zelinski et al., 1984), whereas others did not (Harker et al., 1982; Mandel & Johnson, 1984; Meyer & Rice, 1981a, 1983a; Young, 1983). In addition, our knowledge about the prose learning skills of older adults with deficient verbal skills and grammar school education is extremely limited. One reason for the lack of studies with samples from this group is that these adults rarely volunteer for prose learning experiments; people who perform poorly on verbal tasks avoid experiencing frustration on vocabulary tests and prose learning tasks.

Age

These studies have varied regarding the ages of subjects identified as young and old. These variations may have contributed to the contradictory findings. The average age for most young groups was the twenties, and the average age for most old comparison groups was the sixties. The few studies whose average age groups fell outside of these ranges reported large age deficits: 17-year-olds versus 71-year-olds (Zelinski et al., 1984, Exp. I); 21-year-olds versus 81-year-olds (Spilich, 1983); 19-year-olds versus 76-year-olds and 81-year-olds (Spilich & Voss, 1982). Also see Cohen and Faulkner (Chapter 14, this volume).

Other learner variables

As Bartlett (1932) pointed out 50 years ago, and as the current explosion of interest in cognitive psychology confirms (Anderson & Pearson, 1984), comprehension and recall involve active cognitive processes, and memory for what is read often is not a reproduction, but a reconstruction guided by schematized knowledge. A reader's prior knowledge or "schema" for the topic of a passage has been shown to affect the accuracy as well as the amount of information remembered (Anderson & Pichert, 1978; Anderson, Reynolds, Schallert, & Goetz, 1977; Bower, 1978; Bransford & Johnson, 1972; Bransford & McCarrell, 1974; Dooling & Lachman, 1971; Spilich, Vesonder, Chiesi, & Voss, 1979; Spiro, 1977). Because new information is assimilated with what is already known or believed, if this information does not fit with a person's current understanding or schema, it is quite likely to be forgotten or misunderstood. Recalls of unfamiliar materials often contain a variety of distortions and intrusions that serve to modify the original passage to fit the reader's expectations (Rice, 1980; Steffensen & Colker, 1982). This is true for all adults, but older adults appear to be especially likely to intrude bits of prior knowledge into their recall of new information (Hultsch & Dixon, 1983; Smith et al, 1983). Smith and associates found that the numbers of additions and distortions from learners' prior knowledge that appeared in recall were functions of an age-by-text-organization interaction. Old adults produced more additions and distortions for stories presented in a standard, well-organized story structure, whereas young adults produced more additions and intrusions for stories in a poorly organized, scrambled condition. Old adults added prior knowledge to make their stories more interesting, whereas young adults added prior knowledge to make the unorganized stories more coherent. Different perceptions of the recall task may have led to these differences. However, Surber and associates (1984) found that young adults added more theme-related intrusions in their recall of a long expository text than did old adults.

The Hultsch and Dixon (1983) study is the only one available that systematically investigated the effects of prior knowledge and age on prose learning. Average-verbal, high-school-educated young, middle, and old adults read short biographical sketches about famous entertainment figures of various eras. The results suggested that age differences in recall performance may be present or absent depending on the levels of preexperimental knowledge of the topic possessed by the various age groups.

Perspective (Duell, 1974; Meyer & Freedle, 1984; Owens, Dafoe, & Bower, 1977; Pichert & Anderson, 1977), purpose, and processing style (Dunn, 1985; Spiro, 1978) also have been found to influence the amount and type of information remembered from prose. As suggested by the findings of Smith and associates with respect to differences in intrusions added by the young and old adults with different types of text, differences between age groups in prose recall could result from differences in perspective or purpose related to the social and intellectual contexts of the various age groups. No aging studies involving prose learning have systematically investigated these variables, but the variables may contribute to some of the confusion in the literature.

Task variables

Mode and rate of presentation

Research examining presentation (listening versus reading) with young adults has found that performances are similar after reading and listening when reading time is equal to listening time (Sticht & James, 1984). However, if reading is self-paced, as is the case in most nonlaboratory situations, then recall after reading is superior to recall after listening (King, 1968; Kintsch, Kozminsky, Streby, McKoon, & Keenan, 1975; Taub, 1975, 1976; Taub & Kline, 1976, 1978; Stine, Wingfield, & Poon, Chapter 13, this volume).

Dixon and associates (1982) examined the effects of input modality on immediate recall and delayed recall for short newspaper articles by average-verbal, high-school-educated adults. They found that younger and middle-aged adults benefited more from the opportunity to read material than did older adults. They saw this to be a result of older adults not taking as much advantage of the opportunity to review material during reading as did the younger and middle-aged adults. Taub and Kline's data (1978) from average-verbal, high-school-educated adults also support this explanation that old adults benefit less from an opportunity for review. In their study, short paragraphs were presented to young and old adults to evaluate the effects of three types of input conditions. In the "aloud" condition, subjects read the paragraphs aloud, without review, four times and after each reading verbally recalled the text. In the "silent" condition, the task was identical except that the text was read silently. In the "review" condition, subjects also read silently, but were allowed to review the material. The results indicated that for both age groups, opportunity for review required more reading time and led to significantly better recall than did the silent and aloud conditions, which did not differ. An age-by-trial interaction indicated that age-related differences in recall were not significant until the third trial, with the young subjects outperforming the old. In both the Dixon and associates study and the Taub and Kline study, the adults were average in verbal ability and primarily were high-school-educated. In comparing high-verbal and average-verbal old adults (Meyer, 1984; Rice & Meyer, in press), we have found average-verbal old adults deficient in their use of text structure, recall of logical relationships in text, and ability to find and underline the important ideas in a text. Thus, average-verbal old adults may be unable to take advantage of opportunities to review because of ineffective strategies for finding and utilizing the organization in text. We might not have found these age deficits in utilization of review opportunities if we had studied high-verbal adults, because they are more practiced and more analytical readers than are their average-vocabulary counterparts.

With high-verbal, college-educated adults, Cohen (1981) reported that memory for spoken information was more impaired for old adults than was memory for written information. She found that old adults performed better when they read than when they listened, whereas young adults showed no differences for the two input modes. Cohen (1979) also reported age deficits in free recall for old adults when listening to a passage similar to "Circle Island" (Dawes, 1966) at 120 words per minute (wpm). However, at that presentation rate and at 200 wpm for one-paragraph descriptions (16-, 60-, and 75-word messages with one verbatim question per message), Cohen (1979) did not find age effects on verbatim questions. The presentation rate had no effect for old adults for verbatim questions, but it impaired their performance on inference questions. The rate had no effect on either type of question for young adults.

Table 12.3. *Existence of aging deficits in research studies with controlled presentation times*

Study	Presentation time (words per minute)	Age deficits?
Mandel & Johnson (1984)	102	No
Meyer & Rice (1983b)	120	Yes
Cohen (1979)	120	Yes
Petros et al. (1983)	120	Yes
Surber et al. (1984)	136	Yes
Zelinski et al. (1984)	155	Yes
Petros et al. (1983)	160	Yes

Table 12.3 lists the research studies conducted with controlled presentation times. All but two of those listed used oral presentation without visual exposure to the text. Zelinski and associates had their subjects read the text while it was being read to them at a fast pace. Surber and associates allowed their subjects 11 min and 30 sec to read a 5.5-page text. Petros and associates expected an age-by-rate (120 wpm versus 160 wpm) interaction, but did not find it. The rate impaired the recall performance to equivalent degrees for young and old subjects. As suggested by Table 12.3, a rate between 102 wpm and 120 wpm appears critical for exceeding the optimal level of processing by old adults. In a study with 160 high- and average-verbal old and young adults, we found the average reading speed of old adults to be 121 wpm, but it was 144 wpm for young adults. A pace of 120 wpm is too fast for about half of the old adults, but it is well within the optimal range for nearly all young adults.

One possible explanation for greater age deficits for faster-paced presentations than for slower or self-paced presentations focuses on slowing with aging (Birren, 1974; Salthouse, 1982). Older individuals are said to differ from their younger counterparts primarily in terms of the speed with which they can carry out mental operations, such as encoding, comparison, and response selection and execution (Birren, Woods, & Williams, 1980; Charness, 1983). Another proposed explanation emphasizes a reduction in working memory capacity with increasing age (Cohen, 1979; Hasher & Zacks, 1979; Petros et al., 1983; Spilich, 1983). Having the text to read and review in the self-paced condition should help to reinstate information lost from working memory and serve as a memory aid to compensate for lost capacity. As noted earlier from the findings with average-verbal adults (Dixon et al., 1982; Taub & Kline, 1978), some sophistication in reading skills may be necessary before older adults try to compensate through rereading and review.

Other task variables

On most of the other task variables, such as recall versus recognition and immediate recall versus delayed recall, conflicting results have been found concerning the relative degrees of age deficits (Hultsch & Dixon, 1984). Some studies have found equivalent age deficits for both recall and recognition (Gordon & Clark, 1974; Spilich, 1983); others have found age differences for recall, but not recognition (Spilich & Voss, 1982); still others have found no age deficits for recall and questions or recognition (Labouvie-Vief, Schell, & Weaverdyke, 1981; Meyer & Rice, 1981a). Also, in terms of delay interval, some studies have found greater aging deficits immediately (Dixon et al., 1982; Hultsch & Dixon, 1983; Hultsch et al., 1984), whereas others have found greater deficits 1 week later (Cohen & Faulkner, 1983; Gordon & Clark, 1974; Meyer & Rice, unpublished data).

Most recent studies have employed standard prose learning instructions: Subjects were asked to attend to the passage as they would normally do for a magazine article they wanted to remember, and then they were asked to recall it in their own words or words from the passage. Few studies (Simon et al., 1982; Surber et al., 1984) compared different types of instructions to subjects. Simon and associates found age deficits on incidental tasks, but no age differences with intentional, standard prose learning instructions. Surber and associates found no differences between two types of reading instructions.

Earlier studies (Botwinick & Storandt, 1974; Gilbert, 1941; Schneider, Gritz, & Jarvik, 1975) employing verbatim recall consistently reported age deficits; however, adults rarely need to memorize prose in their everyday activities. In terms of frequency of use in everyday life, our data on daily diaries collected on 60 young, middle, and old adults every other week for 5 weeks indicated that adults rarely read and wrote down what they remembered (Rice, in press). In fact, the adults rarely wrote much of anything, other than letters and tax forms.

Neisser (1982) stated that the textual materials popular in learning-research laboratories today are improvements over nonsense syllables and such of the past, but are not representative of what ordinary people remember. However, his clever study with Hupcey (Neisser & Hupcey, 1974), in which Sherlock Holmes fans were questioned about their memory for content in the Holmes mysteries, clearly supports findings from the laboratory with natural texts; that is, relevance to the organization or plot is the critical factor in predicting which ideas will be well remembered. Free recall of text or even answering questions about one specific text will not reflect the ordinary activities of most people. These activities are no doubt closer to the activities of students than to those of most adults. In studying the memory of middle-aged and older adults, assessing memory through conversation or oral recall would be more ecologically valid than would written free recall. Oral recall may be more naturalistic than written recall, but Harker and associates (1982) found no difference between these two response modes in terms of propositions recalled, although written recall was more concise. Research on aging and prose learning should explore additional dependent measures, such as those used by Mayer (1985) or Stone and Glock (1981), which examine a reader's ability to use the information in the text to solve a problem or assemble an object.

Table 12.4. *Reading habits of young, middle-aged, and old adults*

Parameter	Group		
	Young	Middle	Old
Average hours per week spent reading	13.4	12.6	12.3
Percentage of items read for			
Less than 0.5 hour	30%	34%	19%
Less than 1 hour	57%	57%	46%
Average number of different items listed by each subject	19	14	13
Number of top-20 items read that fall within general types of reading material:			
Newspapers	4	6	4
News magazines	3	2	2
Science magazines	1	1	4
General magazines	3	4	5
Textbooks/technical	5	3	0
Percentage of adults who reported reading Bible (about 2 hours/week)	22%	28%	22%
Reasons for reading:			
Need information	39%	24%	5%
General information	28%	45%	69%
Relaxation	29%	27%	23%
Other (e.g., inspiration)	4%	4%	3%

Text variables

Typicality of text used in the prose learning experiments

Table 12.4 gives some preliminary data from a diary study (Rice, in press). In this study, 18 young, middle, and older adults keep track of what they read and how long they spent reading it over a 5-week period. The table shows that the groups were fairly equal in average hours spent reading each week. However, division of these data into groups with high and low vocabulary scores indicates that older adults with high scores read about the same amount as comparable young adults, whereas middle and older adults with low scores read less than comparable young adults. The average hours per week spent reading by adults with high vocabulary scores were 14.4, 15.1, and 14.6 for young, middle-aged, and older adults, respectively; the average hours per week spent reading by adults with low vocabulary scores were 12.4, 10.0, and 10.1 for young, middle-aged, and older adults, respectively (Rice, in press).

Of the items listed as read by these three age groups of adults, most were read for less than an hour at a time, and about one-third for less than half an hour. The oldest age group spent slightly more time reading each item. The youngest group listed the greatest number of different items read, averaging 19 for each person. The names of the items listed were compiled separately for each age group, and the 20 most frequently read items were identified. As can be seen in Table 12.4, newspapers accounted for 20% of these items for the young group, 30% for the middle, and 20% for the older group. The young and middle group showed greater amounts of technical material than did the old group, reflecting their schooling and career tasks. Magazines were widely read by all age groups, but the largest consumers of these materials appeared to be the older group, for whom 55% of the most frequently read items were magazines. *Time* was the most frequently read magazine: 28% of the old adults read it, 17% of the middle, and 28% of the young group; *Newsweek* was second and was more popular with younger readers: no older participants, 22% of middle-aged adults, and 22% of the young participants. Other widely read magazines were *Reader's Digest* (old = 28% of magazines read; middle = 22%; young = 11%) and *People Magazine* (old = 11% of participants; middle = 28%; young = none). The Bible had a fairly consistent readership across age groups of 22% to 28%.

The subjects tended to give three main reasons for reading: (1) needing the information for one reason or another, (2) for general information, and (3) for relaxation. As shown in Table 12.4, the rate of reading for relaxation remained relatively constant across the age groups at about 25% of items read. Reading because of the need for information decreased with age, clearly reflecting changing activities – from school to career to increased leisure reading. Reading for general interest showed a complementary increase across age groups.

Most of the more recent prose learning studies have used materials adapted from popular magazines or newspapers, and given that finding, it would appear that these materials are appropriate to the typical reading patterns of adults of all ages.

Basics about text structure

A definition. The structure of text is the organization that binds it together and gives it an overall coherence. This structure shows how some ideas are of central importance to the author's message, which is expressed through this overall organization, whereas other ideas are shown to be peripheral. In expository text, the text structure specifies the logical connections among ideas as well as the subordination of some ideas to others. It is this structure of text that primarily differentiates text from simple lists of words or sentences.

Reasons for identification. Because text structure is an essential characteristic of text, educators and psychologists interested in reading comprehension have sought to describe and classify it. This description is necessary in order to examine how readers identify and utilize text structure in the comprehension process. In order to examine what information a reader has processed from a text, the researcher needs to know just what information was presented in the text. Thus, the procedures for analyzing text structure and content have been put to use as scoring templates to evaluate a reader's recall of text.

Moreover, researchers hypothesize that the representation of the text in memory is parallel to their analysis of the text structure. Comparisons of structures identified from the text and those identified from readers' recall assist investigators in attempts to validate their models of the representation of text in memory. Models of memory representation based on procedures for prose analysis usually are posited for certain types of learners (i.e., skilled readers with relatively low prior knowledge of the text topic) under certain types of task conditions (i.e., reading for optimal comprehension and recall of text information, with adequate time and immediate recall). Investigators examine variations between the text structure and analyses of recall protocols when the types of learners and task conditions are varied systematically.

Another reason for specifying text structure concerns the problem of generalizing research findings with a particular passage to other texts. Text structure is a significant dimension along which text selections can be evaluated as to their similarities and differences. Investigators examining prose learning have made some progress in characterizing certain discourse types, such as simple stories (Mandler & Johnson, 1977; Rumelhart, 1977), scientific reports (Kintsch & van Dijk, 1978), and exposition (Meyer, 1977; Meyer & Freedle, 1984). However, discourse types have been considered more by rhetoricians (D'Angelo, 1976) and linguists (Brewer, 1980; Longacre, 1968) than by psychologists. We are beginning to make progress in determining which aspects of text structure are important to consider in differentiating among text selections.

Different analysis systems. Given these reasons for the usefulness of specifying the structure of text, it might be expected that researchers would by now have converged on a simple, universally accepted method. There are at least three reasons for the lack of such a method. First, interest in specifying text structure has historically come from a variety of disciplines, including rhetoric, folklore, linguistics, education, psychology, and artificial intelligence (Meyer & Rice, 1984). These disciplines have had different approaches and goals for analyzing text structure. The multiplicity of disciplines involved serves to diversify the text structures proposed as well as to enrich our understanding of text structure.

A second reason for the variety of text-analysis systems currently used to study reading comprehension concerns the purposes for which they were developed. For example, if the research goal is to ascertain recall of the gist of a passage, the analysis structure may be quite different than when the goal is memory for logical relationships.

The most difficult obstacles to a single unified prose-analysis system are those that are inherent in the complexity of text, the writing process, and the reading process. Part of the problem arises from the complexity of the reading process (Meyer & Rice, 1984). Because the text and reader interact in this process, it is difficult to isolate entirely textual variables. The structure of the information read from a text may appear different to readers with different prior knowledge and purposes. A reasonable escape from this problem is to analyze text from the point of view of the author. However, there are some problems with this approach. If a poorly written exposition is selected that fails to interrelate ideas logically, either explicitly or implicitly, the text analyst may want to identify the potential conceptual structure underlying the topic in order to better score the recalls of more astute readers. Individual differences among analysts in making such inferences can produce variability in the analyses produced.

Most of the prose learning experiments have used the prose-analysis systems of Kintsch (1974) or Meyer (1975). However, two studies (Mandel & Johnson, 1984; Smith et al., 1983) have used systems based on the story grammar of Mandler and Johnson (1977); both studies found no age deficits for well-organized, multi-episode stories with similar subjects under similar task conditions. Two other studies used a procedure developed by Johnson (1970) that does not have a theoretical base in linguistics, but empirically determines structural importance by having groups of subjects delete different amounts of unimportant text. These studies (Petros et al., 1983; Surber et. al., 1984) reported age deficits. Although different methods correspond with different findings for these studies, an examination of most of the prose learning studies points out that different analysis systems cannot explain the discrepant findings. For example, the Kintsch system was used by Dixon and associates (1984) and by Harker and associates (1982). The study of Dixon and associates found that old adults remembered considerably less from expository text than did young adults. In contrast, the Harker and associates study with expository text found no age differences in the amount of information remembered by young and old adults. The Meyer system has been utilized by Meyer and Rice (1981a) and Zelinski and associates (1980). Meyer and Rice found no significant age differences, but Zelinski and associates found significantly poorer recall by old adults.

Meyer (1983, 1985) contrasted the strengths and weaknesses of various prose-analysis systems. A detailed analysis was presented of the procedures for analysis and scoring in the Kintsch and Meyer approaches. Briefly, that analysis revealed a number of differences and similarities between the two approaches. Both approaches yield a hierarchical text structure; the hierarchy is built by repetition of concepts in the Kintsch approach, whereas it is based on the semantic and logical relations in the text in the Meyer approach. Few discrepancies are found when the superordinate nodes selected for both approaches are similar. Repeated words in a text are characteristic of the highest levels in the Kintsch hierarchy, whereas logical relationships and the ideas that they bind are characteristic of the highest levels in the Meyer hierarchy. Large variations in the two hierarchies result when different superordinate nodes are selected for the top of the hierarchy. The Meyer approach defines the superordinate node as the content bound by the top-level structure, the superordinate relation that can encompass the remaining ideas of the text. Selection of the superordinate node in the Kintsch approach is based on intuition. The Kintsch approach appears to require less analysis time. For the text and small sample of data examined by Meyer (1985), the approach based on logical relations predicted recall better than did the approach based on word repetition.

With regard to scoring, differences resulted from the different treatments of relationships in the two systems. They are scored separately in the Meyer approach, whereas they are combined with content in the Kintsch approach. Thus, it is possible to show partial recall and recall of relationships with inaccurate or omitted content in the Meyer approach. The Kintsch scoring system is more efficient for scoring immediate free-recall protocols with close correspondence to text content because the system produces fewer units to score. The Meyer approach is more time-consuming, but more informative with less accurate recall protocols. The following example of the recall protocol for an old adult with 12 years of education will exemplify this difference in scoring. The passage read and recalled was originally selected by Miller and Kintsch (1980) from *Reader's Digest.* First the original text is given, followed by the subject's recall:

In the request to canonize the "frontier priest," John Neumann, bishop of Philadelphia in the 19th century, two miracles were attributed to him in this century. In 1923, Eva Benassi, dying from peritonitis, dramatically recovered after her nurse prayed to the bishop. In 1949, Kent Lenahan, hospitalized with two skull fractures, smashed bones and a pierced lung after a traffic accident, rose from his deathbed and resumed a normal life after his mother had prayed ardently to Neumann.

Recall protocol: They put their faith in prayer. In all three instances they were on their deathbed and after they prayed they attributed getting well to faith and incessant prayer to Bishop Neumann. If you pray faithfully, put faith in it, your prayers are answered. I don't remember exactly each instance, but in each instance they were really sick and the only answer to their hope was prayer.

Three points (10% of the scorable units in the Kintsch analysis structure) were scored from the Kintsch approach, whereas 31 points (34% of the units in the Meyer structure) were given credit using the Meyer approach. In the Meyer system, the correct relationships could be credited even though there were few accurate specifics. For example, in the Meyer system the subject is credited for knowing that someone prayed in some manner (incessantly rather than ardently) to Neumann (credited with 5 points, 1 for each of the following: prayed, manner of praying, agent, range, and Neumann). However, in the Kintsch system, parts of propositions (relations and arguments) are not scored separately, but as whole units. The proposition containing "prayed" in the Kintsch system is "prayed mother John-Neumann"; because the subject did not recall "mother," credit is not given for the proposition. In scoring a protocol from a very accurate and proficient learner, the Kintsch system recorded 76% correct, whereas the Meyer system recorded 88%. The correlation on total recall scores was .96 between the two scoring systems for nine subjects who varied greatly in recall proficiency (Meyer, 1985). However, differences between the recall of the proficient learner and that of the older adult quoted earlier would appear greater utilizing the

Kintsch system (66% difference in amount recalled) than using the Meyer system (54% difference). Thus, age differences may reach statistical significance more easily using the Kintsch system, where partial credit is not given. One study (Smith et al., 1983) found age differences with strict scoring that required recall of every idea in a complex sentence for credit in recalling that sentence, but found no age differences with more lenient scoring. Differences in the types of ideas recalled between old and younger adults can be more sensitively measured with the Meyer system. That is, instead of simply finding a deficiency in recall of propositions, the types of relationships and content present and absent in the recall can be specified. In addition, the underlying logic processed by learners from expository text is better studied with the latter approach; differences in overall organization of the text and recall protocol have been reliably studied with this approach (Meyer, Brandt, & Bluth, 1980; Meyer & Freedle, 1984).

Age differences in the use of the text's top-level organization

Through the Meyer analysis system (Meyer, 1975, 1985), all of the information from a text is represented in a detailed outline or tree structure called the content structure. The content structure shows the text's top-level organization and the interrelationships among its ideas and their relative importance. Figure 12.2 depicts the top-level structure and major logical relationships of a magazine article on the topic of supertankers. This passage (Meyer, 1985) contains 388 words and 244 scorable units in the complete analysis of the text; the content structure arranges the ideas from the passage into nine levels of importance.

Meyer, drawing on linguistics and rhetoric (Meyer, 1975; Meyer & Freedle, 1984), has gathered evidence for five basic ways to organize discourse: collection, description, causation, problem/solution, and comparison. The typology is not intended to be exhaustive or definitive, but there is good evidence that there are significant distinctions among these discourse types. Figure 12.3 specifies the organizational components of the structures that correspond to the five basic types of discourse. The collection structure is a list of elements associated in some manner, such as ordering in time, in the case of a sequence. The description structure gives more information about a topic by presenting an attribute, specification, or setting. The causation organization presents causal relationships, as in the "if/then" antecedent/consequent statements in logic. The problem/solution structure has all the organizational components of causation, with the addition of overlapping content between the problem and solution where the solution blocks a cause of the problem. In contrast, the comparison discourse type does not organize on the basis of time or causality, but on the basis of similarities and differences.

These basic discourse types are familiar in various contexts. Political speeches often are of the comparison type – in particular, its unequally weighted subtype. Newspaper articles often are of the descriptive type, telling us who, where, how, and when. Scientific treatises often adhere to the problem/solution type, first rais-

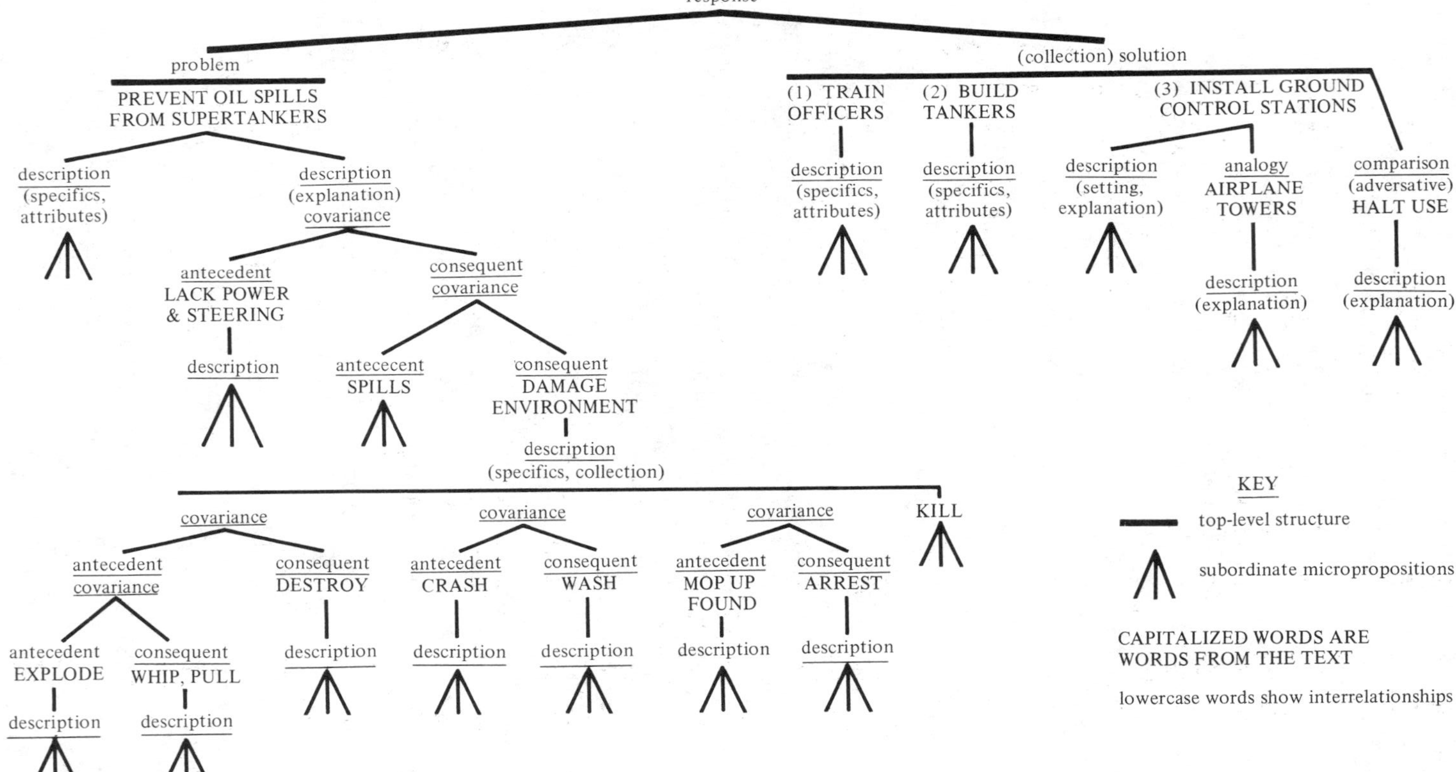

Figure 12.2. The superordinate structure of a passage about supertankers. (From Meyer, 1984.)

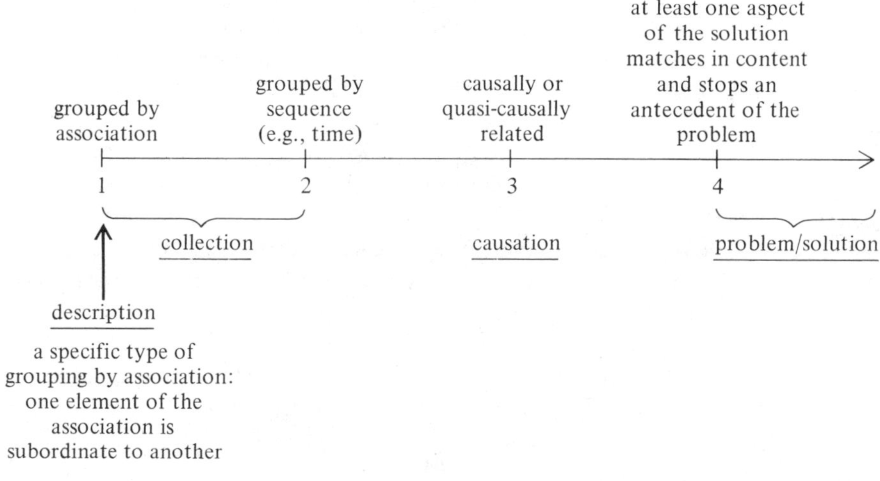

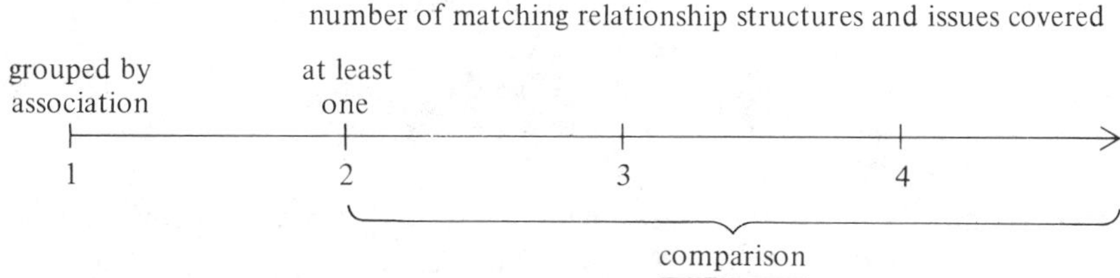

Figure 12.3. Type and number of specified organizational components required for different discourse types. (From Meyer & Freedle, 1984.)

ing a question or problem and then seeking to give an answer or solution. History texts often exemplify the collection structure.

We have used expository texts to probe how these five top-level structures affect reading comprehension. In one study (Meyer et al., 1980) we found that ninth-graders who used the author's top-level structure to organize their recall remembered more, even a week later, than those who did not. Ninth-graders evaluated by reading-comprehension tests and by their teachers as good readers used the text's top-level structure to organize their recalls, whereas those evaluated as poor readers did not. Meyer and Freedle (1984) found that university students remembered more from discourse that was written in a comparison structure than from that written in a description structure. Although other investigators have used Meyer's approach to study developmental changes in the ability to use the text's top-level structure (Taylor, 1980), their investigations have been confined to children or young adults. Thus, only our research is reviewed in this section. First to be discussed is the frequency with which different age groups find and utilize the top-level structure of prose when they write their own recalls. Later we shall focus on the effects of different types of top-level structures on recall of prose by older adults.

Age differences in frequency of use. In a study (Meyer, 1983) with average-verbal adults (48th percentile), the best predictor of their recall from texts was whether or not they used the text's top-level structure to organize their recall protocols. These findings indicate that the ability to identify and utilize the author's top-level organization is a crucial skill in reading comprehension for older adults.

A second interesting finding was an age-and-structure interaction when high-school-educated old adults were compared with ninth-graders of average vocabulary performance. For both groups, use of the top-level structure greatly facilitated recall: The average percentage of ideas recalled from a passage when the author's top-level structure was used by a subject to organize the recall protocol was 31%, but only 14% when it was not utilized. However, the ability to utilize the author's top-level structure was even more crucial to recall for the older group (34% recall when the structure was used, and 13.5% when not used, versus 28% recall when the structure was used by ninth-graders, and 15% when it was not used). The interaction between age and the use of the author's structure was statistically significant at the .01 level. For both the older subjects and the ninth-graders, when the text's structure was not used, the subjects tended simply to list sentences they remembered from the passage, with no attempt to interrelate the sentences; they did not impose a different, well-organized structure, such as we have found when graduate students disagree with an author (Meyer & Freedle, 1984).

In contrast to these finding with average-verbal adults, a study with higher-verbal Arizona State University (ASU) alumni from young, middle, and old groups found no age-related differences in the use of top-level structure; nearly all of the adults from each age group used the same top-level structure as that used in the text to organize their recall (Meyer, Rice, Knight, & Jessen, 1979). More recently, we looked at age and verbal ability and found that high-verbal adults from all age groups used the text's top-level structure more often than did average-verbal adults. More significantly, age interacted with verbal ability. Old and young high-verbal adults did not differ in their use of the text's top-level structure, but average-verbal young adults used the text's top-level structure more than did average-verbal old adults (Meyer & Rice, unpublished data; Rice & Meyer, 1985). Table 12.5 shows these data.

An intervention program (Meyer, Young, & Bartlett, 1986) with average-verbal young and old adults was conducted recently to see if older adults could improve their ability to find and use the top-level structure in magazine and newspaper articles. Findings from that study have shown that older adults can learn this strategy aimed at utilizing the structure in the text and achieve substantial increases in the amount of information remembered.

Effect of discourse type on prose recall. Meyer and Rice (1983b) attempted to determine if older adults would perform better after listening to passages organized with a comparison top-level structure than with a collection of descriptions. Meyer and Freedle (1984) found that graduate students remembered more facts

Table 12.5. *Number of high- and average-verbal young, middle, and old adults who used and did not use the top-level structure (TLS) immediately after reading expository text*

	Verbal ability			
	High		Average	
Age	Recall's TLS same as author's	Recall's TLS different from author's	Recall's TLS same as author's	Recall's TLS different from author's
Young	64	16	55	25
Middle	63	17	56	24
Old	64	16	42	38
	$\chi^2 = .05$, n.s.		$\chi^2 = 6.6$, $p < .05$	

about such topics as dehydration if two views about the topic were compared, rather than simply reading three paragraphs describing the topic. In the Meyer and Rice (1983b) study, 40 young (18–32), 38 middle-aged (40–54), and 40 old (62 and over) adults with above-average scores on the WAIS vocabulary test listened to passages on two topics organized either as a comparison or as a collection of descriptions. The main effects of discourse type and age were statistically significant. The comparative structure yielded superior performance on recall of the same information for all three age groups. In contrast, adults with average scores on the vocabulary subtest of the WAIS did not show facilitation of recall for the comparative structure (Vincent, 1985). This lack of effect for discourse type held for young, middle-aged, and old adults with these lower scores on the WAIS.

Age differences in sensitivity to the hierarchical structure of text

Because studies with list learning have indicated age-related differences in using organization (Craik, 1977), a number of investigators have sought to determine if older adults are deficient in their use of text organization. In addition to looking at the top-level structure of the text and its recall, as discussed earlier, two prevalent methods for investigating age differences in sensitivity to text structure have been (1) to ask subjects to rate the information in the text according to its importance and (2) to examine the proportion of information recalled by the different age groups from high and lower levels in the text structure.

Identification of important information by subjects. Two studies (Mandel & Johnson, 1984; Petros et al., 1983) had subjects judge the importance of the ideas in the text. Both found that young and old adults did not vary in rating the importance of information. The materials used in both studies were stories. Mandel and Johnson had subjects with some college education (14 years of education; 24 of 30 items on the WAIS) rank-order the propositions from the most important to the least important. Petros and associates had subjects rate a Japanese folk tale (Brown & Smiley, 1978) that was evaluated at the fifth-grade readability level (Dale & Chall, 1948). Subjects were told that the individual idea units differed in importance to the theme of the story and that some less important idea units could be eliminated without destroying the main theme. They were first instructed to eliminate the units that they believed to be least important (about one-quarter) by crossing them through with a blue pencil. They then were requested to eliminate the idea units that could still be removed without destroying the main theme (about one-quarter), using a red pencil. Finally, they were asked to repeat this procedure again with a green pencil, leaving one-quarter of the original units intact. It was emphasized that these remaining units should be the most important in the story. Young and old adults in groups with high education (18 years; WAIS vocabulary scaled score = 15) and low education (11.5 years; WAIS vocabulary scaled score = 13) rated the passage; the authors found no differences for either age or education.

These results for the high- and low-education groups of old adults are contrary to findings reported by Meyer (1984); also see Rice and Meyer (1985). We asked older adults to underline the 10 most important ideas from the supertanker passage, a 388-word expository text with a problem/solution top-level structure (Figure 12.2). Twenty of these adults could be classified as high in education; they largely consisted of college-educated professionals (mean years of education = 16.8; 70% professionals). Another 20 could be classified as low in education; this group was composed largely of blue- and white-collar workers with high school educations (mean years of education = 12.22; 24% professionals). The high-education group had extremely high vocabulary skills (Quick mean = 82; WAIS scaled score = 16), whereas the low-education group could be considered average to high average in vocabulary (Quick mean = 45; WAIS scaled score = 12). Fifty percent of the underlining from the high-education group could be mapped on the top levels (1–4) of the content structure, whereas the low-education group underlined ideas from all levels in the content structure equally (four levels examined: 1–4, 5, 6, and 7–9; these divisions were obtained by dividing the structure into fourths based on the number of idea units). When asked to explain their choices, the high-education group was much more likely to use explanations that referred to organizational properties of the text, such as "If you analyzed it, the theme is contained in the first sentence."

These studies suggest that old adults with some college education are as sensitive to the organizational structure in the text as are young adults. However, taken together, they also suggest that the type of text (exposition or narrative), the ability or education level of the older adult, the difficulty of the text, and the nature of the rating task need to be considered in evaluating age-related differences in sensitivity to text structure. Our underlining task and the deficit for average-verbal old adults in using top-level structure reported earlier suggest that this group of old adults may be deficient in their sensitivity to text structure with expository text adapted from magazine articles.

Age differences in recall of main ideas and details: the levels effect. Research in the laboratory has consistently shown that superordinate propositions, main ideas, are more likely to be remembered than subordinate propositions, details (Kintsch & Keenan, 1973; Mandler & Johnson, 1977; Meyer, 1975; Meyer & McConkie, 1973; Thorndyke, 1977). This finding is also evident in more naturalistic situations (Neisser & Hupcey, 1974). The levels effect, in which information high in the hierarchical structure of a passage is better recalled than information low in the structure, is taken as evidence that the reader is sensitive to the relative importance of the ideas in a passage as it is organized by the author. There have been several recent studies that have looked for aging differences in sensitivity to prose structure by examining the levels effect for each age group. These studies have not presented consistent findings with respect to older adults' use of text structure; these studies will be reviewed in this section, and an attempt will be made to understand the reasons for these inconsistent findings.

Mandel and Johnson (1984) presented clearly organized stories, slowly and auditorially, to adults who were above average in verbal ability and education and found no deficits in total recall nor in the levels effect for older adults. Meyer and Rice (1981a) had the same type of subjects read a 641-word expository text without many explicit organizational cues, and they also found no deficits in total recall. However, an age-by-level interaction narrowly missed significance (p = .053). Post hoc multiple-comparison tests showed that the young group's recall of high-level information was significantly greater than their recall of medium- and low-level information, but the levels effect, though in the usual pattern, did not reach significance for middle-aged and old subjects. With respect to answers to questions, the old and middle groups were able to correctly answer significantly more detail questions than was the young group. There were no differences in questions about main ideas. All age groups remembered the main ideas equally well, but young adults recalled more of the logic and major details that supported these main ideas, whereas the older groups recalled more of the minor details at the lowest levels of the content structure. We interpreted these findings as showing that older adults were less sensitive to the hierarchical structure and more sensitive to details. One explanation we considered was different reading strategies for young and older subjects. We reasoned that young adults influenced by the daily requirements of school focused on what the teacher or the text emphasized as important and on the related logic and main ideas. In contrast, we thought that older adults had made up their minds on most of the important issues of life and continued to read primarily for their own interest. We thought that they read to find the author's main idea, then accepted or rejected it, skipped the author's logic, and focused on details of particular interest to them.

However, our recent data (Meyer & Rice, 1982, 1983a; Rice & Meyer, in press, unpublished data) indicate that that explanation is incorrect for the older adults.

Table 12.6. *Mean proportions of information recalled from high and low in the structure by young, middle, and old adults of high and average verbal ability (VA) under different emphasis conditions*

	Emphasis			
	Structure		Details	
Structural level	High VA	Average VA	High VA	Average VA
Young adults				
High	.53	.38	.45	.30
Low	.37	.27	.37	.30
(%high – low)	(16%)	(11%)	(8%)	(0%)
Middle-aged adults				
High	.53	.38	.4	.33
Low	.40	.28	.35	.30
(%high – low)	(13%)	(10%)	(5%)	(3%)
Old adults				
High	.48	.27	.37	.28
Low	.29	.17	.36	.21
(%high – low)	(19%)	(10%)	(1%)	(7%)

In a study with 300 young, middle, and old adults with high or average verbal ability, subjects assigned to different conditions read different versions of two expository texts. In some conditions, the top-level structure, hierarchical structure, and major logical relations were emphasized, whereas in other conditions the structure was deemphasized and the details were emphasized. Overall, we found that old adults performed significantly poorer than did the two younger groups (which did not differ), and those subjects reading the versions with the structure emphasized recalled more than did those reading deemphasized versions. When the structure was emphasized, the subjects' recall protocols reflected a greater levels effect (43% main ideas versus 30% details) than when it was deemphasized (35% main ideas versus 31% details). These different emphasis plans had a greater effect on high-verbal adults than on average-verbal adults, but the patterns were the same for both. However, there was an interesting interaction among the emphasis plans, the level in the content structure, age, and verbal ability. This interaction showed up consistently: immediately, 1 week late, on the free-recall data, and on questions. Table 12.6 shows the immediate free-recall data.

This interaction [$F(2, 228) = 5.72$; $p < .004$] resulted because there was little or no levels effect for the average-verbal young adults (main ideas = 30%; details = 30%) and the high-verbal old adults (main ideas = 37%; details = 36%) under conditions that deemphasized the structure and emphasized the details, in comparison with the other groups, for which larger levels effects were found. In addition, the group of high-verbal old adults showed the greatest changes in the

Table 12.7. *Average percentages of details recalled by young, middle-aged, and old adults of high and average verbal abilities from passages varying in emphasis on structure and details*

		Emphasis	
Age	Verbal ability	Structure	Details
Young	Average	27.2%	26.7%
	High	42.6%	38.6%
Middle-aged	Average	32.2%	28.9%
	High	38.9%	37.5%
Old	Average	19.6%	22.8%
	High	28.8%	37.4%

type of information remembered in response to different emphasis conditions. For this group of subjects, a 19% difference was found in the recalls of high- and low-level information with structure emphasized (main ideas = 48%; details = 29%); as seen earlier, only a 1% difference was found between the two levels without emphasis on the structure. It is interesting to note, in light of the findings of Meyer and Rice (1981a), that the only age comparison not showing age deficits for old adults was recall of details by high-verbal adults under emphasis conditions focused on details and away from structure (young = 37%; middle-aged = 35%; old = 36%).

From these data it is clear that high-verbal old adults can be highly sensitive to the levels in the organization of prose. However, their display of the levels effect is dependent on how clearly the structure of the text is emphasized and signaled. When this structure is not explicitly signaled and emphasis is placed on specific details, the older adults focus on these details and either are drawn away from the main ideas and logical relationships or are unable to identify these logical relationships without explicit cues (Cohen, 1979).

Table 12.7 examines this issue of age differences and details. The emphasis plans contrasted in Table 12.7 vary on signaling. Signaling (Meyer, 1975) is information in the text that does not add new content about a topic, but gives emphasis to certain aspects of the semantic content or points out aspects of the structure of the content. Signaling of the logical structure in a passage explicitly points these relationships out to the reader. Examples of signaling for comparison relationships include the use of phrases such as "in contrast," "however," "but," "on the other hand"; for causal relationships, examples include "therefore," "as a result," and so forth. Such signaling words explicitly signaled the top-level structure and major logical relationships for the reader in the structure-emphasized condition. Both passages were the same except that one signaled these logical relations and the other did not, but instead signaled specific details. The same specific details were contained in both conditions, but they were signaled by pointer words such as "important" or "notable" in the detail-

Table 12.8. *Effects of text variations in signaling and details on high-verbal old adults' recall of logical relations, main ideas, and details*

	Logical relations		Levels effect		
Text manipulation	Free	Cued	Main ideas −	Details =	Difference (%)
Signal structure + specific details	7.45	9.9	.46	.29	17
No signaling + specific details	5.45	5.9	.36	.34	2
No signals + signal specific details	5.55	7.8	.38	.37	1
Signal structure + general details	8.00	8.1	.50	.30	20
No signals + general details	6.15	8.2	.42	.31	11

emphasized condition. As seen in Table 12.7, only the old adults increased their recall of details when details were emphasized in this way. The high-verbal old adults were the only group who improved their recall of details substantially (8.6%) under these conditions varying on signaling. As seen in Table 12.7, young and old adults of high verbal ability were equivalent in their recall of details when they were emphasized, but when they were not emphasized, the old adults' recall of them fell, whereas the emphasis manipulation did not affect the young adults. The passage on parakeets used by Meyer and Rice (1981a) contains little signaling and many specific details (e.g., dates, names, numbers) and is not highly organized (it is a collection of descriptions concerning "Parakeets: Ideal Pets"); of its 641 words, only 14 (2%) are signaling words, and they do not signal logical relationships, but instead summarize the main point. In contrast, 26 (11%) of 242 words in the preceding passages with emphasized structure are signaling words, and they all signal logical relationships. Thus, the findings of Meyer and Rice (1981a) appear to be limited to high-verbal old adults, utilizing passages that contain historical dates, names, and other details, where the structure is not explicitly signaled.

The question remains whether the minimal levels effect exhibited by high-verbal older adults on passages without signaling and with emphasized details results from processing the details at the expense of the main ideas or simply from an inability to comprehend the logical relationships among the main ideas when they are not explicitly signaled. There is research literature on both sides of the latter issue; some studies show age deficits in making inferences (Cohen, 1979, 1981; Cohen & Faulkner, 1981), but others do not (Belmore, 1981; Burke & Yee, 1984). We systematically manipulated signaling of logical structure, signaling of details, and the specificity of details in order to answer this question. The detail manipulation involved substituting general details, such as "early last century," for specific details, such as "1820." We examined the magnitudes of the levels effects for high-verbal old adults (Table 12.8) to see if they processed details at the expense of logical relations and main ideas, thereby reducing the levels effect, or if instead they could not figure out logical relations without signaling, thereby decreasing their recall of main ideas and the magnitude of the levels effect. The data support the first explanation. The free-recall data for both the free condition and particularly the cued condition for logical relations indicate that high-verbal older adults can identify and store these relationships when they are not explicitly signaled (see the last condition listed in Table 12.8, where neither the structure nor the details are emphasized). When specific details are present and text structure is not emphasized, high-verbal old adults appear to process details at the expense of logical relationships and main ideas. The greater effects of these emphasis conditions on high-verbal old adults over high-verbal young adults may result from reduced cognitive capacity with aging (Hasher & Zacks, 1979; Light, Zelinski, & Moore, 1982; Zacks & Hasher, 1982), with the effort of processing details reducing that available for main ideas.

In summary, the three studies reviewed here (Mandel & Johnson, 1984; Meyer & Rice, 1981a, unpublished data) indicate that when the text is clearly organized, with emphasis on the structure and main ideas, young, middle, and old adults are sensitive to text structure. high-verbal adults of all ages show greater levels effects than do lower-verbal adults of all ages; high-verbal adults recall more main ideas and details than do lower-verbal adults, but are particularly superior in their recall of main ideas. Table 12.6 shows that average-verbal young adults and particularly high-verbal old adults show large levels effects (11% difference in percentage of recall of main ideas and details by average-verbal young adults, and 19% difference for high-verbal old adults) when the text structure is emphasized, but no levels effects (zero difference for young, 1% difference for old) when details are emphasized rather than the structure. However, this manipulation of emphasis has the least effect on the average-verbal old (10% differences in levels with structure emphasized versus 7% differences in levels without emphasis of the structure). As shown in Figure 12.4, average-verbal old adults do not show the facilitative effects of signaling for either free or cued recall of logical relations as do the other groups of adults. This, taken with their deficient use of top-level structure, as discussed earlier, suggests that even though they show a levels effect, they are deficient in some aspects of their utilization of text structure. In contrast to average-verbal old adults, high-verbal old adults are very sensitive to the emphasis plans of an author: When specific details in a passage are emphasized over the structure, these older adults appear to use their resources to process the details at the expense of fully processing the main ideas and logical relations. Thus, the different findings with respect to the levels effect for these three studies can be reconciled by examining the clarity of organization and emphasis of the prose and the verbal ability of the learners.

Hultsch and Dixon (1984) also attempted to reconcile the different findings of aging research with respect to the levels effect by examining prose organization and verbal ability. Three studies have examined age-related differences in recall for stories varying in degree of organization. Byrd (1981) had young and old adults listen to a normally organized story and a randomly organized story. For

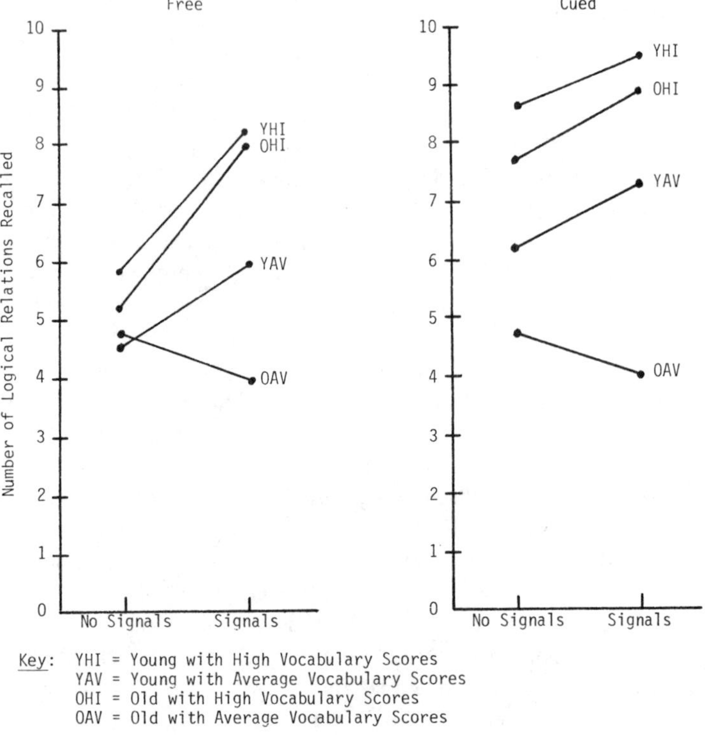

Figure 12.4. Number of logical relationships recalled under free-recall and cued-recall conditions by high- and average-verbal young and old adults from text with signals and without signals. (From Meyer & Rice, 1981b.)

the normal story, older adults recalled as many of the main ideas as did younger adults, but recalled fewer of the details. However, in the random-story condition, younger subjects recalled more of the main ideas of the story than did the older adults. Hultsch and Dixon (1984) interpreted these data as suggesting that with well-structured texts, age differences may be found at the subordinate level, whereas with less well structured texts, they may be found at the superordinate level. This is consistent with the findings for high-verbal adults cited earlier (Meyer & Rice, 1983a, unpublished data) if the passages with emphasized structure are classified as well structured and if those with no emphasis on structure, but specific details, are classified as less well structured.

Similarly, Smith and associates (1983) had young and old adults listen to four simple double-episode stories based on Mandler's story grammar. Three organizations were examined: (1) a normal story, (2) a less well organized interleaved story requiring extra effort to keep track of alternated information, and (3) a random story. No age differences were found for either the normal or random story, but old adults performed worse on the interleaved story. The young adults did as well with the interleaved story as with the standard story, whereas the interleaved story for the old looked like their scrambled versions. Again, this study points to greater age differences with poorly structured text. However, Mandel and Johnson (1984) looked at a similar manipulation for canonical versus noncanonical stories, and although they found inferior recall on the noncanonical stories, similar results were found for all age groups.

In considering verbal ability, Hultsch and Dixon (1984) argued that both their recent study (Dixon et al., 1984) and the literature support the claim that age differences in the use of organization in the text depend on the verbal ability of the subjects. Specifically, they stated that high-verbal college graduates showed greater age deficits for details (low-level information), whereas lower-verbal high school graduates showed greater deficits for main ideas. The study of Dixon and associates asked 108 young (20–39), middle-aged (40–57), and old (60–84) adults to read six short (98-word) passages about health and nutrition at their own paces. Young and middle-aged adults recalled more information than did old adults. The passages had five levels, as analyzed with the Kintsch approach. The five levels were collapsed into four levels: level 1, with 73% recall; level 2, with 48% recall; level 3, with 36% recall; level 4, with 34% recall. All comparisons among the levels were significant except that between levels 3 and 4; this is the typical levels-effect pattern, with high-level information recalled better than lower-level information. They reported an age-by-verbal-ability-by-level interaction. For high-verbal adults, the three age groups did not differ in their recall of level 1, but the young recalled more than did the middle-aged adults, and they both recalled more than did the old on the three lower levels. In contrast, the three lower-verbal groups differed significantly at level 1 and showed clear age deficits; for the other levels, the young and middle-aged subjects did not differ, but were superior to the old adults. Dixon and associates (1984) argued that other research also supports this pattern; Cohen (1979) and Dixon and associates (1982) found greater age deficits on main ideas and are believed to have tested low-verbal adults. That was the case for the Dixon and associates study. However, Cohen reported deficits in gist or main-idea recall for high-verbal adults; recall of details was not reported. Dixon and associates (1984) argued that Byrd (1981), Labouvie-Vief, Schell, and Weaverdyck (unpublished data cited in Dixon et al., 1984), Spilich (1983), and Zelinski and associates (1980) found greater deficits in recall of details and tested high-verbal college-educated adults. However, information on the types of subjects in terms of verbal ability and education is not available for the study of Zelinski and associates.

The one study that those investigators could not incorporate into this interaction was the Meyer and Rice (1981a) study, because in that study, with high-verbal college graduates, older adults recalled details as well as (free recall) or better than (questions) did young adults. Table 12.6 shows that this discrepancy can be clarified by examining the organization and emphasis of the texts. For the texts with emphasized structure, the pattern found by Dixon and associates (1984) held; for high-verbal adults, there was a 5% age deficit in old adults' recall of main ideas as compared with young adults, and the difference between the groups was 8% on details. In addition, the differences between young and old adults yielded an 11% age deficit for main ideas for average-verbal high school graduates, and a 10% age deficit on details. In contrast, on the versions with deemphasized structure and emphasized details, that pattern was reversed. For high-verbal adults, the results were consistent with those of Meyer and Rice (1981a); there was an 8% difference on main ideas, and a 1% difference on details. For the lower-verbal adults, there were greater age deficits on details (9% difference) than on main ideas (2% difference).

In summary, for text in which emphasis was placed on a well-organized structure, high-verbal young and older adults were sensitive to text structure; they exhibited large levels effects, and greater age-related deficiencies were found in recall of details. On these same types of text, old lower-verbal adults showed less sensitivity to text structure and exhibited greater deficits on main ideas. This may have been due to an encoding inefficiency problem similar to that found with list materials (Craik, 1977; Hultsch, 1974; Hultsch & Dixon, 1984). However, with text that deemphasized organization and emphasized details, the opposite pattern was found. For high-verbal adults, less severe age deficits were found for details than for main ideas. This appears to have been due to efforts to focus on details, which placed a greater drain on the resources of old high-verbal adults than on young high-verbal adults. For average-verbal adults, it appears that the greater age deficit for details than for main ideas reflected the young adults' deterioration in performance on main ideas when signaling was removed, whereas that manipulation had little effect on the old average-verbal adults.

The only other studies that have examined aging and the levels effect were conducted by Surber and associates (1984), Petros and associates (1983), and Zelinski and associates (1984). Surber and associates asked young and older adults of above average verbal ability (education levels not known) to read and recall a 1,563-word passage on commercial fishing. Young adults recalled more information overall and more information at the three most important levels than did old adults, but the two groups did not differ on the lowest-level details. Those results fit the pattern for text whose structure and main ideas are not clearly emphasized; perhaps that was the case for that lengthy passage. Petros and associates asked adults with high and low levels of education (no vocabulary data) to listen to two stories; they reported no interaction among age, level, and education, but scores were not available to examine the education groups with respect to age and level. However, when the data were collapsed over education, a pattern similar to that for high-verbal adults on well-structured text was found; greater aging deficits were found on the lowest-level details (young = .49; old = .37) than on the most important ideas (young = .87; old = .81). These authors pointed out that both age groups were sensitive to text structure, because levels effects were found for both groups.

The final study, by Zelinski and associates (1984), does not appear to fit neatly into the age-by-verbal-ability-by-organization interaction outlined earlier. Zelinski and associates (1980, 1984) had subjects recall passages analyzed with the Meyer (1975) prose-analysis procedure. However, Zelinski and associates reported different findings. For example, in a review by Hartley, Harker, and Walsh (1980), it was shown that Meyer and Rice (1981a) and Zelinski and associates (1980) found opposite results using the passage on parakeets. Zelinski and associates reported age deficits in recall of details, but not main ideas. However, this discrepancy was easily resolved, because Zelinski and associates shortened the passage and presented only information at levels 1 to 8, whereas Meyer and Rice presented information at 17 levels. Thus, the two studies showed similar patterns of recall for levels 1 to 8.

However, it appears more difficult to resolve certain differences found in the most recent study of Zelinski and associates (1984). The results from the three experiments in that study showed that there was no evidence for age-related differences in sensitivity to text structure for either essays or stories, regardless of education and verbal ability. In all three experiments, subjects read the passages to themselves as they listened to them spoken at a fast rate (155 wpm; Table 12.2). In the first experiment, juniors and seniors in high school were compared with high-school-educated old adults; age deficits were found in recall of a 209-word version of "Circle Island" (Dawes, 1966), and age did not interact with level (Meyer analysis technique). The samples selected in experiment I may have overestimated aging deficits, because the older adults had lower scores on the vocabulary test. In experiment II, high-verbal, college-educated young and old adults were asked to learn stories adapted from Thorndyke's (1977) "Old Farmer" stories and his version of "Circle Island." Again, age deficits were found, but there were no interactions between age and level.

The final experiment asked high-verbal, college-educated adults to learn and recall short and long versions of two passages from Meyer (1975). One passage was "Parakeets: Ideal Pets"; this is of particular interest because the entire passage was also used by Meyer and Rice (1981a) with similar subjects. Zelinski and associates reported recall from all or nearly all of the levels in the content structure, whereas Meyer and Rice divided the units into equivalent thirds. For the entire parakeet text, age deficits were found, as well as an age-by-level interaction; there were no age deficits at levels 1, 2, 6, 9, 10, and 12, but there were at the other levels. Zelinski and associates dismissed this interaction because it did not follow any pattern predicted or found by others. Figure 12.5 collapses their findings into the same thirds examined by Meyer and Rice and compares the data. The superior recall of low-level details for both young and old adults in the Zelinski and associates study is at variance with the findings for Meyer and Rice's young adults and at variance with most conceptions of the levels effect. Perhaps the differences in the findings can be explained by differences in presentation rate and mode. Meyer and Rice's subjects read the passages at their own rate; a fast presentation (by the reader in the oral presentation of the Zelinski and associates

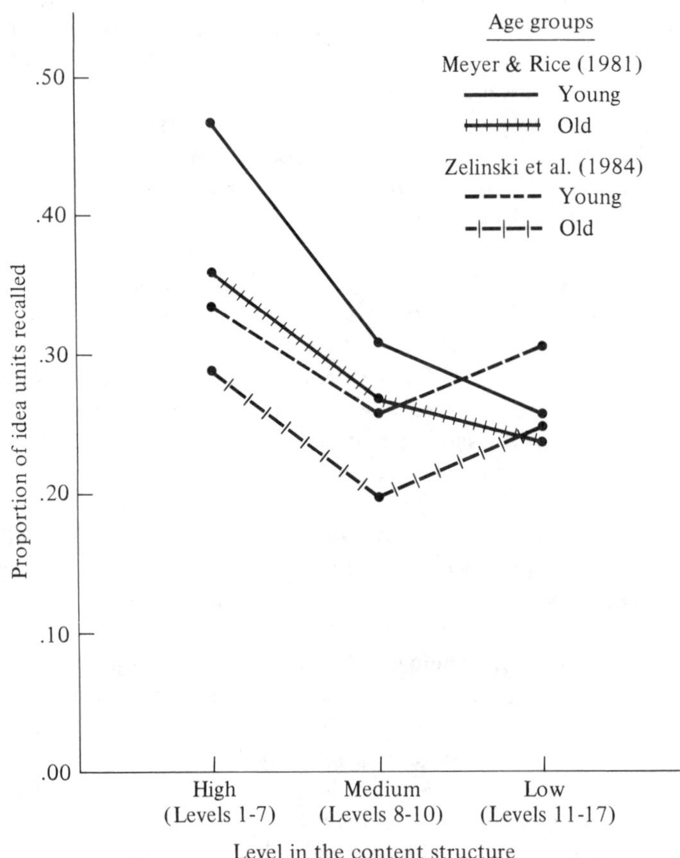

Figure 12.5. Proportion of idea units recalled from high, medium, and low levels in the content structure by young and old adults in studies conducted by Meyer and Rice (1981a) and Zelinski and associates (1984).

study) emphasizing certain low-level facts about parakeets may have been responsible for the differences; Cohen and Faulkner (1986) found stress to influence recall.

Conclusion

Many of the discrepancies in the literature with regard to the magnitudes of age deficits in prose learning can be explained by examining learner, task, and text variables. Some differences can be clarified by looking at the different levels of education and vocabulary skills among the samples of adults in different studies. Age deficits in prose learning were consistently found for adults with average or lower vocabulary scores and no education past high school. However, mixed results came from studies in which adults had high vocabulary scores and no education past high school. However, mixed results came from studies in which adults had high vocabulary scores and college educations. Apparently, vocabulary mediates age effects. In addition, some of the confusion can be clarified by considering the pacing of the prose materials. Greater age deficits were evident for faster presentation speed than for slower or self-paced presentation; a pace of 120 wpm or faster appeared to have an adverse effect on the recall of old adults, much more than for young adults. The materials read in prose learning experiments adequately reflected the everyday reading of adults, although tasks approximating writing a recall protocol rarely occur in everyday life. Everyday tasks requiring reading comprehension may be more practiced by older adults than are the recall tasks and may show lesser age deficits; we need creative ways to study these everyday situations involving reading comprehension among older adults.

Text variables can help to clarify the discrepancies in the literature. Some differences can occur because of the selection of a particular prose-analysis method. Most of the disparate findings concerning older adults' sensitivity to text structure can be understood by considering text organization, age, and verbal ability. The variable of emphasis in the text was shown to correlate with different findings reported by investigators. For text with emphasis placed on well-organized structure, young and old adults with high vocabulary scores were sensitive to text structure; they exhibited large levels effects, and greater age-related deficits were found in recall of details. On these same texts, old adults with average vocabulary scores showed less sensitivity to text structure and exhibited greater deficits on main ideas. However, with text that deemphasized organization and emphasized details, the opposite pattern was found. For highly verbal adults, less severe age deficits were found for details than for main ideas. For average-verbal adults, less severe age deficits were found for main ideas than for details. High-verbal old adults appeared to utilize text structure as well as did young adults. They showed facilitation in recall after listening to text structured with the more organized comparative structure, as compared with the less organized descriptive structure. They were very sensitive to the emphasis plans of an author. When specific details were emphasized over structure, old adults appeared to use their resources to process details at the expense of fully processing main ideas and logical relationships. Although average-verbal old adults showed some sensitivity to text structure by exhibiting a levels effect, they were deficient in other aspects of their use of text structure. These older adults tended to list things they remembered from a passage without attempting to interrelate them. They showed little sensitivity to manipulations of emphasis in the text.

In summary, this chapter has examined text, reader, and task variables that interact in the prose-comprehension process. Certain types of older adults under certain task conditions with certain types of texts can remember as much information from text as can younger adults. However, under the majority of reader, task, and text conditions tested so far in the laboratory, age-related declines in prose processing can be found. Further research will be needed to test the generality of these findings in more naturalistic settings.

References

Anderson, R. C., & Pearson, P. D. (1984). A schema-theoretic view of basic processes in reading. In P. D. Pearson (Ed.), *Handbook of reading research* (pp. 255–291). New York: Longman.

Anderson, R. C., & Pichert, J. W. (1978). Recall of previously unrecallable information following a shift in perspective. *Journal of Verbal Learning and Verbal Behavior, 17,* 1–12.

Anderson, R. C., Reynolds, R. E., Schallert, D. L., & Goetz, E. T. (1977). Frameworks for comprehending discourse. *American Educational Research Journal, 14,* 271–279.

Bartlett, F. C. (1932). *Remembering*. Cambridge University Press.

Belmore, S. M. (1981). Age-related changes in processing explicit and implicit language. *Journal of Gerontology, 36,* 316–322.

Birren, J. E. (1974). Translations in gerontology – from lab to life: Psychophysiology and speed of response. *American Psychologist, 29,* 808–815.

Birren J. E., & Morrison, D. F. (1961). Analysis of the WAIS subtests in relation to age and education. *Journal of Gerontology, 16,* 363–369.

Birren, J. E., Woods, A. M., & Williams, M. V. (1980). Behavioral slowing with aging: Causes, organization, and consequences. In L. W. Poon (Ed.), *Aging in the 1980's: Psychological issues* (pp. 293–308). Washington, DC: American Psychological Association.

Borgatta, E. F., & Corsini, R. J. (1964). *Manual for the Quick Word Test.* New york: Harcourt, Brace & World.

Botwinick, J. (1978). *Aging and behavior.* New York: Springer.

Botwinick, J., & Storandt, M. (1974). *Memory, related functions, and age.* Springifeld, IL: Charles C Thomas.

Bower, G. H. (1978). Experiments on story comprehension and recall. *Discourse Processes, 1,* 211–231.

Bransford, J. D., & Johnson, M. K. (1972). Contextual prerequisites for understanding: Some investigations of comprehension and recall. *Journal of Verbal Learning and Verbal Behavior, 11,* 717–726.

Bransford, J. D., & McCarrell, N. S. (1974). A sketch of a cognitive approach to comprehension. In W. Wiemer & D. S. Palermo (Eds.), *Cognition and the symbolic processes* (Vol. 1, pp. 189–230). Hillsdale, NJ: Lawrence Erlbaum.

Brewer, W. F. (1980). Literary theory, rhetoric, and stylistics: Implications for psychology. In R. J. Spiro, B. C. Bruce & W. F. Brewer (Eds.), *Theoretical issues in reading comprehension* (pp. 221–243). Hillsdale, NJ: Lawrence Erlbaum.

Brown, A. L., & Smiley, N. S. (1978). The development of strategies for studying texts. *Child Development, 49,* 1076–1088.

Burke, D. M., & Yee, P. L. (1984). Semantic priming during sentence processing by young and older adults. *Developmental Psychology, 20,* 903–910.

Byrd, M. (1981). *Age differences in memory for prose passages.* Unpublished doctoral dissertation, University of Toronto.

Charness, N. (1983). Age, skill, and bridge bidding: A chronometric analysis. *Journal of Verbal Learning and Verbal Behavior, 22,* 406–416.

Cohen, G. (1979). Language comprehension in old age. *Cognitive Psychology, 11,* 412–429.

Cohen, G. (1981). Inferential reasoning in old age. *Cognition, 9,* 59–72.

Cohen, G., & Faulkner, D. (1981). Memory for discourse in old age. *Discourse Processes, 4,* 253–265.

Cohen, G., & Faulkner, D. (1983). Memory for text: Some age differences in the nature of information that is retained after listening to text. In H. Bouman & D. Bouwhuis (Eds.), *Attention and performance*. Hillsdale, NJ: Lawrence Erlbaum.

Cohen, G., & Faulkner, D. (1986). Does "elderspeak" work? The effect of intonation and stress on comprehension and recall of spoken discourse in old age. *Brain and Language, 6,* 91–98.

Craik, F. I. M. (1977). Age differences in human memory. In J. E. Birren & K. W. Schaie (Eds.), *Handbook of the psychology of aging* (pp. 384–420). New York: Van Nostrand Reinhold.

Dale, E., & Chall, J. S. (1948). A formula for predicting readability. *Educational Research Bulletin, 11–20,* 37–59.

D'Angelo, F. J. (1976). The search for intelligible structure in the teaching of composition. *College Composition and Communication, 27,* 142–147.

Dawes, R. (1966). Memory and distortion of meaningful verbal material. *British Journal of Psychology, 57,* 77–86.

Dixon, R. A., Hultsch, D. F., Simon, E. W., & von Eye, A. (1984). Verbal ability and text structure effects on adult age differences in text recall. *Journal of Verbal Learning and Verbal Behavior, 23,* 569–578.

Dixon, R. A., Simon, E. W., Nowak, C. A., & Hultsch, D. F. (1982). Text recall in adulthood as a function of level of information, input modality, and delay interval. *Journal of Gerontology, 37,* 358–364.

Dooling, D. J., & Lachman, R. (1971). Effects of comprehension on retention of prose. *Journal of Experimental Psychology, 88,* 216–222.

Duell, O. K. (1974). Effect of type of objective, level of test questions, and judged importance of tested materials upon post-test performance. *Journal of Educational Psychology, 66,* 225–232.

Dunn, B. R. (1985). Bimodal processing and memory from text. In V. M. Rentel (Ed.), *Psychophysiologic aspects of reading.* London: Pergamon Press.

Ekstrom, R. B., French, J. W., Harman, H. H., & Derman, D. (1976). *Manual for kit of factor-referenced cognitive tests.* Princeton, NJ: Educational Testing Service.

Gilbert, J. G. (1941). Memory loss in senescence. *Journal of Abnormal and Social Psychology, 36,* 73–86.

Glynn, S. M., Okun, M. A., Muth, K. D., & Britton, B. K. (1983). Adults' text recall: An examination of the age-deficit hypothesis. *Journal of Reading Behavior, 15,* 31–45.

Gordon, S. K., & Clark, W. C. (1974). Application of signal detection theory to prose recall and recognition in elderly and young adults. *Journal of Gerontology, 29,* 64–72.

Harker, J. O., Hartley, J. T., & Walsh, D. A. (1982). Understanding discourse – a life-span approach. In B. A. Hutson (Ed.), *Advances in reading/language research* (Vol. 1, pp. 155–202). Greenwich, CT: JAI Press.

Hartley, J. T., Harker, J. O., & Walsh, D. A. (1980). Contemporary issues and new directions in adult development of learning and memory. In L. W. Poon (Ed.), *Aging in the 1980's* (pp. 239–252). Washington, DC: American Psychological Association.

Hasher, L., & Zacks, R. T. (1979). Automatic and effortful processes in memory. *Journal of Experimental Psychology, 108,* 356–388.

Hultsch, D. F. (1974). Learning to learn in adulthood. *Journal of Gerontology, 29,* 302–308.

Hultsch, D. F., & Dixon, R. A. (1983). The role of pre-experimental knowledge in text processing in adulthood. *Experimental Aging Research, 9,* 17–22.

Hultsch, D. F., & Dixon, R. A. (1984). Memory for text materials in adulthood. In P. B. Baltes & O. G. Brim, Jr. (Eds.), *Life-span development and behavior* (Vol. 6, pp. 77–108). New York: Academic Press.

Hultsch, D. F., Hertzog, C., & Dixon, R. A. (1984). Text recall in adulthood: The role of intellectual abilities. *Developmental Psychology, 20,* 1193–1209.

Johnson, R. E. (1970). Recall of prose as a function of the structural importance of the linguistic units. *Journal of Verbal Learning and Verbal Behavior, 9,* 12–20.

King, D. J. (1968). Retention of connected meaningful material as a function of modes of presentation and recall. *Journal of Experimental Psychology, 77,* 676–683.

Kintsch, W. (1974). *The representation of meaning in memory.* Hillsdale, NJ: Lawrence Erlbaum.

Kintsch, W., & Keenan, J. M. (1973). Reading rate as a function of number of propositions in the base structure of sentences. *Cognitive Psychology, 6,* 257–274.

Kintsch, W., Kozminsky, E., Streby, W. J., McKoon, G., & Keenan, J. M. (1975). Comprehension and recall of text as a function of content variables. *Journal of Verbal Learning and Verbal Behavior, 14,* 196–214.

Kintsch, W., & van Dijk, T. A. (1978). Toward a model of text comprehension and production. *Psychological Review, 85,* 363–394.

Krauss, I. K. (1980). Between- and within-group comparisons in aging research. In L. W. Poon (Ed.), *Aging in the 1980's* (pp. 542–551). Washington, DC: American Psychological Association.

Labouvie-Vief, G., Schell, D. A., & Weaverdyck, S. E. (1981). *Recall deficit in the aged: A fable recalled.* Unpublished manuscript, Wayne State University, Detroit, MI.

Light, L. L., Zelinski, E. M., & Moore, M. (1982). Adult age differences in reasoning from new information. *Journal of Experimental Psychology: Learning, Memory, and Cognition, 8,* 435–447.

Longacre, R. E. (1968). *Discourse, paragraph, and sentence structure in selected Philippine languages* (Vol. 1). Santa Ana: Summer Institute of Linguistics.

Mandel, R. G., & Johnson, N. S. (1984). A developmental analysis of story recall and comprehension in adulthood. *Journal of Verbal Learning and Verbal Behavior, 23,* 643–659.

Mandler, J. M., & Johnson, N. S. (1977). Remembrance of things parsed: Story structure and recall. *Cognitive Psychology, 9,* 111–151.

Mayer, R. E. (1985). Structural analysis of science prose: Can we increase problem-solving performance? In B. K. Britton & J. Black (Eds.), *Understanding expository text* (pp. 65–87). Hillsdale, NJ: Lawrence Erlbaum.

Meyer, B. J. F. (1975) *The organization of prose and its effects on memory.* Amsterdam: North Holland.

Meyer, B. J. F. (1977). The structure of prose: Effects on learning and memory and implications for educational practice. In R. C. Anderson, R. Spiro, & W. Montague (Eds.), *Schooling and the acquisition of knowledge* (pp. 179–200). Hillsdale, NJ: Lawrence Erlbaum.

Meyer, B. J. F. (1983). Text structure and its use in studying comprehension across the adult life span. In B. A. Hutson (Ed.), *Advances in reading/language research* (Vol. 2, pp. 9–54). Greenwich, CT: JAI Press.

Meyer, B. J. F. (1984). Text dimensions and cognitive processing. In H. Mandl, N. Stein, & T. Trabasso (Eds.), *Learning from texts* (pp. 3–52). Hillsdale, NJ: Lawrence Erlbaum.

Meyer, B. J. F. (1985). Prose analysis: Procedures, purposes, and problems. In B. K. Britton & J. Black (Eds.), *Understanding expository text* (pp. 11–64, 269–304). Hillsdale, NJ: Lawrence Erlbaum.

Meyer, B. J. F., Brandt, D. M., & Bluth, G. J. (1980). Use of the top-level structure in text: Key for reading comprehension of ninth-grade students. *Reading Research Quarterly, 16,* 72–103.

Meyer, B. J. F., & Freedle, R. O. (1984). The effects of different discourse types on recall. *American Educational Research Journal, 21,* 121–143.

Meyer, B. J. F., & McConkie, G. W. (1973). What is recalled from prose after hearing a passage? *Journal of Educational Psychology, 65,* 109–117.

Meyer, B. J. F., & Rice, G. E. (1981a). Information recalled from prose by young, middle, and old adults. *Experimental Aging Research, 7,* 253–268.

Meyer, B. J. F., & Rice, G. E. (1981b). *Organizational strategies in prose comprehension across the adult life span.* Paper presented at a meeting of the American Psychological Association, Los Angeles.

Meyer, B. J. F., & Rice, G. E. (1982). The interaction of reader strategies and the organization of text. *Text, 2,* 155–192.

Meyer, B. J. F., & Rice, G. E. (1983a). Learning and memory from text across the adult life span. In J. Fine & R. O. Freedle (Eds.), *Developmental studies in discourse* (pp. 291–306). Norwood, NJ: Ablex.

Meyer, B. J. F., & Rice, G. E. (1983b). *Effects of discourse type on recall by young, middle and old adults with high and average vocabulary scores.* Paper presented at the National Reading Conference, Austin, TX.

Meyer, B. J. F., & Rice, G. E. (1984). The structure of text. In P. D. Pearson (Ed.), *Handbook of reading research* (pp. 319–352). New York: Longman.

Meyer, B. J. F., Rice, G. E., Knight, C. C. & Jessen, J. L. (1979). *Effects of comparative and descriptive discourse types on the reading performance of young, middle, and old adults.* (Prose Learning Series #7). Department of Educational Psychology, Arizona State University, Tempe.

Meyer, B. J. F., Young, C. J., & Bartlett, B. J. (1986). *A prose learning strategy: Effects on old and young adults.* Paper presented at a meeting of the American Psychological Association, Washington, DC.

Miller, J. F., & Kintsch, W. (1980) Readability and recall of short prose passages: A theoretical analysis. *Journal of Experimental Psychology: Human Learning and Memory, 6,* 335–354.

Neisser, U. (1982). *Memory observed.* San Francisco: Freeman.

Neisser, U., & Hupcey, J. (1974). A Sherlockian experiment. *Cognition, 3,* 307–311.

Owens, J., Dafoe, J., & Bower, G. (1977). *Taking a point of view: Character identification and attributional processes in story comprehension and memory.* Paper presented at a meeting of the American Psychological Association, San Francisco.

Petros, T., Tabor, L., Cooney, T., & Chabot, R. J. (1983). Adult age differences in sensitivity to semantic structure of prose. *Developmental Psychology, 19,* 907–914.

Pichert, J. W., & Anderson, R. C. (1977). Taking different perspectives on a story. *Journal of Educational Psychology, 69,* 309–315.

Poon, L. W., Krauss, I. K., & Bowles, N. L. (1984). On subject selection in cognitive aging research. *Experimental Aging Research, 10,* 43–49.

Rice, G. E. (1980). On cultural schemata. *American Ethnologist,7,* 152–171.

Rice, G. E. (in press). The everyday activities of adults: Implications for prose recall, Part II. *Educational Gerontology.*

Rice, G. E., & Meyer, B. J. F. (1985). Reading behavior and prose recall performance of young and older adults with high and average verbal ability. *Educational Gerontology, 11,* 57–72.

Rice, G. E., & Meyer, B. J. F. (in press). Prose recall: Effects of aging, verbal ability, and reading behavior. *Journal of Gerontology.*

Rumelhart, D. E. (1977). Understanding and summarizing brief stories. In D. LaBerge & S. J. Samuels (Eds.), *Basic processes in reading: Perception and comprehension* (pp. 265–303). Hillsdale, NJ: Lawrence Erlbaum.

Salthouse, T. A. (1982). *Adult cognition: An experimental psychology of human aging.* New York: Springer-Verlag.

Schneider, N. G., Gritz, E. R., & Jarvik, M. E. (1975). Age differences in learning, immediate and one-week delayed recall. *Gerontologia, 21,* 10–20.

Simon, E. W., Dixon, R. A., Nowak, C. A., & Hultsch, D. F. (1982). Orienting task effects on text recall in adulthood. *Journal of Gerontology, 31,* 575–580.

Smith, S. W., Rebok, G. W., Smith, W. R., Hall, S. E., & Alvin, M. (1983). Adult age differences in the use of story structure in delayed free recall. *Experimental Aging Research, 9,* 191–195.

Spilich, G. J. (1983). Life-span components of text processing; Structural and procedural differences. *Journal of Verbal Learning and Verbal Behavior, 22,* 231–244.

Spilich, G. J., Vesonder, G. T., Chiesi, H. S., & Voss, J. F. (1979). Text processing of domain-related information for individuals with high and low domain knowledge. *Journal of Verbal Learning and Verbal Behavior, 18,* 275–290.

Spilich, G. J., & Voss, J. F. (1982). Contextual effects upon text memory for young, aged-normal, and aged memory-impaired individuals. *Experimental Aging Research, 8,* 45–49.

Spiro, R. J. (1977). Remembering information from text: The "state of schema" approach. In R. C. Anderson, R. J. Spiro, & W. E. Montague (Eds.), *Schooling and the acquisition of knowledge* (pp. 137–166). Hillsdale, NJ: Lawrence Erlbaum.

Spiro, R. J. (1978). *Individual differences in discourse processing*. Paper presented at a meeting of the Pacific Region Reading Research Symposium, Tucson.

Steffensen, M. S., & Colker, L. (1982). *Intercultural misunderstandings about health care: Recall of descriptions of illness and treatment* (Technical Report No. 233). Center for the Study of Reading, University of Illinois, Urbana-Champaign.

Sticht, T. G., & James, J. H. (1984). Listening and reading. In P. D. Pearson (Ed.), *Handbook of reading research* (pp. 293–318). New York: Longman.

Stone, D. E., & Glock, M. D. (1981). How do young adults read directions with and without pictures? *Journal of Educational Psychology, 73*, 419–426.

Surber, J. R., Kowalski, A. H., & Pena-Paez, A. (1984). Effects of aging on recall of extended expository prose. *Experimental Aging Research, 10*, 25–28.

Taub, H. A. (1975). Mode of presentation, age, and short-term memory. *Journal of Gerontology, 30*, 56–59.

Taub, H. A. (1976). Method of presentation of meaningful prose to young and old adults. *Experimental Aging Research, 2*, 469–474.

Taub, H. A. (1979). Comprehension and memory of prose materials by young and old adults. *Experimental Aging Reserach, 5*, 3–13.

Taub, H. A., & Kline, G. E. (1976). Modality effects on memory in the aged. *Educational Gerontology, 1*, 53–66.

Taub, H. A., & Kline, G. E. (1978). Recall of prose as a function of age and input modality. *Journal of Gerontology, 33*, 725–730.

Taylor, B. M. (1980). Children's memory for expository text after reading. *Reading Research Quarterly, 15*, 399–411.

Thorndyke, P. W. (1977). Cognitive structures in comprehension and memory of narrative discourse. *Cognitive Psychology, 9*, 77–110.

Vincent, J. P. (1985). *Effects of discourse types on memory of prose by young, middle-age, and old adults with average vocabularies.* Unpublished doctoral dissertation, Arizona State University, Tempe.

Wechsler, D. (1955). *Manual for the Wechsler Adult Intelligence Scale*. New York: Psychological Corporation.

Wingfield, A., Poon, L. W., Lombardi, L., & Lowe, D. (1985). Speed of processing in normal aging: Effects of speech rate, linguistic structure and processing time. *Journal of Gerontology, 40*, 579–585.

Young, C. J. (1983). *Integration of facts across textual distances by young and old adults.* Unpublished thesis, Arizona State University, Tempe.

Zacks, R. T., & Hasher, L. (1982). *Young and elderly adults' memory for explicit and inferential information.* Paper presented at a meeting of the Psychonomic Society.

Zelinski, E. M., Gilewski, M. J., & Thompson, L. W. (1980). Do laboratory tests relate to self-assessment of memory ability in the young and old? In L. W. Poon, J. L. Fozard, L. S. Cermak, D. Arenberg, & L. W. Thompson (Eds.), *New directions in memory and aging: Proceedings of the George A. Talland memorial conference* (pp. 519–550. Hillsdale, NJ: Lawrence Erlbaum.

Zelinski, E. M., Light, L. L., & Gilewski, M. J. (1984). Adult age differences in memory for prose: The question of sensitivity to passage structure. *Developmental Psychology, 20*, 1181–1192.

13 Speech comprehension and memory through adulthood: The roles of time and strategy

Elizabeth Lotz Stine, Arthur Wingfield, and Leonard W. Poon

Comprehension of spoken language involves rapid construction of meaning from a transitory acoustic signal, the complexity of which can easily be overlooked. In ordinary conversation, speech rates may average between 100 and 180 words per minute (wpm), and a speaker reading aloud can easily average over 200 wpm. In addition, the words in spoken discourse often are unclear or garbled (Pollack & Pickett, 1963). In spite of these challenges, phonemic and syntactic structures interact with semantic and contextual contraints to produce the perception of an intelligible message in "real time" (Marslen-Wilson & Tyler, 1980). That is, unlike reading, in which the viewer may backtrack and proceed at a comfortable rate, speech is heard at the rate produced by the speaker. Not only must this complex acoustic signal be understood phonologically at this extraordinary rate, but also the utterances must be further analyzed into the sentences and propositional representations that give rise to meaning.

Whereas older adults often suffer from deficits in auditory processing (Olsho, Harkins, & Lenhardt, 1985), it has also been argued that they have particular difficulty with tasks requiring "deeper," more effortful processing operations (Craik & Simon, 1980) and are slower in performing many cognitive operations (Salthouse, 1980, 1982). For these reasons, it might seem surprising that older adults are not more often noticed to have trouble in understanding everyday speech (e.g., in conversation, from television or radio). We would like to argue that the answer to this paradox lies in the elderly listener's ability to use higher-order contextual structures to frame and interpret lower-order phonological information. In this chapter we attempt to develop this position by reviewing current perspectives on speech and speech processing and considering what is known about how older adults process the information in speech.

The research reported in this chapter was supported by PHS grant AG04517 from the National Institutes of Health. We are grateful to our colleagues both at Brandeis University and at the Mental Performance and Aging Laboratory, Veterans Administration Hospital, Boston, Massachusetts, for their help and advice in all stages of this research.

On-line speech processing

Consider for a moment the interpretive difficulties faced by any listener. As we have indicated, individual words in ordinary conversation are not always optimally pronounced. In a dramatic illustration of this point, Pollack and Pickett (1963) tape-recorded samples of normal conversational speech and then tested the intelligibility of isolated words removed from these tapes. Not only were many of these words unintelligible; in many cases they hardly sounded like words at all. When these words were reinserted into the fluent speech, however, they were again heard to be crystal clear and unambiguously the correct words as intended by the speaker. In the modern idiom, the processing of spoken language represents a complex interaction between "bottom-up" and "top-down" processes.

In the context of speech comprehension, *bottom-up processing* means that the acoustic signal must be processed upward from the level of the acoustic waveform to the level of recognition of word elements and words and then to idea units, which convey meaning. *Top-down processing* means that the context available from the speech already heard, along with one's world knowledge, may facilitate one's perception of speech yet to be heard.

To say that context plays a major role in immediate language processing does not, of course, specify how such top-down and bottom-up processes ordinarily interact. Some of these operations may occur "on-line," affecting perceptual and linguistic decisions as the speech is being heard. Other operations may occur "off-line," in the form of retrospective or interpretive analyses that occur some time after the acoustic signal has been received and has been given preliminary analysis (Bierwisch, 1983; Frazier & Fodor, 1978; Marslen-Wilson & Tyler, 1980). These points can be best illustrated by considering the ordinary demands of reading and listening.

Differential input characteristics of reading and listening

Top-down processing of language input is necessary regardless of modality, but certain features of speech make this even more crucial for the comprehension of spoken language. Everyday reading and listening are ecologically very different, both in the quality of the stimulus input and in the nature of their processing. One striking difference between reading and listening is that the input for listening is *sequential*. Unlike reading, in which the eyes dart between word groups or glance back for missing information, the listener is obliged to hear speech word by word in the order that the message is delivered.

The listener therefore has much less control over the input than does the reader. In the course of everyday conversation, the listener often does have some broad control over the speaker's productions through the use of verbal and nonverbal signals (Bohannon, Stine, & Ritzenberg, 1982; Brown & Yule, 1983; Stine & Bohannon, 1983), but there are many listening situations (e.g., radio, movies, television) in which the listener has no control whatever over the speech input (except perhaps to end it). This can also occur with reading (e.g., subtitles in a foreign-language film), but it is rare. One feature of speech that varies quite naturally in the environment beyond the control of the listener is the rate at which it is spoken.

From the researcher's point of view, another difference between listening and reading is that in listening, the immediate input that the subject experiences is overt. That is, in the course of speech, we can more easily know the exact time of arrival of the stimulus elements.

These characteristics of speech (1, linear input; 2, variable rate; 3, input that is accessible to the researcher) are features that work to the experimenter's advantage in the study of real-world language comprehension. Features 1 and 3 are desirable experimental controls, and feature 2 is a natural independent variable—an experiment designed by God herself.

Brown and Yule (1983) have contrasted the typical uses of speech with those of written text: (1) Speech typically is interactional, whereas written text usually is transactional. That is, whereas written text usually is used to convey information, spoken language often is used to negotiate social relationships. (2) In a variety of ways, speech is less structured. In speech, we do not always complete our sentences; we make repairs and changes as we go (which is absolutely inappropriate in written communication). We also use less rhetorical organization in spoken language (e.g., terms such as "however," "in conclusion"). (3) Because of its predominance of simple declarative statements, its fewer noun phrases with series of premodifiers, and its more repetition of syntactic forms, speech generally is simpler (simpler than this sentence, for example). (4) Speech tends to be less precise, containing more generalized vocabulary (e.g., "things," "stuff," "place"), more prefabricated fillers (e.g., "um," "you know"), and more ambiguous referents that can be inferred from shared context.

Even though reading and listening vary along a number of dimensions, the ultimate representation of knowledge probably is not affected by input modality (Kintsch & Kozminsky, 1977). We reiterate, however, that the ecologies for these two inputs often are very different, and it is these differences that make context especially critical for everyday speech comprehension.

Speech sounds and lexical processing

Numerous studies have supported the contention that higher-level interpretive processing places constraints on and facilitates the perception of lower-level information. For example, a word embedded in noise is more intelligible if it is framed by a normal sentence than if framed by an anomalous sentence (Miller & Isard, 1963). We have already seen an example of the importance of top-down processing in speech comprehension in the work of Pollack and Pickett (1963), in which words were excerpted from tape recordings of fluent conversation. In that case, the ambiguous signal was a naturally occurring phenomenon. As we have indicated, individual words, especially unstressed words, often are poorly articulated in spoken discourse and would be unintelligible if heard in isolation. In the case of Pollack and Pickett's study, the intelligibility of these poorly articulated words increased monotonically with the number of prior words of context listeners were allowed to hear.

Another powerful illustration of the use of linguistic context is the phonemic-restoration effect (Warren, 1970). In this phenomenon, subjects hear the speech as normal even though a phoneme has been replaced by a cough or by "white noise." Not only do subjects experience the illusion of hearing the phoneme; they are even unable to determine the location of the extraneous cough. The strength of this illusion is confirmed by the fact that listeners hear the phoneme even when they are told in advance that a phoneme has been replaced. It would seem, then, that the listener has little choice but to interpret phonemic information in light of surrounding context.

In fact, the listener is so dependent on linguistic context that when this context is not available, perception may become unstable (Warren, 1961a). When a single, clearly pronounced word (e.g., "see") was recorded over and over again and presented to naive listeners, the word seemed to change periodically (e.g., "see," "cease," "beast," "beef," "this," "next please"). This verbal-transformation effect suggests not only that it may be impossible to understand continuous phonemic input that is not framed by context but also that this perceptual transformation may be an attempt by the listener to reorganize stored auditory input in order to find some context.

The use of context is especially important in *rapid* processing of speech. Word recognition in context can occur within 200 msec of a word's onset. This was first demonstrated by Marslen-Wilson (1975), who measured the speed with which subjects would (often unconsciously) correct speech errors when shadowing recordings of spoken prose. This time estimate was subsequently confirmed by Grosjean (1980) in his "gating" studies. Subjects were presented with the first 50 msec of a word and asked to identify it. If the subjects failed to do so, they were given the first 100 msec, then the first 150 msec, and so on, with the size of the "gate" systematically increased until correct recognition was obtained. Grosjean found that words in context could be recognized within 175 to 200 msec of onset—when only half or less of the full acoustic signal had been heard. The average figure for words out of context was 333 msec. To put these figures in perspective, 202 msec would represent the mean duration of a word-initial CV in English (Sorensen, Cooper, & Paccia, 1978).

Furthermore, it has been shown that the number of word-initial segments necessary for correct identification must be increased when the quality of the speech is poor or degraded (e.g., whereas the word *elephant* may ordinarily be recognizable from just *eleph,* the usually redundant *ant* may be necessary under poor listening conditions) (Nooteboom & Doodeman, 1984). Good reviews of the current models suggested to account for how an acoustic waveform triggers categorical identities of words, and how context facilitates this process, have been provided by Marslen-Wilson (1984) and Marcus (1984).

When there are multiple levels of information present, the speech signal contains considerable *redundancy* that is used to facilitate rapid processing. In fact, Miller and Licklider (1950) have shown that as much as 50% of the speech signal can be deleted while still maintaining the intelligibility of monosyllabic words at 90%. Certainly, our ability to comprehend speech does not seem to depend on our ability to understand individual words, because, as we have seen, many words excerpted from everyday conversation and presented individually are totally unintelligible (Pollack & Pickett, 1963). Rather, speech comprehension is a more global process that depends on the extraordinary richness of the acoustic signal.

Working vocabulary contributes to this redundancy. A university-educated adult has a comprehension vocabulary of somewhere between 75,000 and 100,000 words (Oldfield, 1963). However, only a small part of this larger vocabulary is routinely used in ordinary discourse. Clearly, some words are used more frequently than others, and we rarely go beyond 10 or 15 words without repeating a word. In fact, the 50 most commonly used words in English account for about 60% of all the words we speak, and about 45% of those we write (Miller, 1951). The redundancy of English on the lexical level has been estimated to run between 30% and 50% as measured by words that can be totally removed without changing the meaning of a sentence beyond recovery (Chapanis, 1954). These latter figures are based on samples of written text; we know of no comparable data for spoken discourse.

Processing spoken sentences and discourse

At the sentence level, the listener continually makes decisions about the structure of the speech, determining, among other features, clause boundaries that ordinarily complete functional, or semantic, relationships. This process of sentential parsing can seem so automatic that it often goes unnoticed until something goes wrong. The so-called garden-path sentence, such as "The old man the boats," is a good example. On a first pass, one can easily take the word *old* as the modifier of the noun *man,* with *the old man* taken as a full noun phrase. Our discovery of a second *the* instead of an expected verb thus causes major confusion. To comprehend the sentence, we must retrospectively rework the entire sentence to recode *man* as the verb it was intended to be. In this example, we have an off-line reinterpretation correcting an initial on-line error induced by a not unreasonable expectation of a more usual structure than the one actually encountered.

"Basic units" in language processing. One can imagine two possible extremes in the operations required to process spoken discourse. One possibility is that we register and hold in working memory whole sentences or clauses before beginning any serious interpretive processing for deep structure or meaning. The other extreme is represented by a left-to-right word-by-word analysis for meaning in an

ongoing cumulative fashion as each new word is heard. The former would imply inordinate demands on working memory and would deny the fact that we do have momentary expectations about what may be heard at the level of the word. The second alternative, on the other hand, would produce innumerable mistakes in comprehension based on incomplete thoughts and would also imply extraordinarily rapid processing at multiple levels of analysis.

Of course, neither extreme, in the simple form we have put it here, has ever been proposed, although theorists have sometimes emphasized the importance of syntactic or functional clauses as major ''units'' of language perception (Carroll & Tannenhaus, 1978; Fodor, Bever, & Garrett, 1974) and at other times have emphasized the continuous nature of on-line syntactic and semantic analysis of speech as it is being heard (Marslen-Wilson & Tyler, 1980). It is probably the case that there are elements of both strategies in natural language processing, although they may well operate in parallel or overlapping fashion at different levels of analysis.

There is evidence to support the importance of analysis at the level of the linguistic or functional clause in active language processing (Carroll & Tannenhaus, 1978; Fodor et al., 1974; Jarvella, 1973). There also is evidence that listeners continually form hypotheses about the meaning and structure of what they are hearing on a moment-to-moment basis, making predictions about what they have yet to hear (Grosjean, 1983; Marslen-Wilson & Tyler, 1980). In the latter case, of course, these will have to be working hypotheses, either confirmed or denied on the arrival of new information (Wingfield & Nolan, 1980).

The process we find ourselves describing is that of a temporally continuous, on-line analysis of the speech stream, but one that nevertheless involves a knowledge-driven search for completion of functional semantic relationships. These points, invariably sentence and clause boundaries, serve as crucial decision points for higher-level analyses at the propositional and discourse level to further guide the continuing speech analysis. We leave many open questions. Which of these operations are automatic, and which involve higher-level inferential processes? Which are truly on-line operations, and which represent more retrospective, off-line operations? How do these operations array themselves or overlap temporally? The details of such a multilevel organization must be complex and have yet to be fully developed in any single processing model (Frazier & Fodor, 1978; Marslen-Wilson & Tyler, 1980; van Dijk & Kintsch, 1983).

Prosody. It often takes a peculiar case such as a garden-path sentence for us to appreciate our natural tendency to actively parse linguistic input into its linguistic constituents, as well as the supplemental role that prosodic features can play in this process. ''Prosody'' is used here as an inclusive term that can be decomposed into a variety of acoustic features that ordinarily correlate with linguistic structure. One such feature is the overall pitch contour of a sentence, which is essentially the variation in its fundamental frequency (f_0) over time. Other prosodic features include word stress, pauses at the ends of major syntactic elements, and the lengthening of final vowels in words immediately prior to a clause boundary (Cooper & Sorensen, 1981; Lehiste, 1970). Prosody can indicate the semantic focus of a sentence (Jackendoff, 1972), disambiguate an otherwise ambiguous sentence (Wales & Toner, 1979), act as an aid to on-line parsing of a sentence into its constituent elements (Wingfield, 1975a, 1975b), or allow us to predict the entire length of an utterance we have yet to hear in full (Grosjean, 1983).

It would be misleading to suggest that linguistic constituents are parsed on the basis of their prosodic patterns alone. Even when prosodic features and linguistic structure are put in direct conflict, anomalous prosodic marking can be ignored when it is misleading (Wingfield, 1975b). It is safe to say, however, that prosodic marking facilitates correct parsing and adds a sometimes valuable source of redundancy to an already rich acoustic signal. Indeed, prosodic cues are themselves redundant to the extent that the absence of any one prosodic feature can be compensated for (at least partially) by the presence of others (Cutler & Darwin, 1981; Streeter, 1978; Wingfield, Lombardi & Sokol, 1984).

In summary, the transient nature of the speech signal necessitates that it be redundant to some extent. In fact, speech is an extraordinarily rich acoustic signal that the listener interprets on-line at several different levels. Even though lower-level phonemic information may be deficient, the listener constructs a coherent message from syntactic, semantic, and prosodic context.

Age differences in speech comprehension and memory

There are several reasons a priori that we might expect elderly adults to have difficulty with speech processing. As we have already stressed, the on-line nature of the speech signal requires the listener to perform word recognition and parsing operations quickly. These processes can pose problems for the elderly, who have been found to be slower in performing many cognitive operations (Birren, Woods, & Williams, 1980; Salthouse, 1980) and to have difficulty with organization in working memory (Smith, 1980). It is also known that at the most elemental level of speech comprehension, the elderly may have difficulty in simply hearing the signal. In fact, the effects of *presbycusis* are not trivial. There are various changes that occur in the auditory system in older adults that impact on the comprehension of language.

Presbycusis

Presbycusis (literally, "old hearing") has several features, including (1) loss of sensitivity, particularly in the higher frequency ranges of hearing, (2) an increased probability of recruitment, and (3) an increased probability of phonemic regression. Even though it has been estimated that only about 13% of those over age 65 in the United States show symptoms of advanced presbycusis (Corso, 1977), it is important to keep in mind that the physiological bases of these symptoms probably represent continuous changes with aging. That is, most older adults, though not clinically diagnosed as suffering hearing loss, may experience these changes to lesser or greater degrees. To complicate matters further, presbycusis is not a unitary disorder. The extent and type of hearing loss in old age may vary from individual to individual, depending on the extent and location of damage in the auditory system.

The most common feature of presbycusis is a *loss of sensitivity* that is likely to be exaggerated at the higher frequencies. That is, all hearing frequencies must be amplified in order for older adults to detect them, and, on the average, high frequencies must be especially intense. Sensitivity shows a monotonic decline from early adulthood through the life span, although these changes tend to be greatest for frequencies that are less important for speech perception (>3,000 Hz).

As with most aging phenomena, there is no single locus for high-tone loss. The number of hair cells at the basal end of the organ of Corti is known to decrease with age; because this is the area on the basilar membrane that is maximally displaced by high frequencies, it is probable that their deterioration is partly responsible. A stiffening of the basilar membrane and other mechanical changes, as well as metabolic changes in the inner ear, may also contribute. With advancing age also come numerous changes in middle-ear function, such as a loss of tissue elasticity in the ligaments holding the ossicles together and in the drum membrane. It is unclear, however, whether or not these changes really do contribute to sensitivity loss. A final factor that may contribute to sensitivity loss is the environment, with many studies showing a causal relationship between exposure to noise and high-tone loss (Kryter, 1970).

A second problem with sensitivity encountered by the elderly is *recruitment,* the abnormal increase in perceived loudness with an increase in stimulus intensity. This typically involves an abrupt transition in loudness as a function of intensity, such that increases in intensity produce little or no change in perceived loudness at lower intensities, until some point at which loudness increases dramatically. This corresponds to the common experience of raising one's voice a number of times to an older person who is having difficulty hearing, only to be told finally not to shout. Explanations for loudness recruitment have centered on differential changes in sensitivity among inner and outer hair cells (Davis, 1978) and bioelectric and biochemical changes in the endolymphatic fluid of the cochlea (Corso, 1977).

Another form of hearing impairment that is likely to occur in later adulthood is *phonemic regression*. Phonemic regression is a loss in intelligibility of speech stimuli that cannot be accounted for by the loss of sensitivity to tones alone. This is typically measured in a speech-discrimination test in which the subject listens to and repeats a series of phonemically balanced, one-syllable words of varying intensities. Such performance often is lower among older adults (Feldman & Reger, 1967). Furthermore, older adults do not show the same gain in intelligibility with increased intensity that one sees in younger adults (Punch & McConnell, 1969).

The cause of phonemic regression is not clearly understood, but, as suggested earlier, its locus probably is at the level of the cortex (Davis, 1978). Corso (1977) has hypothesized that the general decrease in speech discrimination in later adulthood is partly due to an increase in the processing time required by the higher auditory centers of older adults.

It is important to note that the term "phonemic regression" is a clinical term that carries no explanatory force. It merely describes the fact that older adults sometimes are noticed to be unable to understand words (or short word strings) in spite of their ability to hear pure tones at that intensity. Although earlier researchers tended to regard phonemic regression as a symptom found predominantly among clinical populations as a specific abnormality (Feldman & Reger, 1967), a loss of speech intelligibility is more recently thought of as a typical concomitant of aging (Corso, 1977).

The loss of intelligibility in later adulthood seems to be exacerbated by almost any condition that in any way distorts the speech. Bergman (1971) found that elderly adults hearing short test sentences showed very little decline in intelligibility when there were no speech distortions, but the performances of elderly adults showed steeper declines when the speech signal was reverberated, was regularly interrupted, or contained overlapping words.

The intelligibility of single words also was found to decrease differentially for older adults when the speech was accelerated (Konkle, Beasley, & Bess, 1977; Sticht & Gray, 1969). Younger and older adults with diagnosed sensorineural hearing loss, however, did not show such an increased difficulty with accelerated speech, as compared with younger and older adults with normal hearing (Sticht & Gray, 1969). Thus, the negative effects of accelerated speech are increased by age, but not by sensorineural hearing loss. Although it is possible among younger adults to ameliorate the effects of rapid speech by increasing the intensity of the speech, Calearo and Lazzaroni (1957) found that this did not occur to the same degree among the elderly. Such data suggest that older adults' difficulty with the processing of rapid speech may have more do to with a central slowing than with peripheral hearing loss, a point that will be useful to us in our later discussions.

To summarize, the principal effect of presbycusis is loss of sensitivity that can be remedied through sound amplification, though there are other effects (e.g., on speech intelligibility) that are less well understood. Clearly, it is the case that the causal locus of presbycusis includes both peripheral and central factors (Corso, 1977). For a more comprehensive treatment of the physiological bases and psychophysical effects of presbycusis, the interested reader is directed to reviews by Corso (1977, 1981, 1982), Davis (1978), and Olsho and associates (1985).

Memory for spoken discourse in later adulthood

Research studies that have examined age differences in memory for spoken material have yielded mixed results. Cohen (1979) examined the ability of older adults of varying educational levels to make inferences, detect anomalies, and preserve gist information from spoken text. Whereas highly educated older adults were no different from highly educated younger adults in answering questions about surface meaning, they were less accurate in the more integrative aspects of text comprehension. Among subjects with less education, an age deficit was apparent in extracting surface meaning as well, but as Cohen mentioned, these groups were not well matched on other factors such as health. This study suggests that among well-educated adults, speech comprehension shows little decline with age, provided that constructive integration is not required. Farrimond (1968) has also reported stability over age in recall of a list of short spoken sentences for subjects of high and low verbal ability. Age differences in that study, however, may have been suppressed by a floor effect.

As suggested by the Cohen results (1979), integrative processing may pose special problems for elderly listeners. Moreover, Cohen (1981) found that older adults had particular difficulty in inferential reasoning when the logical problems were spoken.

Several other studies have shown clear deficits in the ability of older adults to process spoken material. For younger and older adults matched on vocabulary and educational level (about 13 years), Taub (1975) found the recall of short spoken prose passages and recipes to be poorer among older adults. As part of a larger study, Dixon, Simon, Nowak, and Hultsch (1982) asked subjects (with educational levels of about 12 years) to listen to short newspaper articles and simply to recall them. They, too, reported age differences in performance favoring the younger subjects. Similarly, Petros, Tabor, Cooney, and Chabot (1983) found recall of Japanese folk tales to be poorer among elderly adults of varying educational levels. Unlike Cohen (1979), Petros and associates found their highly educated older subjects (with about 18 years of formal education) to be at the same disadvantage as their less well educated counterparts (who had about 12 years).

Cohen and Faulkner (1981) asked younger and older adults of equally high verbal ability to listen to passages of spoken text and then identify changes in written versions of the passages. Older adults generally were less able to detect differences between the spoken and written versions. When the delay between the spoken text and written test was manipulated, older adults were found to be particularly impaired at detecting semantic changes (as opposed to changes that preserved the meaning of the spoken passage) at the longest delay (40 sec). Thus, older adults were less able to recognize the meaning of spoken text, and their disadvantage increased with the delay between encoding and retrieval.

It seems that most (but not all) studies have found that older adults are less able to comprehend and remember spoken language than are younger adults, even when the speech materials consist of such ecologically relevant content as folk tales or news items. It is probably the case that, as with reading (J. Hartley, Chapter 11, this volume; Meyer & Rice, Chapter 12, this volume), educational level, verbal ability, text difficulty, and mode of retrieval all play roles in determining the presence of age differences in memory for speech.

Rate, context, and sentence processing. Several aging studies have provided a more specific focus on the characteristics of speech processing, with emphasis given to rapid on-line processing of a speech signal that occurs in context. In this section, we examine several such studies and their implications for understanding language processing among the elderly.

The use of speech context by the elderly in overcoming the effects of sensory loss has been demonstrated by Cohen and Faulkner (1983, Experiment 3). In their experiment, the participants' task was to listen to a series of target words and write each word down as it occurred. Each of these target words either occurred alone or came at the end of a short sentence that provided a predictable context for the word. In order to mimic the effects of a decline in stimulus quality, target words and sentences were presented simultaneously, with varying levels of noise. The ability of older adults to understand the target words was differentially facilitated by the sentence context. Furthermore, the age difference in target recognition differentially decreased when going from low to medium noise levels when targets were embedded in context, suggesting that the elderly were making greater use of context as the signal became noisier. Age differences increased dramatically, however, at the highest noise level, probably because the context itself had become so degraded as to be no longer useful. These results suggest that older listeners may be particularly dependent on the use of alternative top-down strategies.

Support for this position came from work in our own laboratory. We were particularly interested in how a slowing of mental processes (Birren et al., 1980; Cerella, Poon, & Williams, 1980; Salthouse, 1980, 1982) might impact on speech recall in later adulthood and the extent to which such effects might vary with the degree of linguistic context. If older adults were slower in on-line processing of speech, they would be expected to show disproportionate declines if the processing time were removed, as is the case with rapid speech. Ordinarily this might not be evident in everyday speech processing because of the great redundancy inherent in the speech signal. The data reported here are taken from a larger study reported by Wingfield, Poon, Lombardi, and Lowe (1985).

The speech rate in this experiment was varied by the sampling method of time compression (Foulke & Sticht, 1969). In this procedure, small segments (20 msec each) of the speech signal are removed periodically, and the remaining speech segments are abutted in time. Because the typical duration of a syllable is 180–300 msec, such deletions do not substantially distort the speech. The result is speech that is faster, but it is not changed in pitch.

Certainly the presence of coherent syntax and meaning of an utterance should facilitate performance under difficult listening conditions (Wingfield et al., 1984). Our question was whether or not these constraints would be particularly

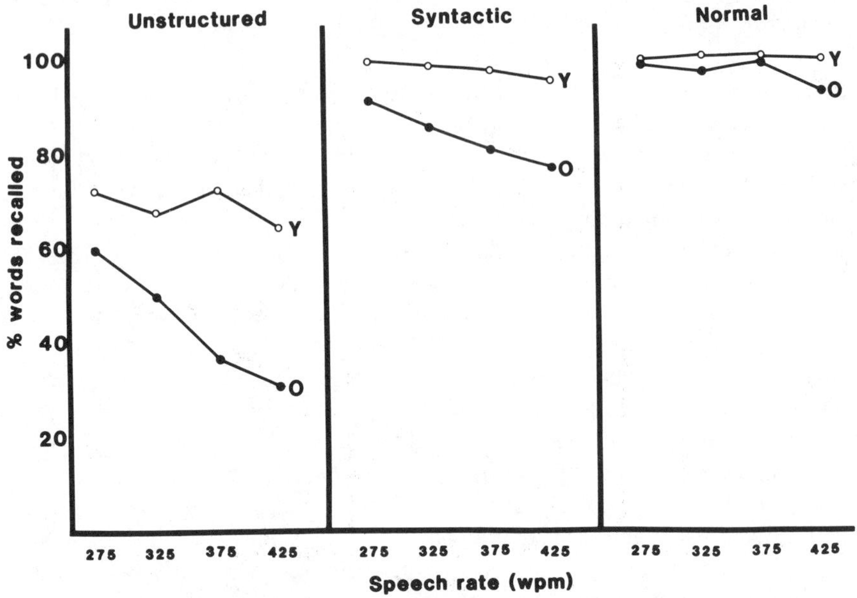

Figure 13.1. Percentages of words recalled as functions of age, speech rate, and degree of linguistic constraint.

useful to the elderly, such that their presence would decrease the difficulty of processing rapid speech more for the elderly than for the young.

Participants were tested on a baseline of recall for short lists of random words (*unstructured,* e.g., "clear drank dogs water frisky"). Against this baseline, we examined the recall of these same words when they were ordered so as to follow normal syntactic constraints, but without semantic constraints (*syntactic,* e.g., "frisky water drank clear dogs"). Finally, words were reordered to produce fully meaningful sentences with both semantic and syntactic constraints (*normal,* e.g., "frisky dogs drank clear water"). Such materials have received wide use in the psycholinguistic literature (Marks & Miller, 1964).

Twelve younger adults (18–22 years) and 12 older adults (65–73 years) similar in educational level and verbal ability listened to a total of 36 eight-word strings for immediate recall. Of this full set, 12 were normal sentences, 12 were syntactic strings, and 12 were unstructured strings. Because all of the words for the syntactic and unstructured strings were taken from the original normal sentences, the 36 speech strings were thus automatically equated for such features as word length and frequency.

Each subject heard the same number of strings of each type at each of four speech rates: 275, 325, 375, and 425 wpm. The subject's task was to listen to each string and immediately report aloud as accurately as possible as much of the string as possible.

The proportions of words recalled as functions of speech rate and age for the three degrees of linguistic constraint are shown in Figure 13.1. Performance decreased as a function of increasing age, increasing speech rate, and decreasing linguistic constraint. Whereas the performances of both younger and older adults were affected by speech rate and by the degree of linguistic constraint, the performances of the elderly group were differentially depressed by increasing the speech rate and by decreasing the linguistic constraints. In addition, the performances of the elderly were especially disrupted by the combination of very fast speech and less linguistic structure.

We take these results to support the contention that older adults rely on the redundancy of language and on linguistic constraints to facilitate processing in a slower system. The elderly were found to be at a differential disadvantage with the removal of ordinarily available processing time, or to look at it another way, they gained disproportionately by the availability of additional processing time. At the same time, as we contrast their performance for unstructured materials with the results from syntactic strings and normal sentences, it is clear that they make good use of linguistic constraints to overcome the effects of rapid speech.

We did find a significant age effect, but it was one that diminished as the speech materials more closely paralleled everyday natural speech in both rate and structure. Thus, our results support the slowing hypothesis, but also show that processing deficits can have minimal effects when normal linguistic constraints are present.

The normal sentences used in this experiment were short in length and simple in structure. We wanted to examine the ability of older adults to recall time-compressed speech using somewhat more naturally occurring speech materials that had varying levels of difficulty (which would also be typical of everyday speech). This would also give us the opportunity to put the slowing hypothesis to an even stronger test.

Salthouse (1982) has extended Birren's notions of "generalized slowing" (Birren et al., 1980) to show how this might account for a differential decline of abilities with age. He proposes that when more component processes are involved in a task, slowing will produce cumulative errors (e.g., by a contingent process not acting quickly enough on a fading trace). Thus, cognitive performance requiring more processing steps will be expected to show steeper age declines. If one assumes that performance with more processing steps is more difficult, then these notions have found some support (Cerella et al., 1980).

A strong test of the Salthouse slowing hypothesis as applied to speech processing would require that in addition to manipulating the rate of the speech materials, one vary the number of processing steps necessary to comprehend the speech. One option for accomplishing this would be to create speech materials containing different numbers of propositions, or idea units, in the text (Kintsch, 1974).

It is now well established (Graesser, Hoffman, & Clark, 1980; Kintsch & Keenan, 1973) that, other things being equal, reading time for text increases lin-

Table 13.1. *Sample stimulus materials showing variations in propositional density*

Four-proposition sentence
The economy in the region of the Caribbean islands is based on farming that is done on plantations.
1 (of Caribbean islands, economy)
2 (base on, economy, 3)
3 (farm, $)
4 (loc: on, 3, plantations)

Ten-proposition sentence
In many Greek coffee houses, men spend hours reading foreign newspapers or playing backgammon for small stakes.
1 (loc: in, 8, coffee houses)
2 (Greek, coffee houses)
3 (many, 2)
4 (duration: for, 8, hours)
5 (read, men, newspapers)
6 (foreign, newspapers)
7 (play, men, backgammon)
8 (or, 5, 7)
9 (for stakes, 7)
10 (small, stakes)

early with the number of propositions it contains. Therefore, the number of propositions used to represent a text seems to be a psychologically real way of estimating the amount of processing a text will require. Thus, given two sentences that have the same numbers of words, it will take longer to read the one with more propositions (Kintsch & Keenan, 1973). One would predict, then, if one were listening to these same two sentences, that the one that was more propositionally dense (i.e., the one with more propositions for a given number of words) might require more processing steps and hence be more difficult to comprehend and recall.

The following experiment was conducted as a specific test of that hypothesis (Stine, Wingfield, & Poon, 1986). Text bases for the sentences were constructed according to the guidelines in Turner and Greene (1977) and Kintsch and van Dijk (1978). Table 13.1 illustrates two such sentences of approximately the same length in words, one containing 4 propositions and the other 10. The sentences in this experiment contained 4, 6, 8, or 10 propositions.

In addition, the speech rate was varied (200, 300, or 400 wpm) and factorially combined with propositional density. Thus, the rate of information input was manipulated in two ways: via the rate of the speech (words per minute) and via the density of propositions.

University undergraduates (17–32 years; $n = 24$) and community-dwelling older adults (61–80 years, $n = 24$) participated in this study. All participants were highly verbal, with the older group somewhat higher in verbal ability than

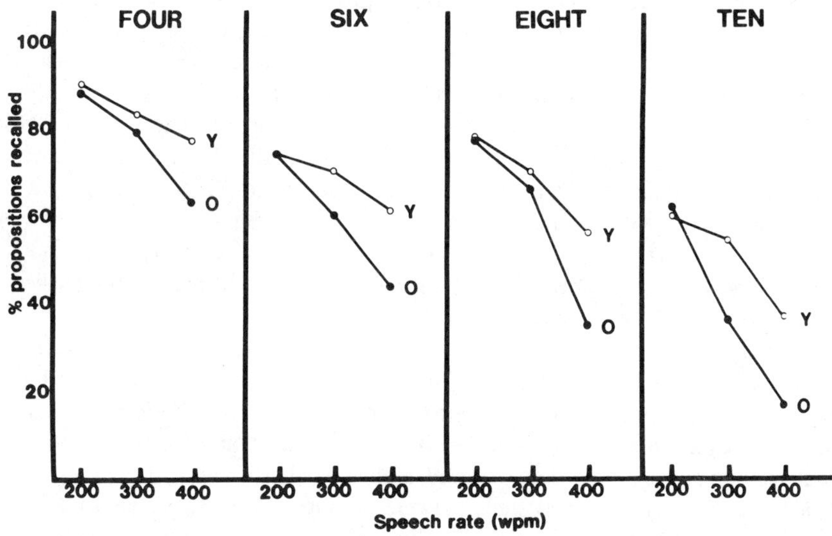

Figure 13.2. Percentages of propositions recalled as functions of age and speech rate for sentences with 4, 6, 8, and 10 propositions.

the younger group. The older adults were also particularly well educated (mean years of education = 16.1), though the effects we describe here were similar to those seen when older adults of average ability were tested.

The subject's task was to listen to each sentence and immediately recall as much of it as possible. Given that it takes time to process propositions, the speech rate and propositional density should have cumulative effects in compromising performance, and according to the slowing hypothesis proposed by Salthouse, these two variables should interact with age.

As illustrated in Figure 13.2, increases in age, speech rate, and propositional density all had adverse effects on the ability to recall the sentences. As in the previous experiment, an increase in speech rate was more detrimental to the performances of elderly adults than those of younger adults. An increased speech rate was also found to be more difficult when sentences were more propositionally dense.

The fact that speech rate interacted with both age and propositional density suggests that both age and propositional density exert effects on the time course of speech processing. However, neither the age-by-propositional-density interaction nor the three-way interaction among age, propositional density, and speech rate reached significance. In spite of the fact that both age and propositional density are known to increase the time required for processing (and hence decrease encoding accuracy in the present experiment), we failed to find these effects cumulative (in the interaction). One possibility is that older adults could have been compensating for a decrease in processing rate by processing the incoming propositions in a qualitatively different way. It is also possible that listening to speech for immediate recall or utilization is such an overlearned skill (e.g., in conversation) that, as with many practiced tasks (Denney, 1982), there is little deterioration in propositional processing with age. In any case, it is clear that at least within the densities tested, informationally dense text presented no particular problems for the elderly, as would be predicted if older adults are generally slower in working memory processing. It is important to note, however, that even among these exceptional older adults, increasing speech rates had serious adverse effects on comprehension. Thus, listening skill may facilitate the processing of complicated speech, but not rapid speech.

Although recall, in principle, might be possible without comprehension, this would not ordinarily be the case with meaningful natural language (van Dijk & Kintsch, 1983). Indeed, in this experiment, we analyzed recall performance in terms of levels in a coherence graph (Kintsch & van Dijk, 1978) and found that both younger and older adults showed higher recall for the more important sentence ideas, suggesting that subjects were attempting to comprehend the speech rather than simply to give rote recall. For a discussion of how this "levels effect" was influenced by other variables, see Stine and associates (1986).

Therefore, research examining immediate memory for speech suggests that the elderly are able to use the linguistic context to facilitate comprehension and recall and that this ability comes into play particularly when listening conditions are difficult, as is the case with noisy or fast speech. It has also been shown that the ability to understand informationally dense speech is preserved in later adulthood, even under adverse listening conditions. These findings are consistent with the argument that as some cognitive skills decline in old age, others are maintained or even continue to improve in order to compensate for the concomitant declines (Labouvie-Vief & Schell, 1982; Szafran, 1968).

Construction of contexts. We have shown in a limited way how older adults use their knowledge of language context to overcome some of the effects of slowing. The question remains how this context is constructed. That is, speech is rarely presented to us in "bite-sized" pieces. Rather, it is a continuous stream that must be parsed by the listener into meaningful chunks, with each chunk providing context for lower-level phonemic information.

We have already discussed the illusion of verbal transformation (Warren, 1961a) among younger adults when a meaningful context for speech is not available. Warren (1961b; Warren & Warren, 1966) has also examined this effect among elderly adults and has shown that they are less susceptible to this illusion. They perceive not only fewer transformations but also fewer different forms; thus, the elderly adult's perception shows greater stability. Warren argues that the decline in the verbal-transformation effect in the later years is indicative of the older adult's reduced capacity for recoding operations, which the younger adult appears to use in order to construct context. Thus, it may be that the older adult is more dependent on linguistic context because it has become more difficult to construct one.

Another age difference in this effect is that whereas younger adults are likely to report hearing strings consisting of nonsense words, older adults are not – even when the "word" being repeated is, in fact, nonsense. The older adult's speech perception is, in this case, more veridical than that of the younger adult, providing that the stimulus is meaningful. Warren considers these subjects' reports as evidence of the kind of organization employed by the listener. For example, unlike young adults, young children report hearing phonemic combinations that do not occur in English, suggesting that their organizational unit is the phoneme rather than the phonemic sets used by young adults. Similarly, because older adults report only meaningful English words, it would seem that their organizational unit, the whole word, is larger than that used by young adults.

In everyday language comprehension, construction of a linguistic context is quite different from that required for a repeating stimulus. We can, however, illustrate the same principle of context utilization by elderly adults in a more natural speech setting. In a recent experiment, we specifically examined the ability of older adults to use their knowledge of the language to control linguistic input for recall of language varying in its degree of linguistic constraint.

As discussed previously, the receipt of verbal information can be a highly interactive process. Most noticeable is the way one often self-paces verbal input by periodically interrupting a speaker, through either eye movements or verbal interruption, when the speaker has said too much too rapidly. These periodic interruptions may allow time for processing and retention of what has been heard prior to the arrival of yet more information (Chodorow, 1979).

One laboratory technique used elsewhere to assess such linguistic knowledge among younger adults is *spontaneous segmentation* (Wingfield & Butterworth, 1984). In this methodology, the listener hears running speech and is allowed to stop this input as often as desired in order to recall the speech, segment by segment. The subject controls the rate of input by pressing the pause button to stop and start the tape play. Research with younger adults has demonstrated that listeners stop predominantly at major syntactic boundaries. In order for such selection to occur, the listener must predict syntactic structure in advance of the boundary. Thus, this task requires both (1) on-line formation of predictive hypotheses about the syntactic structure of incoming speech and (2) simultaneous monitoring of current memory capacity in order to select meaningful segments that do not exceed memory capacity.

In the experiment described next, we used the spontaneous-segmentation paradigm to examine the ability of older adults to segment speech and to recall the resulting speech segments. Our special interest was to determine not only the accuracy of their recall but also the points at which they chose to segment the passages in order to facilitate that recall.

University undergraduates (18–21 years; $n = 18$) and community-dwelling older adults (66–77 years; $n = 18$) comparable in educational level and verbal

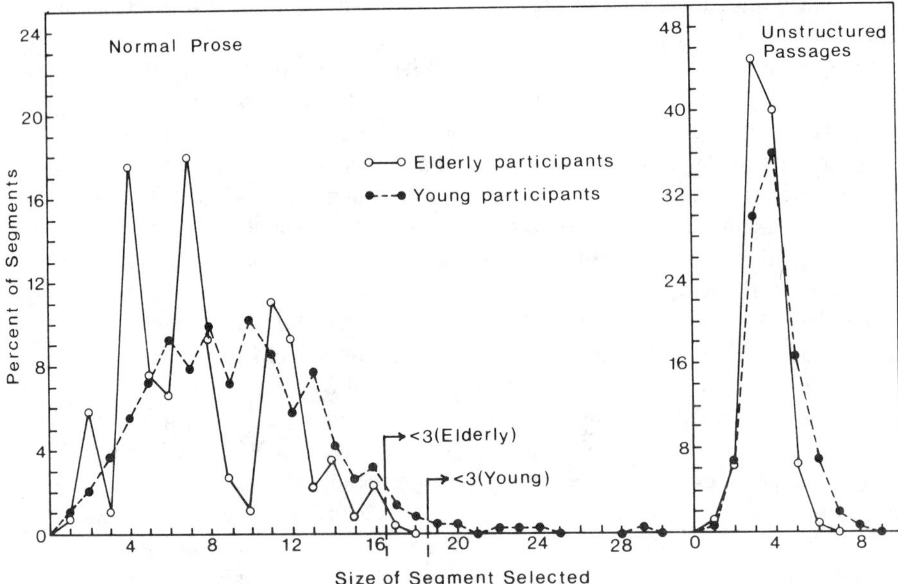

Figure 13.3. Percentages of segments of each size chosen for intermediate recall of normal prose (left panel) and unstructured passages (right panel) for young and elderly participants (note change of scale on ordinate). Segment sizes in normal prose with fewer than three examples are indicated by vertical lines on the abscissa.

ability participated in this study. The tape-recorded passages to which subjects listened were either normal or unstructured. Normal passages were taken from popular magazines and averaged 125 words in length; they were chosen to be easily comprehensible samples that contained a variety of syntactic forms. Unstructured passages were constructed by rearranging the normal passages so as to be devoid of semantic and syntactic constraints. The left-hand panel in Figure 13.3 shows the full distribution of segment sizes selected for intermediate recall of normal prose by the elderly and younger participants. Although there is overlap in the two distributions, the elderly participants tended to select shorter segments (mean = 7.6 words for the older group, and 8.8 for the younger group). The right-hand panel in Figure 13.3 shows the elderly and young participants' segment size distributions for the unstructured passages. Both groups showed a marked shift in strategy to the selection of fairly short segments, with a relatively narrow range of segment sizes. Again, segments selected by the elderly were shorter (mean = 3.2 words for old, and 3.9 for young).

Although the finding that older adults took shorter segments than did younger adults is potentially interesting, this particular result, as we shall see, is not always found. This should not be surprising, because the segmentation interval is under strategic control and thus may be influenced by a variety of subject and text factors.

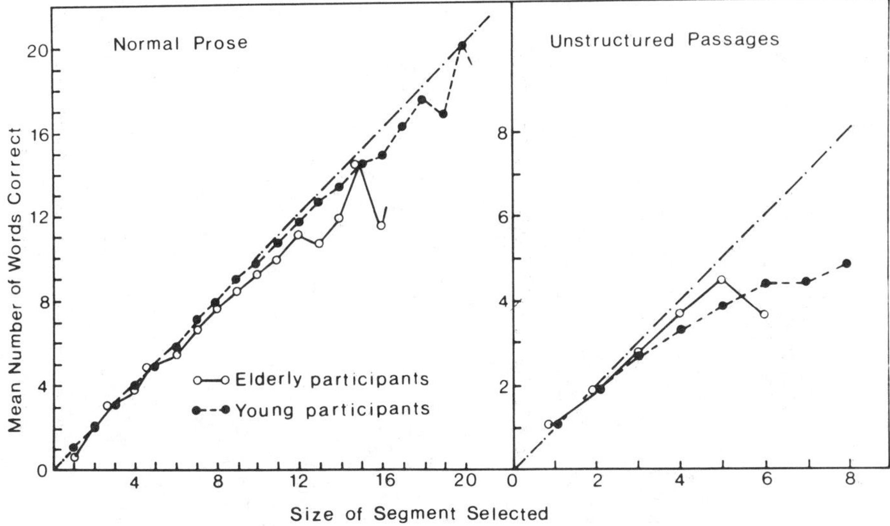

Figure 13.4. Mean numbers of words correctly recalled as a function of the sizes of segments selected by young and elderly participants for normal prose (left) and unstructured passages (right). The broken line represents perfect recall (note change of scale).

If the segment sizes selected reflect participants' estimates of their memory capacity, their recall performance for these segments should be indicative of their metamemory ability, which would be important in controlling speech input. Immediate-recall performance in all cases was excellent. Figure 13.4 shows the mean number of words recalled as a function of segment size for normal (left panel) and unstructured (right panel) passages. Only those cases for which there were at least three examples per mean are plotted; the dotted line along the diagonal represents perfect possible recall.

As can be seen, recall of normal prose by both age groups kept good pace with the size of the segments selected. The slope constants for elderly participants represent an additional 0.83 word correct for each one-word increment in selected segment size, and 0.94 word for younger adults. This small difference appears as a very slight departure in their performance curves at the larger segment sizes. It should be emphasized, however, that in absolute terms, the performances of both groups were excellent.

The data for the unstructured passages also show an excellent level of recall and further illustrate the effectiveness of the elderly participants' more conservative strategy. This strategy allowed them to maintain an overall slope constant of 0.72 word. By contrast, the younger adults tended to take longer segments even though performance had clearly begun to reach an asymptote at shorter segment lengths. This yielded an overall slope constant of only 0.54 word. Thus, both groups spontaneously adjusted their segmentation strategies to the type of speech material, selecting segment sizes that they could handle.

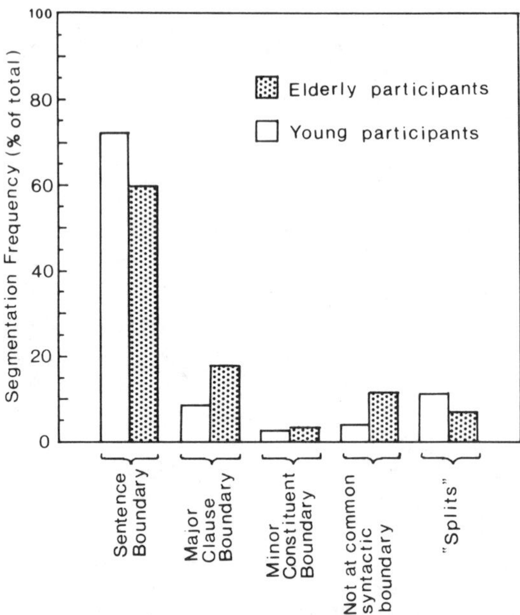

Figure 13.5. Percentages of segments that occurred at various types of syntactic boundaries for young and elderly participants segmenting normal prose.

In the case of normal prose, participants' interruptions were clearly based on natural linguistic constituents. Figure 13.5 shows the percentages of all segments for the young and elderly participants as functions of the type of syntactic boundary at which these segmentations occurred. For both age groups, the majority of segmentations occurred at sentence boundaries. Syntactically driven segmentations (i.e., those at sentence, major-clause, or minor-constituent boundaries) accounted for 84.0% of all segmentations for the young participants, and 81.1% for the elderly participants, a difference that was not significant. A small proportion of segmentations occurred at points not corresponding to a commonly recognized syntactic boundary. Finally, some segmentations were "splits," in which input was interrupted in the middle of a word.

Whether one considers segmentation strategies or recall accuracy, one sees strikingly parallel results for the elderly and younger participants. Older adults were as skilled as younger adults in monitoring their own memory operations and controlling linguistic input in order to keep recall performance high. Thus, the construction of local linguistic context as measured by parsing ability seemed to be preserved in later adulthood.

Because we have seen that elderly subjects have special difficulties with rapid input rates, we wondered if older adults would still be able to use effective parsing strategies under such conditions of rapid speech. An increase in speech rate not only might put a strain on linguistic processing but also might make the monitoring of working memory more difficult.

University undergraduates (17–32 years; *n* = 16) and community-dwelling older adults (65–80 years; *n* = 16) participated in this study (Wingfield & Stine, 1986). Subjects listened to and segmented, as described previously, four 80-word passages of normal prose (two at 200 wpm and two at 350 wpm). Comparing segment sizes selected at the slower rate with those from the previous experiment, the mean segment sizes selected by both age groups were longer (9.5 words for young, and 9.7 words for elderly). These differences in segment length may be reflecting differences in passages; for example, the syntactic complexity could change the overall interruption rate. The participants in this experiment were somewhat higher in educational level than those in the other experiment, and that also could have contributed to the difference. The mean segment size did not vary between age groups (as it did in the previous study).

Both younger and older adults tended to select even longer segments when the speech rate was faster (9.7 words per segment for young, and 11.0 words per segment for old). This corroborates the observations of Chodorow's subjects (1979) (and our own), who reported a feeling of "falling behind" in listening to time-compressed speech. That is, there is not sufficient time to make parsing decisions, and the tendency is to let the speech run past the normal, more optimum segmentation points. In this case, older adults tended to select slightly longer segments than did younger adults.

In spite of the small age difference in segment size at the faster speech rate, an increase in speech rate seemed to affect the parsing strategies of younger and older adults in the same way. The faster speech rate disrupted the more effective parsing strategies used by subjects at the slower rate (both in the previous experiment and in this one). Whereas younger and older adults segmented the slower speech at syntactic boundaries 75.6% and 79.9% of the time, respectively, these percentages dropped to 53.9% and 57.6% at the faster rate. This syntactic analysis suggests that participants tended to let rapid speech run past syntactically optimal segmentation points, though older adults did not do this more often than did younger adults. Thus, a decrease in processing time had no particular age-related effects on the predictive hypotheses of sentence structure. Also, because older adults' parsing strategies were similar to those of younger adults at fast rates, this would suggest that the longer segments taken by older adults were not due simply to a longer response time in pressing the pause button.

In the previous experiment, subjects' conservative strategies produced virtually perfect recall. In this experiment, subjects were induced (for whatever reason) to select longer segments. There is a subtle advantage here in that it enables us to examine segmental recall when the listener is pushed beyond memory capacity. There is a further advantage in the fact that the segmentation strategies used by younger and older adults, though producing fewer well-formed segments, were for all practical purposes matched. Thus, in the previous experiment, segmentation strategies were matched between age groups (generally producing syntacti-

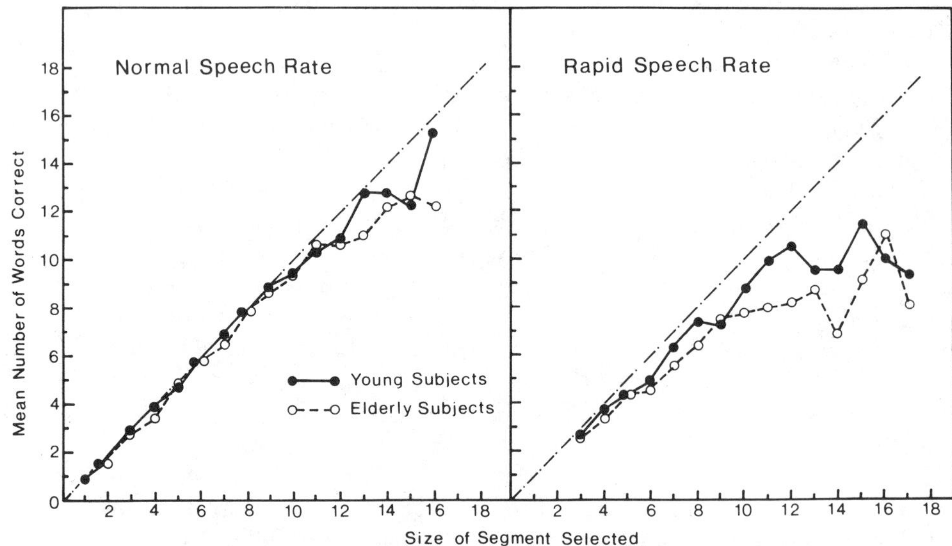

Figure 13.6. Mean numbers of words correctly recalled as a function of the sizes of segments selected by young and elderly adults for slow (left) and fast (right) speech rates.

cally coherent segments); in this experiment, segmental strategies were again matched (but were not syntactically coherent).

Figure 13.6 shows segmental recall as a function of segment size selected at slower (left panel) and faster (right panel) speech rates. As in the previous experiment, segmental recall at slower speech rates is seen to be very high for younger and older adults. At the faster rate, however, segmental recall shows some decline, especially among the elderly subjects.

It would seem that although the segmentation strategies for younger and older adults were similar at the faster rates, younger and older adults were not equally successful in estimating their memory capacities. As we have shown (Wingfield et al., 1985), language comprehension among older adults is particularly disrupted when speech lacks syntactic structure. Because rapid speech induced selection decisions at nonsyntactic boundaries, older adults were at a particular disadvantage.

These results suggest that metamemory processes (like other memory processes) take time, and when time is not available for their execution, there can be adverse effects on memory performance. Thus, when time was removed for the segmentation decision by increasing the speech rate, performance deteriorated, in part because poor selection decisions were made. The impact of these poor selection decisions was shown to be greater for elderly adults. When time was available, however, as was the case at normal speech rates, older adults were able to control input rates strategically to keep immediate-recall performance high.

Summary

Many skills related to speech processing, which involves bottom-up input of phonemic information constrained by top-down analysis of context, show some decline in the later years. The extent of that decline, however, may depend on a variety of factors. The older adult is hindered in bottom-up processing by a failing auditory system and a reduced capacity to process information efficiently in working memory, both of which appear to be associated with an age-related slowing in information processing. Top-down facilitation, however, may to some extent ameliorate these deficits by allowing older adults to infer lower-level information from context. Elderly adults' effective use of language knowledge is further illustrated by their ability to process informationally dense speech and to control speech input, when given the opportunity.

Conclusions

Research in cognitive aging has traditionally followed the dominant trends in the general psychological literature. The past few years have seen a dramatic evolution in the classes of memory activities that psychology has considered to be theoretically important for study. Crowder (1976), for example, reminds us that Ebbinghaus himself did at one time dabble with memory for prose. In one instance, he found that lines from Byron's *Don Juan* required only a tenth of the effort required for lists of nonsense syllables, concluding that the difference lay in "rhyme, rhythm, meaning, and the natural language" (Crowder, 1976, p. 464). Nevertheless, Ebbinghaus's conviction that the "molecule" of memory was the simple association and that one's goal should be the study of "pure" memory did, as we know, develop its own history. Bartlett's voice (1932) for many years remained a cry in the wilderness.

The rise of modern psycholinguistics extended the scientific study of verbal memory from nonsense syllables and word lists to full sentences, complete with their "rhythm, meaning, and the natural language" (Clark & Clark, 1977; Fodor et al., 1974). Even here, however, the level of study was rigidly restricted to the syntax, and later the semantics, of single sentences in isolation. As van Dijk and Kintsch (1983) have noted, generative grammarians were slow to see the relevance of discourse to the study of language processing. It is only in recent years that full discourse processing has begun to assume a central role in memory theory, with highly developed models of on-line interpretive processes for discourse understanding as it is being heard or read (van Dijk & Kintsch, 1983).

The work reported in this chapter has focused on what might be called the middle stage of discourse processing – a level beyond lexical access (Marcus, 1984; Marslen-Wilson, 1984), but short of full discourse analysis. Our focus has been on young and elderly adults' input parsing strategies and immediate processing capabilities, only slightly probing the representation of meaning in memory.

Our goal has been to explore age-sensitive limitations and compensatory strategies in this early stage of spoken-discourse processing.

Regardless of the listener's age, proficiency in speech processing depends on continuous processing in working memory to interpret rapidly arriving phonemic information in light of linguistic knowledge and surrounding context. The work we have summarized suggests that whereas lower-level phonemic information may be particularly degraded for the elderly listener, top-down processing strategies help to ameliorate what might otherwise be a devastating handicap in language processing.

There are numerous new directions for research on speech processing in later adulthood. Task demands (e.g., verbatim recall versus "getting the gist of it"), speech characteristics (e.g., rate, complexity, qualitative content), and listener characteristics (e.g., verbal intelligence, educational level) will surely prove to be relevant in understanding the relationships among age, speech comprehension, and memory. It is particularly important to consider the world knowledge and the knowledge of linguistic organization that elderly adults use in the everyday listening situation.

References

Bartlett, F. C. (1932). *Remembering: An experimental and social study.* Cambridge University Press.

Bergman, M. (1971). Hearing and aging. *Audiology, 10,* 164–171.

Bierwisch, M. (1983). How on-line is language processing? In G. B. Flores D'Arcais & K. J. Jarvella (Eds.), *The process of language understanding* (pp. 113–168). New York: Wiley.

Birren, J. E., Woods, A. M., & Williams, M. V. (1980). Behavioral slowing with age: Causes, organization, and consequences. In L. W. Poon (Ed.), *Aging in the 1980s: Psychological issues* (pp. 293–308). Washington, DC: American Psychological Association.

Bohannon, J. N., Stine, E. L., & Ritzenberg, D. (1982). The "fine-tuning" hypothesis of adult speech to children: Effects of experience and feedback. *Bulletin of the Psychonomic Society, 19,* 210–214.

Brown, G., & Yule, G. (1983). *Discourse analysis.* Cambridge University Press.

Calearo, C., & Lazzaroni, A. (1957). Speech intelligibility in relationship to the speed of the message. *Laryngoscope, 67,* 410–419.

Carroll, J. M., & Tannenhaus, M. K. (1978). Functional clauses and sentence segmentation. *Journal of Speech and Hearing Research, 21,* 793–808.

Cerella, J., Poon, L. W., & Williams, D. (1980). Age and the complexity hypothesis. In L. W. Poon (Ed.), *Aging in the 1980s: Psychological issues* (pp. 332–342). Washington, DC: American Psychological Association.

Chapanis, A. (1954). The reconstruction of abbreviated printed messages. *Journal of Experimental Psychology, 48,* 496–510.

Chodorow, M. S. (1979). Time-compressed speech and the study of lexical and syntactic parsing. In W. E. Cooper & E. C. T. Walker (Eds.), *Sentence processing: Linguistic studies presented to Merrill Garrett.* Hillsdale, NJ: Lawrence Erlbaum.

Clark, H. H., & Clark, E. V. (1977). *Psychology and language.* New York: Harcourt, Brace & Jovanovich.

Cohen, G. (1979). Language comprehension in old age. *Cognitive Psychology, 11,* 412–429.

Cohen, G. (1981). Inferential reasoning in old age. *Cognition, 9,* 59–72.

Cohen, G., & Faulkner, D. (1981). Memory for discourse in old age. *Discourse Processes, 4,* 253–265.

Cohen, G., & Faulkner, D. (1983). Word recognition: Age differences in contextual facilitation effects. *British Journal of Psychology, 74,* 239–251.

Cooper, W. E., & Sorensen, J. M. (1981). *Fundamental frequency in sentence production.* New York: Springer-Verlag.

Corso, J. F. (1977). Auditory perception and communication. In J. E. Birren & W. K. Schaie (Eds.), *Handbook of the psychology of aging* (pp. 535–553). New York: Van Nostrand Reinhold.

Corso, J. F. (1981). *Aging sensory systems and perception.* New York: Praeger.

Corso, J. F. (1982). Sensory processes and perception in aging. In A. Viidik (Ed.), *Lectures on gerontology. Vol. 1: On biology of aging* (pp. 441–480). New York: Academic Press.

Craik, F. I. M., & Simon, E. (1980). Age differences in memory: The role of attention and depth of processing. In L. W. Poon, J. L. Fozard, L. S. Craik, D. Arenberg, & L. W. Thompson (Eds.), *New directions in memory and aging: Proceedings of the George A. Talland memorial conference* (pp. 95–112). Hillsdale, NJ: Lawrence Erlbaum.

Crowder, R. G. (1976). *Principles of learning and memory.* Hillsdale, NJ: Lawrence Erlbaum.

Cutler, A., & Darwin, C. J. (1981). Phoneme-monitoring, reaction time and preceding prosody: Effects of stop closure duration and fundamental frequency. *Perception and Psychophysics, 29,* 217–224.

Davis, H. (1978). Abnormal hearing and deafness. In H. Davis & S. R. Silverman (Eds.), *Hearing and deafness* (pp. 83–139). New York: Holt, Reinhart & Winston.

Denney, N. (1982). Aging and cognitive changes. In B. B. Wolman (Ed.), *Handbook of developmental psychology.* Englewood Cliffs, NJ: Prentice-Hall.

Dixon, R. A., Simon, E. W., Nowak, C. A., & Hultsch, D. F. (1982). Text recall in adulthood as a function of level of information, input modality, and delay interval. *Journal of Gerontology, 37,* 358–364.

Farrimond, T. (1968). Retention and recall: Incidental learning of visual and auditory material. *Journal of Genetic Psychology, 113,* 155–165.

Feldman, R. M., & Reger, S. N. (1967). Relations among hearing, reaction time, and age. *Journal of Speech and Hearing Research, 10,* 479–495.

Fodor, J. A., Bever, T. G., & Garrett, M. F. (1974). *The psychology of language.* New York: McGraw-Hill.

Foulke, E., & Sticht, T. G. (1969). Review of research on the intelligibility and comprehension of accelerated speech. *Psychological Bulletin, 72,* 50–62.

Frazier, L., & Fodor, J. D. (1978). The sausage machine: A new two-stage parsing model. *Cognition, 6,* 291–325.

Graesser, A. C., Hoffman, N. L., & Clark, L. F. (1980). Structural components of reading time. *Journal of Verbal Learning and Verbal Behavior, 19,* 131–152.

Grosjean, F. (1980). Spoken word recognition processes and the gating paradigm. *Perception and Psychophysics, 28,* 267–283.

Grosjean, F. (1983). How long is the sentence? Prediction and prosody in the on-line processing of language. *Linguistics, 21,* 501–529.

Jackendoff, R. S. (1972). *Semantic interpretation in generative grammar.* Cambridge, MA: M.I.T. Press.

Jarvella, R. J. (1973). Syntactic parsing of connected speech. *Journal of Verbal Learning and Verbal Behavior, 10,* 409–416.

Kintsch, W. (1974). *The representation of meaning in memory.* Hillsdale, NJ: Lawrence Erlbaum.

Kintsch, W., & Keenan, J. (1973). Reading rate and retention as a function of the number of propositions in the base structure of sentences. *Cognitive Psychology, 5,* 257–274.

Kintsch, W., & Kozminsky, E. (1977). Summarizing stories after reading and listening. *Journal of Educational Psychology, 69,* 491–499.

Kintsch, W., & van Dijk, T. A. (1978). Toward a model of text comprehension and production. *Psychological Review, 85,* 363–394.

Konkle, D. F., Beasley, D. S., & Bess, F. (1977). Intelligibility of time-altered speech in relation to chronological aging. *Journal of Speech and Hearing Research, 20,* 108–115.

Kryter, K. (1970). *The effects of noise on man.* New York: Academic Press.

Labouvie-Vief, G., & Schell, D. (1982). Learning and memory in later life. In B. B. Wolman (Ed.), *Handbook of developmental psychology.* Englewood Cliffs, NJ: Prentice-Hall.

Lehiste, E. (1970). *Suprasegmentals.* Cambridge, MA: M.I.T. Press.

Marcus, S. M. (1984). Recognizing speech: On the mapping from sound to word. In H. Bouma & D. G. Bouwhuis (Eds.), *Attention and performance* (Vol. X). Hillsdale, NJ: Lawrence Erlbaum.

Marks, L. E., & Miller, G. A. (1964). The role of semantic and syntactic constraints in the memorization of English sentences. *Journal of Verbal Learning and Verbal Behavior, 3,* 1–5.

Marslen-Wilson, W. D. (1975). Sentence perception as an interactive parallel process. *Science, 189,* 226–228.

Marslen-Wilson, W. D. (1984). Function and process in spoken word recognition. In H. Bouma & D. G. Bouwhuis (Eds.), *Attention and performance* (Vol. X). Hillsdale, NJ: Lawrence Erlbaum.

Marslen-Wilson, W. D., & Tyler, L. K. (1980). The temporal structure of spoken language understanding. *Cognition, 8,* 1–71.

Miller, G. A. (1951). *Language and communication.* New York: McGraw-Hill.

Miller, G. A., & Isard, S. (1963). Some perceptual consequences of linguistic rules. *Journal of Verbal Learning and Verbal Behavior, 2,* 217–228.

Miller, G. A., & Licklider, J. C. R. (1950). The intelligibility of interrupted speech. *Journal of the Acoustical Society of America, 22,* 167–173.

Nooteboom, S. G., & Doodeman, G. J. N. (1984). Speech quality and gating paradigm. In M. P. R. van den Broecke & A. Cohen (Eds.), *Proceedings of the Tenth International Congress of Phonetic Science.* Dordrecht: Foris.

Oldfield, R. C. (1963). Individual vocabulary and semantic currency: A preliminary study. *British Journal of Social and Clinical Psychology, 2,* 122–130.

Olsho, L. W., Harkins, S. W., & Lenhardt, M. L. (1985). Aging and the auditory system. In J. E. Birren & K. W. Schaie (Eds.), *Handbook of the psychology of aging* (2nd ed., pp. 332–377). New York: Van Nostrand Reinhold.

Petros, T., Tabor, L., Cooney, T., & Chabot, R. J. (1983). Adult age differences in sensitivity to semantic structure of prose. *Developmental Psychology, 19,* 907–914.

Pollack, I., & Pickett, J. M. (1963). Intelligibility of excerpts from conversation. *Language and Speech, 28,* 97–102.

Punch, J. L., & McConnell, F. (1969). The speech discrimination function for elderly adults. *Journal of Auditory Research, 9,* 159–166.

Salthouse, T. A. (1980). Age and memory: Strategies for localizing the loss. In L. W. Poon, J. L. Fozard, L. S. Craik, D. Arenberg, & L. W. Thompson (Eds.), *New directions in memory and aging: Proceedings of the George A. Talland memorial conference* (pp. 47–66). Hillsdale, NJ: Lawrence Erlbaum.

Salthouse, T. A. (1982). *Adult cognition.* New York: Springer-Verlag.

Smith, A. D. (1980). Age differences in encoding, storage, and retrieval. In L. W. Poon, J. L. Fozard, L. S. Craik, D. Arenberg, & L. W. Thompson (Eds.), *New directions in memory and aging: Proceedings of the George A. Talland memorial conference* (pp. 23–46). Hillsdale, NJ: Lawrence Erlbaum.

Sorensen, J. M., Cooper, W. E., & Paccia, J. E. (1978). Speech timing of grammatical categories. *Cognition, 6,* 135–153.

Sticht, T. G., & Gray, B. B. (1969). The intelligibility of time-compressed words as a function of age and hearing loss. *Journal of Speech and Hearing Research, 12,* 443–448.

Stine, E. L., & Bohannon, J. N. (1983). Imitations, interaction, and language acquisition. *Journal of Child Language, 10,* 589–603.

Stine, E. L., Wingfield, A., & Poon, L. W. (1986). How much and how fast: Rapid processing of spoken language in later adulthood. *Psychology and Aging, 86,* 303–311.

Streeter, L. A. (1978). Acoustic determinants of phrase boundary perception. *Journal of the Acoustical Society of America, 64,* 1582–1592.

Szafran, J. (1968). Psychophysiological studies of aging in pilots. In G. A. Talland (Ed.), *Human aging and behavior* (pp. 37–79). New York: Academic Press.

Taub, H. A. (1975). Mode of presentation, age, and short-term memory. *Journal of Gerontology, 30,* 56–59.

Turner, A., & Greene, F. (1977). The construction of a propositional text base. In *JSAS catalog of selected documents in psychology.* Washington, DC: American Psychological Association.

van Dijk, T. A., & Kintsch, W. (1983). *Strategies of discourse comprehension.* New York: Academic Press.

Wales, R., & Toner, H. (1979). Intonation and ambiguity. In W. E. Cooper & E. C. T. Walker (Eds.), *Sentence processing: Psycholinguistic studies presented to Merrill Garrett.* Hillsdale, NJ: Lawrence Erlbaum.

Warren, R. M. (1961a). Illusory changes of distinct speech upon repetition: The verbal transformation effect. *British Journal of Psychology, 52,* 249–258.

Warren, R. M. (1961b). Illusory changes in repeated words: Differences between young adults and the aged. *American Journal of Psychology, 74,* 506–516.

Warren, R. M. (1970). Perceptual restoration of missing speech sounds. *Science, 167,* 392–393.

Warren, R. M., & Warren, R. P. (1966). A comparison of speech perception in childhood, maturity, and old age by means of the verbal transformation effect. *Journal of Verbal Learning and Verbal Behavior, 5,* 142–146.

Wingfield, A. (1975a). Acoustic redundancy and the perception of time-compressed speech. *Journal of Speech and Hearing Research, 18,* 96–104.

Wingfield, A. (1975b). The intonation-syntax interaction: Prosodic features in perceptual processing of sentences. In A. Cohen & S. G. Nooteboom (Eds.), *Structure and process in speech perception* (pp. 146–160). New York: Springer-Verlag.

Wingfield, A., & Butterworth, B. (1984). Running memory for sentences and parts of sentences: Syntactic parsing as a control function in working memory. In H. Bouma & D. G. Bouwhuis (Eds.), *Attention and performance* (Vol. X). Hillsdale, NJ: Lawrence Erlbaum.

Wingfield, A., Lombardi, L., & Sokol, S. (1984). Prosodic features and the intelligibility of accelerated speech: Syntactic vs. periodic segmentation. *Journal of Speech and Hearing Research, 27,* 128–134.

Wingfield, A., & Nolan, K. A. (1980). Spontaneous segmentation in normal and time-compressed speech. *Perception and Psychophysics, 28,* 97–102.

Wingfield, A., Poon, L. W., Lombardi, L., & Lowe, D. (1985). Speed of processing in normal aging: Effects of speech rate, linguistic structure and processing time. *Journal of Gerontology, 40,* 579–585.

Wingfield, A., & Stine, E. L. (1986). Organizational strategies in immediate recall of rapid speech by young and elderly adults. *Experimental Aging Research, 12,* 79–83.

14 The effects of aging on perceived and generated memories

Gillian Cohen and Dorothy Faulkner

The origins of memories

Chapters 11, 12, and 13 are concerned with age differences in memory for spoken and written information and focus mainly on the processes of encoding and comprehension. This chapter is concerned with the nature of the memory representation and with wider issues arising out of the distinction between perceived and generated memories. This distinction applies to memory for all kinds of information, including scenes, events, and actions as well as discourse.

However, many memories are for things that never happened. This statement seems paradoxical because we tend to assume that memory representations originate from perceived events. We overlook the fact that memories may also be for events that never actually occurred, but have only been thought of or dreamed about. They may be memories of actions that were never performed, but only planned, considered, or intended. They may be memories of words that were never heard or read, but only imagined or inferred. The distinction between externally derived memories that originate from perceptions and internally derived self-generated memories is not always clear-cut. According to current cognitive theories, the sensory information derived from external events is interpreted, elaborated, or transformed by the application of stored prior knowledge and rules. So a perceived memory representation is a joint product comprising some elements that originated internally and some elements that originated externally.

In spite of this intermingling, people usually know how a particular memory originated and are able to distinguish between perceived and generated memories. The ability to make this distinction between real and imagined events, between fact and fantasy, has been called "reality monitoring" (Johnson & Raye, 1981).

Obviously, this ability is of crucial importance in everyday life. For example, being able to plan actions and evaluate their consequences without actually performing them allows us to act more efficiently and to avoid unnecessary effort and costly errors. But these advantages would be nullified if we were unable to distinguish between memories of overt actions and memories of covert plans.

Normally, we take this ability for granted, becoming aware of its importance only when reality monitoring breaks down.

Failures of reality monitoring

Failures of reality monitoring are characteristic of schizophrenia, dementia, delirium, and conditions of mental abnormality that involve hallucinations, obsessions, or thought disorders. In early childhood, also, the borderline between what is real and what is imaginary appears to be blurred (Flavell, Flavell, & Green, 1983), but failures of reality monitoring are not confined to the abnormal and the immature. Imperfect reality monitoring is also quite common in normal, healthy adults and is an important source of errors in judgment, in action, and in belief.

Slips of action

Errors in action can result if the memory of an action performed is confused with the memory of an action planned. Examples of this kind of error come readily to mind. Sometimes it is difficult to remember whether we have added salt to the soup or only thought of doing so; this error has the unfortunate consequence that we add it twice over or not at all. Sometimes it is difficult to remember if we really did lock the door, or turn off the light, and we have to go and check up to see whether the action was actually performed or only planned. Misplacing objects results from a similar type of confusion. We may think we put the missing car key, diary, or other object in its place, but in fact we only planned the action and never actually performed it. We all have these experiences.

Reason (1979) collected diary records of slips of action and categorized the types of errors that were described. Many of the slips he recorded involved this kind of confusion between plan and action, between the self-generated memory and the perceived memory. Norman (1981) reported similar examples. It is worth noting that the direction of the confusion affects the type of error that is made. When a plan is misidentified as an action, the consequence is that the action is omitted: the door left unlocked, the letter unposted, because the agent thinks that he or she has already performed the action. When an action is misidentified as a plan, a different consequence ensues. The action is repeated, or an attempt is made to perform it a second time. The agent goes to perform the action, thinking it has not yet been performed, and does it again or finds that it has been done already. Both kinds of confusion may have inconvenient results. Repetitions are a waste of time and effort, whereas omissions can have serious consequences.

Confusing implications and assertions

Reality monitoring is also involved in memory for spoken and written information of the kind discussed in Chapters 11, 12, and 13.

Failure to remember the origin of verbal information can produce distortions and inaccuracies in belief and judgment. Bartlett (1932) demonstrated how remembered stories are changed to conform to the preconceptions of the listener. In everyday life we encounter cases of tales that improve with each retelling. The original experience or original story is imaginatively embellished until even the narrator is unable to distinguish truth from fiction. The kind of confabulation that is symptomatic of senile dementia and some forms of mental illness represents the same sort of confusion in a more extreme form.

The kinds of mistakes that can distort eyewitness testimony (Loftus, 1979) are rather different: Witnesses can confuse the memory of a visually perceived event with false information about the event that is presented verbally at a later time. In this case, the confusion is between information from two different external sources, the visual and the verbal, rather than between information from an internal and an external source. However, both kinds of confusion involve mistaking the origin of a memory, and both result in believing that something happened when it did not happen.

Most of us have also experienced situations in which we have said the same thing to the same person more than once, or we believe that we have said something when we intended to say it but never did so. The confusion of verbal intentions with verbal utterances, like the confusion of plans and actions, produces omissions or repetitions in performance.

Whereas our knowledge of these kinds of confusions between speech and thought in conversation rests mainly on informal observations, the tendency to confuse implications with assertions has received more formal investigation. Bransford, Barclay, and Franks (1972) showed how readily people would claim that information was explicitly stated when in fact it was only implied. There is a tendency to claim an external origin for information that was generated internally. Similar findings have been reported by Harris and Monaco (1976). In an experiment by Harris (1978), subjects served as "jurors" and listened to simulated courtroom testimony. In a subsequent recognition test, implications were persistently misclassified as assertions, in spite of the fact that the subjects in one condition were specifically instructed to avoid making this mistake.

Frequency judgments

Another consequence of defective reality monitoring is that judgments about the number of times an event has occurred are inaccurate. Johnson, Taylor, and Raye (1977) and Johnson, Raye, Wang, and Taylor (1979) have shown that estimates of the frequency of occurrence of an event can be inflated by imagined repetitions. For example, if an event actually occurs 6 times and the same event is thought about or imaginatively reconstructed 4 more times, the judged frequency of occurrence of the event is likely to be nearer 10 than 60. Experimentally, this effect has been demonstrated by having subjects listen to a list of words or view a set of pictures: The presentation of each word or each picture is repeated a variable number of times, and presentation trials are interspersed with trials in which the subject is required to imagine hearing one of the words or seeing one of the pictures. The judged frequency of actual occurrence is influenced by the number of times the item was imagined. In this situation, people are again unable to distinguish between memories of real events and memories of imagined events.

A particularly interesting aspect of these findings is again the direction of the error. Given that perceived and generated memories are confused, it is logically quite possible to misidentify the real perceived memories and classify them as imaginary generated memories. An error of this kind would produce an underestimate of the frequency of actual occurrence. But this is not what happens. Instead, the generated memories are misclassified as perceived memories, with the result that real occurrences are overestimated. The same sort of bias is also evident in the tendency to treat implications as assertions. Explicit assertions are not mistaken for implications; internally generated representations are misclassified as real external occurrences. It seems as if there is a bias toward reification. People may mistake the fantasy for the fact, but not fact for fantasy. However, although this bias in the direction of error appears both in the frequency judgments and in the recognition of implications, it is not apparent when plans and actions are confused. Among the slips of action recorded by Reason, 40% were repetition errors, and only 18% omission errors. But these errors do not necessarily reflect confusions of perceived and generated memories. Repetition errors may arise either because the memory of a performed action is mistaken for the memory of an imagined action or because one simply forgets that an action has been performed. Omission errors may arise either because an imagined action is mistaken for a performed action or because one simply forgets to carry out a plan.

Johnson (1985) has suggested that in everyday life, the judged frequency of events may be influenced by the frequency with which the events are thought about, in the same way that such judgments were influenced in the experimental situation. She suggests, for example, that our subjective estimates of how happy we have been are affected not only by the frequency of happy occasions but also by the frequency with which we imagine or remember happy or miserable times. If Johnson's suggestion is correct, it is easy to see how inaccuracies may creep into subjective estimates of the frequency of episodes of illness, misfortune, or depression.

Temporal judgments

It has been pointed out (A. Wingfield, personal communication) that apparent failures of reality monitoring in everyday life may sometimes more properly be described as errors in temporal dating. When an action is one that is routinely performed frequently (e.g., brushing one's teeth), the problem may lie in deciding whether a memory representation of performing the action is a memory of doing it half an hour ago or a memory of doing it yesterday. The difficulty

Table 14.1. *Attributes of perceived and generated memories.*

Parameter	Perceived	Generated
Contextual attributes (place and time)	+[a]	−
Sensory attributes (visual, auditory, tactile)	+	−
Detail and complexity	+	−
Coherence	+	−
Schematic	−	+
Cognitive operations (search, reasoning, and decision processes)	−	+

[a]Plus signs indicate attributes more strongly represented; minus signs indicate attributes less strongly represented.

lies in the temporal dating of a perceived memory. In this case, the agent is not trying to distinguish between the memory of a plan and the memory of an action, and it is not, strictly speaking, a reality-monitoring decision. Nevertheless, performance errors that resemble failures of reality monitoring can arise out of temporal-dating confusions. Failure to brush one's teeth may be due to mistaking yesterday's memory for today's memory.

In summary, errors in reality monitoring occur quite commonly in everyday life. People confuse the memory of actions with the memory of plans, so that they do not know whether or not a given action has been performed. They confuse the memory of verbal information they have perceived in speech or writing with the memory of verbal information they have generated in thought. They overestimate the frequency with which events have occurred by conflating the memories of actual and imagined occurrences.

The theoretical distinction between perceived and generated memories

According to Johnson and Raye's model (1981), there are two ways in which perceived and generated memories can be discriminated. The first method is to evaluate the characteristics of the memory trace. The differences between perceived and generated memories have been listed by Johnson and Raye, as shown in Table 14.1. Perceived memories are characterized by being relatively richer in sensory attributes, such as sound, color, and texture; perceived events are set in a context of time and place and are more detailed. Generated memories are relatively more schematic, less rich in sensory attributes, and lacking in context, but they are more likely to incorporate traces of the cognitive operations that engendered them. Accordingly, it is claimed, the origin of a memory can be determined by the extent to which it possesses these characteristics. Johnson and her colleagues have confirmed this account to some extent by experiments manipulating the attributes of perceived and generated memories, with the predicted effects on reality-monitoring judgments.

The extent to which perceived and imagined representations are different has been questioned. Shepard (1984) argues on logical grounds that the representations generated for prospective planning and anticipation *must* be accurate and veridical in all salient respects if they are to serve their purpose. He also cites the results of empirical studies showing that internally generated representations obey the same constraints as externally derived perceptions (Podgorny & Shepard, 1978). Failures of reality monitoring confirm that the two kinds of memory representations are not always readily distinguishable.

When the origin of a particular memory cannot easily be identified by its qualities, other criteria can be invoked. Perceived memories are expected to make sense in terms of knowledge of the world. A second method for evaluating the origin of a memory is therefore in terms of its coherence with other knowledge. Generated memories, such as fantasies and dreams, often can be detected because they violate natural laws; so we may test a memory trace against the criteria of coherence and plausibility. A memory of being able to fly or of conversing fluently in an unfamiliar language, for example, can be recognized as a dream, on the basis of the plausibility criterion. The two methods of evaluation may be employed together, with the final decision based on the joint outcome.

Doubtful cases may arise in various ways. If an event is imagined in unusually vivid detail, and the memory is also coherent and plausible, it may seem like a memory of a real event. If a memory of a real event is vague and sketchy, it may seem like an imagined memory. These considerations suggest some possible reasons why the slips of action that result from confusion between plans and actions seem to occur most often for actions that are frequently repeated and highly automatic. As shown in Table 14.1, actions that are actually performed ought to produce memories rich in sensory details, but automatic actions may lack the sensory information that should characterize them, because little attention is paid to the circumstances and context in which they are performed. On the other hand, when the planned action is one that has been performed on many previous occasions, the plan is likely to be more detailed and less schematic than a novel plan would be. Reality-monitoring decisions are therefore likely to be much more fallible for frequently repeated actions. It is also a plausible assumption that temporal-dating confusions are more common when events are frequently repeated.

In everyday life, people report various strategies for resolving doubtful cases. A memory representation may be tested by searching for distinctive spatiotemporal or contextual details. A memory of locking the door may be identified as "real" if prior and subsequent actions can be reconstructed, or if further details (the cat waiting to be let out, or the letter in the mail slot) are recalled. In the last resort, the agent may be forced to determine if the action was really performed, by checking the consequences (whether or not the door is locked, the toothbrush is wet, the pills are still in the bottle, or the kettle is switched off).

Some individuals have more difficulty than others in reality monitoring. Johnson and associates (1979) showed that good imagers are more likely to confuse imagined occurrences with perceived occurrences. They concluded that vivid imagery carries the disadvantage of being more difficult to distinguish from reality.

Age differences in reality monitoring

There are several bases for hypothesizing that the ability to distinguish between perceived and generated memories declines with age and that the incidence of confusion errors is likely to increase. There is experimental evidence, extensively reviewed by Burke and Light (1981), that elderly people are less likely to encode and remember contextual information. A deficiency of this kind would have the effect that perceived memory representations would lack the contextual and sensory attributes that should distinguish them.

On the basis of everyday experiences we can suggest several factors that would tend to make reality monitoring more difficult for the elderly. As activity is reduced and more time is spent at rest, it seems likely that the amount of time spent in reflection might increase. More time might be devoted to mentally reviewing, considering, planning, and envisaging. As a result, the balance between perceived and imagined events would shift in old age, with an increasing proportion of events being self-generated. Surprisingly, though, results obtained from a questionnaire study by Giambra (1977) indicate that daydreaming declines significantly in both frequency and intensity after the age of 65. It is unlikely, therefore, that a decline in reality-monitoring ability is linked to an increase in daydreaming.

It is probably a more important factor that elderly individuals are less exposed to novel perceptual events. With a less mobile existence, events are more routine, and the environment is more unchanging. Because the real external events that make up daily life for the older person are liable to be familiar, routine, frequently repeated, they will produce memory traces that lack distinctiveness. It is tempting to speculate that this is why people who are institutionalized become confused. The uniformly routine nature of real events may blur the distinction between perceived and generated memories and may also increase the problems of temporal dating. Zelinski and Light (personal communication) have reported an age-related decline in the accuracy of frequency judgments and temporal-dating judgments.

Stine, Wingfield, and Poon (Chapter 13, this volume) review evidence for an age-related decline in auditory sensitivity. If sight and hearing become less acute in old age, reality monitoring is likely to be affected, because perceived memories will then be correspondingly less rich in sensory information.

The hypothesis that there is an age-related reduction in reality-monitoring ability has received some support from anecdotal evidence and from self-assessments of everyday behavior. Cohen and Faulkner administered a memory-lapse questionnaire to young, middle-aged, and old subjects. Included in this study were questions asking them to rate how often they were uncertain whether they had actually performed an action, such as locking the door, or had only intended to do so, and how often they were uncertain whether they had said something in conversation or had only thought of saying it. The age differences were small, but elderly people reported slightly more frequent experiences of this kind of confusion of reality monitoring.

In summary, perceived memories are distinguished by being richer in sensory and contextual details. Generated memories are more schematic. Reality-monitoring decisions can be made by evaluating the characteristics of a memory trace or by assessing its plausibility. Elderly people may have more difficulty in making reality-monitoring judgments because they encode less contextual and sensory detail, and the unchanging nature of their everyday routine makes real memory traces less distinctive.

Methodological issues

Any attempt to study age differences in reality monitoring is bound to run into methodological problems. For practical purposes of assessment, diagnosis, and care, the most appropriate approach is to study naturally occurring instances of errors in reality monitoring; yet there are obvious drawbacks with this method. If people are asked to record details when they experience a failure of reality monitoring, any age differences may be either obscured or inflated by confounding factors: The accuracy of the record may be affected by reluctance to expose cognitive failure; older people who suffer from memory deficits may forget or never detect the errors they make; cohort differences in life style may give rise to differences in the allocation of time to action and reflection and thus affect the opportunity for reality monitoring; the elderly may be more anxious about the consequences of errors in reality judgments and seek to minimize them by obsessive checking; age differences in general alertness, health, and sensory acuity may underlie changes in reality-monitoring ability. Moreover, naturally occurring errors are relatively infrequent, and so it would take a long time to gather a substantial amount of data; the circumstances in which unforced natural errors occur are so difficult to specify and so variable that it would be difficult to draw general conclusions from observations of this kind.

Some doubts have accumulated about the suitability of questionnaires and diaries as methods of studying age differences in cognitive abilities (Herrmann, 1984; Morris, 1984). There are, of course, exceptions to this generalization. J. Hartley (Chapter 11, this volume) reports significant correlations between self-assessed reading habits, elicited by questionnaire, and prose memory. But questionnaires have not always proved to be good predictors of performance either in formal laboratory tests or in everyday settings.

An experimental approach of studying induced errors in reality monitoring in the laboratory has its own disadvantages. Although the nature of the errors and the circumstances that evoke them can be specified much more carefully, the validity of extrapolating from the experimental situation to what happens in everyday life must be doubtful. Even when care is taken to make the laboratory task as naturalistic as possible, the degree of control required is necessarily incompatible with complete verisimilitude. Nevertheless, the experimental approach is likely to be more fruitful than self-report. The studies described next relied mainly on naturalistic experiments, but attempts were also made to validate the results by examining self-ratings of performance in everyday life.

Confusing perceived and imagined actions: An experimental study of age differences

We designed an experiment to test the hypothesis that elderly people have more difficulty than young people in distinguishing among what they actually did (performed actions), what they watched someone else do (watched actions), and what they only thought about doing (imagined actions). It follows from Johnson and Raye's model that it should be difficult to distinguish between performed actions and imagined actions, because both are self-generated, and both leave traces of cognitive operations. Similarly, people might tend to confuse watched actions and performed actions because both leave traces of visual information. Watched and imagined actions should be most distinct from each other because they share few, if any, attributes. If elderly people do not encode sensory and contextual information effectively, they will more easily confuse actions of all kinds.

Subjects

Three groups of subjects were compared: a young group (n = 24; mean age 31; age range 24–39), a young-old group (n = 18; mean age 65; age range 60–68), and an old-old group (n = 18; mean age 76; age range 72–83). The elderly subjects were divided into the young-old and old-old groups because previous studies and pilot testing showed a consistent tendency for age deficits to be quite small in the 60–70 age range, but considerably more marked for those older than 70. Meyer and Rice (Chapter 13, this volume) list a number of studies in which the age differences conformed to this pattern. The groups were matched for social and educational background. The older subjects were retired professional people living at home and recruited by advertisements asking for volunteers.

Method

The task consisted of 36 actions involving moving everyday objects arranged on a grid. Three different arrays were used, with a new array being presented after the 12th and 24th actions. Examples of the actions are "Put the spoon next to the toothbrush" and "Put the stamp on the book." A given object was never involved in more than one action.

Subjects were seated in front of the array and given a pack of cards to turn over one by one. Written on each card was an action and a command. The com-

Table 14.2. *False Alarms and Misses (as percentages of all error responses)*

Age	False Alarms (%)	Misses (%)
70+	35.5	17.7
60–70	32.7	16.4
24–40	15.3	17.3

mand was either Perform, Watch, or Imagine, and these different commands were randomly mixed through the pack. On Perform trials, the subject performed the designated action; on Watch trials, the experimenter performed the action, the subject being instructed to watch carefully; on Imagine trials, the subject was told to look at the objects involved and imagine performing the action. The particular combinations of actions and commands were varied across subjects in a balanced fashion. After the series was completed, there was a 10-min delay during which subjects read a magazine article, followed by a recognition test. Subjects were given a written checklist of all 36 actions randomly reordered and mixed with 18 new distractor items. These were generated by recombining the old actions and objects into combinations that had not been included in the original series. These distractor items are hereafter called Nonevents. Subjects were asked to identify the origin of each item on the checklist as Performed, Watched, Imagined, or Nonevent.

Results

Correct classifications. Correct responses in this analysis were those in which the origin of the action described in the checklist was correctly identified as Performed, Watched, Imagined, or Nonevent. The mean percentages of correct identifications of origin are shown in Figure 14.1 for each age group. A mixed-design analysis of variance was carried out on the number of correct responses with age as the between-groups factor and origin as the within-groups factor. There were significant main effects of age [$F(2, 57) = 13.38$, $p < .001$] and of origin [$F(3, 171) = 24.9$, $p < .001$]. The interaction of age and origin was also significant [$F(6, 171) = 2.71$, $p < .01$]. Post hoc analysis by the Newman-Keul test showed that the old-old group made fewer correct identifications of Imagined actions than did the other age groups, and both old-old and young-old were less accurate than the young in identifying Nonevents. Age differences were not significant for actions that were Watched or Performed.

Misclassifications: false alarms and misses. The pattern of errors can be characterized by focusing on the distribution of False Alarms (misclassifying Nonevents as actions Imagined, Watched, or Performed) and Misses (missclassifying actions that were Imagined, Watched, or Performed as Nonevents). Table 14.2 shows the age differences in this distribution. The differences are significant ($X^2 = 21.8$, df

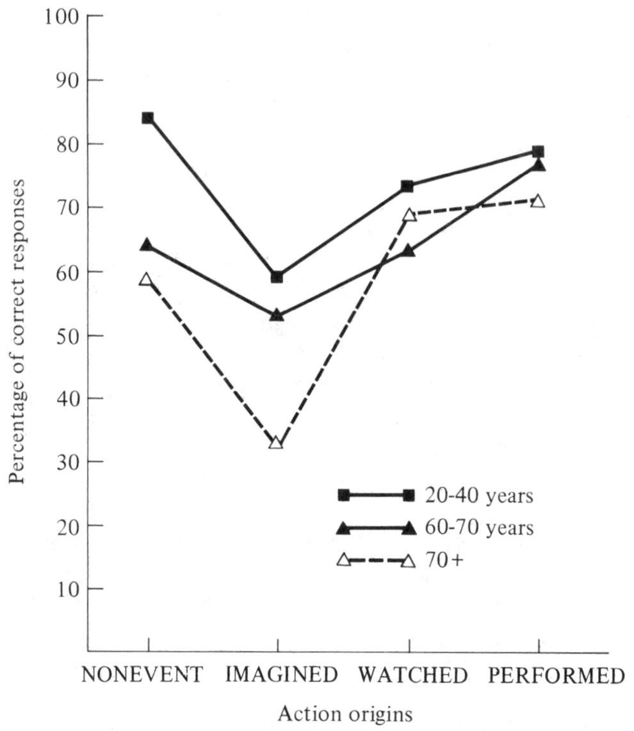

Figure 14.1. Mean percentage of correct identifications of origin for each age group.

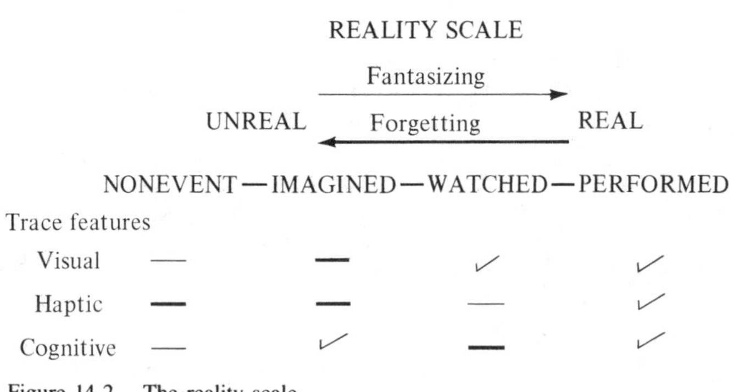

Figure 14.2. The reality scale.

= 2, $p < .001$), with both old groups making more False Alarm errors than the young.

A signal-detection analysis was carried out to see how far age differences in sensitivity and bias contributed to the results. Hits consisted of responses identifying any actions that had occurred as either Performed, Watched, or Imagined.

Table 14.3. *Mean values of* d′ *and* β *for each age group for each action origin*

	d'			β		
Age	Performed	Watched	Imagined	Performed	Watched	Imagined
70+	1.7	1.4	1.0	1.5	1.3	2.6
60–70	2.3	1.5	1.2	2.2	1.7	1.7
20–40	2.5	2.1	2.0	3.2	2.3	4.5

False Alarms consisted of responses identifying Nonevents as either Performed, Watched, or Imagined. Table 14.3 shows the mean values for d' and β for each age group. Separate analyses of variance were performed on the values calculated for d' and β. In the analysis of d', there was a significant effect of age [$F(2, 51) = 13.7$, $p < .001$] and of action origin [$F(2, 102) = 30.4$, $p < .001$]. There was no interaction between age and origin. The value of d' was higher for the young group, and for all age groups d' was highest for Performed actions, next highest for Watched actions, and lowest for Imagined actions.

In the analysis of β, again there were significant effects of age [$F(2, 51) = 3.94$, $p < .025$] and of origin ($F(2, 102) = 6.3$, $p < .002$]. There was no interaction between age and origin. The value of β was higher for the young group. For all groups, β was lower for Watched actions than for Imagined or Performed actions.

Misclassifications: types of error. Actions with different origins can be roughly ordered in terms of the extent to which the memory trace should possess the detailed sensory information characteristic of real events. For Nonevents there can be no memory trace at all, and Imagined events should be lacking in sensory detail. The trace of Watched events should include visual information, and the trace of Performed actions should contain both visual and haptic information. Accordingly, a reality scale can be constructed as shown in Figure 14.2. Errors can be characterized according to the direction of misclassification on the reality scale. Rightward-shifting errors attribute greater reality to the event than it actually had and can be described as fantasizing or reifying errors. A leftward-shifting error, such as misclassifying a Performed action as a Nonevent, attributes less reality and can be described as a forgetting error, because the subject has forgotten that he or she performed the action.

Fantasizing errors include the following misclassifications:

Nonevents misclassified as Imagined
Nonevents misclassified as Watched
Nonevents misclassified as Performed
Imagined actions misclassified as Watched
Imagined actions misclassified as Performed
Watched actions misclassified as Performed

Table 14.4. *Percentages of fantasizing and forgetting errors for each age group (as percentages of all errors)*

Age	Fantasizing (%)	Forgetting (%)
70+	66.1	33.9
60–70	59.6	40.4
20–40	44.3	55.7

Forgetting errors include the following misclassifications:

Performed actions misclassified as Watched
Performed actions misclassified as Imagined
Performed actions misclassified as Nonevents
Watched actions misclassified as Imagined
Watched actions misclassified as Nonevents
Imagined actions misclassified as Nonevents

Age differences in the incidences of fantasizing and forgetting errors are shown in Table 14.4. The young made more forgetting errors, but the old-old displayed the opposite bias and made more fantasizing errors ($X^2 = 29.1$, df $= 2$, $p < .001$). In the young-old group there was a smaller difference in the incidences of both kinds of errors. The nature of the errors made by each age group can be examined in more detail by calculating the incidence of each type of misclassification, as shown in Figure 14.3. For all kinds of actions there were significant age differences in the incidences of different sorts of confusion. For Performed actions, $X^2 = 9.01$; for Watched actions, $X^2 = 22.8$; for Imagined actions, $X^2 = 16.5$; for Nonevents, $X^2 = 14.4$. These differences can be summarized as follows:

1. The young group more often misclassified Performed actions as never having happened at all (i.e., as Nonevents). These were Misses or false negatives.
2. The old-old were more likely to misclassify Performed actions as Watched, and Watched actions as Performed, than were the other two age groups.
3. The old-old were more likely to misclassify Imagined actions as Performed or Watched than was either of the other two groups.
4. The old-old misclassified more Nonevents as Performed actions, and both old groups misclassified more Nonevents as Watched than did the young. These were False Alarms or false positives.

All these comparisons were significant by X^2 tests, with at least $p < .05$.

Discussion

The main focus of interest lies in the age differences in this task. The absence of any age decrement for Performed actions conforms to the findings reported by Bäckman (Chapter 28, this volume). Bäckman found no age differences for recall of subject-performed actions, though there was an age effect in

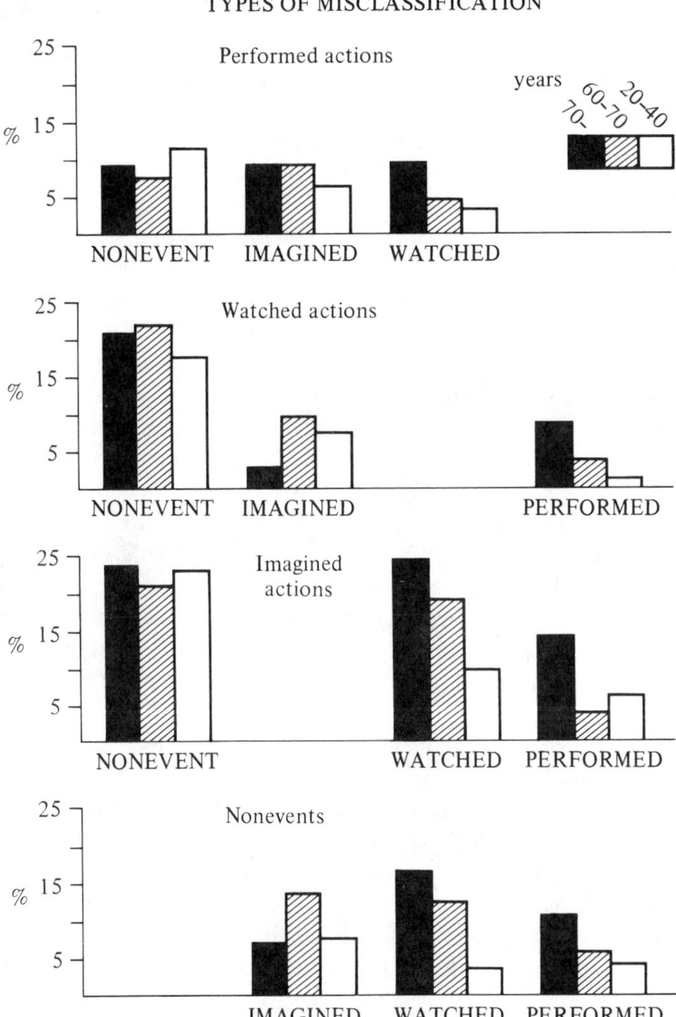

Figure 14.3. Incidences of different types of misclassifications made by each age group.

recall of the same actions when these were verbally presented and imagined by the subjects. In our study, the elderly made more errors in classifying Imagined actions and Nonevents, and there were marked age differences in the directions of errors.

The elderly were more likely to make False Alarm fantasizing errors, attributing more reality to events than they actually had. This reifying bias contrasts with the findings for the young, who made more forgetting errors. The elderly were also particularly prone to misclassify actions as Watched.

When the young did make false positive responses, these were in line with what Anderson (1984) called the "it had to be you" effect, whereby her young subjects attributed falsely recognized items to an external (other-generated) source rather than to themselves. Similarly, other-generated actions (watched and nonevents) were very rarely attributed to a self-generation. Young people were very clear about what they had or had not done themselves. In the elderly, this distinction between self-generated and other-generated actions was less clear-cut. The elderly group also appeared to use the Watched category as a kind of default category for items that lacked compelling evidence of origin.

There are several possible explanations for the observed patterns of results:

1. Age differences in memory trace: It might be argued that the elderly make more false positive errors because they have unusually vivid traces of Imagined actions that are therefore easily confused with the traces of real Performed or Watched actions. Foley and Johnson studied reality monitoring in young children and found that they also had difficulty in distinguishing between Performed and Imagined actions. Foley and Johnson suggested that in young children, Imagined representations have not yet acquired the distinctively schematic character that they assume later. They cited the tendency of the young child to subvocalize as an indication of the detailed and veridical nature of children's imaginal representations. Perhaps in old age imaginal memory representations again become less abstract and schematic and therefore more similar to "real" memory representations. This suggestion seems unlikely in view of Giambra's finding (1977) that elderly people rate their daydreams as less vivid than young people rate theirs. Also, in our experiment, the old subjects were also more likely to misclassify Nonevents (which can have no memory trace) as Performed or Watched. This observation suggests that the age differences cannot be due entirely to differences in the quality of the memory trace, but must also stem from differences in strategy or bias. Nevertheless, there is some evidence that memory traces are qualitatively affected by age. Young people made relatively few confusions between Performed and Imagined actions and Watched actions. For them, the memory of a self-generated action is distinct from the memory of an other-generated action, but the elderly subjects were clearly much less able to distinguish memory traces on this basis.

2. Age differences in strategy: It is possible to explain the age differences in the directions of errors as reflecting differences in confidence. If young subjects are generally confident that their memories are reliable, they will tend to assume that if they do not remember something, then it did not happen; so forgetting will produce false negative responses. Old people may be less confident in the reliability of their memories. In this case, if they have no clear memory of an event, they may assume that it did happen and they have forgotten it. This strategy will produce false positive responses.

To test this explanation, our experiment was rerun exactly as before. This time, however, when subjects classified the origin of each action on the recognition checklist, they were required to give a confidence rating for the judgment on this

Table 14.5. *Mean confidence ratings for each age group*

	Performed		Watched		Imagined		Nonevent	
Age	Correct[a]	Error	Correct	Error	Correct	Error	Correct	Error
70+	3.7	3.5	3.5	2.6	3.2	2.8	3.2	2.5
60–70	3.8	2.9	3.5	2.9	3.1	2.7	3.1	2.6
20–40	3.6	3.2	3.6	2.5	3.2	2.4	3.3	2.4

[a]Correct responses identify the action origin correctly; error responses are those incorrectly attributing that origin to an action.

scale: 4 (very sure); 3 (sure); 2 (not very sure); 1 (just guessing). The pattern of errors replicated the findings in the original experiment, but there was no sign of the expected age difference in levels of confidence. As can be seen in Table 14.5, for all age groups the level of confidence was highest for Performed actions, followed by Watched actions, Nonevents, and Imagined actions. The hypothesis that the elderly make false positive errors because of lack of confidence was not supported. Instead, it was surprising and somewhat disquieting to note that when the old made erroneous responses, such as misclassifying Nonevents as actions they had performed themselves, they did so with a high level of confidence.

3. Age differences in criterion: The signal-detection analysis suggests another possibility. The elderly had a significant reduction in d', suggesting that their memory traces contained less evidence, and they also had a significantly lower value of β, indicating a lower criterion. If less evidence were required for an item to be classified as real, this would produce the greater incidence of False Alarm responses and the greater readiness to misclassify items as Watched or Performed that was observed. Whereas the age-related reduction in d' can be ascribed to reduced sensitivity or increased neural noise, it is more difficult to understand why there should be an age-related lowering of criterion. Such a criterion shift would be a useful compensatory change if the cost of making false negative errors (Misses) were higher than the cost of False Alarms (the consequences of denying that something happened when it did happen are more damaging than the consequences of saying that something did happen when in fact it did not). In terms of slips of action in everyday life, a bias to classify Imagined actions (plans) as Performed would produce omission errors, because the action would not actually get done. We can think of some examples in which this might be less damaging than the repetition errors that the opposite bias would produce. It is probably better to put no salt in the soup than to put it in twice; better to take no medicine than to take double the dose. But in other cases it seems clear that omission errors would have more serious consequences than repetitions: Not turning off the gas is more costly than trying to turn if off a second time.

The findings that emerge from this study are broadly similar to those reported by Anderson (1984). Her investigation was confined to young subjects. She tested their ability to remember whether they had traced line drawings, imagined tracing them, or only looked at them. As in our experiment, she found that memory for imagining was more susceptible to confusion than was memory for tracing or looking. Her subjects' responses resembled those of our young group in that performing (tracing) and imagining were more often confused than were performing and watching. Although she did not carry out a signal-detection analysis, she found some evidence that different criteria were adopted in identifying different types of actions. As in our study, the least strict criterion was used for assigning items to the Watched category. The similarity between her findings and ours lends support to our results.

Kausler and Lichty (1985), however, compared young and older adults' memories for planned and performed actions. They found that although the frequency of planning had no effect on the estimated number of times performed, performing an action did inflate the estimate of number of times planned. There was no sign of any age difference in this pattern of results. Our findings would predict that older people would tend to misclassify planning as performance and thus overestimate the frequency of performance. One possible explanation of this discrepancy is that in Kausler and Lichty's experiment, ''planning'' consisted of reading and listening to instructions for the task. This is not quite equivalent to imagining doing the action and may entail that the memory representation of the plan is not very similar to the representation of the action.

In summary, our experimental study showed that an old-old (70+ years) group of subjects made more errors in reality monitoring. They made more false positive errors and were more likely to decide that actions that had never occurred or had only been imagined had been watched or even performed by themselves. A signal-detection analysis revealed age differences in both d' and β.

Age differences in confusing perceived and imagined actions in everyday life

To what extent can we say that the tendency to confuse real and unreal actions displayed in this experiment is also characteristic of older people in everyday life?

There are two sources of information available: self-assessments and observations of performance on naturalistic tasks set by the experimenter, but carried out in everyday settings.

Self-assessments

Self-assessments suffer from the drawbacks already outlined. In fact, of the considerable number of self-assessment questionnaires that have been in use in recent years (Herrmann, 1982), many do not examine age differences, and few ask questions designed to reveal lapses in reality monitoring. When such questions are posed, they may relate either to actions or to speech. Subjects are asked to rate the frequency of repetition errors ("How often do you find that you do/say something when you have already done/said it?") or of omission errors ("How often do you find you have failed to do/say something you intended to do/say?"). However, failures of these kinds are not always due to confusion between imagined and perceived events. An action may be omitted because the intention is simply forgotten, not because the intention is confused with performance. And an action may be repeated because the performance is simply forgotten, not because the performance is confused with the intention. This may explain why these self-assessments do not conform to the findings in the reality-monitoring experiment. Zelinski, Gilewski, and Thompson (1980) and Harris and Sunderland (1981) both found that the young reported a higher frequency of verbal-omission errors (forgetting to tell somebody something) than did the old. Harris and Sunderland also found that the young reported a slightly higher incidence of action-omission errors (forgetting to carry out an intended action). For both verbal- and action-repetition errors, no age differences have been noted.

However, Cohen and Faulkner (1984) asked the subjects who participated in the reality-monitoring experiment the following: "How often do you feel uncertain whether you have actually done something, like turning off the lights or locking the door, or only planned to do it?" This question does relate closely to failures and reality monitoring that involve confusions between real and imagined events, and the over-70 age group reported a slightly higher incidence ($p < .06$).

Naturalistic tasks

In several recent studies, subjects were asked to carry out specified actions at specified times, and compliance was monitored. Wilkins and Baddeley (1978) studied performance on a simulated pill-taking regimen. Their subjects were all under age 50; so no conclusions about age effects can be drawn. It is of interest, though, that there were many omission errors, but very few repetition errors. So, clearly, people do not often make the mistake of confusing the performed act of taking the pill with the imagined intention to take it. Moscovitch (1982) asked subjects of different ages to telephone the experimenter at a stated time of day. On this task, the performances of the elderly were superior, but this was attributed to the use of external reminders. So far, none of these naturalistic tasks has been well suited to assess age differences in reality monitoring.

This conclusion is reinforced by the results of studies by Sinnott (1984) and West (1984). In prospective memory tasks, such as remembering to make telephone calls or send postcards, the elderly usually outperform the young. Sinnott has suggested that old people compensate for declining memory ability by focusing their resources on the fulfillment of daily tasks and by using external reminders extensively and efficiently. A point that has been neglected is the extent to which people rely on cancelling their reminders in order to have a record of whether or not a task has actually been performed. Does the elderly shopper, for example, need to strike out each item on the shopping list as it is bought in order to avoid duplicating purchases? Such a strategy would be an effective way of avoiding the consequences of reality-monitoring failure.

In a study assessing the accuracy and credibility of elderly witnesses, Yarmey (1984) reported that elderly people made 20% more mistakes, misidentifying foils as targets in recognizing both victims and assailants. The high proportion of erroneous responses appeared to result from an unwillingness to respond "don't know." These findings conform to the age-related increase in False Alarms found in our reality-monitoring experiment.

Age differences in confusing implications and assertions

In memory for verbal information, are elderly people more prone to confuse the generated memories of implications with the perceived memories of assertions? Although there is evidence (e.g., from studies of memory for courtroom testimony, such as that by Harris, 1978) that people do tend to misremember implications as having been explicitly asserted, there have been no studies to compare the incidences of this type of confusion in different age groups. However, numerous experiments have indicated that memory for self-generated verbal information (such as implications and inferences) is more impaired by aging than is memory for perceived verbal information (explicit statements that have been heard or read).

There have been several studies that have examined age differences in memory for inferences as compared with memory for information that has been explicitly stated. Several of these found evidence of an age-related deficit in memory for inferences, whereas memory for explicit information was not affected by aging, but in some cases it was apparent that the elderly were failing to construct inferences rather than failing to remember them (Cohen, 1979, 1981; Light, Zelinski, & Moore, 1982). In Belmore's study (1981), older people did remember implicit information as well as explicit information, but the task was an easy one, with a low memory load. In a study of memory for texts, Cohen and Faulkner (1984) reported an age deficit in answering some kinds of multiple-choice questions after a delay. When the correct choice involved recognition of an inference, there was an age deficit, but when the correct answer required recognition of material reproduced verbatim from the original text, there was no age difference. This age-related failure to recognize inferences after a delay indicates that generated memories are less durable in old age. In another experiment, Cohen and Faulkner (1981) studied age differences in memory for deep structure and surface structure of texts. They found that old people made more errors in recognizing the deep structure from a text they had previously heard, but were as good as young adults in recognizing the surface structure. Because surface structure is directly perceived, whereas deep structure has to be generated by the listener, this finding also conforms to the view that age differences are greater for generated memories.

So the general trend of these experiments (in spite of some discrepant results) is to show that perceived memories are unimpaired by aging, whereas generated memories are more vulnerable to age effects. In old age, the cognitive operations involved in generation may be defective, so that memories that are constructed are not robust. Alternatively, old subjects may employ text-processing strategies (as outlined in Chapters 11 and 12) that are not so appropriate for generating information. Although there are indications that in old age, implications are poorly remembered, none of the studies has examined the possibility that the tendency to misremember implications as assertions increases with age, as our experimental results would predict.

Rabbitt (1981) did show that elderly people had difficulty in remembering the sources of information in multilateral conversations, such that utterances were attributed to the wrong speakers, but more direct experimental evidence for age differences in reality monitoring of verbal information is not available at present.

Conclusions

The combined weight of evidence from experimental testing, self-assessment, and formal observations supports the conclusion that in old age, generated memories are less distinctive and less robust and sometimes are liable to be confused with perceived memories. The experimental results reported here revealed a bias whereby the elderly were particularly prone to make reifying errors, believing that what was only imagined or never occurred at all was actually perceived. Naturalistic observations have not, thus far, shown much indication of this bias operating in everyday behavior, but this may be due to the fact that they have not been designed to capture the directional aspects of confusions between perceived and generated memories. It is important, though, that future research address this issue, because it has many practical implications. Changes in the ability to discriminate between memories of imagined and perceived events affect the reliability of eyewitness testimony and of autobiographical memories, the efficiency with which everyday tasks are performed, and the ability to comply with advice and instructions.

An age-related deficit in memory for imagined events can be theoretically linked to Rabbitt's suggestion (1982) that conceptually driven processes are impaired by aging, whereas data-driven processes are unaffected. Craik (1984) restated the same view that "age differences are slightest when processes are driven by the stimulus or are strongly determined or supported by the environment. Age differences are greatest, on the other hand, when the task requires the subject to go beyond the information given, where the processes must be self-initiated." Applied to the phenomena of reality monitoring, this theoretical distinction predicts the finding that the conceptually driven representations of imagined events are vulnerable to aging, whereas the data-driven representations of watched or performed events resist the effects of age. Of course, not all real-time actions are data-driven. Routine automatic actions become detached from environmental influence and are controlled by learned rules and habits. It is these automatic actions, therefore, that are most liable to be confused with conceptually driven plans and imaginings.

References

Anderson, R. E. (1984). Did I do it or did I only imagine doing it? *Journal of Experimental Psychology: General, 113,* 594–613.

Bartlett, F. A. (1932). *Remembering*. Cambridge University Press.

Belmore, S. M. (1981). Age related changes in processing explicit and implicit language. *Journal of Gerontology, 36,* 316–322.

Bransford, J. D., Barclay, J. R., and Franks, J. H. (1972). Sentence memory: A construct versus interpretive approach. *Cognitive Psychology, 3,* 193–209.

Burke, D. B., & Light, L. L. (1981). Memory and aging: The role of retrieval processes. *Psychological Bulletin, 90,* 513–546.

Cohen, G. (1979). Language comprehension in old age. *Cognitive Psychology, 11,* 412–429.

Cohen, G. (1981). Inferential reasoning in old age. *Cognition, 9,* 59–72.

Cohen, G., & Faulkner, D. (1981). Memory for discourse in old age. *Discourse Processes, 4,* 253–265.

Cohen, G., & Faulkner, D. (1984). Memory for text: Some age differences in the nature of the information that is retained after listening to texts. In H. Bouma & D. G. Bouwhuis (Eds.), *Attention and performance. Vol. X: Control of language processes.* Hillsdale, NJ: Lawrence Erlbaum.

Craik, F. I. M. (1984). Age differences in the acquisition and use of verbal information—a tutorial review. In H. Bouma & D. G. Bouwhuis (Eds.), *Attention and performance. Vol. X: Control of language processes.* Hillsdale, NJ: Lawrence Erlbaum.

Flavell, J. H., Flavell, E. R., & Green, F. L. (1983). Development of the appearance-reality distinction. *Cognitive Psychology, 15,* 95–120.

Giambra, L. M. (1977). Adult male day-dreaming across the life-span: A replication, further analyses and tentative norms based upon retrospective reports. *International Journal of Aging and Human Development, 8,* 197–228.

Harris, J. E., & Sunderland, A. (1981). *Effects of age and instructions on an everyday memory questionnaire.* Paper presented to the British Psychological Society conference on memory, Plymouth.

Harris, R. J. (1978). The effects of jury size and judge's instructions on memory for pragmatic implications from courtroom testimony. *Bulletin of the Psychonomic Society, 11,* 129–132.

Harris, R. J., & Monaco, G. E. (1976). Psychology of pragmatic implication: Information processing between the lines. *Journal of Experimental Psychology: General, 107,* 1–22.

Herrmann, D. J. (1982). Know thy memory: The use of questionnaires to assess and study memory. *Psychological Bulletin, 92,* 434–452.

Herrmann, D.J. (1984). Questionnaires about memory. In J. E. Harris & P. E. Morris (Eds.), *Everyday memory, actions and absentmindedness* (pp. 133–152). London: Academic Press.

Johnson, M. K. (1985). The origin of memories. In P. C. Kendall (Ed.), *Advances in cognitive behavioural research and therapy* (Vol. 4). New York: Academic Press.

Johnson, M. K., Raye, C. L., Wang, A., & Taylor, T. (1979). Fact and fantasy: The role of variability in confusing imaginations with perceptual experiences. *Journal of Experimental Psychology: Human Learning and Memory, 5,* 116–122.

Johnson, M. K., & Raye, C. L. (1981). Reality monitoring. *Psychological Review, 88,* 67–85.

Johnson, M. K., Taylor, T., & Raye, C. L. (1977). Fact and fantasy: The effects of internally generated events on the apparent frequency of externally generated events. *Memory and Cognition, 5,* 116–122.

Kausler, D. H., & Lichty, W. (1985). Adult age differences in recognition memory and frequency judgements for planned versus performed activities. *Developmental Psychology, 21,* 647–654.

Light, L. L., Zelinski, E. M., & Moore, M. (1982). Adult age differences in inferential reasoning in episodic memory. *Journal of Experimental Psychology: Learning, Memory and Cognition, 8,* 435–447.

Loftus, E. F. (1979). *Eyewitness testimony.* Cambridge, MA: Harvard University Press.

Morris, P. E. (1984). The validity of subjective reports on memory. In J. E. Harris & P. E. Norris (Eds.), *Everyday memory, actions and absentmindedness* (pp. 153–172). London: Academic Press.

Moscovitch, M. (1982). A neuropsychological approach to memory and perception in normal and pathological aging. In F. I. M. Craik & S. Trehub (Eds.), *Aging and cognitive processes.* New York: Plenum Press.

Norman, D. A. (1981). Categorization of action slips. *Psychological Review, 38,* 1–15.

Podgorny, P., & Shepard, R. N. (1978). Functional representations common to visual perception and imagination. *Journal of Experimental Psychology: Human Perception and Performance, 4,* 21–35.

Rabbitt, P. M. A. (1981). Talking to the old. *New Society, 22,*

Rabbitt, P. M. A. (1982). Cognitive psychology needs models for changes in performance with old age. In J. Long & A. Baddeley (Eds.), *Attention and performance. Vol. IX: Stress and aging* (pp. 555–579). Hillsdale, NJ: Lawrence Erlbaum.

Reason, J. T. (1979). Actions not as planned: The price of automatization. In G. Underwood & R. Stevens (Eds.), *Aspects of consciousness* (Vol. 1). New York: Academic Press.

Shepard, R. N. (1984). Ecological constraints on internal representation: Resonant kinematics of perceiving, imagining, thinking and dreaming. *Psychological Review, 91,* 417–446.

Sinnott, J. D. (1984). *Prospective/intentional and incidental everyday memory: Effects of age and the passage of time.* Paper presented to the American Psychological Association, Toronto.

West, R. L. (1984). *An analysis of prospective everyday memory.* Paper presented to the American Psychological Association, Toronto.

Wilkins, A. J., & Baddeley, A. D. (1978). Remembering to recall in everyday life: An approach to absentmindedness. In M. M. Gruneberg, P. E. Morris, & R. W. Sykes (Eds.), *Practical aspects of memory.* New York: Academic Press.

Yarmey, A. D. (1984). Accuracy and credibility of the elderly witness. *Canadian Journal on Aging, 3*(2), 79–90.

Zelinski, E. M., Gilewski, M. J., & Thompson, L. W. (1980). Do laboratory tests relate to self-assessment of memory ability in young and old? In L. W. Poon, J. L. Fozard, L. S. Cermak, D. Arenberg, & L. L. Thompson (Eds.), *New directions in memory and aging* (pp. 519–550). Hillsdale, NJ: Lawrence Erlbaum.

15 Aging and word retrieval: Naturalistic, clinical, and laboratory data

Nancy L. Bowles, Loraine K. Obler, and Leonard W. Poon

A common complaint among older people is their increasing difficulty in finding common words and proper names with which they are familiar in everyday speaking and writing (e.g., Zelinski, cited in Burke & Light, 1981). At the same time, vocabulary scores indicate that knowledge of word meanings is well maintained with increasing age (Botwinick, 1977; Kramer & Jarvik, 1979). Tulving and Thomson (1973) distinguished between semantic memory (i.e., the store of knowledge about words and concepts, their properties and interrelations) and episodic memory (i.e., the store of knowledge about personally experienced events). Standard laboratory tests have suggested that semantic memory is retained well into old age (Eysenck, 1975; Smith & Fullerton, 1981), in contrast to episodic memory, which shows impairment with age (Craik & Simon, 1980; Perlmutter, 1979). Bowles and Poon (1985a) suggested that the laboratory tasks that have been used to measure semantic-memory functioning are not sensitive to the deficits of which older people complain.

Word retrieval is of special interest in this context because it has been studied in the naturalistic setting (Cohen & Faulkner, 1986; Reason & Lucas, 1983), in the clinical setting (Goodglass, 1980; Nicholas, Obler, Albert, & Goodglass, 1985), and in the laboratory setting (Bowles & Poon, 1985a, 1985b; Brown, 1979). In this chapter it is argued that the research goals differ in these settings, and each makes its own contribution to our understanding of behavior. It will be shown that despite the fact that each line of research appears to be relatively independent of the others, there has been a convergence toward a common conceptual model of word-retrieval processing.

A two-component model of semantic memory of the sort proposed by Collins and Loftus (1975) will be adopted to provide a common framework for the present discussion. This model is characterized by the separation of lexical information (word names) and semantic information (concepts). The lexical component contains the names of the words known to an individual and phonemic

Preparation of this chapter was supported by National Institute on Aging grant 1 R01 AG05972–01 and by the Medical Research Service of the Veterans Administration.

(sound) and orthographic (spelling) information about the items. The semantic component is a complex system of interconnected concepts or categories. Word-retrieval tasks, for the purposes of this discussion, are those in which a stimulus activates a concept in the semantic network, and the response requires accessing the concept name in the lexical network (or lexicon). Such a stimulus might be an object or a picture, a verbal definition or description, or internally generated activation of a concept, among many other possibilities. This word-retrieval (or naming) type of memory task provides a special opportunity to compare the approaches taken in the naturalistic, clinical, and laboratory environments and to observe how each has contributed to our understanding of behavior.

This chapter summarizes some of the major findings in each setting and attempts to understand what each tells us about the processing involved in successful and unsuccessful word retrieval and about how this processing might be affected by cognitive changes associated with aging. What follows is a selective review that illustrates the common themes that recur in the study of naming. Changes in automatic and controlled retrieval processes, in activation of semantic memory, and in the structure and organization of the semantic network are postulated to account for naming impairment in aging, aphasia, and dementia.

Although there seems to have been little cross-fertilization among word-retrieval investigations in naturalistic, clinical, and laboratory settings, one seminal study has been cited in virtually all publications on word retrieval: the "tip-of-the-tongue" study by Brown and McNeill (1966). Briefly, in that study, college students were presented with definitions of target words of low normative frequency that were expected to be on the fringes of their accessible vocabularies (e.g., *apse, nepotism, cloaca*). The task was to write down the name of the target word that was defined. Whenever a student believed that he or she knew the word, was close to retrieving it, had it "on the tip of the tongue," but was unable to produce it, the task was to write down as much as possible about the word. Students in this state were able to produce more information than would be produced by chance concerning some of the letters of the word (most frequently the initial or terminal letters), the number of syllables, and the stress patterns. These results have provided a common background for virtually all investigators interested in word retrieval.

In order to account for their partial-recall results, Brown and McNeill (1966) proposed a card-sorting model in which a concept is accessed on the basis of a definition by sorting on salient features in the definition. According to this model, word-name information associated with the concept is not always completely "legible." That is, partial information, such as the initial letter, may be available when the rest of the features are too "faint" to recall. Further retrieval efforts can be based on the concept that has been identified, yielding words that are semantically related to the target word, or they can be based on the partial orthographic and phonemic information, yielding words that share these features with the target word. Although their model does not provide for separation of the word name from conceptual information, it does encompass the possibility that a concept can be retrieved without recall of its associated word name.

Studies in a naturalistic setting

Two means used to study word retrieval in the naturalistic setting have been the diary and the questionnaire. This type of study is concerned with failures in word retrieval, or word-retrieval blocks, recorded as they occur in the course of daily living. Subjects are asked to record occurrences of failures to retrieve a word or name whenever they occur, along with information about the event. Studies of this type with young adult subjects were reported by Reason and Lucas (1983). They carried out two diary studies to investigate the tip-of-the-tongue (TOT) experience as it occurs in a natural setting. The first study was intended to test for the presence of incorrect blocking stimuli during the TOT state. An incorrect blocking stimulus was defined as an incorrect name or word that repeatedly came to mind instead of the correct target word or name. Such a word or name was labeled a ''recurrent blocker.'' Young adult volunteers were asked to record over a period of 4 weeks the occurrences of those TOT experiences that were eventually resolved and to provide specific information about each experience and its resolution. The experience was found to be relatively rare, with an average of 2.5 TOT states reported per participant in the 4-week period. The investigators divided the reported TOT states into those that were blocked by a recurring word or name that was known to be wrong and those in which no recurrent blocker occurred. They found that about half of the TOT states were characterized by recurrent blockers and that the resolution for these states differed from the resolution for those without such blocks. That is, blocked states were more likely than unblocked states to be resolved by the use of external strategies (e.g., consulting other people or using a reference book). This was true even though more features of the target word were available in the blocked state because a recurrent blocker generally shared features with the target word. Unblocked states were more likely to be resolved by internal strategies (e.g., an alphabetical search or recalling contextual information). The two types of states were equally likely to be resolved by later spontaneous access to the target word or name.

Reason and Lucas (1983) saw the retrieval of words and names as a largely automatic process that becomes conscious only when it has failed by activating an incorrect target or no target. In their view, the conscious system does not have access to the more efficient automatic retrieval schemata. A recurrent blocker inhibits retrieval because once it has been brought into consciousness, the additional activation of the recent event (the recurrent blocker) makes it difficult for the correct target to gain attention.

Aging

Cohen and Faulkner (1986) reported a questionnaire study of memory blocks for proper names, comparing old, middle-aged, and young adults. Each participant was requested to fill out the questionnaire the next time a name block occurred in the course of daily living. The results for the young and middle-aged groups were quite similar to those obtained by Reason and Lucas (1983), whose studies included blocks for both words and proper names. Cohen and Faulkner found that partial phonological information about a blocked target name was significantly less available for the older adults than for the younger and middle-aged adults. Consistent with this lack of phonological information, the older adults experienced significantly fewer recurrent blockers than did the other groups. They often described the experience in terms like "my mind was a complete blank." Finally, when a blocking name did occur, older adults were less certain about whether it was or was not the sought-after target name. These authors interpreted these results in terms of a reduced level of activation of concepts in semantic memory among the elderly.

In summary, accessing desired words and names is rarely a problem for young adults; when there is a retrieval failure, they often have some partial information about the target word or name. Older adults report more retrieval failures and less information about targets they cannot retrieve.

The diary and questionnaire studies have yielded some potential sources of naming impairment. For example, the results have been interpreted in terms of automatic and conscious processing, inhibition by related blockers (Reason & Lucas, 1983), reduced activation of concepts in semantic memory, and reduced access to phonological information in the lexicon (Cohen & Faulkner, 1986), notions that will appear again as we discuss other approaches to the study of word retrieval.

Studies in a clinical setting

Meanwhile, there has long been interest in word retrieval in the diagnosis and study of neurological disorders such as the aphasias (Goodglass, 1980) and the dementias (Obler & Albert, 1984). The most widely used task in this setting is confrontation naming in which an object or picture is presented, and the task is to provide its name. The Boston Naming Test (Kaplan, Goodglass, & Weintraub, 1976) is a standard diagnostic and research tool consisting of a series of line drawings of objects whose names vary in frequency of occurrence (e.g., *tree, comb, abacus*). Patients are asked to name the object pictured in each drawing. The clinical studies of word retrieval are distinguished from other laboratory studies by their common interest in comparing the performances of subgroups differing in clinical presentation. As we examine some of the word-retrieval studies that have been carried out with patients with aphasia or dementia, we shall see how inferences about processing can be made based on the differences in performance between populations with specific clinical diagnoses.

The conceptual model of confrontation naming that is shared by a number of clinical researchers generally includes several stages of processing, such as a perceptual stage in which the stimulus is recognized, a lexical stage in which the phonological characteristics of the word name are located, and an articulatory stage in which the motor program necessary to produce the word is activated (Goodglass, 1980). An underlying theme of this research has been the determination of which stage is affected in different clinical populations.

Aphasia

Patients with aphasia typically are classified into one of several categories. Patients with pure anomic aphasia are characterized by difficulty with naming (anomia) exclusively. Patients with other sorts of aphasia evidence anomia as part of their syndrome. In addition to anomia, Wernicke's aphasia is characterized by fluent speech that is lacking in meaningful content; Broca's aphasia is characterized by limited, nonfluent speech consisting largely of content words; conduction aphasia is characterized by difficulty in the production of speech. It is thought that patients with either anomic aphasia or Wernicke's aphasia have a problem in the association between an activated concept in semantic memory and the phonological characteristics in lexical memory. Broca's aphasics and those with conduction aphasia exhibit a problem in the motor programs required to produce the target word (Goodglass, 1980).

Selected experiments from a series carried out by Goodglass and his colleagues demonstrated how the study of naming in aphasics can illuminate our understanding of possible sources of naming impairment. Goodglass, Kaplan, Weintraub, and Ackerman (1976) used the Brown and McNeill (1966) paradigm to learn how much information about a word was available when the word could not be named, for four different types of aphasic groups. Both Broca's aphasics and conduction aphasics were significantly above the chance level of performance in identifying the initial sounds of words that they were unable to produce. In contrast, anomic and Wernicke's aphasics showed no evidence of partial knowledge about the words that they could not retrieve. However, it was shown that the types of word associations elicited in response to the stimulus pictures did not differ across groups, and all groups were able to select the correct target word in a multiple-choice test virtually without error. The word-association results suggest similar structures of the semantic network for the four groups. The nearly perfect recognition results indicate that the word names are present in the lexicon for all groups. There appears to be impairment in accessing the word name that is most severe for the anomic and Wernicke's aphasics.

Goodglass and Stuss (1979) compared naming in response to picture stimuli and in response to verbal descriptions in anomic, Wernicke's, and Broca's aphasics. They assumed that picture stimuli led to immediate and direct access to the response word, whereas verbal descriptions relied on indirect peripheral associations to locate the correct word. They found that Broca's aphasics were superior to the other groups in naming under both stimulus conditions. Wernicke's aphasics showed the greatest impairment in response to verbal descriptions, and this was true even after covarying for oral comprehension ability.

To account for these data, Goodglass (1980) proposed that anomic and Wernicke's aphasics depend largely on automatic retrieval processes, being limited in controlled retrieval processing. Both automatic and controlled retrieval processes are assumed to be available to Broca's aphasics, as they are to normal adults. Some of the supporting data can be summarized as follows: Broca's aphasics can sometimes consciously access partial information in the lexicon when they are unable to produce a word, and they are helped by cues that support controlled lexical access (phonological cues). Wernicke's aphasics, on the other hand, have little partial lexical information available to consciousness when they cannot retrieve a word, and they are helped relatively little by cues that support controlled retrieval processing. They are differentially benefited by stimuli (pictures) that foster more rapid responses. One can speculate, as Goodglass did, that these aphasic groups represent differential impairments of controlled processes in word retrieval.

Another possible source of naming impairment in aphasia might be changes in the organization of the semantic network. Lhermitte, Desrouesné, and Lecours, cited by Goodglass and Baker (1976) speculated that naming impairment might in part be due to semantic-field breakdown. Evidence for such a breakdown is seen in a study by Zurif, Caramazza, Myerson, and Galvin (1974) in which Wernicke's aphasics performed almost randomly in a semantic sorting task. Goodglass and Baker (1976) studied the relationship of naming to the availability of associative information about target words in aphasic patients varying in comprehension ability. Subjects were first asked to name pictured objects and then to recognize words that were related to the target objects in a variety of ways. They found that impaired naming in the low-comprehension aphasics (equivalent to Wernicke's) was related to reduced ability to recognize associates of the target concept. This result was interpreted as supporting the notion that naming impairment in some aphasics reflects a breakdown of semantic fields.

Based on these studies and a large body of other work with aphasic patients, Goodglass (1980) proposed several hypotheses about word retrieval. The evidence supports the notion that there is a separation between a concept in memory (labeled the "semantic field" in Goodglass's work) and the lexical information necessary to identify its name (its phonological features). The difference between Wernicke's and Broca's aphasics in partial knowledge about words they were unable to retrieve led to the suggestion that there are two ways in which a target word can be accessed. One is a direct connection between the concept and the articulatory program necessary to produce its name. This results in a rapid and automatic response when it is successful. The second type of retrieval occurs when the direct association fails, and it involves a search process that depends on semantic and phonological associations. The first type of retrieval appears to occur for all aphasic types, as well as for normal subjects. The search process, however, according to Goodglass, may be less readily available to patients with anomic or Wernicke's aphasia.

Additional support for the hypothesis that automatic semantic processing is preserved in aphasics comes from a study of semantic priming in lexical decision.

It is well established that healthy adults can decide whether or not a letter string is a word more quickly if it is preceded or accompanied by a semantically related word, rather than an unrelated word (Meyer & Schvaneveldt, 1971). This facilitation typically is attributed to automatic activation of words that are semantically related to the prime, which is assumed to make them more accessible (Collins & Loftus, 1975). Milberg and Blumstein (1981) demonstrated automatic semantic priming for aphasic patients who were unable to identify related words in a sorting task.

Naming might also be impaired by inadequate arousal of the concept (Goodglass, 1980). This could account for the improvement in naming for aphasics when both pictures and verbal stimuli are presented (Goodglass & Stuss, 1979). However, such a result would also be consistent with impairment of the representation of concepts in semantic memory. This idea received support from the results of the Goodglass and Baker (1976) study showing that low-comprehension aphasics were deficient in associative information about concepts they could not name.

In summary, the results of studies of aphasic patients suggest that there are several possible sources of impairment in the naming process: Conscious search processes may be less available. Activation of the semantic field may be inadequate. The associations between the semantic field and the phonological information necessary to identify its name may be less accessible. Finally, the connection between the phonological information and the articulatory program necessary to produce the sounds may be impaired.

Dementia

Impairment of naming is reported to be an early symptom of senile dementia of the Alzheimer type (SDAT) and has been shown to occur before other language changes associated with SDAT are measurable (Kirshner, Webb, & Kelly, 1984). Researchers have been interested in identifying which stage or stages of the naming process are likely to be affected in dementia. In particular, studies have addressed whether the naming failure associated with dementia is in the perceptual stage or in the lexical-access stage.

Barker and Lawson (1968) used a picture-naming task with demented patients. They showed that demonstration of the use of a pictured object reduced naming errors. Demonstration of function was assumed to facilitate the perception of the object pictured. The results were therefore interpreted as showing that the perceptual stage was impaired in dementia.

Rochford (1971) compared mixed-etiology demented patients to aphasic patients in a naming task, with body parts and line drawings of objects as stimuli. Perceptual demands were assumed to be less for body parts than for line drawings. The demented patients were more successful at naming body parts than at naming line drawings, whereas the aphasic patients performed at the same level with both types of stimuli. Furthermore, errors for the demented patients were more likely to be for the names of visually similar objects, whereas errors for aphasics were more likely to be either a failure to respond or an erroneous description of the object or its use. Rochford concluded that the naming deficits of dementia were primarily perceptual.

Kirshner and associates (1984) used a confrontation naming task in which they varied the degree of perceptual difficulty, word frequency, and word length. Perceptual difficulty was assumed to affect stimulus identification. Word frequency and word length were assumed to affect the search stage. Subjects had progressive dementia of at least 1 year's duration, assumed to be Alzheimer's dementia by exclusion of other causes. A normal age-matched control group was also tested. The performances of demented patients were significantly worse than those of normal controls in all conditions. Naming deficits were found even for those demented patients who were normal in language performance on subtests of the Boston Diagnostic Aphasia Examination (Goodglass & Kaplan, 1972). Naming, then, is affected early in dementia, before changes in other language functions are apparent. In addition, there were group-by-perceptual-difficulty and group-by-word-frequency interactions. Demented patients were significantly affected by perceptual difficulty and by word frequency, whereas normal controls were not. Kirshner and associates concluded that both the perception and word-search stages of naming are impaired in demented patients.

Obler and her colleagues studied naming in patients with a diagnosis of SDAT, ranging from very mild to moderately severe. Ten of the patients completed the Action Naming Test (Obler & Albert, 1978), in which the stimuli are drawings depicting actions (e.g., *sleeping, raking, knighting*). The SDAT patients were significantly less accurate and slower on the Action Naming Test than were healthy control subjects in their seventies. Both groups benefited from phonological cues when unable to retrieve a target word. Of interest with respect to the question of perceptual difficulties as a source of naming impairment in dementia, the demented patients gave proportionally fewer perceptually related responses than did the normal older adults. One possible reason that some investigators (Barker & Lawson, 1968; Rochford, 1971) have found more perceptual errors by demented patients than by healthy age-matched subjects, whereas the data from Obler and her colleagues showed the opposite, may be a difference in the identification of perceptual errors. In agreement with Bayles and Tomoeda (1983) and Goodglass (1980), it can be argued that not all errors that are called perceptual errors are truly perceptual in nature. Many things are both semantically related and visually similar (e.g., acorn and walnut). It is necessary to distinguish between errors resulting from shared visual features alone and those resulting from both shared visual features and shared semantic features. Based on a strict definition of perceptual errors, the data of Obler and associates do not suggest that naming problems associated with dementia are based on perceptual difficulty.

A later analysis of the data from the Action Naming Test (Obler & Albert, 1978) revealed a subset of SDAT patients who were indistinguishable from the healthy older adults in number of words correctly retrieved, but who gave significantly more error responses prior to correct responses. These patients were able to access appropriate response candidates, but had difficulty in selecting among them. In effect, they responded with all of the words that seemed plausible and let the experimenter decide when a correct response had been given. Such a problem in identifying the correct response could be due to loss of distinguishing features in semantic representations or to reduced ability to use semantic information in the decision-making process.

Grober, Buschke, Kawas, and Fuld (1985) addressed these alternatives in studies of semantic organization in SDAT. In two experiments the task was to identify semantic attributes that were associated with stimulus concepts. It was assumed that loss of features in the semantic representations of concepts would be reflected in failure to associate attributes with their target concepts. Although demented patients made more errors than did healthy older adults, they were nonetheless quite accurate in identifying associated attributes (a hit rate of 95% in Experiment 1). Grober and associates proposed that semantic representations are relatively intact in dementia, but that the salience of attributes is altered. In a third experiment, the task was to rank attributes associated with a concept in order of their importance to its meaning. Those with dementia were less successful than healthy older adults in correctly ranking essential features (e.g., "fly" for the concept "airplane"). These authors suggested that dementia may result in reductions in the relative weights assigned to essential attributes in semantic representations of concepts in memory; semantic memory may no longer be organized in terms of attributes ordered according to their relative importance to associated concepts, but rather in terms of equally weighted attributes. Thus, dementia is seen to affect the organization of the semantic network, rather than its underlying content.

Schwarz, Marin, and Saffran (1979) extensively studied language function in a patient with a progressive dementia. The patient (W. L. P.) was able to name only one object from a set of 70 color photographs of common household objects. She did not benefit from phonological cues. She was, however, able to demonstrate by gestures that she recognized the objects. A multiple-choice naming test for these objects provided as response alternatives the correct name of each object and three distractors that were semantically related, phonologically related, and unrelated to the correct name. The results showed considerable impairment even though the target word was present among the response alternatives. In the earlier stages of the disease (the first 15 months of testing), her errors almost always consisted in selection of the semantically related distractor. Based on this and other experiments related to naming, Schwarz and associates concluded that W. L. P.'s naming difficulty preceded lexical access and was associated with a "dedifferentiation" between concepts in the semantic network. This process was thought to be systematic and characterized by loss of distinguishing characteristics, whereas general aspects of meaning were preserved. The fact that W. L. P. was able to demonstrate the use of stimulus objects showed that she did perceive the differences between them. She was, however, unable to use those differences conceptually in order to classify and name those objects.

Another line of research relevant to naming impairment in dementia is the investigation of automatic activation in SDAT patients. Nebes, Martin, and Horn (1984) reported automatic priming by semantically related words for SDAT patients in a word-reading task. They concluded that semantic memory was spared in dementia and could be accessed through automatic processes. Nebes and Boller (in press) confirmed that automatic processes were intact in dementia by showing equivalent context effects for demented patients and healthy older adults in a visual letter-search task. On the other hand, Grober and Kawas (1986) reported reduced automatic activation in patients who were considered to be at risk for developing dementia, based on scores on the mental-status test of Blessed, Tomlinson, and Roth (1968). Interference in a modified version (Warren, 1972) of the Stroop (1938) task and incidental memory for spatial location were used to assess automatic processing. Impairment in automatic processing, seen in the absence of the standard interference effect, was observed only in those patients who later were diagnosed as having dementia. These same patients were also deficient in incidental memory for spatial location of stimulus words, also thought to depend on automatic processing. Grober and Kawas proposed that even in the preclinical stage of dementia, processes that are normally carried out automatically begin to make demands on the limited-capacity attentional system. A deficiency in automatic processing would indeed lead to the impairment in semantic encoding and retrieval seen in demented patients. Resolution of the conflicting results concerning the fate of automatic processing in dementia remains an important area in current research.

In summary, studies of naming in dementia indicate that there is impairment both in identification of concepts in the semantic network and in access to word names in the lexicon. Current research is concerned with uncovering the sources of problems in concept identification. There are conflicting interpretations concerning the contribution of perceptual problems to naming impairment in SDAT. Naming failure due to difficulty in distinguishing between related response candidates is attributed to changes in the content and/or organization of semantic representations. Reduction in automatic semantic activation is proposed as a possible source of word-retrieval deficits in dementia, although there are contradictory data on this issue.

Aging

Growing out of the clinically oriented research, there have been two studies that have direct relevance to naming effects associated with normal aging. One was the work of Borod, Goodglass, and Kaplan (1980), which provided normative data for the Boston Naming Test. These results showed little age-related change in naming ability until 70 years of age.

Nicholas and associates (1985) studied naming in healthy elderly adults using the Boston Naming Test (Kaplan et al., 1976) and the Action Naming Test (Obler & Albert, 1978). Their subjects represented four age groups: 30–39 years, 50–59 years, 60–69 years, and 70–79 years. There were significant age-related effects on both tests in accuracy as well as latency. In accuracy, the seventies group was significantly poorer in performance than the other three groups. In latency, the thirties group was significantly faster than the other three groups. For those trials on which cues were given (trials on which the subject was unable to name the stimulus), there were no age differences in the percentages of target words correctly retrieved. There were, however, significantly more such trials for the older group. Semantic cues were given only when the subject did not correctly perceive the stimulus. Such cues led to successful retrieval less than 50% of the time for any age group, and the proportions of successful retrievals after semantic cues did not differ with age. The error analysis showed that the younger adults produced a higher proportion of semantically related responses, and the older groups produced more circumlocutions. This study demonstrated that healthy older adults take longer to retrieve words in response to picture stimuli and fail to name them correctly more often than do younger adults. These authors suggested that the increased use of circumlocutions by older adults reflects a compensatory mechanism for the inability to retrieve word names.

In summary, healthy older adults are impaired in naming relative to younger adults, but significantly less so than are patients with aphasia or dementia. Their difficulty appears to involve retrieval of words in the lexicon.

Naming impairment is an early symptom of SDAT, even preceding other signs of language impairment. It is also, of course, a primary symptom of aphasia. Patients with either kind of disorder are significantly impaired in naming relative to age-matched control groups. Deficits typically are viewed in terms of perceptual failure, failure at the level of concept recognition, failure in lexical access, or failure at the level of motor realization. Very broadly, it appears that aphasics suffer from inability to retrieve the word name, given that a concept has been identified (anomics and Wernicke's aphasics), or suffer from inability to retrieve the motor program to speak the word (conduction and Broca's aphasics). There is some evidence that Wernicke's aphasics may also have some loss of information in the conceptual network. Patients with SDAT appear to be impaired both in the ability to identify concepts in the semantic network and in the ability to retrieve concept names. Hypotheses are being tested concerning the availability, accessibility, and organization of information in semantic memory in aphasia and dementia. In addition, the fate of automatic activation processes in aphasia and dementia is under investigation.

Studies in a laboratory setting

A. S. Brown (1979) introduced a modified version of the Brown and McNeill (1966) paradigm that appears to be a very productive approach to the study of word retrieval in the experimental laboratory setting. He presented young adult subjects with definitions of words, preceded by priming stimuli, and measured the latency to produce the target word as a function of the relationship of the prime to the target word. The primes were semantically related (e.g., *thim-*

ble for the target word *needle*), orthographically related (e.g., *noodle* for *needle*), unrelated (e.g., *closet* for *needle*), or neutral with respect to the target words. This paradigm emphasizes the nature of the factors that influence successful word retrieval, rather than those that are relevant to failures in word retrieval (the typical approach in the studies we have considered so far). Brown found that for young adults, primes that began with the same letters (and same phonemes) as the target words had no effect on retrieval latency relative to neutral primes; semantically unrelated primes inhibited retrieval latency relative to neutral primes; unexpectedly, semantically related primes also inhibited retrieval latency relative to neutral primes, at least as much as unrelated primes and in one study significantly more than unrelated primes. Brown suggested that unrelated words led to conscious selection of the inappropriate category to be searched, whereas semantically related words inhibited the automatic within-category search, presumably because the prime word was more highly activated than the target word. According to Baddeley (1982), the word-retrieval system is devised to inhibit the retrieval of related concepts in order to prevent interference between their names in fluent speech.

Bowles and Poon (1985b) recently proposed that Brown's data (1979) can better be understood in terms of orthographic and phonemic facilitation and inhibition, rather than in terms of semantic facilitation and inhibition. They demonstrated that initial-letter primes (the first two letters of the target words) significantly speeded retrieval. In addition, they pointed out that although orthographically related prime words in Brown's studies did not lead to significantly faster responses than did neutral primes, responses were significantly faster than for the semantically unrelated primes, although the orthographically related primes were also semantically unrelated to the targets. This was seen as indicating that retrieval was benefited by orthographic relatedness. Furthermore, both the semantically related and unrelated primes were orthographically unrelated to the targets, and both showed inhibition of response latencies relative to neutral primes. Bowles and Poon concluded that orthographic priming is important in word retrieval when orthographically related primes are present. This conclusion, though somewhat of a departure from Brown's interpretation, certainly would not surprise the investigators who have presented phonological cues after failures in picture naming.

The distinction between automatic and controlled processes in word retrieval, raised earlier by Reason and Lucas (1983), by Goodglass (1980), and by Brown (1979), has recently been addressed experimentally. Goodglass, Theurkauf, and Wingfield (1984) varied stimulus difficulty in a picture-naming task with young adult subjects. They analyzed the response distributions of naming latencies to test the possibility that the mean (or median) response time in a naming task, typically used as the dependent measure in the analysis of response latencies, encompasses a population of rapid responses, representing automatic retrieval, and another of slow responses, reflecting voluntary (conscious) processes. The analysis showed that stimulus difficulty, determined empirically and by normative word frequency, affected rapid responses, but not slow responses, confirming that the two sets of responses reflect different processes. Bowles and Poon (1985b) also raised the issue of automatic and controlled processes in word retrieval. They argued that providing partial orthographic information in a word-retrieval task affects controlled retrieval processing. The argument was based on data showing both facilitation by orthographically related primes and inhibition by unrelated primes. The presence of inhibition was taken to indicate that controlled processing was involved (Posner & Snyder, 1975). This was confirmed in another word-retrieval study in which inhibition was eliminated when subjects knew that the primes would be unrelated.

Roediger, Neely, and Blaxton (1983) showed that when a correct prime (the target word itself) was sometimes presented (which was true in the 1979 Brown studies), semantically related primes resulted in longer responses than did semantically unrelated primes. When there were no correct primes, there was no difference in response latency between semantically related and unrelated primes. These authors proposed that when correct primes were sometimes presented, subjects first made a decision whether or not the prime was the correct target word, and then, if it was not, initiated a search for the correct word. Collins and Quillian (1972) showed that the time to make such a decision is increased as semantic relatedness is increased. When the correct target word never occurs as a prime, no such decision is required, and the search for the target word can begin immediately.

The priming paradigm is interesting in the ways that it differs from other approaches to the study of word retrieval. First, it is concerned with factors that affect successful retrieval, rather than those that affect retrieval after a failure has occurred. The primes are presented before word retrieval can be attempted, rather than after a retrieval failure. Second, subjects do not typically know the relationship of the prime to the target word on any trial, because the prime types are randomly mixed. Third, according to Goodglass and Stuss (1979), the use of a verbal definition, rather than a picture stimulus, elicits more indirect, controlled retrieval processing. The primed word-retrieval paradigm shares with picture-naming studies a stimulus that is presumed to access the conceptual representation of a concept in memory and a response that requires access to the lexicon in the absence of reliable orthographic or phonemic information in the stimulus. The results are consistent with those of the picture-naming paradigm in showing an advantage for orthographic (and/or phonemic) cuing over semantic cuing.

Aging

Bowles and Poon (1985a) adopted Brown's paradigm (1979) to study word-retrieval processes in healthy older adults. The goal was first to determine if a deficit could be measured in the laboratory consistent with reports of increased difficulty associated with aging in word and name retrieval. The second goal was to identify specific sources of such difficulty in older individuals.

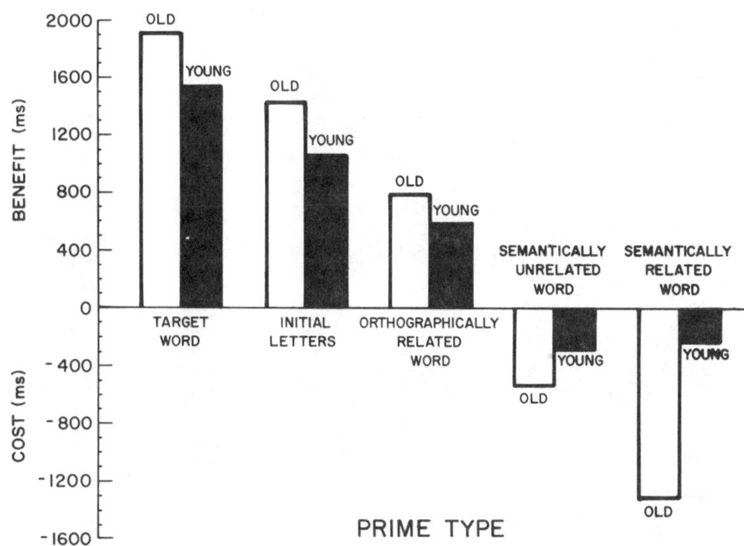

Figure 15.1. Mean facilitation (benefit) and inhibition (cost) of response latency relative to latency in the neutral condition for older and younger adults as a function of prime type.

Subjects were presented with a stimulus definition displayed on the screen of a video monitor. For example, "a mythical animal with one straight horn on its head" served as the definition for the target word, *unicorn*. Each definition was preceded by a priming stimulus that could be the correct target word (*unicorn* for the foregoing definition), an orthographically related word (*uniform*), a semantically related word (*dragon*), an unrelated word (*candle*), the initial letters of the target word (*un*), or a neutral prime (*xxxxxx*). The task was to say the word that was defined as quickly as possible.

The overall pattern of results replicated that of Brown (1979) for young adults. Response latencies are shown in Figure 15.1 in terms of mean cost or benefit for each prime condition relative to the neutral prime condition. Performance was facilitated by orthographically related primes and inhibited by both semantically related and unrelated primes, which were also orthographically unrelated, for both older and younger adults. As can be seen in Figure 15.2, the pattern of priming effects on number of successful retrievals paralleled that for response latency. There were significant deficits for older adults both in number of successful retrievals and in speed of retrieval, and there were significant age-by-prime-type interactions for both measures. For number of successful retrievals, the interaction was due to the fact that the old and young groups did not differ in the correct prime condition or in the initial-letters prime condition, but did differ

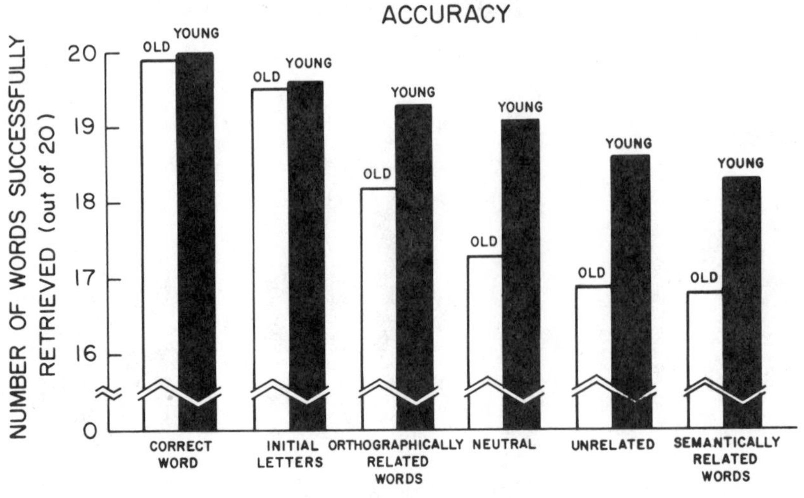

Figure 15.2. Mean numbers of words successfully retrieved (out of a possible 20) for older and younger adults as a function of prime type.

in all other conditions. The old were just as successful as the young in recognizing the prime as the correct word and just as successful at retrieving the correct word when reliably provided with the initial two letters. This suggested that the age-related problem in word retrieval is one of activation of orthographic and phonemic information in the lexical network.

Whereas the latency analysis showed the overall slowing typical of older adults in all conditions, the interaction was due to a tendency for older adults to take longer in the semantically related condition than in the unrelated condition; the young showed no difference in latency between the unrelated and the semantically related conditions. In two other studies of young adults in which correct primes were sometimes used, young adults also showed greater inhibition by semantically related primes than by semantically unrelated primes (Brown, 1979, Study 2; Roediger et al., 1983, Experiment 1). As was discussed earlier, Roediger and associates (1983) attributed this inhibition to a strategy of first rejecting the prime as the correct target word and then searching for the target. The Bowles and Poon (1985a) results suggested that older adults were more likely to adopt such a strategy and/or take longer to reject the prime as the correct target word. In support of this possibility, older subjects were more likely to incorrectly accept a semantically related prime as the correct target word. This could have been due to changes in the content or organization of semantic representations in healthy older adults similar in kind to those suggested by Goodglass (1980) in aphasics and by Schwarz and associates (1979) and Grober and associates (1985) in demented patients. Such a possibility requires further testing.

A second word-retrieval study was carried out in our laboratory (identical with the first except that we used no correct primes) to test the account of Roediger and associates (1983) of inhibition by semantically related primes relative to semantically unrelated primes. According to Roediger's explanation, there should be no inhibition by semantically related primes relative to unrelated primes in the absence of any correct primes. There was no suggestion of any difference in response latency between the semantically related and semantically unrelated prime conditions for the young adults. For the older adults, there was a large but nonsignificant increase in latency in the semantically related condition as compared with the unrelated condition, even in the absence of any correct primes. In this study, only 10 of 20 older subjects showed this effect, and the apparent difference between the two conditions was largely due to a subset of subjects who had exceptionally large effects. Some of these older adults insisted that the semantically related primes were the correct target words, even though the correct words never appeared as primes. A longitudinal study is needed to determine if this effect reveals early breakdown of the semantic fields, which might signal more serious problems to come, or if this simply represents a difference in criterion or style of no significance with respect to memory function.

In summary, interpretation of word-retrieval experiments concerned with healthy older adults relies on the same themes that we have encountered in naturalistic investigations and in work with clinical populations: The distinction is made between automatic and controlled processes in understanding the sources of priming effects (Bowles & Poon, 1985b; Goodglass et al., 1984); older adults are seen to have a deficit in activation of orthographic information in the lexical network (Bowles & Poon, 1985a); at least some apparently healthy older adults have difficulty in selecting between related words, which is seen as a possible breakdown at the level of semantic representation.

Conclusions

Age-related deficits in word retrieval

Lexical access. The Bowles and Poon (1985a) results, along with those of Nicholas and associates (1985), established that the word-finding difficulty about which older adults complain is measureable in the laboratory in terms of the ability to provide word names and the speed of retrieval. These results, along with those of others (Chapters 11–13, this volume), contradict the traditional view that semantic-memory processing is relatively unaffected by cognitive changes associated with normal aging. Two tasks that are commonly cited to support this view are lexical-decision tests and vocabulary tests. In lexical decision, the stimulus is a string of letters, and the task is to decide whether or not the letter string forms a real word. Older adults are just as accurate as younger adults at this task, and the age differences in response latency are relatively small (Bowles & Poon,

1985a; Howard, McAndrews, & Lasaga, 1981). The stimulus letter string provides complete orthographic information about the target word, which apparently assures access to its representation in the lexicon. The success of older adults in lexical decision indicates that the lexicon is intact and access to it is unimpaired, given the complete target word as a retrieval cue. In the standard vocabulary test, the stimulus word also provides the complete orthographic information that facilitates direct lexical access. Further retrieval required by the task is from the word name in the lexicon to the concept in the semantic network. The fact that healthy older adults perform this task as well as younger adults indicates that the semantic network is maintained and that connections from the word name to the concept are as accessible for older adults as for younger adults. Further support for this view was the observation that in word retrieval, there was no age difference in the ability to recognize the correct target word when it was given as a prime (Bowles & Poon, 1985a). In addition, the age difference observed in word retrieval was significantly reduced when partial orthographic information was provided in the prime (Bowles & Poon, 1985a) or when partial phonological information was given as a cue (Nicholas et al., 1985). In the naturalistic setting, older adults were shown to be lacking in partial orthographic information about words that they were unable to retrieve, whereas younger adults often had such partial information (Cohen & Faulkner, 1986). All of these results are consistent with the notion that the word-retrieval deficit associated with healthy aging lies, at least in part, in access from a concept in a conceptually organized store to a word name in an orthographically and phonemically organized store in the absence of orthographic or phonemic stimulus information.

Stimulus identification. In dementia, particularly as the disease progresses, there is evidence that naming impairment occurs prior to lexical access: in identification of the stimulus concept in the semantic network (Schwarz et al., 1979). A similar suggestion has been made to account for naming impairment in some aphasic patients (Goodglass, 1980). Inability to identify a stimulus concept implies a loss of information in the semantic network, a change in its organization, or reduced ability to access, or use, available information in the semantic network. There is mixed evidence concerning such changes in the semantic network in healthy older adults (Burke & Light, 1981). Bowles and Poon (1985a) showed relatively large inhibition of response latency by semantically related primes for some older adults. This inhibition can be seen as an indication of difficulty in discriminating between related concepts. Such inhibition might reflect some loss of features, or change in organization, in the semantic network for a subset of older adults, who otherwise have no apparent symptoms of a memory disorder. Further support comes from the observation by Cohen and Faulkner (1986), in a questionnaire study, that older adults were less certain whether a recurrent blocker was or was not the target word they were seeking. Again, this result suggests that a reduction in the discriminability between related concepts in the semantic network may contribute to word-retrieval impairment in some apparently healthy older adults.

Hypothesis testing and naturalistic research

Several testable hypotheses concerning the underlying processes involved in word-retrieval failure have been suggested by the foregoing work in the naturalistic, clinical, and experimental laboratory settings. First, semantic activation may be reduced, with lower activation leading to difficulty in accessing the pathway to the lexical information (Cohen & Faulkner, 1986; Goodglass, 1980; Grober & Kawas, 1986). Seemingly contrary evidence comes from experiments showing that healthy older adults (Bowles & Poon, 1985a; Howard et al., 1981), aphasics (Milberg & Blumstein, 1981), and patients with mild dementia (Nebes et al., 1984) benefit as much as control subjects from activation by semantically related primes in a lexical-decision task or a reading task. These results indicate that the magnitudes of semantic activation of related concepts by word stimuli are comparable for these groups that vary widely in word-retrieval abilities. However, there have been few tests reported that have been concerned with the relative speed or duration or scope of such activation for older and younger adults; but see Howard, Shaw, and Heisey (1986) for one such experiment. Differences in these properties of activation in semantic memory could account for some of the age differences in word-retrieval processing. Furthermore, it is activation of orthographic and phonemic information that appears to be impaired in healthy older adults. Little is known about this type of activation, which may differ from semantic activation and may differ for old and young adults. These suggestions concerning semantic and orthographic activation can be tested.

Reason and Lucas (1983), Goodglass (1980), Baddeley (1982), and others have proposed that there are two types of word-retrieval processes: automatic and controlled. Processing may typically be automatic and come to our attention only when it has failed. The controlled system is assumed to be slower and less efficient than the automatic system. Impairment of word retrieval could be the result of reduced access to the controlled retrieval system, as Goodglass suggested might be the case for anomic and Wernicke's aphasics. Alternatively, it could also result from an increased dependence on the less efficient controlled processes. These are testable hypotheses.

Goodglass (1980), Schwarz and associates (1979), and Bayles and Tomoeda (1983), among others, have implicated the concept-identification stage as a source of word-retrieval failure in aphasia and in dementia. Evidence has been discussed showing that some healthy older adults may also have problems at this stage. Such problems could be due to a loss of features in the semantic network, changes in the organization of the semantic network, a reduction in access to semantic features, or changes in decision criteria. These, too, are testable hypotheses.

An important problem in attempting to test such hypotheses by using diary studies, questionnaires, or observation in natural settings is that important aspects of word-retrieval processing are likely to be, at least to some extent, automatic and not subject to either introspection or observation. Laboratory experiments will be essential to achieve the task control required to test hypotheses about underlying mental processes at this level. We would argue that observation and introspection in natural settings will be necessary to identify the phenomena that are important and to validate laboratory findings. Studies in a clinical setting can take advantage of a unique opportunity to relate more or less well known abnormalities to cognitive performance. Experimental studies will be necessary to provide means to elucidate processes that are not subject to direct observation. The issue should never be to choose among naturalistic, clinical, and experimental studies, but rather to increase the communication between those involved in these separate research strategies in order that our understanding of any particular aspect of memory can be informed by the widest possible knowledge base.

References

Baddeley, A. D. (1982). Domains of recollection. *Psychological Review, 89*, 708–729.

Barker, M., & Lawson, J. (1968). Nominal aphasia in dementia. *British Journal of Psychiatry, 114*, 1351–1356.

Bayles, K. A., & Tomoeda, L. K. (1983). Confrontation naming impairment in dementia. *Brain and Language, 19*, 98–114.

Blessed, G., Tomlinson, B. E., & Roth, M. (1968). The association between quantitative measures of dementia and of senile change in the cerebral grey matter of elderly subjects. *British Journal of Psychiatry, 114*, 797–811.

Borod, J. C., Goodglass, H., & Kaplan, E. (1980). Normative data on the Boston Diagnostic Aphasia Examination, Parietal Lobe Battery, and the Boston Naming Test. *Journal of Clinical Neuropsychology, 2*, 209–215.

Botwinick, J. (1977). Intellectual abilities. In J. E. Birren & K. W. Schaie (Eds.), *Handbook of the psychology of aging* (pp. 580–605). New York: Van Nostrand Reinhold.

Bowles, N. L., & Poon, L. W. (1985a). Aging and retrieval of words in semantic memory. *Journal of Gerontology, 40*, 71–77.

Bowles, N. L., & Poon, L. W. (1985b). Effects of priming in word retrieval. *Journal of Experimental Psychology: Learning, Memory, and Cognition, 11*, 272–283.

Brown, A. S. (1979). Priming effects in semantic memory retrieval processes. *Journal of Experimental Psychology: Human Learning and Memory, 5*, 65–77.

Brown, R., & McNeill, D. (1966). The "tip of the tongue" phenomenon. *Journal of Verbal Learning and Verbal Behavior, 5*, 325–337.

Burke, D. M., & Light, L. L. (1981). Memory and aging: The role of retrieval processes. *Psychological Bulletin, 90*, 513–546.

Cohen, G., & Faulkner, D. (1986). Memory for proper names: Age differences in retrieval. *British Journal of Developmental Psychology, 4*, 187–197.

Collins, A. M., & Loftus, E. F. (1975). A spreading-activation theory of semantic processing. *Psychological Review, 82*, 407–428.

Collins, A. M., & Quillian, M. R. (1972). Experiments on semantic memory and language comprehension. In L. W. Gregg (Ed.), *Cognition in learning and memory* (pp. 117–138). New York: Wiley.

Craik, F. I. M., & Simon, E. (1980). Age differences in memory: The roles of attention and depth of processing. In L. W. Poon, J. L. Fozard, L. S. Cermak, D. Arenberg, & L. W. Thompson (Eds.), *New directions in memory and aging: Proceedings of the George A. Talland memorial conference* (pp. 95–112). Hillsdale, NJ: Lawrence Erlbaum.

Eysenck, M. W. (1975). Retrieval from semantic memory as a function of age. *Journal of Gerontology, 30,* 174–180.

Goodglass, H. (1980). Disorders of naming following brain injury. *American Scientist, 68,* 647–655.

Goodglass, H., & Baker, E. (1976). Semantic field, naming, and auditory comprehension in aphasia. *Brain and Language, 3,* 359–374.

Goodglass, H., & Kaplan, E. (1972). *The assessment of aphasia and related disorders.* Philadelphia: Lea & Febiger.

Goodglass, H., Kaplan, E., Weintraub, S., & Ackerman, N. (1976). The "tip-of-the-tongue" phenomenon in aphasia. *Cortex, 12,* 145–153.

Goodglass, H., & Stuss, D. T. (1979). Naming to picture versus description in three aphasic subgroups. *Cortex, 15,* 199–211.

Goodglass, H., Theurkauf, J. C., & Wingfield, A. (1984). Naming latencies as evidence for two modes of lexical retrieval. *Applied Psycholinguistics, 5,* 135–146.

Grober, E., Buschke, H., Kawas, C., & Fuld, P. (1985). Impaired ranking of semantic attributes in dementia. *Brain and Language, 26,* 276–286.

Grober, E., & Kawas, C. (1986). Early identification of dementia: An information processing approach. In *Proceedings and Abstracts of the Annual Meeting of the Eastern Psychological Association.* New York.

Howard, D. V., McAndrews, M. P., & Lasaga, M. I. (1981). Semantic priming of lexical decisions in young and old adults. *Journal of Gerontology, 36,* 707–714.

Howard, D. V., Shaw, R. J., & Heisey, J. G. (1986). Aging and the time course of semantic activation. *Journal of Gerontology, 41,* 195–203.

Kaplan, E., Goodglass, H., & Weintraub, S. (1976). *The Boston Naming Test* (experimental edition). Boston.

Kirshner, H. S., Webb, W. G., & Kelly, M. P. (1984). The naming disorder in dementia. *Neuropsychologia, 22,* 23–30.

Kramer, N. A., & Jarvik, L. A. (1979). Assessment of intellectual changes in the elderly. In A. Raskin & L. A. Jarvik (Eds.), *Psychiatric symptoms and cognitive loss in the elderly.* Washington, DC: Hemisphere Publishing.

Meyer, D. E., & Schvaneveldt, R. W. (1971). Facilitation in recognizing pairs of words: Evidence of a dependence between retrieval operations. *Journal of Experimental Psychology, 90,* 227–234.

Milberg, W., & Blumstein, S. E. (1981). Lexical decision and aphasia: Evidence for semantic processing. *Brain and Language, 14,* 371–385.

Nebes, R. D., & Boller, F. (in press). The use of language structure by demented patients in a visual task. *Cortex.*

Nebes, R. D., Martin, D. C., & Horn, L. C. (1984). Sparing of semantic memory in Alzheimer's disease. *Journal of Abnormal Psychology, 93,* 321–330.

Nicholas, M., Obler, L. K., Albert, M. L., & Goodglass, H. (1985). Lexical retrieval in healthy aging. *Cortex, 21,* 595–606.

Obler, L. K., & Albert, M. L. (1978). *Action Naming Test* (experimental edition). Boston.

Obler, L. K., & Albert, M. L. (1984). Language in aging. In M. L. Albert (Ed.), *Clinical neurology of aging* (pp. 245–253). New York: Oxford University Press.

Perlmutter, M. (1979). Age differences in adults' free recall, cued recall, and recognition. *Journal of Gerontology, 34,* 533–539.

Posner, M. I., & Snyder, C. R. R. (1975). Attention and cognitive control. In R. L. Solso (Ed.), *Information processing and cognition: The Loyola symposium* (pp. 55–86). Hillsdale, NJ: Lawrence Erlbaum.

Reason, J., & Lucas, D. (1983). Using cognitive diaries to investigate naturally occurring memory blocks. In J. E. Harris & P. E. Morris (Eds.), *Everyday memory, actions and absentmindedness* (pp. 53–70). London: Academic Press.

Rochford, C. (1971). A study of naming errors in dysphasic and in demented patients. *Neuropsychologia, 9,* 437–443.

Roediger, H. L., III, Neely, J. H., & Blaxton, T. A. (1983). Inhibition from related primes in semantic memory retrieval: A reappraisal of Brown's (1979) paradigm. *Journal of Experimental Psychology: Learning, Memory, and Cognition, 9,* 478–485.

Schwarz, M. F., Marin, O. S. M., & Saffran, E. M. (1979). Dissociations of language function in dementia: A case study. *Brain and Language, 7,* 277–306.

Smith, A. D., & Fullerton, A. M. (1981). Age differences in episodic and semantic memory: Implications for language and cognition. In D. S. Beasley & G. A. Davis (Eds.), *Aging and communicative disorders.* New York: Grune & Stratton.

Stroop, J. R. (1938). Factors affecting speech in serial verbal reactions. *Psychological Monographs, 50,* 38–48.

Tulving, E., & Thomson, D. M. (1973). Encoding specificity and retrieval processes in episodic memory. *Psychological Review, 80,* 352–373.

Warren, R. E. (1972). Stimulus encoding and memory. *Journal of Experimental Psychology, 102,* 151–158.

Zurif, E. G., Caramazza, A., Myerson, R., & Galvin, J. (1974). Semantic feature representations for normal and aphasic language. *Brain and Language, 1,* 167–187.

16 Acquisition and utilization of spatial information by elderly adults: Implications for day-to-day situations

Kathleen C. Kirasic

Spatial activities form such an integral part of everyday life that they are rarely noticed as phenomena unto themselves. However, we are reminded of the critical roles that spatial thought and behavior play in the quality of life when problems occur in the course of these activities, as, for example, when we search for but cannot find a desired object or when we become disoriented in an unfamiliar part of town. Relatively little is known about the effects of aging on human spatial abilities, especially those cognitive skills involved in spatial activities. Consequently, we can make only the most general of inferences regarding the impact of spatial cognition and behavior on the quality of life for elderly adults.

Clearly, additional research is needed in this area, but in order to be of optimal value, this research should be guided by a general conceptual framework that can be used to evaluate previous empirical work and point to promising avenues for future inquiry. The purpose of this chapter is to delineate a potentially valuable approach to the scientific study of spatial cognition and behavior in elderly adults, with particular emphasis on the spatial tasks that confront them in the course of their daily lives. Fundamental to this approach is the proposition that meaningful research in this area should be based on an understanding of real-world situations, that is, psychological events in their ecological context.

Cohen (1985) has suggested that there is something special about spatial cognition and behavior. Those researchers who make reference to the term "spatial cognition" share a general assumption that thinking about the spatial attributes of objects and events is phenomenologically different from other types of thought and that underlying this unscientific sense of difference are unique, scientifically discernible modes of acquiring and utilizing information. There is no consensus concerning the boundaries of this uniqueness (i.e., the similarities between spatial and nonspatial cognitive activities). However, psychometric evidence (Guilford, 1967; McGee, 1979) and psychoneurological evidence (De Renzi, 1982;

During the preparation of this chapter, the author was supported by grant AG05169-02 from the National Institute on Aging.

Luria, 1973) of the distinctiveness of spatial cognition are sufficient to support the basic assumption that it is a unique, useful area of inquiry.

Spatial cognition and behavior are involved in a wide range of human activities. Despite this variety, however, certain spatial activities may be assumed to be common to individuals across age groups and life-styles. Everyone is faced with the task of navigating to and from necessary and desired destinations using some means of transportation, and everyone must rely on spatial memory for the day-to-day activity of locating objects in the home or place of work. These problems represent reasonable foci for researchers interested in studying the role of spatial cognition in everyday life.

Identification of spatial activities that are particularly relevant to older adults represents a worthwhile enterprise. One approach to this objective entails simply asking individuals to keep track of their activities. I employed this approach as an exploratory exercise: Three elderly women in different geographic settings and rather different life circumstances were asked to keep track of their spatial activities for a period of 1 week. The three participants were Pauline K., a 72-year-old lifetime resident of a northeastern industrial community, Anna V., who was 83 years old and a 10-year nursing-home resident in a midwestern college town, and Jean B., a 68-year-old retiree who had resided in a ''sunbelt'' retirement community for only 2 months. Each woman was asked to pay particular attention to (1) spatial activities within the confines of her private living space (i.e., house, apartment, or room), (2) spatial activities outside of her private living space, (3) accompanied and unaccompanied travel away from home, and (4) problems related to spatial tasks (e.g., difficulty in locating objects or in navigating to destinations).

The logs of these three women indicated a number of spatial activities during a 1-week period. Most of the spatial tasks within the immediate living space involved well-established patterns of movement within rooms or from one room to another. It should be pointed out that the private living space of the nursing-home resident was limited to one room. As might be expected, she spent much less time in that area than the other two women spent in their private residences. All women reported engaging in tasks requiring them to remember the locations of objects. For example, Pauline K. engaged in a search for bills to be paid and for information needed to complete tax forms.

All three women spent a great deal of time traveling to destinations outside of their private spaces. For Anna V., this movement involved visiting friends within the nursing home, going to chapel, visiting the activity room (where she played video games), and going to the dining hall. She was unaccompanied in all of her travel with the exception of one trip to the physical therapist, during which she was accompanied by an orderly. Pauline K. followed well-known routes through her urban area to visit the homes of friends and relatives and to shop at several grocery stores, a pharmacy, and a shopping mall. Similarly, Jean B.'s activities included trips to friends' houses, the local supermarket, shopping malls in the vicinity of her new home, and a hospital where she works as a volunteer. During these travels, both Pauline K. and Jean B. drove their own automobiles and were unaccompanied. None of the women reported visiting a new place or taking a new route to a familiar destination during the week.

Given the activities reported, it is a straightforward matter to anticipate the types of spatial problems encountered by these women. As suggested previously, remembering the locations of objects in the home environment was problematic in some instances. When memory failed, search procedures were employed to find objects, as in the case of Pauline K.'s misplaced glasses. None of the women became disoriented in the familiar surroundings of their own homes, but occasionally Pauline K. would find herself in a room without remembering exactly what she had intended to do there.

No one reported becoming lost or disoriented in her travels outside the home environment, which is not too surprising, because they visited no novel places during the week and used familiar routes. However, remaining oriented in large-scale environments such as shopping malls was mentioned as a potential problem. Specifically, Jean B. reported the problem of remembering the location of her automobile in the shopping-mall parking lot, a problem she sought to overcome by parking next to the same landmark (a broken lightpost) on every visit. The effectiveness of this strategy was tested when she emerged from the mall by a different exit than she had planned. Interestingly, Pauline K., too, volunteered information regarding past difficulties in recalling parking locations in large lots. She also related a particularly upsetting incident several years earlier: After multiple stops on an extended shopping trip, she had become disoriented and could not spontaneously recall the spatial relationship between the shopping center where she stood and her home neighborhood.

These three informal case studies provide a small, unscientific sample rather than an exhaustive account. Nevertheless, this type of anecdotal evidence permits us to infer that several types of spatial activities are common for most older people. These activities include remembering the locations of objects, searching for missing objects, maintaining orientation in large-scale environments, and navigating routes to desired destinations.

The scope of these spatial activities suggests the need for a comprehensive approach to the scientific study of spatial cognition and behavior, an approach that is activity-oriented rather than methodologically oriented. In the absence of a general framework for conceptualizing a research area, studies that focus on a specific problem (e.g., spatial memory) and that employ a particular methodology (e.g., psychometric testing) may yield findings that will be difficult to relate to other findings and to issues of real-world relevance. A broad conceptual framework can help to remedy these problems by transforming real-world activities into scientifically approachable problems and by relating empirical findings to everyday circumstances.

An ecological framework for studying spatial cognition and behavior

The conceptual framework described by Kirasic and Allen (1985) offers an ecological approach to examining critical issues in spatial cognition. This framework has been influenced to some extent by a contextualistic philosophical position (Pepper, 1965), with emphasis on activity within a defined context. In this instance, the activities primarily involve the acquisition and utilization of spatial information, and the context includes the multitude of behavior settings that compose the physical environment.

Dimensions of the framework

The framework involves three major dimensions, representing the characteristics of the individual, adaptive processes, and situations (Kirasic & Allen, 1985). Rather than being unified or unitary categories, each of these dimensions includes a variety of phenomena studied by psychologists.

Characteristics of the individual. Under this broad dimension fall the many psychological variables that differentiate individuals from each other. This includes the basic perceptual, motor, cognitive, and personality domains that immediately come to mind, as well as factors such as physical and neurological status. Also considered part of this dimension are demographic variables such as sex, socioeconomic status, life-style, and means of transportation. Differences in spatial or geographic knowledge gained through travel and residential experience provide another important basis for distinguishing among individuals.

Adaptive processes. The term "process" is used in a number of ways in the psychological literature, but in this case it is used to refer to activities that facilitate achievement of spatial objectives or accomplishment of spatial tasks. Learning (in virtually all of its connotations), remembering, and problem solving are general cognitive phenomena that fit this description; map interpretation, orientation maintenance, and comprehension of verbal directions are examples of specialized adaptive processes in the spatial domain. This dimension also covers the use of strategies, coping mechanisms, and assorted remedial or therapeutic measures.

Situations. As Sjoberg (1981) pointed out, the concept of situations has generated more debate than research. Despite problems of definition and conceptual rigor (Magnusson, 1981; Scheidt & Schaie, 1978), it will be difficult to gain an accurate picture of spatial cognition and behavior in elderly adults without considering contextual influences. Behavior occurs only in relation to a situation and thus cannot be adequately explained or understood in isolation from it (Magnusson, 1981). This seems particularly true in the case of spatial behavior. However, spatial situations have yet to be cataloged, classified, and analyzed into components. An adequate classification system presumably would include distinctions among tasks (i.e., what the individual must do to achieve the desired objective) and among task settings (i.e., when and where these demands must be met). Tasks can be presented in terms of specific perceptual, cognitive, and behavioral demands, and task settings can be differentiated on the basis of function (e.g., home environment versus occupational setting), scale of space (e.g., room-sized area versus geographic area), complexity, and familiarity.

Heuristic value of the framework

The purpose in identifying the three dimensions of the framework is not simply to provide another set of rubrics for classifying variables of interest. Instead, the framework is designed to focus attention on the interactive influences of variables composing the three dimensions. As Siegel (1981) pointed out, the key to progress in a research area lies largely in the ability to ask better research questions. Questions relating to the extent of individual differences in spatial abilities are important, but questions concerning the interactions of these differences with the cognitive demands of a cognitive task (e.g., map reading) provide richer insight into everyday cognitive functioning. Situational factors (e.g., reading a subway map in an unfamiliar city) present a third interactive dimension that brings ecologically based influences on cognition and behavior into sharper focus.

This three-dimensional framework will prove useful if it assists researchers in establishing direct links between scientific studies, on the one hand, and real-world spatial activities, on the other. One way of establishing such links retrospectively is to relate past research on spatial cognition and behavior in elderly adults to the three general dimensions constituting this framework. Accordingly, the next section of this chapter consists of a summary of the spatial literature. Another way of establishing links between scientific research and everyday problems using this framework involves the development of a prospective research agenda, and the final section of this chapter is concerned with this endeavor.

Research on the acquisition and utilization of spatial information

The literature on aging and spatial cognition can be divided into three parts on the basis of methodology employed: research in the psychometric tradition, research in the experimental tradition, and research in the ecological tradition (Kirasic & Allen, 1985). Most of the work in the psychometric tradition concerns individual differences and thus corresponds to the dimension of the characteristics of the individual in the framework; most of the experimental work has been process-oriented and thus corresponds to the adaptive-processes dimension; most of the ecologically based studies have been concerned with environmental effects and thus correspond loosely to the situation dimension.

Assessment of individual characteristics

For decades, psychologists have relied on standardized psychometric instruments to assess the basic capabilities and characteristics of the individual. In a majority of studies, test scores have yielded evidence of general age-related decrements in cognitive and perceptual-motor abilities with increasing age (Botwinick, 1977; Horn & Cattell, 1966; Levison, 1981). Corresponding to these general decrements, profiles of performances on psychometric tests have indicated similar age-related declines in measures of spatial aptitude (Arenberg, 1978; Bilash & Zubeck, 1960; Fozard & Nuttall, 1971).

Most intelligence tests have spatial subtests or components, and age-related differences in performance on these subtests provide some information concerning the stability of spatial abilities into late adulthood. The Object Assembly, Picture Completion, Block Design, and Picture Arrangement subtests, for example, are WAIS subtests with spatial components. In a review, Salthouse (1982) noted that the data suggest a 5% to 10% decline per decade in performance on these subtests after age 30. Performance on the Space test of the Primary Mental Abilities Tests, one of five tests composing that instrument, also provides evidence of age-related changes in late adulthood. For example, the massive data set gathered by Schaie and his colleagues (Schaie & Labouvie-Vief, 1974; Schaie, Labouvie-Vief, & Buech, 1973) included evidence that spatial abilities declined slightly after the fifth decade of life.

Studies involving tests of distinct spatial abilities, or factor-referenced spatial tests, have also indicated a decline in such abilities beginning in the fourth or fifth decade of life. Just how many visuospatial abilities can be identified through factor-analytic techniques is a matter of debate (Lohman, 1979; McGee, 1979; Werdelin & Stjernberg, 1969). However, four factors that have received considerable attention from researchers are highlighted in this summary: *Visualization* is the ability to manipulate or transform the images of spatial forms or patterns (Ekstrom, French, & Harman, 1976). It is assessed using tests that require the visual structuring of objects from components, such as the Form Board Test or the Surface Development Test. *Spatial orientation,* also known as "spatial relations," is the ability to maintain orientation with respect to objects in space (Ekstrom et al., 1976), primarily by anticipating changes in appearance that result from varying the viewing angle. This ability is assessed using tests such as the Cube Comparison Test. *Speed of closure* refers to the ability to integrate apparently unrelated spatial elements into a single perceptual pattern (Ekstrom et al., 1976). The Gestalt Completion Test is an example of a test designed to measure this ability. *Flexibility of closure* refers to the ability to differentiate or disembed a figure from its perceptual background (Ekstrom et al., 1976). Tests such as the Hidden Figures Test have been used to assess this ability.

In their comprehensive treatment of age-related change in cognitive functioning, Horn and Cattell (1966) presented evidence that different spatial abilities peak in the 20–40-year age range and decline thereafter. With reference to Horn and Cattell's oldest age group (40–61 years old), the greatest decline was shown for the spatial-orientation factor (approximately 19%), followed by speed of closure (approximately 11%), visualization (approximately 6%), and flexibility of closure (approximately 5%). This pattern of age-related decline is characteristic of fluid abilities (Cattell, 1963; Cunningham, Clayton, & Overton, 1975; Horn &

Cattell, 1967); that is, those cognitive abilities pressed into service in the face of novel, abstract tasks.

In general agreement with this pattern of age-related decrements were other studies of speed of closure involving variations on the Gestalt Completion Test (Basowitz & Korchin, 1957; Danziger & Salthouse, 1978). Studies concerned with performance on tests for flexibility of closure have also produced evidence of age-related declines (Botwinick & Storandt, 1974; Lee & Pollack, 1978).

In addition to psychometrically assessed spatial abilities per se, perceptually based characteristics may play important roles in the acquisition and use of spatial information. Depth perception, visual tracking, and perceptual-motor coordination are examples. Despite the fact that distance perception may be presumed to play a very basic role in spatial cognition and behavior, little research has been done on age-related differences in visually perceived depth. Elderly adults appear to be less sensitive to stereopsis than are younger adults (Bell, Wolf, & Bernholtz, 1972; Hoffman, Price, Garrett, & Rothstein, 1959), but as Kline and Schieber (1985) pointed out in their review, stereopsis is but one source of depth information. Age-related changes in sensitivity to other sources of depth information (e.g., texture gradient, linear perspective, motion parallax) have not been well explored. Age-related decrements in the speed and effectiveness of visual tracking (i.e., keeping the eyes focused on a target object moving across the visual field) have also been documented (Sharpe & Sylvester, 1978), but as in the case of depth perception, the issue has not received a great deal of attention.

In contrast to the dearth of research on individual and age-related differences in perception, a great deal of scholarly attention has been directed toward the effects of aging on perceptual-motor coordination, particularly in reference to skilled behavior. Two aspects of perceptual-motor coordination have apparent implications for spatial behavior in real-world environments. The first of these is the pervasive phenomenon of behavioral slowing, which is well documented but not very well understood (Birren, Woods, & Williams, 1980; Salthouse, 1985). Limitations in processing and execution speed no doubt exert significant influences on the efficiency of spatial behavior. The second aspect of perceptual-motor coordination that should be considered is the presence of highly developed skills applied to spatial tasks (e.g., typewriting, mechanical drawing, map reading). Motor skills appear to be relatively robust into late adulthood (Welford, 1977). There is also evidence indicating that psychometrically assessed spatial abilities may be considered trainable skills (Willis & Schaie, 1985).

As an additional consideration, it is appropriate to mention psychoneurological status as a characteristic of the individual. Aging is not a pathologic condition, but pathologic conditions do tend to appear with age. Accordingly, any damage to those brain structures involved in spatial perception, spatial thought, or topographic memory will profoundly impact everyday spatial activities (De Renzi, 1982).

Summary. Most of the research concerned with individual characteristics relevant to spatial cognition and behavior has consisted of psychometric studies of spatial abilities, and the majority of this work has been dedicated to addressing the question of age-related decline in cognitive functioning. The consensus of this literature indicates that spatial abilities increase during adolescence, reach their peak during the second or third decade of life, and decrease rather steadily thereafter. Decrements have also been found in spatial perception and in perceptual, motor, and perceptual-motor speed.

Although it is important to document the relative stability of abilities through the life-span, it would also be worthwhile to focus attention on individual differences within the elderly population. Indeed, psychometric instruments have been designed primarily for the purpose of examining such individual differences. Recognition of individual abilities and liabilities and consideration of how they affect psychological functioning in various settings can contribute to a better understanding of spatial cognition and behavior in everyday life.

Experimental investigation of adaptive processes

Within the Kirasic and Allen (1985) framework, adaptive processes are described as those psychological activities necessary in the performance of spatial tasks. Although this description is intentionally broad, these activities can conveniently be discussed in terms of traditional experimental areas. Experimental research on spatial cognition and behavior in elderly adults has been directed toward three major problems: memory for spatial location; orientation; problem solving. In the following discussion, memory for spatial location and memory for orientation in large-scale space are considered research areas distinct from research on these same phenomena in small-scale space. Large-scale space is defined as an area whose structure cannot be perceived in its entirety from a standpoint within the boundaries of the space itself (Kirasic & Allen, 1985). Consequently, cognitive tasks involving large-scale space require the spatial and temporal integration of information typically achieved by means of actual or simulated locomotion within the area. Tasks in small-scale space (e.g., a tabletop array, a one-room environment, a photograph of an abstract figure) usually have no such requirement.

The literature addressing memory for spatial location in small-scale space can be summarized in a straightforward manner. Evidence pointing to an age-related decline in spatial memory performance is provided by studies involving memory for locations of features on a map (Light & Zelinski, 1983; Perlmutter, Metzger, Nezworski, & Miller, 1981), buildings in a model town (Bruce, 1983), matrices of letters, words, and objects (Pezdek, 1983; Schear & Nebes, 1980), and objects in random arrays (Waddell & Rogoff, 1981). However, there is evidence suggesting that this decline is attenuated when verbal mediation is available to aid in encoding spatial locations (McCormack, 1982) or when objects are organized into meaningful contexts (Waddell & Rogoff, 1981).

Recently, there has been considerable interest in the issue of automatic versus effortful processing of spatial information (Hasher & Zacks, 1979). The question of automatic encoding of spatial location has been addressed in a number of investigations involving older subjects. In general, these studies indicated that younger subjects performed with greater accuracy than did elderly subjects and that intentional spatial memory was superior to incidental spatial memory regardless of subjects' ages (Light & Zelinski, 1983; Park, Puglisi, & Lutz, 1982). Evidence suggesting lack of automatic encoding of spatial information has been found for both visual memory (Park et al., 1982) and haptic memory (Moore, Richards, & Hood, 1984).

These findings should be viewed in light of the fact that automaticity, whether it involves encoding or some other process, is developed over the course of repeated experience. Various aspects of spatial information processing become automatic for people who repeatedly engage in specific spatial tasks. Thus, it is important to note that in tasks such as target detection, which involves spatial components, elderly adults have been found to move toward automaticity at a rate comparable to that for younger adults (Madden & Nebes, 1980; Salthouse & Somberg, 1982).

Several studies have addressed the issue of memory for spatial locations in large-scale environments. Weber, Brown, and Weldon (1978) and Herman and Bruce (1981) investigated elderly residents' spatial knowledge of their nursing-home environments. Weber and associates (1978) found that elderly residents were not very accurate at placing photographed scenes from their nursing home in their correct locations on a map of the environs. Furthermore, these investigators were surprised to find that elderly residents performed significantly poorer on this task than did young adults who merely visited the home. In Herman & Bruce's study (1981), no difference was found between ambulatory residents and those confined to wheelchairs in the ability to specify locations of nursing-home scenes.

In a comparison of young and elderly adults' knowledge of urban landmarks in the subjects' hometown, Evans, Brennan, Skorpanich, and Held (1984) found that elderly adults were less accurate than younger residents in their verbal recall of landmarks and in their placement of landmarks in a grid representing the urban area. Elderly adults' memory for landmarks tended to be influenced by accessibility, uniqueness of appearance, and symbolic significance to a greater extent than did younger adults' memory.

Experimental study of orientation in small-scale space has attracted almost as much attention from researchers as has investigation of spatial memory. For the purpose of this presentation, studies of perspective-taking ability and mental rotation skills fall under the rubric of spatial-orientation studies. Perspective-taking ability (i.e., the ability to determine the appearance of a spatial array from a viewpoint other than the one perceived through either self-movement or array movement) involves a generic procedure developed for use with children (Piaget & Inhelder, 1967), but a number of studies have been conducted with elderly subjects. Surprisingly, there appears to be only one general finding on which researchers agree, namely that young adults perform perspective-taking tasks with greater accuracy and speed than do elderly adults (Herman & Coyne, 1980; Looft & Charles, 1971; Ohta, Walsh, & Krauss, 1981; Papalia & Bielby, 1974).

Little agreement can be found elsewhere in this literature. For example, asking subjects to imagine a viewing position by means of imagined array rotation rather than imagined self-movement led to improved performance for elderly adults in one study (Herman & Coyne, 1980), poorer performance in another study (Kirasic, 1980), and no difference in other studies (Krauss & Quayhagen, 1977; Krauss, Quayhagen, & Schaie, 1980). Similar discrepancies appeared in studies that allowed subjects to preview arrays from various positions. Again, some found previewing to be a facilitating activity (Herman & Coyne, 1980), and others did not (Ohta et al., 1981).

The picture obtained from studies of mental rotation is a little clearer. Such studies typically involve a chronometric analysis of the process required to determine whether or not two abstract stimuli viewed from different perspectives are identical. Generally, analyses have indicated a linear relationship between the time needed to determine similarity and the angle of disparity between stimuli (Cooper & Shepard, 1973; Shepard & Metzler, 1971). Studies involving elderly adults have supported this general finding, in addition to demonstrating that the time/angle function decreases with age, so that elderly adults are considerably slower at rotation than are younger adults (Berg, Hertzog, & Hunt, 1982; Cerella, Poon & Fozard, 1981; Gaylord & Marsh, 1975). Jacewicz and Hartley (1979) reported the one exception to this pattern. They found no differences between the rotation rates for young and elderly subjects when letters (English and Greek) rather than abstract figures were used as stimuli. The lack of an age difference in that case may have been attributable to the special status of the elderly subjects and the nature of the stimuli; both the young and the elderly subjects were college students, and familiar symbols such as letters (perhaps even Greek letters for more highly educated individuals) tend to be processed differently than abstract stimuli in matching tasks.

Little work has been done on elderly adults' orientation in large-scale space. Kirasic (1980) examined perspective-taking abilities in young, middle-aged, and elderly adults, using the subjects' hometown and a mock town as two test settings. In the case of the hometown setting, subjects were instructed to imagine themselves at one location (depicted in a photograph) and then indicate the direction and distance to another location (also depicted in a photograph). In the case of the mock town, subjects first learned an array of photographed buildings and subsequently performed the perspective-taking task. Age decrements in perspective-taking ability were found in the mock-town setting, but no difference between age groups was found in the hometown setting.

Bruce and Herman (1983) used photographs of environmental features taken from various perspectives to examine age differences in the ability to anticipate perceptual experience from an unseen perspective. Results from this study suggested that elderly adults had more difficulty than did younger adults in imagining the appearances of environmental features from alternate viewing positions.

Although the general topic of elderly adults' problem-solving skills has received some attention (Charness, 1985), little work has been done specifically on spatial problem solving. An interesting exception was a study by Ohta (1981) in which he initially posed a verbal scenario of a spatial risk-taking situation, similar to the verbal risk-taking scenarios of Botwinick (1966). The results with these dilemmas replicated the pattern of elderly subjects' reluctance to choose a risky solution. However, when they were later placed in an actual dilemma involving the unavailability of a familiar route and were asked to choose between backtracking along a lengthy but familiar route (conservative strategy) or attempting a shortcut through unfamiliar territory (risky strategy), these same older adults tended to select the less certain, more risky alternative.

Summary. Experimental studies of spatial cognition and behavior in elderly adults correspond rather nicely to the real-world problems of remembering spatial locations and maintaining orientation in large-scale spaces. The evidence from studies of spatial memory indicates that elderly adults do have more memory failures than do younger adults. Future research should continue to focus on specific process failures (e.g., encoding failures, retrieval failures) and remediational prospects (i.e., memory strategies).

Studies of mental rotation skills in elderly adults have served to illustrate a general slowing of visual information processing over the course of aging. This slowing is important to note, but its implications for real-world spatial effectiveness are not clear. A link between reduced speed in visual information processing and impaired spatial behavior is missing. The implications of studies of perspective-taking ability seem to be a little clearer. On the basis of studies using small-scale spatial arrays, one might expect elderly adults to be susceptible to disorientation in unfamiliar settings. Nevertheless, the available evidence suggests little susceptibility in familiar surroundings.

Much work remains to be done on elderly adults' spatial problem-solving skills. For example, there is an impressive literature on search behavior, but little research involving elderly adults has been done on this problem.

Research on spatial situations

Despite the fact that research on spatial situations per se is uncommon, data concerned with this topic can provide a basis for coordinating laboratory research with the needs of the elderly population. Typically, studies of spatial situations have focused on a particular community or on a comparison of communities that vary with regard to an attribute of interest. In Windley and Vandeventer's examination (1982) of elderly individuals' knowledge of and activities in small rural towns, the size of the community was an attribute of interest. It was found that residents of small rural towns (population less than 500) considered their neighborhoods to include larger portions of their hometown than did residents of larger towns (population 1,500 to 2,500). They also could list fewer town amenities and types of amenities than could the individuals in larger towns (Windley & Vandeventer, 1982). The amenities and services mentioned by the elderly residents were not cataloged in the article; however, those data included most of the spatial situations confronting the residents in those communities.

One of the few studies to focus specifically on the task of classifying situations confronting elderly citizens was reported by Scheidt and Schaie (1978). The social and nonsocial situations confronting elderly adults in a western Los Angeles neighborhood were classified according to three dimensions: activity level, commonness, and supportiveness. Four of the activities classified according to this scheme had prominent spatial features; not surprisingly, each of these was high on the activity dimension. Shopping at a busy supermarket was identified as a nonsocial task high on the commonness dimension and high in supportiveness. In contrast, driving in heavy traffic was identified as a nonsocial task low in commonness and low in supportiveness. The same status was given to moving into a new, unfamiliar residence; however, looking for a new residence was considered a social task low in commonness but high in supportiveness.

In general, elderly individuals reported feeling more competent in low-activity situations than in high-activity situations, in common situations than in uncommon ones, and in supportive situations than in unsupportive ones. In addition to these main effects, the three dimensions interacted in complex but rather sensible ways that will not be elaborated here. Relevant to the present discussion was the finding that within the realm of high-activity nonsocial situations, grocery shopping was representative of the type of activity (common but supportive) that resulted in elderly adults' highest ratings of ability, whereas driving in heavy traffic was representative of the type of activity (uncommon and depriving) that resulted in their lowest ratings of ability.

Summary. Little work has been done specifically on structuring a taxonomy of the spatial situations occurring in the everyday lives of elderly adults. Nevertheless, the research that has been done points to the fact that such studies are of considerable value in identifying the tasks facing older individuals and gaining insight into how these tasks are perceived by the population under discussion. In particular, the work of Scheidt and Schaie (1978) reflects the important contribution that the concept of situations makes to the ecological study of aging and spatial cognition.

Ecological research

An ecological approach to studying psychological phenomena requires consideration of (1) qualities or properties of the individual, (2) qualities or properties of the environmental setting, and (3) the systematic interaction of the individual and that setting (Bronfenbrenner, 1979). In applying the ecological approach, consideration of real-life activities necessarily precedes the formulation of research questions. The focus of an ecologically based study is typically on a specific subject, sample, or population engaged in some activity of interest within a particular temporal and spatial context.

With these criteria in mind, two studies will be discussed. A comprehensive interdisciplinary research effort at the Andrus Gerontology Center at the University of Southern California was designed to examine the relationships among spatial abilities, macrospatial knowledge, and neighborhood use in selected samples of elderly adults from two urban neighborhoods (Krauss, Awad, & McCormick, 1981; Walsh, Krauss, & Regnier, 1981). An extensive data set was accumulated in this study. Cononical correlational analyses indicated that spatial abilities were significant predictors of neighborhood knowledge; in turn, neighborhood knowledge was a significant predictor of the use of goods and services in the neighborhood. However, the relationship between spatial abilities and neighborhood use was found not to be significant.

In this project, "spatial abilities" referred to performance on experimental tasks as well as on pencil-and-paper psychometric tests; thus, this group of variables included measures of what would be called "characteristics of the individuals" and "adaptive processes" within the Kirasic and Allen (1985) ecological framework. "Neighborhood knowledge" referred to performance on map-construction tasks. These distinctions are important to consider, because these findings constitute the strongest evidence to date of a relationship between laboratory-based results and environmentally based knowledge and behavior.

The second study presented as an example of ecologically based research is a smaller-scale effort by Kirasic (1981). At the heart of this study was a common activity, namely, shopping in a supermarket. From an empirical (Scheidt & Schaie, 1978; Walsh et al., 1981) and commonsense point of view, grocery shopping is a regular and important activity for most adults. In addition, the supermarket is an excellent environment for the examination of spatial skills.

The study was designed to contrast subjects' performances in their usual supermarket with their performances in a novel supermarket after a brief exploratory period. Psychometric data were obtained using tests designed to assess visualization, spatial orientation, and visual memory, as were experimental-task data from recognition, route-planning, and landmark-placement tasks and from a behavioral task in which subjects planned and executed the most efficient shopping route. The results indicated that young adults' performances on the experimental and behavioral tasks were not affected by the familiarity of the task setting. In contrast, elderly adults performed more accurately and efficiently on tasks in the familiar store than on the same tasks in the unfamiliar store. The only exception to this pattern was the experimental task of landmark placement, which required subjects to place pictures of items in their proper locations on a floor plan of the store. Neither age nor familiarity affected performance on this task, with all subjects exhibiting moderate accuracy.

Multiple-regression analysis revealed psychometric tests of visualization, spatial orientation, and visual memory to be poor predictors of behavioral efficiency in the shopping tasks for both age groups in both stores. Performance measures from the experimental tasks yielded an asymmetric pattern of results. Performances on these tasks were related to behavioral efficiency only in the novel supermarket for the elderly adults and only in the familiar supermarket for the young adults. Perhaps the experimental tasks represented unusual or unexpected activities for the elderly adults in the supermarket setting. If so, it is consistent that performances on these novel tasks were related to behavior in the novel setting only. In contrast, perhaps the tasks were more or less what the experiment-wise college students were expecting. Accordingly, their task performances in the familiar setting may have been a clearer reflection of the spatial information used during the actual shopping exercise.

Still, this account leaves unexplained the not insignificant relationship between experimental-task performance and behavioral performance for young adults in the novel setting. This and other unanswered questions might be answered by additional studies focused on young and elderly adults' acquisition of spatial information in a novel supermarket setting. Such studies are currently being done by our research team.

Summary. By definition, ecologically based studies have direct implications for everyday spatial cognition and behavior. Unfortunately, few studies have utilized this approach. The available evidence suggests that elderly adults are at no particular disadvantage when they seek to remember the locations of objects and execute efficient routes in a familiar spatial context. These activities are subject to performance decrements, however, when they take place in a novel real-world setting. Interestingly, performances on psychometric tests and, to some degree, experimental tasks were not closely related to real-world performances of spatial tasks. These findings suggest the need for more careful consideration of the relationship between cognitive processes as studied in the laboratory and cognitive tasks as experienced in everyday situations.

Conclusion

The potential benefit of the ecological framework for the study of spatial abilities described in this chapter is that it may serve to facilitate integration of the spatial literature while maintaining a focus on real-world spatial activities. What this approach may add to the field is a way of coordinating research design with practical questions.

The four basic spatial objectives and activities described earlier as being common to elderly adults provide a case in point. Investigations of spatial memory, spatial search, orientation maintenance, and spatial navigation can be organized in such a way as to allow for an integration of approaches. For example, Pauline K.'s search for her glasses can be transformed into a program of research. In the search for a missing object, the spatial objective obviously is to locate the missing object, presumably as efficiently as possible. Some characteristics of the individual could be of interest, particularly visuospatial information-processing skills, memory abilities, and knowledge of search strategies. With regard to the situation, particular attention should be paid to task demands and task setting. A search in a familiar home setting may differ from a search in unfamiliar surroundings in important ways.

Intervening between the individual and the task are adaptive processes, referring in this case to cognitive operations such as information retrieval, search strategies, and general problem-solving routines. Several interesting issues could be raised for empirical investigation. For example, are the individual differences in cognitive abilities or cognitive style (characteristics of the individual) related to the production and utilization of effective search strategies (adaptive processes)? What are the effects of specifying familiarity, complexity, and size (situation) on the probability of a successful search (adaptive processes)? How can the environmental design (situation) or the use of mnemonics when putting objects in particular places originally (adaptive processes) reduce the frequency of lost objects and facilitate efficient search?

Similarly, the three other spatial activities mentioned as being important in the lives of elderly adults can lead to important research questions when viewed within the three-dimensional framework. Studies of orientation in large-scale environments could be designed to examine the relationships among orientation and visualization abilities (characteristics of the individual), the use of spatial frames of reference (adaptive processes), and environmental size and complexity (situation). The effectiveness of environmental design (situation) and orientation strategies (adaptive processes) on orientation and maintenance would constitute another beneficial line of inquiry.

To date, a number of studies have been conducted in the area of spatial cognition, and findings from these studies have helped to identify some of the important issues to be addressed in future research. However, it may no longer be profitable to take a piecemeal approach to such a multifaceted domain. It would be unlikely for an integrated picture of spatial cognition and behavior in elderly adults to emerge if researchers were actually fitting pieces from different puzzles together. Currently, the different-puzzles metaphor is something of a hyperbole. Nevertheless, it may be time to consider how microanalytic approaches to cognitive and behavioral phenomena can be linked more directly to approaches that afford clearer insight into the collage of abilities, cognitions, motivations, and situations that contribute to everyday spatial knowledge and behavior. An integrated, ecologically oriented view of the problem area can serve to highlight scientifically important issues and the ways in which they can be investigated – without wandering too far afield from the reality experienced by elderly adults.

References

Arenberg, D. (1978). Differences and changes with age in the Benton Visual Retention Test. *Journal of Gerontology, 33,* 534–540.

Basowitz, H., & Korchin, S. J. (1957). Age differences in the perception of closure. *Journal of Abnormal and Social Psychology, 54,* 93–97.

Bell, B., Wolf, E., & Bernholtz, C. D. (1972). Depth perception as a function of aging. *Aging and Human Development, 2,* 77–81.

Berg, C., Hertzog, C. K., & Hunt, E. (1982). Age differences in the speed of mental rotation. *Developmental Psychology, 8,* 95–107.

Bilash, I., & Zubeck, J. P. (1960). The effects of age on factorially "pure" mental abilities. *Journal of Gerontology, 15,* 175–182.

Birren, J. E., Woods, A. M., & Williams, M. V. (1980). Behavioral slowing with age: Causes, organization, and consequences. In L. Poon (Ed.), *Aging in the 1980's* (pp. 293–308). Washington, D.C.: American Psychological Association.

Botwinick, J. (1966). Cautiousness in advanced age. *Journal of Gerontology, 21,* 347–353.

Botwinick, J. (1977). Intellectual abilities. In J. E. Birren & K. W. Schaie (Eds.), *Handbook of the psychology of aging* (2nd ed.). New York: Van Nostrand Reinhold.

Botwinick, J., & Storandt, M. (1974). *Memory, related functions, and age.* Springfield, IL: Charles Thomas.

Bronfenbrenner, U. (1979). Ecological factors in human development in retrospect and prospect. In H. McGurk (Ed.), *Ecological factors in human development.* Amsterdam: North Holland.

Bruce, P. R. (1983). *Adult age differences in spatial memory.* Paper presented at meeting of the American Psychological Association, Anaheim, CA.

Bruce, P. R., & Herman, J. F. (1983). Spatial knowledge of young and elderly adults: Scene recognition from familiar and novel perspectives. *Experimental Aging Research, 9,* 169–173.

Cattell, R. B. (1963). Theory of fluid and crystallized intelligence: A critical experiment. *Journal of Educational Psychology, 54,* 1–22.

Cerella, J., Poon, L. W., & Fozard, J. L. (1981). Mental rotation and age reconsidered. *Journal of Gerontology, 36,* 620–624.

Charness, N. (1985). Aging and problem solving performance. In N. Charness (Ed.), *Aging and human performance.* New York: Wiley.

Cohen, R. (1985). What's so special about spatial cognition? In R. Cohen (Ed.), *The development of spatial cognition.* Hillsdale, NJ: Lawrence Erlbaum.

Cooper, L. A., & Shepard, R. N. (1973). Chronometric studies of the rotation of mental images. In W. Chase (Ed.), *Visual information processing,* (pp. 75–176). New York: Academic Press.

Cunningham, W. R., Clayton, V., & Overton, W. (1975). Fluid and crystallized intelligence in young adulthood and old age. *Journal of Gerontology, 30,* 53–55.

Danziger, W. L., & Salthouse, T. A. (1978). Age and the perception of incomplete pictures. *Experimental Aging Research, 4,* 67–80.

De Renzi, E. (1982). *Disorders of space exploration and cognition.* New York: Wiley.

Ekstrom, R., French, J. W., & Harman, H. (1976). *Manual for kit of factor-referenced cognitive tests.* Princeton, NJ: Educational Testing Service.

Evans, G. W., Brennan, P. L., Skorpanich, M. A., & Held, D. (1984). Cognitive mapping and elderly adults: Verbal and location memory for urban landmarks. *Journal of Gerontology, 39,* 452–457.

Fozard, J. L., & Nuttall, R. L. (1971). General aptitude battery scores for men differing in age and socioeconomic status. *Journal of Applied Psychology, 55,* 372–379.

Gaylord, S. A., & March, G. R. (1975). Age differences in the speed of a spatial cognitive process. *Journal of Gerontology, 30,* 674–678.

Guilford, J. P. (1967). *The nature of human intelligence.* New York: McGraw-Hill.

Hart, R. A., & Moore, G. T. (1973). The development of spatial cognition: A review. In R. Downs & D. Stea (Eds.), *Image and environment* (pp. 246–288). Chicago: Aldine.

Hasher, L., & Zacks, R. T. (1979). Automatic and effortful processes in memory. *Journal of Experimental Psychology: General, 108,* 356–388.

Herman, J. F., & Bruce, P. R. (1981). Spatial knowledge of ambulatory and wheelchair-confined nursing home residents. *Experimental Aging Research, 7,* 491–496.

Herman, J. F., & Coyne, A. C. (1980). Mental manipulation of spatial information in young and elderly adults. *Developmental Psychology, 16,* 537–538.

Hoffman, C. S., Price, A. C., Garrett, E. S., & Rothstein, W. (1959). Effect of age and brain damage on depth perception. *Perceptual and Motor Skills, 9,* 283–286.

Horn, J. L., & Cattell, R. B. (1966). Age differences in primary ability factors. *Journal of Gerontology, 21,* 277–299.

Horn, J. L., & Cattell, R. B. (1967). Age differences in fluid and crystallized intelligence. *Acta Psychologica, 26,* 107–129.

Jacewicz, M. H., & Hartley, A. A. (1979). Rotation of mental images by young and old college students: The effects of familiarity. *Journal of Gerontology, 34,* 396–403.

Kirasic, K. C. (1980). *Spatial problem-solving in elderly adults: A hometown advantage.* Paper presented at a meeting of the Gerontological Society, San Diego, CA.

Kirasic, K. C. (1981). *Studying the "hometown advantage" in elderly adults' spatial cognition and spatial behavior.* Paper presented at a meeting of the Society for Research in Child Development, Boston, MA.

Kirasic, K. C., & Allen, G. L. (1985). Aging, spatial performance, and spatial competence. In N. Charness (ed.), *Aging and performance.* London: Wiley.

Kline, D. W., & Schieber, F. (1985). Vision and aging. In J. Birren & K. Schaie (Eds.), *Handbook of the psychology of aging* (2nd ed. pp. 296–331). New York: Van Nostrand Reinhold.

Krauss, I. K., Awad, Z.A., & McCormick, D. J. (1981). *Learning, remembering, and using spatial information as an older adult.* Paper presented at a meeting of the Society for Research in Child Development, Boston, MA.

Krauss, I. K., & Quayhagen, M. (1977). *Components of spatial cognition.* Paper presented at a meeting of the Gerontological Society, San Francisco, CA.

Krauss, I. K., Quayhagen, M., & Schaie, K. W. (1980). Spatial rotation in the elderly: Performance factors. *Journal of Gerontology, 35,* 199–206.

Lee, J. A., & Pollack, R. A. (1978). The effects of age on perceptual problem-solving strategies. *Experimental Aging Research, 4,* 37–54.

Levison, W. H. (1981). A methodology for quantifying the effects of aging on perceptual motor capability. *Human Factors, 23,* 87–96.

Light, L. L., & Zelinski, E. M. (1983). Memory for spatial information in young and old adults. *Developmental Psychology, 19,* 901–906.

Lohman, D. F. (1979). *Spatial ability: A review and reanalysis of the correlational literature* (Technical Report No. 8). Aptitude Research Project, School of Education, Stanford University. Stanford, CA.

Looft, W. R., & Charles, D. C. (1971). Egocentrism and social interaction in young and old adults. *Aging and Human Development, 2,* 21–28.

Luria, A. R. (1973). *The working brain.* New York: Basic Books.

McCormack, P. D. (1982). Coding of spatial information by young and elderly adults. *Journal of Gerontology, 37,* 80–86.

McGee, M. G. (1979). Human spatial abilities: Psychometric studies and environmental, genetic, hormonal, and neurological influences. *Psychological Bulletin, 86,* 839–918.

Madden, D. J., & Nebes, R. D. (1980). Aging and the development of automaticity in visual search. *Developmental Psychology, 16,* 377–384.

Magnusson, D. (1981). Wanted: A psychology of situations. In D. Magnusson (Ed.), *Toward a psychology of situations: An interactional perspective* (pp. 9–36). Hillsdale, NJ: Lawrence Erlbaum.

Moore, T. E., Richards, B., & Hood, J. (1984). Aging and the coding of spatial information. *Journal of Gerontology, 39,* 210–212.

Ohta, R. J. (1981). Spatial problem solving: The response selection tendencies of young and elderly adults. *Experimental Aging Research, 7,* 81–84.

Ohta, R. J., Walsh, D. A., & Krauss, I. K. (1981). Spatial perspective-taking in young and elderly adults. *Experimental Aging Research, 7,* 45–63.

Papalia, D. E., & Bielby, D. D. V. (1974). Cognitive functioning in middle and old age adults: A review of research based on Piaget's theory. *Human Development, 17,* 424–443.

Park, D. C., Puglisi, J. T., & Lutz, R. (1982). Spatial memory in older adults: Effects of intentionality. *Journal of Gerontology, 37,* 330–335.

Pepper, S. C. (1965). *World hypotheses.* Berkeley: University of California Press.

Perlmutter, M. (1978). What is memory aging the aging of? *Developmental Psychology, 14,* 330–345.

Perlmutter, M., Metzger, R., Nezworski, T., & Miller, K. (1981). Spatial and temporal memory in 20 and 60 year olds. *Journal of Gerontology, 36,* 59–65.

Pezdek, K. (1983). Memory for items and their spatial locations by young and elderly adults. *Developmental Psychology, 19,* 895–900.

Piaget, J., & Inhelder, I. (1967). *The child's conception of space.* New York: Norton.

Salthouse, T. A. (1982). *Adult cognition: An experimental psychology of human aging.* New York: Springer-Verlag.

Salthouse, T. A. (1985). Speed of behavior and its implications for cognition. In J. Birren & K. Schaie (Eds.), *Handbook of the psychology of aging* (2nd ed. pp. 400–426). New York: Van Nostrand Reinhold.

Salthouse, T. A., & Somberg, B. L. (1982). Skilled performance: The effects of adult age and experience on elementary processes. *Journal of Experimental Psychology: General, 111,* 176–207.

Schaie, K. W., & Labouvie-Vief, G. (1974). Generational versus ontogenetic components of change in adult cognitive behavior: A fourteen-year cross-sequential study. *Developmental Psychology, 10,* 305–320.

Schaie, K. W., Labouvie-Vief, G., & Buech, B. V. (1973). Generational and cohort-specific differences in adult cognitive functioning: A fourteen-year study of independent samples. *Developmental Psychology, 9,* 151–166.

Schear, J. M., & Nebes, R. D. (1980). Memory for verbal and spatial information as a function of age. *Experimental Aging Research, 6,* 271–282.

Scheidt, R. J., & Schaie, K. W. (1978). A taxonomy of situations for an elderly population: Generating situational criteria. *Journal of Gerontology, 33,* 848–857.

Sharpe, J. A., & Sylvester, T. O. (1978). Effects of aging on horizontal smooth pursuit. *Investigative Ophthalmology and Visual Science, 17,* 465–468.

Shepard, R., & Metzler, J. (1971). Mental rotation of three-dimensional objects. *Science, 171,* 702–703.

Siegel, A. W. (1981). The externalization of cognitive maps by children and adults: In search of ways to ask better questions. In L. Liben, A. Patterson, & N. Newcombe (Eds.), *Spatial representation and behavior across the lifespan* (pp. 167–194). New York: Academic Press.

Sjoberg, L. (1981). Life situations and episodes as a basis for situational influence on action. In D. Magnusson (Ed.), *Toward a psychology of situations: An interactional perspective* (pp. 259–274). Hillsdale, NJ: Lawrence Erlbaum.

Waddell, K. J., & Rogoff, B. (1981). The effect of contextual organization on the spatial memory of middle aged and older women. *Developmental Psychology, 17,* 878–885.

Walsh, D. A., Krauss, I. K., & Regnier, V. A. (1981). Spatial ability, environmental knowledge, and environmental use: The elderly. In L. Liben, A. Patterson, & Newcombe (Eds.), *Spatial representation and behavior across the life span* (pp. 321–360). New York: Academic Press.

Weber, R. J., Brown, L. T., & Weldon, J. K. (1978). Cognitive maps of environmental knowledge and preference in nursing home patients. *Experimental Aging Research, 3,* 157–174.

Welford, A. T. (1977). Motor performance. In J. Birren & K. Schaie (Eds.), *Handbook of the psychology of aging* (pp. 450–496). New York: Van Nostrand.

Werdelin, I., & Stjernberg, G. (1969). On the nature of the perceptual speed factor. *Scandinavian Journal of Psychology, 10,* 185–192.

Willis, S. L., & Schaie, K. W. (1985). *Training the elderly on the ability factors of spatial orientation and inductive reasoning.* Paper presented at a meeting of the Gerontological Society, New Orleans, LA.

Windley, P. G., & Scheidt, R. J. (1980). Person–environment dialectics: Implications for competent functioning in old age. In L. Poon (Ed.), *Aging in the 1980's* (pp. 407–423). Washington, D. C.: American Psychological Association.

Windley, P. G., & Vandeventer, W. H. (1982). Environmental cognition of small rural towns: The case of older residents. *Journal of Environmental Psychology, 2*, 285–294.

17 Inner-city decay? Age changes in structure and process in recall of familiar topographical information

Patrick Rabbitt

Until recently, cognitive psychologists had interpreted memory changes in old age in terms of "process" models for information flow. A meticulously detailed exemplar is the "working memory" model first proposed by Baddeley and Hitch (1974) and since extensively developed (Baddeley, Grant, Wight, & Thompson, 1975; Baddeley & Lieberman, 1980). Information from the sense organs is "encoded" into characteristic "representations" in one or more modality-based subsystems (the visual "scratch pad" and the auditory "articulatory loop"). Besides its own characteristic representation code, each of these subsystems has characteristic temporal holding characteristics, which may depend on rate limitations to a dynamic process (the refreshment cycle time of the articulatory loop) or on capacity limitations of unknown provenance (the capacity of the scratch pad). Each subsystem also has its characteristic place in an information-routing diagram for the total "memory system."

In this framework, the study of cognitive aging has become an investigation of the differential vulnerability of subsystems and of their linkages. Thus, among other excellent recent reviews, Erber (1982) discusses changes in the efficiency of "sensory memory," "primary memory," "secondary memory," and dynamic read-in and read-out processes (encoding and retrieval). Kausler (1982) uses a similar "bottom-up" hierarchical description of changes in hypothetical "primary memory" and "episodic memory" systems. Craik (1976) suggests a framework for interpreting age changes in memory in terms of a hierarchical scheme of progressively "deeper" processing stages. Salthouse (1985) accepts similar conventional "process" models for memory, but interprets age changes in terms of an overall reduction in the efficiency of a single system parameter common to all: the maximum rate of information processing, with entailed inefficiency of encoding, rehearsal, and retrieval.

The value of this conceptual framework has recently been questioned. Attention has shifted from specification of "processes" (which perhaps can be defined only in terms of transitory patterns of system limitations) to the "structure" of specific knowledge systems that, once acquired, apparently transcend these limitations. Theoreticians such as F. C. Keil (1985) now question that process models are necessary if structure is understood: "It is surprising how little unambiguous evidence has been found in support of complex processing routines that are not derived from a specific knowledge base. From syntax to pattern perception few models with multiple intermediate steps have held up" (p. 91). One example of such a failure in a study of primary memory was Ericssen, Chase, and Faloon's demonstration (1980) that an individual could develop a complex encoding structure for a list of digits from knowledge of a particular data base (running times). His "process-model" limit for memory span (which has been invoked as evidence for the articulatory loop and other subprocesses) was thereby extended from 7 to 9 to over 70 items. This improvement was very specific to the particular knowledge base that supported it. His span for letters was not improved.

A more moderate view is that distinctions between structure models and process models for memory are, at present, very unclear. This is particularly the case in aging studies, where assumptions of losses in the efficiency of particular processes have been premised on experiments in which people have been given very little practice, and no opportunity to develop appropriate special-purpose knowledge bases. We do not know if there are any changes in memory efficiency in old age, where performance depends on detailed knowledge structures that have been built up and maintained over a lifetime.

Introductory taxonomies of knowledge structures (Kail & Pellegrino, 1985; Klatzky, 1980) distinguish between "declarative" knowledge bases, which specify entities in the real world in terms of their properties and mutual relationships (Collins & Quillian, 1972; Kail & Bizantz, 1982), and "procedural" bases, incorporating knowledge of how to achieve effects on the world, such as the TOTE systems described by Miller, Galanter, and Pribram (1960) or the production systems described by Anderson (1983).

One common body of "expert knowledge" that individual humans build up and share with each other is detailed information about a common environment in which they live, but in this case a distinction between declarative and procedural knowledge structures is unclear. How far is it useful, or meaningful, to make a distinction between our declarative knowledge about the environment (e.g., color, size, shape, and function of buildings and other landmarks, and their spatial relationships to one another) and the procedural knowledge that we employ when we find our way about, plan routes, draw maps, or try to give directions to others? Further, in order to use our knowledge to frame procedures to guide others, we must appropriately select, edit, and organize the information we give them. Must descriptions of how we do this necessarily predicate information-handling processes as well as structures?

There seem to be three questions for aging studies: Is there any age change in the efficiency with which detailed knowledge structures, acquired over a lifetime, continue to be used? Are some types of knowledge structures more vulnerable to age changes than others? Must we make a distinction between the integrity of "knowledge structures" and the "processes" that allow flexible deployment of this knowledge in the world, and does aging have greater effects on structures or on processes?

We conducted two experiments to explore these questions. Experiment 1 (parts A and B) asked whether or not, as age advances, even comprehensive knowledge of a particular environment, acquired, used, and adequately updated over many years, would become less accessible in old age, in particular, whether or not one or two different sets of relationships used to access information from such a knowledge base would become less efficient than the other. Experiment 2 looked for possible age changes in the efficiency with which correctly recalled topographical information could be organized for communication to others as "routes" between specified points.

Experiment 1A

This experiment compared the relative accuracy with which middle-aged and elderly people could use two different cuing systems to recall details of two main thoroughfares, the High Street and the Cornmarket, in Oxford, a city in which they had all lived continuously for at least 30 years.

In one cuing condition, volunteers recalled locations on one of these streets by carrying out a "mental walk" along one sidewalk and back up the other, describing and identifying each location as they "passed" it. To remove any load from working memory, and to ensure that errors were not due to failures to correctly update the points they successively reached on their mental walk, the experimenter repeated each location aloud as they mentioned it, and used it to cue their next response. No other help or information was given at this stage. Responses were tape-recorded and annotated by an experimenter on a simple sketch map of the street. Immediately after this mental walk, the experimenter made no comment on the accuracy of any of their statements, but merely cued recall of each location that they had omitted by asking a question about its function or by a general question about the class of building or shop to be found there. Thus, if they had omitted to recall a dry-cleaning establishment, the experimenter would ask, "Are there any dry cleaners in the street? Only 50% of these cues were valid. The others were lures referring to classes of establishments not found on the street currently under discussion (shoe shops, Post Offices, etc.). In the other cuing condition, volunteers were simply given valid and invalid cues or "probes," as described earlier, until all possible locations had been exhausted. The order in which the two streets and the cuing conditions were used was counterbalanced.

Two groups of 60 volunteers, 50 to 59 years of age ($\bar{X} = 54.3$) and 70 to 79 years ($\bar{X} = 77.5$), were drawn from the Oxford and Bucks volunteer panel of 1,700 persons 50 to 86 years of age. The criterion for selection was at least 30

Table 17.1. *Percentages of all possible locations correctly identified in two streets in Oxford by groups of 60 middle-aged (50–59) and 60 elderly (70–79) long-term (30 years plus) Oxford residents when prompted by two kinds of retrieval cues*

Retrieval cue	Middle-aged	Elderly
Function cuing	94.6%	92.1%
Mental walk	76.5%	60.8%

consecutive years of residence in Oxford for the middle-aged group, and 40 years for the elderly group. The groups were matched for sex and socioeconomic status. To ensure, as far as possible, that the two groups had been equally competent at learning locations in the city when they were young, they were also matched on Mill-Hill vocabulary test scores (50–59-year-olds, $\bar{X} = 23.4$, question $\sigma = 6.1$; 70–79-year-olds, $\bar{X} = 24.2$, $\sigma = 4.3$). This was done because Mill-Hill scores are known to be invariant with age in this population as discussed later. In populations of young adults, Mill-Hill scores correlate well ($r < 0.7$) with performance I.Q. test scores. Thus, matching on current Mill-Hill scores provided a reasonable retrospective index that the two groups had closely similar performance I.Q. test scores when they were young adults. Scores on a simple performance I.Q. test, the AH4, were also available for the two groups (50–59, $\bar{X} = 31.4$, $\sigma = 7.5$; 70–79, $\bar{X} = 20.2$; $\sigma = 83.$). As expected, AH4 test scores were significantly lower for the older group ($T = 14.5$) confirming once again that whereas vocabulary test scores remain constant with age, performance I.Q. declines.

Results

Because there were different numbers of locations on the two streets, correct responses were computed as percentages of possible locations. These are shown in Table 17.1.

In both conditions, only two volunteers made "false positive" errors (i.e., identified locations not actually present in the street). No volunteer ever incorrectly gave a previous location instead of a current location, though many in both groups spontaneously gave, with some satisfaction, short lists of several establishments that had occupied a given site in turn. Thus, all errors were omissions (i.e., locations that individuals could not identify at all).

Table 17.1 shows that performance in the function-cuing condition was close to ceiling for both groups. A Mann-Whitney U test detected no significant difference. In contrast, in the mental-walk condition, the middle-aged again approached performance ceiling, but the older group performed significantly worse (Mann-Whitney U, $p < 0.001$).

In the mental-walk condition, omission of a site from a mental walk did not mean that all information about it had been lost from memory, because when "missing sites" were subsequently prompted by function cues, the younger group successfully recalled 97% of them, and the older group 98.4% of them (no significant difference on Mann-Whitney). Volunteers were then asked to describe the precise spatial location for each of these twice-probed sites (i.e., to give the locations on either side of them and opposite them). The younger group successfully did this for 78%, and the older group for 64% of previously omitted sites (Mann-Whitney, $p < 0.01$). In the overwhelming majority of these cases (86% for the young and 91% for the older group), an adjacent establishment described when successfully retrieving a site in response to a probe had also previously been correctly included as part of the description of the mental walk. This makes two points: Two bits of information about what a site is and where it is in relation to other sites may be simultaneously available in memory, but differentially accessible by different retrieval cues. Second, retrieval cue systems are not necessarily transitive. Remembering shop A may not allow one to recall its neighbor, shop B, but function-cued recall of B may subsequently allow correct recall of its spatial relationship to A. In brief, even when we sometimes fail to recall "what" from "where," we often can subsequently correctly recall "where" from "what." Similar findings of nontransitivity of memory access routes (i.e., that whereas information accessed through one retrieval cue system can be used to access information available through another cue system, the converse is not invariably true) form the basis of Anderson's critique (1983) of schema theory.

In this experiment, the greater difference between cuing conditions shown by the elderly group may have been an artifact consequent to the fact that both groups performed at ceiling in the function-cued condition. Accordingly, the experiment was replicated with residents of another city, Newcastle-upon-Tyne, which has longer and more complex thoroughfares than any available in Oxford.

Experiment 1B

Two groups of 60 volunteers, aged 50 to 59 years ($\bar{X} = 56.3$) and 70 to 79 years ($\bar{X} = 75.5$), were selected for long continuous residence in Newcastle (30 and 40 years, as before). Groups were matched for sex and socioeconomic status and for Mill-Hill vocabulary scores (middle-aged, $\bar{X} = 20.6$, $\sigma = 4.3$; elderly, $\bar{X} = 21.2$ $\sigma = 3.1$). AH4 scores were also available (middle-aged, $\bar{X} = 28.4$, $\sigma = 6.3$; elderly, $\bar{X} = 16.2$, $\sigma = 6.9$). Experiment 1A was exactly replicated using two much longer and more complex thoroughfares, Northumberland Avenue and Grainger Street. Only the percentages of locations correctly recalled were computed and compared. These are shown in Table 17.2. It can be seen that recall was far from ceiling for either group in either condition. A two-way analysis of variance showed main effects for group age (df = 1:59; $F = 12.3$; $p < 0.01$) and cuing condition (df = 1:59; $F = 14.6$; $p < 0.01$) and an interaction between age and condition (df = 1:59; $F = 4.5$; $p < 0.01$). It seems that the

Table 17.2. *Percentages of all possible locations in two complex streets in Newcastle-upon-Tyne correctly reported by 60 middle-aged and 60 elderly long-term (30 years plus) Newcastle residents*

Retrieval cue	Middle-aged	Elderly
Function cuing	80.9%	66.2%
Mental walk	69.1%	41.4%

elderly recalled locations less well than did the middle-aged under both cuing conditions, and this shortfall was significantly more marked in the mental-walk condition than in the function-cuing condition.

Discussion

Middle-aged and elderly volunteers were matched on Mill-Hill scores. Data on the 1,700 Oxfordshire and 2,052 Newcastle residents aged 50 to 85 years from which these groups were recruited showed that not only means but also precise characteristics of Mill-Hill distributions did not change within this age range. This robust invariance of Mill-Hill scores across decade samples, and the high correlations in young adults between Mill-Hill scores and scores on performance I.Q. tests ($r > 0.7$), indicates that current Mill-Hill scores are reasonably good retrospective indices of young-adult I.Q. This fact, with the selection of groups for very long continuous residence in Oxford and Newcastle, reassures us that the elderly groups probably had once possessed a data base for Oxford as accurate and as detailed as that of the middle-aged. There also was no evidence that the elderly had continued to update this data base less efficiently, because even our oldest volunteers never made mistakes by reporting obsolete data.

In one respect, Experiment 1A demonstrates this continued comparability, because both groups performed at ceiling (i.e., both showed nearly perfect maintenance of a restricted data base when cued by function). Moreover, even when elderly volunteers failed to retrieve particular items of information in response to self-generated location cues during a mental walk, subsequently they could do so when cued for function. Once a location had been cued by function, its position in respect to neighboring buildings usually was retrievable. Thus, though location cues sometimes did not work for the elderly in particular cases, there was no evidence that location information had become completely unavailable.

Experiment 1B repeated the comparison with longer and more complex thoroughfares in a much larger city. Ceiling effect disappeared, and under both cuing conditions the elderly showed clear decrements relative to the middle-aged. Both groups were less efficient with location cuing, and there still was some evidence that the elderly were differentially disadvantaged. Taken together, the experiments suggest that the elderly perform worse with either cue system, but may perform differentially worse with the location cuing system (mental walk), which volunteers of all ages found more difficult.

The experiment answered two of the questions we set out to test: There does seem to be a reduction in efficiency of access to long-term, continuously updated knowledge structures in old age. As well as overall loss of efficiency, the elderly may lose flexibility in their access to information and show differentially greater decrements in the use of some cue systems than of others. But our interpretation of the change involved rests on the answer to a further theoretical question: Is it useful, or possible, to distinguish between the "structure of information" held in memory and "retrieval cues" that guide the processes by means of which it can be accessed? In early experiments comparing the relative efficiency of retrieval cue systems (Tulving & Pearlstone, 1966), the implicit model seems to have been that of retrieval from digital-computer hardware storage: Learned paired associates provided "addresses" for the "locations" in which target words were "stored." In terms of such (rather arbitrary and exceptional) models, it is possible to make distinctions among age effects due to absolute loss of all information from memory (i.e., of addresses and the contents of locations), partial degradation of information (loss of some data from location), and specific retrieval problems, which might be described as changes in ratios of surviving addresses or headings to surviving contents.

In terms of the recent "distributed parallel-process" models discussed by Anderson and Hinton (1981) and Hinton (1981), such distinctions are unnecessary and clumsy. In these models, any degradation of mnemonic representations will both reduce the amount of detailed information that can be elicited from the memory representation by an input and limit the range of different inputs that will elicit any particular body of information. In the framework of such models there are no clear predictions for relative degradation of previously "easy" and "difficult" schemes of access. The only point that Experiment 1 can make is that a particular body of information, once presumably equally available to both groups, has begun to degrade in the elderly, with the consequence that the range of alternative inputs (cues) that will elicit any of this information is correspondingly reduced.

One's knowledge of one's local environment is, surely, built up by solving a variety of practical problems within it: where to get milk, how far one must go to get a particular newspaper, the driest way to get from X to Y when it rains. When topological details are frequently learned as partial answers to particular functional questions, it does not seem sensible to regard the topological and structural components of this data base as forming a separate structure, a hypothetical "inner city" that we can inspect to retrieve different kinds of information by altering our direction of gaze or the focus of an "inner eye." Though this charming idea has found serious expression (Shepard & Cooper, 1982), it now seems likely that distinctions between the "map" and the "eye," the "knowledge" and the "questions" that guide its acquisition and evoke its retrieval (i.e., distinctions between separately definable "structure" and "processes" that act on these structures), are artificial dichotomizations within a single dynamic system. If this is part of what Craik (1985) meant by his zen-koan-like aphorisms on the nature of memory systems (Rabbitt, 1985), he has already made this point better and more concisely.

However, it may be premature to abandon all structure–process distinctions and to relax into a nirvana model of memory. In a critique of Keil's extreme adoption of structuralism (Keil, 1985), R. J. Sternberg (1985) made the useful point that an "expert" must learn to interrogate actively and use his or her "expert system," and a description of that requires process models. A simple practical example is the use of a system of expert knowledge of a very familiar city to direct a stranger. Here it is not enough to evoke adequate information from long-term memory. This information must be translated into usable directions. To do this, many different aspects of the human cognitive system are necessary. For example, apart from the obvious necessity for selecting appropriate words and constructing intelligible sentences, in order to know what to tell someone next, we have to remember what we have just told him. It is also necessary to edit information so as to select salient landmarks to guide choice points. Thus, at least two classes of errors that occur in route description may have nothing to do with the integrity or accessibility of information in long-term memory: on the one hand, "editing errors," or "pragmatic errors," which represent inappropriate selection or presentation of essentially accurate information; on the other, "updating errors," in which failure to update information about a route may result in confusion of otherwise valid directions. Therefore, we carried out an experiment to determine if the efficiency with which people can exploit their expert systems of local environmental knowledge changes as they grow old.

Experiment 2

This experiment was carried out to determine how accurately and efficiently people between 50 and 79 years of age could describe to a stranger routes that they knew very well. To provide plausible questions, 12 different pairs of locations were selected on a map of the Oxford city center such that the route between the two ends of a location pair would never overlap another route, though routes might at points intersect. Volunteers were asked to describe the shortest route between the two termini of each pair of locations in turn. The total naiveté of this imaginary interlocutor was stressed before each route description was attempted. The experimenter tape-recorded each route description and followed it, without comment, and out of sight of the volunteer, on a sketch map of the city. Omissions and mistakes were marked on the map and subsequently checked again against the recording. During six of these descriptions the experimenter recorded routes without comment or feedback of any kind, but during the remaining route descriptions the experimenter interrupted volunteers twice, at

Table 17.3. *Total numbers of metamemory errors made by nine groups of volunteers in describing six simple routes when sketch maps were and were not used*

	AH4 score		
Age band (years)	Low (15–25)	Medium (26–35)	High (36–60)
Without sketch maps			
50–59	49	28	6
60–69	56	37	5
70–79	53	22	9
With sketch maps			
50–59	20	3	1
60–69	24	1	0
70–79	16	0	0

preset points along the route, with preset questions that were intended to distract attention briefly from the task. These questions were tangential, rather than completely irrelevant, to the route under discussion. For example, a distracting question might be, "Can you see the Martyrs Memorial from there?" The answer given by the volunteer was recorded without comment, and the volunteer was left to complete the description as well as possible from the point at which it had been interrupted. This was done to test the accuracy with which the volunteer could remember where the description had been broken off and return the listener to the last point mentioned on the route in order to efficiently continue the description.

Orthogonally to the interruption/no-interruption conditions, in six cases volunteers were given no visual aids, and in the remaining six they were allowed to accompany their route descriptions by producing a simple sketch map without location names.

The volunteers were nine groups of 15 people who had not served in Experiment 1A, selected to match across the three age ranges 50 to 59 years, 60 to 69 years, and 70 to 79 years, within three bands of AH4 test scores (low, 15–25; medium, 25–35; high, 35–60). Mill-Hill scores were also available for all volunteers (50–59, $\bar{X}$ = 24.3, σ = 11.2; 60–69, $\bar{X}$ = 25.7, σ = 12.3; 70–79, $\bar{X}$ = 26.2, σ - 10.9). Volunteers were tested one at a time for 30 min each. They were paid £2 each for travel expenses and for their time.

Results

No volunteer ever failed to indicate a feasible route for each pair of locations, but they did not in every case follow the stressed instructions to describe the shortest route. Over all 12 routes, 43 diversions from the shortest routes oc-

Table 17.4. *Numbers of instances of omission of significant information during descriptions of six different routes by groups of 15 volunteers when sketch maps were and were not used*

	AH4 score		
Age band (years)	Low (15–25)	Medium (26–35)	High (36–60)
Without sketch maps			
50–59	15	1	0
60–69	12	0	0
70–79	11	0	0
With sketch maps			
50–59	3	0	0
60–69	4	0	0
70–79	2	0	1

curred. All were made by volunteers who had low AH4 scores. There was no suggestion that the incidence of such errors varied with age.

The term "metamemory errors" was used for cases in which volunteers describing routes gave directions that, though factually accurate, depended for their correct interpretation on information that the hypothetical naive tourist did not have and could not infer from the information already given (e.g., "You walk toward the park," when the latter had not yet been mentioned and would not be visible from the point along the route that had currently been established). A breakdown of these errors by age and AH4 score is given in Table 17.3. Errors for routes described with and without the opportunity to draw sketch maps are given separately. Low-AH4 groups made more of these errors than did high-AH4 groups (Mann-Whitney, $p < 0.01$ for all comparisons), but there was no suggestion of an age effect independent of AH4 score. Across all groups, the incidences of metamemory errors dropped sharply and significantly (Wilcoxon's matched, paired, signed rank test, $p < 0.01$) when sketch maps were used. This suggests that the incidence of metamemory errors is increased by an increasing load on working memory.

A second category of errors comprise omissions of significant choice points or necessary directions (e.g., turn left or turn right). From Table 17.4 we see that whereas those with high and medium AH4 scores made no such errors or very few such errors, all those who scored low on AH4 made many errors of this kind. Again, there was no sign of an age effect independent of current AH4 score. Again, the use of sketch maps significantly reduced the incidence of such errors (Wilcoxon's test, $p < 0.01$).

A final class of errors comprised repetitions of parts of routes, in different words, and without any indication that the same ground was being covered twice. Thus, a naive and unwary listener might assume that the repetition of a section produced a description of two different and successive stages of the route. Here

Table 17.5. *Errors of unannounced repetitions of route sections during descriptions of six simple routes, with and without the use of sketch maps, by nine groups of 15 volunteers*

	AH4 score		
Age band (years)	Low (15–25)	Medium (26–35)	High (36–60)
Without sketch maps			
50–59	5	3	2
60–69	9	4	3
70–79	4	4	0
With sketch maps			
50–59	0	0	0
60–69	1	1	0
70–79	0	0	0

again, Table 17.5 shows that there was a nonsignificant tendency for those with low AH4 scores to make more errors of this kind, but there was no sign of an age effect. Once again, however, significantly fewer such errors were made when sketch maps were permitted (Wilcoxon's test, $p < 0.01$).

Distracting questions were asked to determine if they affected the incidence of lapses that might be attributed to failures of working memory. Each route was selected to have six choice points at which directions to move left or right were necessary. On 6 of the 12 routes, distracting questions were asked at two of these choice points. In three cases, volunteers were using sketch maps, and in three cases they were not. These mean probabilities for each age group and AH4 score group are shown in Table 17.6.

Groups with high and medium AH4 scores made so few errors that shifts in error probabilities associated with interruptions were negligible and nonsignificant. But within the low-AH4 groups there were significant increases in error probability immediately after interruptions (Wilcoxon's test, $p < 0.01$). Again, there was no apparent effect of age independent of AH4 score. When sketch maps were allowed, these errors disappeared for all groups.

All classes of errors certainly had some "metamemorial" components, because volunteers' understanding of the pragmatics of the task determined the demands they recognized and tried to meet. In everyday life, the nature of the information required is typically "negotiated." For example, it is useful to ascertain what general knowledge an interlocutor has, because it may be efficient to frame directions in terms of invisible destinations (e.g., "Then you keep going on toward the river"). With complete strangers, this cannot work. Partial repetitions, and some omissions, will not confuse native, but may mislead strangers. All the errors in communication that we logged may be, at least partially, attributable to failures of metamemorial empathy (or to carelessness about, or forgetfulness of, the "rules of the game" defined by the experimenter, or even of

Table 17.6. *Performance without sketch maps*[a]

Age band (years)	AH4 score Low (15–25)	Medium (26–35)	High (36–60)
50–59			
After interruption	$p = 0.32$	—[b]	—
No interruption	$p < 0.1$	—	—
60–69			
After interruption	$p = 0.28$	—	—
No interruption	$p < 0.1$	—	—
70–79			
After interruption	$p = 0.21$	—	—
No interruption	$p < 0.1$	—	—

[a]Nine groups of volunteers were asked to describe six routes, on each of which six different choice points had to be described. On two of these choice points in each route, volunteers were interrupted by questions. Three routes were described with use of sketch maps. For these, the numbers of errors at choice points were negligible, whether or not interruptions occurred. These data are for the remaining three routes for which sketch maps were not used, and they contrast the probabilities of errors following and not following interruptions.
[b]Only the low-I.Q. groups made enough errors for comparisons to be meaningful.

''Gricean maxims'' of effective discourse management). Bearing all this in mind, the only point this analysis seeks to make is that in order to keep their shifting positions on the routes they described updated correctly to correctly retain the ''rules of the game'' and the current state of the hypothetical interlocutor's information about the route, volunteers had to hold in mind (more formally, to hold in ''working memory'') all these disparate kinds of information simultaneously. Distractions that might be expected to impair the efficiency of working memory increased the numbers of errors. The use of sketch maps as working aide-mémoires reduced all these kinds of errors. All these errors, apparently associated with the integrity of the working memory, were more commonly made by groups with low AH4 scores. But there was no evidence that chronological age, separate from AH4 score, had any effect.

Discussion

Taken together, Experiments 1A and 1B suggest that there may be two distinct, though probably correlated, changes in the efficiency of long-term recall in old age: Some information once available in long-term memory may become entirely inaccessible, and such information as can still be retrieved may be accessed in fewer different ways.

It has been argued that it is unnecessary to conceptualize retrieval of information from long-term memory in terms of two distinct functional entities, a structured data base (e.g., the "inner city") and a variety of retrieval processes that can "access" information from this base in different ways. Following Craik (1985), it has been suggested that a better framework for this discussion is a system in which "memories" cannot be distinguished from the processes that evoke them any more than "percepts" can be distinguished from "perceptual processes." The parallel-distributed models for memory suggested by Anderson and Hinton (1981) and Hinton (1981) provide such a framework. In this context, the age changes observed in Experiment 1 would not be discussed as the gradual loss of integrity of a mnemonic data base ("inner-city decay"), nor in terms of differences in the relative preservation of different access routes to an extant data base. Rather, loss of integrity of the data base would necessarily imply a reduction in the range of different inputs that would evoke any part of it to solve specific everyday problems. Note that, in one sense, this state of affairs could be taken to be a loss of "crystallized" intelligence in old age.

The results of Experiment 1 present no challenge to Keil's view (1985) that appropriate structural models render some classes of process models redundant. However, Experiment 2 gives some support to Sternberg's critique (1985) of Keil's view (1985) on the grounds that an "expert" must, after all, learn to exploit his "expert system," and process models may be necessary to describe how this is done. In Experiment 2, all volunteers had available in memory all the necessary information to describe the simple routes required. But in order to do so, they had to organize this information into a linear series of instructions. They never gave incorrect information, but made errors involving failures of updating that resulted in omission or repetition of necessary details. These errors are precisely consistent with demonstrations of other age-related failures to correctly update sequences of successive operations under distraction from a secondary task (Rabbitt, 1982) and can be very well described in terms of the process model for working memory developed by Baddeley and Hitch (1974). In Experiment 2, these working memory failures were associated with low scores on performance I.Q. tests rather than with age per se. Again, this agrees with findings that individual differences in scores on measures of working memory capacity, on which effective comprehension of text depends, are directly predicted by performance I.Q. tests (Lansman, Donaldson, Hunt, & Yantis, 1983).

A second class of errors comprised failures of the "pragmatics" of communication, in which volunteers failed to select the most appropriate information, or presented inappropriate information, because they did not take account of the needs of the hypothetical naive stranger whom they were attempting to guide. At first sight, these errors would seem to represent failures in previous learning or current use of pragmatic rules for effective discourse management. Consistent with this view is the fact that they were made by volunteers with low AH4 scores. However, ignorance or loss of pragmatic rules could not have been the only factor involved, because, within individual volunteers, these errors were driven by distracting interruptions.

This suggests that it is not enough to know the appropriate rules for giving instructions. Effective use of rules depends on the integrity and efficiency of a working memory system in which information about routes, permanently available in memory, can be "edited" in conformity with pragmatic rules to produce instructions useful to a naive listener.

Experiments 1 and 2 made some general points about the relationships among memory efficiency, chronological age, and psychometric measures of intelligence. In Experiment 2, middle-aged and elderly groups were matched in terms of their current raw scores on a test of performance I.Q. (AH4). When this was done, middle-aged and elderly groups performed equally well. Performance varied only with current AH4 scores. To confirm this, a multiple regression was used to compare the predictions of the total numbers of all errors made by all groups by chronological age and by AH4 score. When variance due to differences in chronological age had been partialled out the AH4 score remained a significant negative predictor of errors (T = 4.32), but when all effects due to differences in AH4 score had been partialled out, age gave no significant prediction of performance (T = 0.98). An equivalent multivariate analysis showed that both chronological age and Mill-Hill scores remained significant predictors when variance due to the other had been taken into consideration (T = 2.4 and T = 2.8, respectively). The same analyses were carried out for errors made in Experiments 1A and 1B. In Experiment 1A, age was again not a predictor when AH4 scores were taken into account (T = 0.87 and T = 5.7, respectively), but both age and Mill-Hill scores were significant when assessed as independent predictors (T = 2.9 and T = 3.1, respectively).

Finally, scores on AH4 and the Mill-HIll vocabulary test were compared as predictors of performance in both experiments. In Experiment 1 AH4 remained a significant predictor when Mill-Hill scores had been taken into account (T = 3.6), but the reverse was not the case (T = 0.7). The same was true in Experiment 2 (AH4, T = 2.9; Mill-Hill, T = 0.79).

We have noted that Mill-Hill vocabulary scores did not change with age within two populations of 1,700 (Oxford) and 2,052 (Newcastle) individuals aged 50 to 86 years from which these subgroups were drawn. This agrees with many previous findings that scores on vocabulary tests change little, or not at all, in old age. However, scores on performance I.Q. tests, similar to the AH4, are known to decline markedly with age. Thus, it is probable that matching of elderly and middle-aged volunteers for current AH4 scores ensured selection of an elderly group whose AH4 scores would have been much the higher of the two had the groups been compared as young adults. By the same token, by matching groups in terms of age-weighted I.Q. norms for the AH4, we could have selected an elderly group whose young-adult scores would have matched those of the middle-aged groups – but their current raw, unadjusted AH4 scores would then have been much lower. With these comparisons in mind, we can interpret the results of the I.Q. comparisons as follows: Surprisingly, scores on the AH4, a simple pencil-and-paper test, picked up all age-associated changes in performance in both experimental tasks. In contrast, the Mill-Hill vocabulary test gave weak predictions for performance in both tasks, but did not pick up all the variance associated with age differences. When variance due to differences in AH4 scores had been partialled out, Mill-Hill scores did not predict performance. Thus, the predictive component in Mill-Hill was completely absorbed in the variance picked up by the AH4. Moreover, the AH4 seemed to pick up all the age-related changes that affected performance of individuals in both these tasks.

These results are not quite what we would expect in terms of at least one well-documented psychometric model for age changes in cognition (Horn, 1982) that distinguishes problem-solving processes based on the use of information and procedures learned and maintained over many years (''crystallized intelligence'') from problem-solving processes requiring discovery and use of previously unknown relationships in a new knowledge domain (''fluid intelligence''). Vocabulary test scores are good measures of crystallized intelligence, which, Horn suggests, is comparatively age-invariant. Performance I.Q. tests such as the AH4 are good measures of fluid intelligence, which, like scores on these tests, declines with age. Fluid intelligence is also correlated with performance on perceptual motor tasks such as visual search and short-term memory scanning. Thus, this model would predict that AH4 scores should be better predictors of performance in Experiment 2 than should Mill-Hill scores, because working memory efficiency is regarded as an important component of fluid intelligence. Indeed, demonstrations of correlations between other performance I.Q. tests and other measures of working memory capacity have been reported (Lansman et al., 1983). But Experiment 1, which tested the efficiency of retrieval of information acquired and updated over a period of 30 or 40 years, appears to have been a paradigmatic test of crystallized intelligence. Yet here, the Mill-Hill, another test of crystallized intelligence, gives no residual prediction when variance associated with scores on a test of fluid intelligence have been taken into consideration. An attractively simple model for interpreting these relationships might formerly have been based on a distinction between (1) stable, long-acquired memory ''structures'' that constitute crystallized intelligence and remain relatively unaffected by age and (2) relatively labile ''processes'' of perceptual coding, interpretation of information, and its handling by a working memory system that collectively constitute fluid intelligence and that decline with age. Alas, this now seems too rigid and simplistic. These and many other experiments (Rabbitt, 1983) now set us a different problem: Although tests of general intelligence, such as AH4, are only crude predictors of performance, they still seem to pick up the entire range of age-related changes in a variety of cognitive tasks – now including tasks of effective retrieval from long-term memory. What makes these tests so good? And are there any age changes in general cognitive skills that are *not* associated with concomitant changes in these simple tests?

References

Anderson, J. L. (1983). *The architecture of cognition.* Cambridge, MA: M.I.T. Press.

Anderson, J. L., & Hinton, G. E. (1981). Models of information processing in the brain. In G. E. Hinton & J. L. Anderson (Eds.), *Parallel models of associative memory* (pp. 9–48). Hillsdale, NJ: Lawrence Erlbaum.

Baddeley, A. D., Grant, S., Wight, E., & Thomspon, N. (1975). Imagery and visual working memory. In P. M. A. Rabbitt & S. Dornic (Eds.), *Attention and performance* (Vol. 5). London: Academic Press.

Baddeley, A. D., & Hitch, G. J. (1974). Working memory. In G. A. Bower (Ed.), *The psychology of learning and motivation (Vol.* 8). New York: Academic Press.

Baddeley, A. D., & Lieberman, K. (1980). Spatial working memory. In R. Nickerson (Ed.), *Attention and performance* (Vol. 8, pp. 521–540). Hillsdale, NJ: Lawrence Erlbaum.

Collins, A. M., & Quillian, M. R. (1972). How to make a language user. In E. Tulving & W. Donaldson (Eds.), *Organization of memory.* New York: Academic Press.

Craik, F. I. M. (1976). Age differences in human memory. In J. E. Birren & K. W. Schaie (Eds.), *Handbook of the psychology of aging.* New York: Van Nostrand Reinhold.

Craik, F. I. M. (1985). Age differences in remembering. In L. R. Squires & N. Butters (Eds.), *Neuropsychology of memory.* New York: Guilford Press.

Ericssen, K. A., Chase, W. G., & Faloon, S. (1980). Acquisition of a memory skill. *Science, 208,* 1181–1182.

Erber, J. T. (1982). Memory and age. In T. M. Field & A. Huston (Eds.), *Review of human development* (pp. 569–585). New York: Wiley.

Hinton, G. E. (1981). Implementing semantic networks in parallel hardware. In G. E. Hinton & J. A. Anderson (Eds.), *Parallel models of associative memory* (pp. 161–188). Hillsdale, NJ: Lawrence Erlbaum.

Horn, J. L. (1982). The theory of fluid and crystallized intelligence in relation to cognitive psychology and concepts of aging in adulthood. In F. I. M. Craik & Trehub (Eds.), *Aging and cognitive processes,* New York: Plenum Press.

Kail, R., & Bizantz, T. (1982). Information processing and cognitive development. In H. W. Reese (Ed.), *Advances in child development and behavior* (Vol. 17). New York: Academic Press.

Kail, R., & Pellegrino, J. W. (1985). *Human intelligence: Perspectives and prospects.* San Francisco: Freeman.

Kausler, D. H. (1982). *Experimental psychology and human aging.* New York: Wiley.

Keil, F. C. (1985). Mechanisms of cognitive development and the structure of knowledge. In R. J. Sternberg (Ed.), *Mechanisms of cognitive development* (pp. 81–100). San Francisco: Freeman.

Klatzky, R. L. (1980). *Human memory structures and processes* (2nd ed.). San Francisco: Freeman.

Lansman, M., Donaldson, G., Hunt, E., & Yantis, S. (1983). Ability factors and cognitive processes. *Intelligence, 6,* 347–386.

Miller, G. A., Galanter, E., & Pribram, K. (1960). *Plans and the structure of behaviour.* New York: Holt.

Rabbitt, P. (1982). Breakdown of control processes in old age. In T. M. Field & A. Huston (Eds.), *Review of human development* (pp. 540–550). New York: Wiley.

Rabbitt, P. (1983). How can we tell whether human performance is related to chronological age? In D. Samuel & S. Algeri (Eds.), *Aging of the brain.* New York: Raven Press.

Rabbitt, P. (1985). A sense of the past. *Nature, 319* (6052), 365.

Salthouse, T. A. (1985). *A theory of cognitive aging.* Amsterdam: North Holland.

Shepard, R. N., & Cooper, L. (1982). *Mental images and their transformations.* Cambridge, MA: M.I.T. Press.

Sternberg, R. J. (1985). *Beyond I.Q.: A triarchic theory of human intelligence.* Cambridge University Press.

Tulving, E., & Pearlstone, Z. (1966). Availability versus accessibility of information in memory for words. *Journal of Verbal Learning and Verbal Behavior, 5,* 381–391.

18 The cognitive ecology of problem solving

Alan A. Hartley

Discussions of perception or memory seldom begin by defining a percept or a memory. Discussions of problem solving, however, almost always begin by attempting to define a problem. Yet the term "problem" is in the everyday vocabulary of virtually every adult. When a term that is commonly used must be explicitly defined, usually it is because the meaning that is intended differs from the common usage. The difference may be connotative. For example, the term "relativity" has almost completely different connotations for the theoretical physicist and for the layperson. The difference may also be denotative. For example, the term "flu" denotes different sets of disorders for the epidemiologist and for the layperson. It seems unlikely that two concepts would denote the same things but have different connotations. It is likely, then, but not assured, that the scientific and the lay concepts of a problem denote different things. It is an open question whether or not the two concepts have similar connotations. If the connotations are similar, then we must ask if the problems we, as scientists, study are sufficiently similar to the problems people experience that we can generalize what we learn about how problems are solved and how to assist the process. If the connotations are not similar, the questions are more serious: If our problems are not like people's problems, to what aspect of human experience do they generalize? What fields of scientific inquiry do address problems that people experience?

There are two plausible goals for the study of everyday problem solving: to understand real-world problem-solving performance and to predict real-world problem-solving performance. If the goal is to understand real-world problem solving, the tasks chosen must have external validity. They must adequately represent problems that are actually encountered. In addition, it must be possible to identify factors that contribute to performance either through experimental manip-

Support was provided by grant AG01073 from the National Institute on Aging and by a Faculty Research Grant from Scripps College. I am grateful to Heidi Cover and James Kieley for their extensive assistance with the study reported here and to Joellen Hartley for her conceptual and material contributions to the work.

ulations of the problems or through correlations of problem-solving performance with performance on other tasks that are reliable, valid indicators of basic abilities or processes. If the goal is to predict real-world problem solving, the tasks chosen must have predictive validity. They must correlate well with some measures of real-world performance. The tasks should be easy to administer; they should translate easily to the laboratory or testing situation. The tasks do not have to be representative; that is, they do not have to have face validity. For example, the Raven Progressive Matrices and subtests of the WAIS do not resemble problems that most people face in their everyday lives, but they do predict real-world performance. The two goals are not inconsistent. If contributing processes can be identified, then problem solving performance can both be understood and be predicted. At the same time, valid, easily administered tests that do predict real-world performance are of considerable value even if they are not representative or do not allow clear identification of underlying processes. Denney describes several examples of such tests in the next chapter.

This chapter examines the first goal: understanding real-world problem solving. It is particularly concerned with issues of representativeness and what has been called ecological validity (Hartley, Harker, & Walsh, 1980). In addition, because there is considerable evidence that there are differences across the adult life span in solving problems, as reviewed by Botwinick (1978), Giambra and Arenberg (1980), and Rabbitt (1977), it will be important to ask whether or not age is an important qualifier to the conclusions that are reached. The first section discusses the problems people actually face and reviews the paradigms used in scientific investigations to represent problems, including studies of age differences and changes in problem solving. The second section explores the extent to which the lay and scientific domains overlap and finds that there is little overlap. The final section describes an exploratory study of problems representative of those people report facing in everyday life.

In the next chapter, Denney devotes more attention to the second goal – predicting real-world problem-solving performance – in the context of a broad discussion of task validity and performance stability. The evidence for the contributions of age and experience is then synthesized into a comprehensive developmental model of problem-solving performance. Suggestions for future research are drawn from review of prior work and from the model.

Problems and problem solving

The natural ecology of problems

The most straightforward way to learn what constitutes a problem in everyday life is to ask. Therefore, 96 individuals ranging in age from 18 to 89 years were asked to "think of someone you know who is good at solving problems" and to "describe what kinds of problems this person is good at solving." The most frequent categories of responses are given in Table 18.1. The modal response, given by 52% of all respondents, was that the person was good at dealing with social and interpersonal problems, often involving emotional conflict. Technical, scientific, or mathematical problems were also mentioned frequently, most often by middle-aged adults. In addition, older adults mentioned financial or home-repair problems. Most commonly, then, the term ''problem'' referred to difficulties in human relationships, but it also comprised other situations at school, at work, or in professional activities for younger and middle-aged individuals, or situations in the home for older individuals. The age-group differences likely reflect age differences in the situations in which individuals find themselves. To generalize from the specific responses that were given, ''problem'' connotes for the layperson a situation in which there are one or more goals to be achieved, and it is not immediately clear what steps to take to achieve those goals.

To explore the denotative definition of ''problem,'' the individuals surveyed were given the following description that defined a problem broadly without using the term:

> Everyone encounters situations in which they have to figure something out. These situations may be big challenges or they may be little challenges, but they are all situations in which you don't know exactly what to do right away. Sometimes it takes just a few seconds of thought to figure out what to do; sometimes it can take much longer.

They were asked to think of and describe particular incidents of such challenging situations in several facets of everyday life: (a) work, professional activities, or school; (b) hobby, volunteer work, sports, or recreational activities; (c) around home; (d) in interacting with or dealing with other people; (e) in puzzles, board games, or card games. The responses are summarized in Table 18.1.

To generalize, there were again clear age differences, but for adults of all ages reporting on their own experiences, a problem was most likely to be a difficult personal choice or a difficulty in interpersonal relations. Less often, it was a difficulty in managing the routine or special demands of school, home, or the workplace. Rarely, it was a challenge of mathematics, science, or formalized games or puzzles. For younger adults, but not older adults, it was the challenge of acquiring the skills of a sport.

In addition to probing for the everyday concept of ''problem,'' it was also of interest to explore people's understanding of the processes of problem solving. Consequently, once respondents had identified someone who was good at problem solving and described the problems that person was good at, they were also asked to explain ''what you think makes him or her good at'' solving problems. The most common answers at all ages were that good problem solvers were good listeners who could look at a problem from many ''angles'' or ''viewpoints.'' Good problems solvers were also persistent, patient people who could concentrate well and who had substantial experience. Other traits mentioned at least once were intelligence, common sense, logic, and level-headedness.

Table 18.1. *Frequently reported problem types (percentages of respondents reporting)*

Problem type	Younger (18–25 years)	Middle (26–64 years)	Older (65–89 years)	Total sample
"Good problem solver"				
Interpersonal	56	33	53	52
Technical/scientific	44	67	20	38
Finance/home management	–[a]	–	27	11
Self				
Work or school				
Time management	47	–	–	25
Low grades	20	–	–	10
Interpersonal	–	73	–	13
Work-related				
Technical/logistical	–	18	36	13
New responsibilities	–	–	45	13
Hobby, volunteer, recreation				
Learning skills	82	33	–	33
Sports participation	–	–	24	12
Time management	–	33	–	5
Interpersonal	–	22	29	18
Home				
Family	100	64	26	60
Friends/others	–	–	9	5
Home repair/maintenance	–	27	48	26
Other people				
Friends	92	9	32	52
Family	–	36	21	15
Co-workers	–	45	5	9
Others	–	9	22	11
Puzzles and games				
Board games	30	40	33	33
Card games	10	10	33	20
Crosswords	–	–	40	20

[a]No response.

The respondents to this survey generally were well educated as well as intellectually and physically active. They tended to be retired from, engaged in, or headed toward professional, relatively well paid employment (or were from families in which the main income earner was professional). No claim is made that the sample was representative of the wider population. It is likely, though, that if any individuals face problems resembling those studied in the laboratory, this sample included them.

The general conclusions from this survey are supported by converging evidence from three very different lines of research. In the first, Kanner, Coyne, Schaefer, and Lazarus (1981) constructed instruments to elicit the hassles and uplifts experienced in everyday life. Hassles are "irritants that can range from minor annoyances to fairly major pressure, problems, or difficulties" (pp. 24–29); uplifts are "events that make you feel good. They can be sources of peace, satisfaction, or joy" (pp. 30–35). It is clear that the classes of hassles and uplifts include but are broader than the class of problems. Hassles can include problems in getting along with fellow workers and having too many things to do, but they also include such things as the weather and nightmares. Uplifts include using skills to solve a problem, but also being lucky. Among the most frequently mentioned hassles and uplifts were relationships with family and friends, time management, health, job responsibilities, and others closely similar to the problems reported by the survey respondents in our study. Kanner and associates (1981) also found differences between college students and middle-aged individuals. The students reported problems of time management and meeting academic standards; the middle-aged adults reported problems of home and financial management. These findings are similar to those presented in Table 18.1.

The second line of research, by Sternberg, Conway, Ketron, and Bernstein (1981), found that the strongest factor in lay judgments of intelligence comprised a cluster of behaviors labeled "practical problem solving." The cluster included many items similar to those ascribed to good problem solvers in our survey (e.g., reasons logically, sees all aspects of a problem, keeps an open mind, gets to the heart of problems, listens to all sides of an argument) (Sternberg et al., 1981, p. 45).

The final line of research was carried out by Charlesworth (1979), who took an ethological approach to the study of intelligence. He observed two 22-month-old children for 16 hours each in order to determine the kinds of problems to which intelligence is applied in real life. He defined a problem as an instance in which ongoing behavior was disrupted by someone or something or in which there was a deficit, a need, or a want for something that was not available. He found that 89% of the problems were social or interpersonal, 6% were physical, and 4% were cognitive. Of course, these were infants, not adults, and observations of infants make the presence of cognitive problems difficult to infer. Nonetheless, Charlesworth's findings are consistent with the assertion that most problems are interpersonal.

The laboratory ecology of problems

There is reasonable consistency in the connotative definitions of "problem" with which most discussions of problem solving commence (Anderson, 1980; Glass, Holyoak, & Santa, 1979; Mayer, 1983). A problem is characterized as having some givens (an initial state), a goal or goals to be achieved, and a set of operations that will transform the current state. The critical features are, first, that there is (or may be) a sequence of operations that will transform the initial state into the goal state and, second, that the problem solver does not initially know what that sequence is. The agreement on the definition may reflect general adoption by researchers in problem solving of the information-processing metaphor. Earlier researchers proposed more restrictive definitions consistent with their own paradigms, such as those of the Gestalt psychologists (Duncker, 1945) and the associationists (Maltzman, 1955).

The scientific concept of a problem is denotatively defined by the problems that are studied. There is no agreed-on taxonomy of problems or problem-solving processes, and reviews of the literature reflect this. The review may be organized around the particular problem or paradigm (Giambra & Arenberg, 1980; Rabbitt, 1977) or, still focused on the problem but at a somewhat deeper level, organized around whether or not the initial state or the final state or both are well defined (Glass et al., 1979). The review may be historical, organized around the broad point of view within which the problems were introduced or extensively studied (Mayer, 1983). Finally, the organization may be based on the processes or abilities that are called for to solve the problems (Greeno, 1978). Although none of the approaches that have been taken is completely satisfactory, the one that will be used here is organization by the presumed processes, following Greeno (1978). The general format of the review will be a summary of work on a particular problem or class of problems with younger adults, followed by a description of efforts to extend the findings to include later states in the adult life span. For problems that have received considerable attention, such as concept identification, no attempt will be made to give an exhaustive list of studies. Rather, a few exemplary studies will be listed. Kausler (1982) provides a particularly thorough review of age differences in problem solving.

Induction problems. The first class of problems comprises those that require the problem solver to induce the structure, that is, to understand. These include analogy problems such as those studied by Mulholland, Pellegrino, and Glaser (1980), Rumelhart and Abrahamson (1973), and Sternberg and Gardner (1983). The problem solver must extract the relevant features and induce the relationship on which the analogy is based; errors increase as the complexity of the relationship increases, presumably because holding and manipulating the information in working memory increases the load on general processing resources. In an unpublished study, Hartley used the same stimuli as Mulholland and associates (1980) and found not only that older adults made more errors but also that the age differences increased as the number of transformations that had to be held in working memory increased. Series extrapolation or completion problems are very similar to analogies. Again, as the complexity of the information that must be held in working memory increases, so do errors (Holtzman, Glaser, & Pellegrino, 1976; Kotovsky & Simon, 1973; Simon & Kotovsky, 1963). Hartley also used the same stimuli as the earlier investigators and found that age differences were larger on series that imposed a more severe burden on working memory. One set of problems in analogical reasoning that has been used extensively in studies of age differences is the Raven Progressive Matrices Test (Raven, 1974). Although age differences are reliable and well documented (Cunningham, Clayton, & Overton, 1975), the test has been used more for its psychometric properties than to explore processes of problem solving [but see the theoretical assault by Hunt (1974)].

One class of inductive-reasoning problems that has been extensively investigated comprises concept learning or acquisition tasks. These tasks are well understood, and powerful models have been developed to describe the strategies individuals adopt both with simple versions of the task (Trabasso & Bower, 1968) and with complex versions (Bourne, 1966; Bruner, Goodnow, & Austin, 1956). Older adults reliably performed less well than did younger adults (Giambra & Arenberg, 1980; Rabbitt, 1977), although there were suggestions that the age differences might be reducible through training (Sanders, Sterns, Smith, & Sanders, 1975). The differences were particularly large when the amount of irrelevant information was large (Hoyer, Rebok, & Sved, 1979) or when the relevant information was not salient (Hartley, 1981; West, Odom, & Aschkenasy, 1978). Problems in deductive logic might also be included under this rubric. For example, Dickstein (1978) and Johnson-Laird and Steedman (1978) investigated evaluation of syllogisms. Wright (1981) and Light, Zelinski, and Moore (1982) found age differences on linear syllogisms or linear-order problems that they attributed to limitations of working memory in older adults.

Transformation problems. The second category of problems comprises those that require transformation of the initial state. The difficulty in these problems is thought to result from two burdens on memory. One is that of holding subgoals in mind while selecting and executing moves; the other is that of mentally transforming the current state to determine whether or not goals or subgoals can be achieved. Such problems include the "towers of Hanoi" or pyramid puzzle (Egan & Greeno, 1974; Karat, 1982; Simon, 1975) and the missionaries–cannibals or Hobbits–Orcs problem (Greeno, 1974; Jeffries, Polson, Razran, & Atwood, 1977; Thomas, 1974). Age differences on the towers-of-Hanoi problem have been found in unpublished studies by Charness and by Hartley. Hartley also found that older adults performed less well than did younger adults on an isomorph of the missionaries–cannibals problem. On both the towers-of-Hanoi and missionaries–cannibals, Hartley found that older adults made more moves that violated the rules or regressed to previous problem states, as would be expected if working memory were more taxed in older adults. Performance is also a function of working memory load in mental arithmetic tasks (Hitch, 1978), and Wright (1981) has reported results generally consistent with the interpretation that age differences increase as memory load increases.

Water-jug tasks also can be considered transformation problems. In these problems, the individual must discover a sequence of transfers that will result in a specified quantity. After several trials that require the same sequence, many individuals will fail to realize when a much simpler sequence will do (Luchins, 1942). This failure is more pronounced in older adults than in younger adults (Heglin, 1956).

Finally, Greeno (1978) includes the proving of geometry theorems in the category of transformation tasks (Newell & Simon, 1972). Age differences in theorem proving have not been investigated. Algebra word problems (Mayer, 1982) and physics problems (Larkin, McDermott, Simon, & Simon, 1980) have also received considerable attention, perhaps because of the difficulty they pose for students. Again, the performance of older adults on these problems has not been assessed.

There is another group of transformation tasks that has been widely used with children and to some extent with older adults, but seldom with young adults (Chance, Overcast, & Dollinger, 1978). These are tasks used by Piaget or those in the Piagetian tradition to assess stages of cognitive development. A number of investigators have used these tasks to evaluate the hypothesis that decline in abilities in adulthood may mirror the acquisition of abilities in childhood; see Papalia and Bielby (1974) for a review of this work. The results are generally consistent with the hypothesis, but they have been criticized for possible confounds such as problem difficulty (Rabbitt, 1977) and extraexperimental factors (Hornblum & Overton, 1976).

Arrangement problems. The third class of problems comprises those requiring arrangement. The anagram is a type of arrangement problem that was widely studied by researchers influenced by the associationist tradition (Mayzner & Tresselt, 1966). The relative frequency of occurrence of the solution or of the anagram and its components could be varied, providing an easy operationalization of the habit family hierarchy. Hayslip and Sterns (1979) found no age differences in the numbers of anagrams solved. The numbers solved were positively correlated with measures of both fluid intelligence and crystallized intelligence within young, middle-aged, and older groups. See Horn and Cattell (1967) for a discussion of the fluid–crystallized distinction. The matchstick and card-trick problems studied by Katona (1940) were arrangement problems. It appeared that persons prompted to discover general problem structures and to think productively showed better long-term retention and transfer, though this conclusion was questioned (Hilgard, Irvine, & Whipple, 1953). The cryptarithmetic problems studied by Newell and Simon (1972) also involved arrangement, though both these and Katona's tasks might better be thought of as involving constraint satisfaction or constraint propagation. None of these tasks has been replicated with older adults.

One very simple type of problem that could be classified as an arrangement or constraint problem and that has been extensively studied with older adults includes variants of the 20-question game in which one of many possible objects must be identified by asking questions that can be answered yes or no (Denney, 1974; Denney & Denney, 1974). In an early study with children (Mosher & Hornsby, 1966), and in studies conducted by Denney and her colleagues, the task was to identify one pictured object from among 42 objects in a six-by-seven array. The reliable finding was that older adults were more likely than younger adults to ask hypothesis-testing questions (e.g., "Is it this one?") and less likely to ask constraint-seeking questions (e.g., "Is it living?").

Within the class of arrangement problems, Greeno (1978) distinguishes those that also involve inducing structure. Such problems include the insight or recentering problems popularized by the Gestalt psychologists, such as the candle problem, the two-string problem, the hat-rack problem, the horses-and-riders problem, and the nine-dot problem. These and related problems are described and illustrated by Scheerer (1963). These problems have not been studied with older adults, but given their lower likelihood of recentering in the water-jugs task (Heglin, 1956), it seems likely that there would be age differences in solving these set, or functional-fixity, problems. Arrangement problems also include design and invention tasks, such as the composition of a musical fugue (Reitman, 1965). Planning in general has been subjected to theoretical investigation, but that work has been more within the tradition of artificial intelligence than the psychological study of problem solving (Sacerdoti, 1975). An exception is a study by Meyer and Rebok (1985), who examined planning for a simple task of sorting a shuffled deck of playing cards and found that older adults produced less fully elaborated plans that were more likely to be insufficient.

Decision making and expert judgment. There are two additional areas of research that do not fit comfortably within Greeno's taxonomy (1978). Neither paradigm is usually considered problem solving, but both appear relevant to everyday problem solving as described by our survey respondents. These two areas are decision making and expert judgment.

Early studies of decision making examined choices of monetary gambles to determine if choices conformed to the prescriptions of economic theory, as reviewed by Payne (1973, 1982). More recent studies have examined decisions in a number of domains (often consumer commodities, because it is relatively easy to specify and manipulate component attributes) and have identified a variety of decision strategies (Einhorn, 1970; Jacoby, Szybillo, & Busato-Schach, 1977; Lussier & Olshavsky, 1979; Payne, 1976; Svenson, 1979). The strategy that is adopted for information search and decision making is a function of the importance of the decision and the pressures under which it must be made. In an unpublished study, Hartley, Anderson, and White compared the information-search patterns of young, middle-aged, and older adults and inferred the decision rule that was used. Older adults were more likely to organize their searches around the different objects under consideration (in this case, small appliances), whereas younger adults were more likely to organize their searches around the attributes of the objects.

Decisions under uncertainty or risk might also be included in this category; the volume edited by Kahneman, Slovic, and Tversky (1982) reprints many of the relevant studies. When people are asked to judge the likelihood or relative likelihood of events (e.g., "Which is more likely, that someone will die of spider bite or lightning strike?"), the judgments are distorted by failure to take base-rate information into account and by heuristics that lead to biased judgment. One such heuristic is representativeness; a representative outcome (such as heads-tails-heads-tails in flipping a coin) is judged more likely than a nonrepresentative outcome (such as heads-heads-heads-heads). Another heuristic is availability; it is more likely that one will have heard or read reports in the news media about a death due to lightning strike than a death due to spider bite, and the differential familiarity is used as the basis for judgment. The occurrence of these biases in judgments by older adults has not been determined. There have been several studies directed at the hypothesis that there is a conservative bias in the decisions of older adults (Okun, 1976). A conservative bias has been found in responses to the Choice Dilemmas Questionnaire, but it may be an artifact of the instrument.

The final area is expert judgment. Much of this work has been concerned with implementing expert systems on the computer. An example is Shortliffe's successful system for diagnosing and prescribing for infectious diseases (MYCIN) that was constructed by representing the knowledge of experienced specialists in internal medicine and developing a natural-language-like interface for querying the knowledge base (Shortliffe, 1976). Other investigations of expertise have been more in the psychological tradition, although computer models of human thought and behavior have played central roles. One of these was chess playing (Chase & Simon, 1973; Newell & Simon, 1972); the other was learning to use a computer text editor (Card, Moran, & Newell, 1983). The general finding was that, with experience, the individual builds a "vocabulary" of situations that occur in his or her field of expertise and appropriate responses to them. The individual learns how best to structure the situation or represent the information in a particular domain. The result is that situations that would pose very difficult or impossible problems for novices no longer even meet the definition of a problem for experts; the solution or the way to get the solution is immediately available.

Charness (1981a, 1981b) studied expert chess players ranging from young adulthood to late middle age. Although he found a decline with age in memory ability, he found that skill at rapidly sizing up a situation and selecting the best move improved. Hartley, Hartley, and Johnson (1984) monitored younger and older adults as they acquired expertise in the use of a computer text editor. Age differences in recalled knowledge were significant, but small – much smaller than differences in standard measures of memory from comparable samples. Older adults, however, performed significantly less well in applying acquired knowledge to editing tasks. Some of the differences simply reflected slowing of responses in older adults. Other differences in errors and number of steps required to achieve a goal suggested that older adults maintained a less complete and accurate model of the current state of the edited text.

Matching laboratory to life

Are laboratory paradigms representative of real-world problem solving? The connotative definitions of problems in everyday life and in the laboratory match reasonably well. There are, however, substantial differences in the specific situations and events that are denoted as problems. This can be made apparent by contrasting two different mappings: first, from the laboratory to the real world; second, from the real world to the laboratory.

From the laboratory to the real world

The matching can be approached by selecting laboratory tasks and seeking real-world analogues. With this approach, laboratory tasks match rather well with real-world problems for the simple reason that the real-world problems have been imported into the laboratory. Problems in formal systems of thought, such as algebra, geometry, and physics problems, have been studied in the laboratory. Similarly, puzzles such as the towers-of-Hanoi and games such as chess and even 20-questions were entertaining laypersons long before they were entertaining researchers and perplexing their subjects.

The study of expert problem solving has also been imported from the real world, though it is clear that there are enormous numbers of domains of expertise that have not been examined in the laboratory. Technical expertise appears to be an important source of problems for younger and middle-aged adults. Newell and Simon (1972) believe that the same general problem-solving processes underlie most domains of expertise. Nonetheless, because it is possible that there are domain-specific processes, just as there is domain-specific knowledge, it will be important not to jump to premature conclusions. Just as important, researchers have barely begun to explore age differences, and it is unwarranted to assume without empirical test that age differences in the acquisition and application of cognitive skill are independent of the domain of expertise.

One class of tasks that originated in the laboratory (e.g., tasks such as concept identification) is a good analogue for inductive-reasoning tasks in the real world, such as scientific investigations. Perhaps because of the name given to the paradigm, these tasks have unfortunately been dismissed as invalid representations of the acquisition of semantic concepts (Medin & Schaffer, 1978; Rosch, 1978).

From the real world to the laboratory

If the matching is approached by selecting the everyday experiences of people of all ages in the real world and attempting to find laboratory analogues, the laboratory study of problems and problem solving is virtually irrelevant. Personal and interpersonal choices and dilemmas are reported to be ubiquitous and important problems. Their study has most often been the province of personality psychologists and clinicians, not cognitive psychologists.

The problems most commonly mentioned by our survey respondents concerned interpersonal relations. Do these situations satisfy the scientific connotative definition of a problem? Consider the problem of a friend making inconsiderate demands for one's time and attention. That is the initial state. There is also a goal state – a situation without the demands. It is, however, very likely that one will know a course of action. In fact, one might well conceive of several courses of action in such situations – talk to the friend, avoid the friend for a time, end the friendship, or continue to endure the demands. What one does not know immediately is which course of action is most likely to achieve the goal without incurring unacceptable costs. It might be argued that this does not meet the definition of problem solving because one has a choice to make rather than a problem to solve. But if one does not know which sequence of operations to select, then the final component of the connotative definition of a problem has been satisfied. The choice is a problem because each alternative has both positive and negative implications. The implications vary on many dimensions, and it is not clear how to make them commensurable. Further, one cannot be certain of the outcome of any alternative one chooses. These situations are modeled better by the choice and decision paradigms than by any of the conventional problem-solving paradigms. Techniques are available for assessing utility and subjectively determining likelihoods, and procedures have been developed to monitor the information that is considered. The fact that previous investigations often have used consumer goods as the objects to be chosen need not prevent the development of scenarios involving interpersonal decisions. It is an open question whether or not the cognitive processes that have been revealed by these methods are sufficient to account for decisions with interpersonal content. An even more important question is whether or not there are age differences in the processes, because very little is known about decision making in older adults. Systematic study of the processes of choice has not been extended to older adults even in the domain of consumer behavior; see Phillips and Sternthal (1977) for a review of the issues and statements of hypotheses.

There was an interesting difference between the problems our respondents mentioned when asked to describe the kinds of problems at which good problem solvers were good and those they mentioned when describing challenging situations they themselves had experienced. In several instances, the good problem solvers were singled out as adepts at solving technical problems or problems related to their work that were not interpersonal problems. Yet there were very few cases in which individuals described such problems as challenges for themselves. If we speculate about the daily lives of people such as these survey respondents, it seems likely that they would have faced a variety of challenges that they could plausibly have called problems. One who sews might have to ease a bloused sleeve into a shoulder. A lawyer might have to develop a theory of what occurred consistent with the client's statements. A computer engineer might have to design an operating system that will fit into a 64K chip. If these situations are common, why were they only occasionally described as problems, and then only for others, not for the respondent?

It seems likely that the layperson makes a distinction very similar to one made by cognitive psychologists between problem solving and exercising cognitive skill. Fitting an operating system into 64K is a complex design problem, but if one has faced that task a number of times, one will already be aware of the different approaches that can be taken and the questions that will need to be addressed – of algorithms for subtasks such as handling a priority queue of actions for the system to take, of heuristics for other tasks such as memory support for both computation and video display. There are decisions to be made, but even the decisions reflect the sophisticated representation of the problem that the skilled designer has available. In most cases that representation is created even as the individual is listening to the problem specifications.

Turning to an example from a very different domain, Sherlock Holmes, in *The Red-Headed League,* has determined that a crime is planned, that it very likely involves tunneling, and even the probable identity of the criminal well before the befuddled pawnbroker, Jabez Wilson, has completed his description of the events that have transpired. There are a few points to be resolved – such as the target of the tunnel – but Holmes knows precisely how to collect the needed information at the outset of the problem. Both the design engineer and Sherlock Holmes are more appropriately described as exercising a cognitive skill than solving a problem (Anderson, 1980; Card et al., 1983). Both have a substantial body of relevant knowledge. The knowledge is more than specific instances; it incorporates a set of rules or a vocabulary (Simon & Gilmartin, 1973) that allows the person to parse the situation and formulate an appropriate course of action. Exercise of a cognitive skill shares with problem solving an initial state, a goal state, and a sequence of operations that will transform the initial state into the goal state. There is a problem to be solved rather than a skill to be applied, however, only when the individual does not know what the sequence of operations is or how to find that sequence. One respondent said that he found bridge enjoyable, but that it posed no real problems; it is likely that he was making a distinction between exercising a cognitive skill and solving a problem.

In the early stages of acquiring a skill, individuals clearly engaged in problem solving. The expert vocabulary is either nonexistent or in primitive form, and the problem representations often are inadequate or inappropriate. Holmes's roommate, Watson, also sees the red-headed pawnbroker and hears his story, but despite his efforts to carry out a Holmesian analysis, he infers far less than the great consulting detective. As novices solve more problems in a domain, they gain expertise, and it becomes less appropriate to describe their efforts as problem solving. If laypersons make the same distinction, they will describe the situations they encounter as problems only when they are novices. Most people will not remain novices for long; they will either become more expert or abandon the field. It is not surprising, then, that so few people described such situations as problems for themselves. Why would they describe them as problems for others, for the good problem solvers? For the same reason that Watson marveled at Holmes's deductions: because a situation that is easily comprehensible to an expert may seem a difficult problem to one without the skill to deal with it.

Applications of cognitive skill by experts range from situations that simply require recall of an appropriate response to situations in which a problem must be solved. A skilled chess player playing a standard opening can select the next move from a thoroughly memorized table of openings. In other cases there are uncertainties, but the problem solver knows what the alternatives are and how to choose among them. For example, a rheumatologist described the process of diagnosing a famous football player with the symptoms of skin rash, areas of dead skin, and arthritis of the hands (Weisman, 1985). He knew that the combination of these three symptoms narrowed the diagnosis to one of three possibilities. The available information did not allow a choice among the three, but he knew that simply observing the individual over several months would provide disambiguating evidence. It did. Increasingly severe muscle weakness eliminated two of the possibilities, leaving the third as the most probable cause. There were points at which the physician did not know the solution, but at every point he knew how to proceed to arrive at an eventual solution. At the other extreme from simple recall are situations in which an expert is faced with a true problem. This occurs when expertise fails and the individual has an inappropriate representation of the problem. For example, this occurs to Sherlock Holmes in *The Adventure of the Lion's Mane*. He incorrectly represents the information as evidence of a murder when in fact the individual has died from an accidental jellyfish sting. Only after being blocked and recentering his thinking does Holmes find the solution that might have been obvious to one less accustomed to dealing with criminal behavior. Thus, expert applications of cognitive skill range from simple recall to actual problem solving. The frequency of occurrence, though, varies systematically over the range. Most situations require only recall; only a few require that a problem be solved. The important conclusion is that the study of problem solving is only one component of the study of expertise.

Studies of expertise, as reviewed by Charness (Chapter 24, this volume), address the classes of tasks in which cognitive skill is truly exercised. Those studies typically have imported into the laboratory a real-world domain such as bridge (Charness, 1979), chess (Charness, 1981a, 1981b, 1981c; Newell & Simon, 1972), or word processing (Card et al., 1983; Hartley et al., 1984; Mikaye & Norman, 1979). Relatively few domains have been investigated. Studies of expertise at bridge, chess, and word processing have been extended to the later life span, but such investigations have been uncommon.

Matches and mismatches

If we tally the matches and mismatches, scientific and everyday problems match principally for games and puzzles. Yet these compose only a small subset of the problems faced in everyday life. The obvious conclusion is that we must direct our research attention toward paradigms that capture everyday problems. Calling for more representative research, though, is both simplistic and misleading. Simply importing everyday problems into the laboratory is not enough. If the goal is to understand the processes by which problems are solved, the attention must be directed to the strategies that are selected, the contributions of abilities and personal characteristics, and the ways in which those things change or remain stable with age. Representative tasks are important because the processes of solving everyday problems may well differ from the processes of solving the games and puzzles that have been studied in the laboratory. What we already have available in the laboratory are the tools to begin the enterprise. We can co-opt decision paradigms and use them to explore representative choice scenarios. We can adopt the techniques for studying expert judgment, expanding the domains to which they have been applied. We can use individual-difference approaches to gain leverage on problems that do not lend themselves to manipulation or intervention. And we can make more use of hypothesis-formulating approaches, such as think-aloud protocol analysis, to explore everyday problems in vivo. We must explicitly address the contributions of knowledge and experience to the problem-solving process.

Exploratory study

From our review of problems faced by laypersons and the problem-solving literature it was concluded that research should be directed toward problems that are representative of those faced in everyday life, particularly toward discovering the antecedents of performance on those problems. There have been few studies that have met those criteria. Consequently, a preliminary investigation of problem solving using tasks modeled on the problems reported in the survey was designed and carried out. The goals were to explore possible paradigms, to draw parallels to research using standard problems, and to produce hypotheses for future research. The general approach was to select representative or ecologically valid problem-solving situations and to include them in a battery of other measures to explore cognitive abilities, health, and current activities. These tasks were given to 44 individuals ranging in age from 19 to 84 years. Thus, it was possible to investigate relations between problem-solving performance and age, as well as other personal characteristics, and also between performance and cognitive abilities. In addition, to extend the study of laypersons' conceptions of problem solving begun with the survey described earlier, relations were explored between performance and self-report measures of problem-solving experience and style.

Problem-solving tasks

The tasks were selected to simulate situations that require choosing a course of action either to meet a person's own needs or to meet the expressed needs of someone else. The situations included a health-related choice, consumer advice to others, and personal advice to others.

Medicare-supplement insurance choice. In this task, the participant's problem was to gather information about four different Medicare-supplement insurance policies that varied on eight features. The goal was to select the best of the four policies. The different policies were identified simply as A, B, C, and D. The participant gained information by specifying a policy and a feature. An interactive computer program provided the information, for example, "The annual premium for policy C is $495." The information remained available until the next question was asked. The participant continued to gather information until ready to make a decision. At that point, the program asked for the policy that had been selected and called a research assistant, who asked the participant to explain why that policy had been chosen.

Two simple measures are available that reflect the decision process: (1) the number of questions asked and (2) the proportion of those questions that are redundant, repeating an earlier question. The sequence of questions can also reveal the individual's information-gathering strategy. The questions can be organized around the different policies, gaining information about several features of one policy, then another, and then another; this can be inferred from a sequence in which a high proportion of the questions concern the same policy as the preceding question, but a different feature. Alternatively, strategies that involve comparing the different policies on one feature, then on another feature, and then another can be inferred from sequences in which a high proportion of the questions concern the same feature as the preceding question, but a different policy. Unsystematic strategies can be inferred from sequences in which a high proportion of questions change both policy and feature from the preceding question. It is possible to make very specific identifications of the decision rules used by examining the type of question-to-question transition and the depth of search (Svenson, 1979). That was not done here; the analysis focused on the general characteristics of the search process (Payne, 1976).

Automobile purchase. In this task, the participant was given a written description of an individual who wished to purchase an automobile. Descriptions of six possible automobiles were also provided. The participant was to rank-order the six cars according to how well each met the described needs of the individual. The task was repeated with descriptions of four different buyers. Again, the task simulated a consumer choice. In this case the choice was for another person, whereas the choice of an insurance policy was based on one's own standards. The descriptions of buyers and of automobiles were constructed so that an overall measure of goodness of fit between car and buyer could be computed. The dependent measure was the nonparametric correlation between the ranks given for the six automobiles and the computed values, averaged over the four descriptions of buyers.

Personal advice. Two requests for advice were taken from published letters to a syndicated advice columnist. One asked for advice in a situation in which the mother of a bride had stricken members of the groom's family from the list of wedding invitees. The other described an elderly man in failing health who was becoming increasingly dependent on his son's former wife. The man's own family had assumed no responsibility for his care, and the former wife was seeking advice on how to ask her former husband, with whom she did not communicate, to provide help for his father. The participants' task was to read each item and to suggest any courses of action they would recommend to the writer (the columnist's response was not provided). After the participant finished providing suggestions, he or she was asked to recall the contents of that letter. Verbatim recall was not required – only the gist of the message. The first three suggestions were rated for their appropriateness, probable effectiveness, and ingenuity or unusualness. The recall was scored for the number of idea units correctly recalled from the requests.

Measures of cognitive ability

These measures fell into two categories. The first included measures of basic cognitive abilities. The second category included tasks that assess cognitive performance but that are not pure measures of a particular ability. Rather, these tasks probably require higher-level combinations of basic cognitive abilities.

The measures of basic abilities were primarily memory tasks. This choice was made because both Charness and Hartley, in unpublished studies, found that measures of memory were powerful predictors of individual differences in performance on standard problem-solving tasks. Memory is also given a central role in theoretical analyses of problem solving (Simon, 1975; Simon & Gilmartin, 1973; Simon & Kotovsky, 1963). Measures of short-term memory and working memory included the forward and backward digit span from the Wechsler Adult Intelligence Scale–Revised (WAIS-R). The reading-span measure of Daneman and Carpenter (1980) was also included. The final measure was the recency component of the free recall of four 12-word lists. For two of the lists, recall was immediate; for the other two, 30 sec of counting backward by threes preceded recall. The recency component was operationally defined as the number of items recalled from the last third of the list in immediate recall less the number recalled from the last third in delayed recall. To assess longer-term memory, the number of words correctly recalled on delayed-recall trials was tallied. Finally, to assess very long term, lexical memory, the Quick Word Test (Borgatta & Corsini, 1964) was administered.

The higher-level cognitive tasks all required that critical information be extracted from a complex stimulus. The tasks used were the Group Embedded Figures Test (Witkin, Oltman, Raskin, & Karp, 1971), the Picture Completion subtest from the WAIS-R, and a shortened version of the Davis Reading Test. The Embedded Figures Test (EFT) requires that simple line figures be located within more complex figures. Pilot research had shown that the EFT was a powerful predictor of performance at a variety of problem-solving tasks. The Picture Completion task requires that the missing element be identified in pictures of common scenes. Again, in pilot research this was found to be a significant predictor of problem-solving performance. The Davis Reading Test is a commonly

Table 18.2. *Items on the questionnaire for problem-solving style*

1.	I compromise.	18.	I am smart.
2.	I have patience	19.	I am logical.
3.	I am open-minded.	20.	I am disciplined.
4.	I am persistent.	21.	I am analytical.
5.	I am organized.	22.	I am level-headed and rational.
6.	I set priorities.	23.	I draw on past experience.
7.	I decide between alternative solutions.	24.	I am creative.
8.	I can leave a difficult problem and come back to it.	25.	I consult others.
9.	I use common sense.	26.	I have a positive self-image.
10.	I treat problems as a challenge.	27.	I break the problem into pieces.
11.	I remain unbiased and objective.	28.	I concentrate on the problem and solve it piece by piece.
12.	I consider all the options.	29.	I remain calm.
13.	I am sympathetic.	30.	I approach the problem from different angles.
14.	I consider conflicting ideas.	31.	I have a good memory.
15.	I listen carefully.	32.	I remain unemotional.
16.	I look at the pros and cons.	33.	I am motivated to solve the problem.
17.	I have a good attitude.		

used test of reading comprehension. Information must be extracted from a short passage in order to answer questions about it. The questions concern both directly stated facts and inferences that can be drawn.

The three tasks selected tap the ability to locate critical information in abstract visual displays, in meaningful visual displays, and in verbal materials. Skill at these tasks probably is dependent on a variety of basic abilities – attention and search, short-term memory, symbol decoding – as well as general cultural knowledge.

Self-report measures of problem solving

The responses to the survey described previously were used to create two instruments that each participant completed. The first concerned problem-solving style. Thirty-three items were constructed that described the characteristics and approaches to problems attributed to good problem solvers by respondents. The participant was asked to rate how descriptive each item was of him or her using a five-point scale from "definitely like me" to "definitely not like me." The items are listed in Table 18.2. The measure derived from these items was termed "problem-solving style." The second instrument concerned types of problems the person actually faced. Twenty-five items were constructed from the challenges that the survey respondents reported facing. Two responses were requested for each item: first, how frequently this sort of problem had been encountered (using a five-point scale from "very often" to "very seldom"; second, how good the individual was at solving this kind of problem (using a five-point scale from

Table 18.3. *Items on the questionnaire for problem-solving skill/frequency*

1.	Budgeting time	14.	Card games, board games, puzzles
2.	Doing well at work or school	15.	Managing investments
3.	Making a decision	16.	Relations with employer/employee
4.	Priority conflicts	17.	Auto repair
5.	Choosing between work and social activity	18.	Home improvements or repair
6.	Handling family responsibilities	19.	Technical problems
7.	Doing well at a sport or hobby	20.	Math or science problems
8.	Your own health	21.	Financial affairs
9.	Health of someone close to you	22.	Fitting into a new situation
10.	Independence from family or relatives	23.	Boredom
11.	Relations within your family	24.	An emergency
12.	Dealing with inconsiderate friends	25.	Dealing with business and professional people
13.	Relations with the opposite sex		

"very good" to "not very good"). The items on this instrument are listed in Table 18.3. The measure derived from the first set of responses was termed "problem-solving frequency"; that derived from the second set was termed "problem-solving skill."

The three sets of item responses were subjected to reliability analysis. Coefficient *d* was .90 for problem-solving style, .82 for problem-solving frequency, and .89 for problem-solving skill. Because the reliabilities were acceptably high, single scores were obtained by averaging the responses within each of the three sets. Intercorrelations of the scores showed that problem-solving style and problem-solving skill were strongly related (r = .64), providing some evidence of concurrent validity; individuals who reported being good problem solvers had the qualities attributed to good problem solvers. Problem-solving frequency was uncorrelated with either style, (r = .15) or skill (r = −.08), indicating that that scale assessed a different aspect of self-perceptions concerning problem solving.

Health and activities measures

It also seemed desirable to assess the participant's health and current level of activity, because it could be argued that age differences in performance are really attributable to poorer health and limited activity.

Health status was assessed by asking about the presence and severity of any current problems in eight areas: blood pressure, systemic infections, heart disease, pulmonary disease, vision, hearing, other. The eight responses were combined into a single index of health status.

To assess activity level, a questionnaire was constructed asking the individual how frequently he or she engaged in a variety of common physical, intellectual, recreational, and social activities. There were nine possible responses ranging

Table 18.4. *Items from the activity questionnaire*

1. I engage in recreational sports such as golf, swimming, tennis, jogging, walking, dancing, or fishing.
2. I travel away from my home in California (other than for daily activities).
3. I travel outside California in the USA or in a foreign country.
4. I do volunteer work for a political organization or for a hospital, church, school, or similar organization.
5. I work crossword puzzles, acrostics, or anagrams.
6. I repair a car.
7. I do woodworking, carpentry, or furniture refinishing.
8. I play word games such as Scrabble.
9. I attend films (travel films, commercial movies, etc.).
10. I watch television.
11. I read books or magazines as part of my job, career, or formal education.
12. I read books or magazines for leisure.
13. I give a public address.
14. I engage in business activities, such as investments or real estate transactions, not related to my job or career.
15. I engage in sewing, knitting, or needlework.
16. I engage in painting, sculpting, ceramics, drawing, etc.
17. I engage in creative writing, writing poems, writing newspaper articles, etc.
18. I write a letter.
19. I play a musical instrument.
20. I act or participate in a theatrical activity.
21. I go to a concert or to the theater.
22. I attend an educational course (including nonacademic courses such as yoga or cooking).

from "never" to "daily." The items are listed in Table 18.4. To obtain an overall activity level for an individual a *z* score was calculated for each item, and the *z* scores were averaged for all 22 items.

Procedure

Forty-four persons were recruited for the study from nearby senior-citizens' centers, college campuses, and the general community. Their ages ranged from 19 to 84 years. Eleven were 25 years of age or younger; 15 were between 26 and 64 years; 18 were 65 years or older. Education ranged from 10 years to 21 years. The self-report measures were completed at home; the other tasks were completed in the laboratory during one session lasting from 2 to 4 hours. Participants were paid $20.00 for their participation.

Results

Age and performance. The correlations between chronological age and problem-solving performance are given in Table 18.5. Correlations between age and cognitive and self-report measures are also given. There were no significant correlations between age and performance on the insurance-purchase task. Age did not affect the organization of the search or the frequency of redundant questions. In the automobile-purchase task, the fit between the participant's rank-

Table 18.5. *Correlations with chronological age*

Measure	r
Problem-solving measures	
Insurance-policy-choice task	
Number of questions	−.260
Proportion same-policy transitions	−.048
Proportion same-feature transitions	−.158
Proportion different-policy/different-feature transitions	.100
Proportion redundant questions	.058
Automobile-purchase task	
Nonparametric correlation	−.473[a]
Personal-advice task	
Number of suggestions	−.298[b]
Appropriateness of suggestions	.197
Probable effectiveness of suggestions	.235
Unusualness of suggestions	.101
Number of idea units recalled	−.383[c]
Cognitive measures	
Measures of basic abilities	
Forward digit span (WAIS-R)	−.366[c]
Backward digit span (WAIS-R)	−.447[c]
Reading span	−.563[a]
Recency in free recall	−.272
Delayed free recall	−.546[a]
Quick Vocabulary Test	−.194
Measures of complex abilities	
Embedded Figures Test	−.838[a]
Picture Completion (WAIS-R)	−.707[a]
Davis Reading Test	−.703[a]
Personal characteristics	
Self-report problem-solving scales	
Problem-solving style	.015
Problem-solving frequency	.542[a]
Problem-solving skill	.009
Health index	−.070
General activity index	−.123

[a] $p < .001$.
[b] $p < .05$.
[c] $p < .01$.

ordering of the automobiles and the objectively determined ordering declined with increasing age. In the personal-advice task, there was no correlation between age and the quality of the suggestions – their appropriateness, effectiveness, or unusualness. The number of idea units recalled from the letters declined with age, however, and there was a tendency for older adults to offer fewer suggestions. Denney and Palmer (1981) have also examined age differences in suggested courses of action for everyday problems. They found a nonlinear relation in which the rated quality of the suggestions was higher in the middle years and lower for both young and elderly respondents. To search for nonlinear relations between age and performance in the present tasks, the sample was split approximately into thirds by age, and analyses of variance were carried out with the age group as the independent variable. Post hoc comparisons were done using the Newman-Keuls test with the overall *d* set at .05. The only variables for which the results of analyses of variance diverged from those of the linear-correlation analyses were measures of the quality of solution on the personal-advice task. There were significant age-group differences for appropriateness [$F\ (2, 41) = 3.59$, $p < .05$] and unusualness [$F\ (2, 41) = 3.61$, $p < .05$]. The differences for effectiveness fell short of significance [$F(2, 41) = 2.90$, $p = .07$]. In each case, the ratings were somewhat higher for the older group than for the younger group, but both were higher than the middle group. These differences were significant for appropriateness and unusualness.

In contrast to the varied relations between age and problem performance, there were strong linear correlations between age and most of the cognitive-ability measures. Only vocabulary scores and the recency component of free recall were not significantly correlated with age. Age was unrelated to either problem-solving style or problem-solving skill, but self-reported frequency of encountering problems did increase with age.

Predicting problem-solving performance. A hierarchical regression approach was employed to explore the extent to which individual differences in problem solving could be predicted by cognitive abilities and other characteristics. At the first step in the regression, predictors that tapped basic abilities were entered in a block. These included forward and backward digit span, reading span, and recency in free recall (short-term and working memory), delayed free recall (longer-term memory), and vocabulary (long-term lexical memory). At the second step, the higher-level cognitive measures were entered. This provided an indication of the contribution of the integrated ability to draw out critical information beyond contributions of memory alone. At the third step, the computed measures of health and general activity were entered. If current health status and life style account for variance in problem solving not explained by cognitive status, these variables should significantly improve the prediction equation. Finally, chronological age was entered at the last step. If age makes a significant contribution, this indicates that there are other important variables covarying with age that have yet to be identified.

There were five criterion measures from the insurance-policy-choice task. For three of them there were no significant predictors, and the prediction equations never achieved significance – the number of questions, the proportion of redundant questions, and the proportion of same-policy question transitions. The regression analyses for the other two measures – proportion of same-feature question transitions and proportion of different-policy/different-feature transitions – are summarized in Table 18.6. In both cases, the block of basic cognitive abilities led to a significant prediction equation, but the higher cognitive abilities,

Table 18.6. *Hierarchical regressions of abilities and characteristics on problem-solving performance*

Criterion	Predictor	R^2	F(change)	F(equation)
Insurance-policy-choice task				
Proportion same-feature transitions	Basic cognitive	.294	2.574[a]	2.574[a]
	Complex cognitive	.365	1.252	2.168[a]
	Health & activity	.413	1.331	2.050
	Age	.425	0.621	1.909
Proportion different-policy/ different-feature transitions	Basic cognitive	.288	2.491[a]	2.491[a]
	Complex cognitive	.335	0.805	1.903
	Health & activity	.373	0.959	1.727
	Age	.398	1.325	1.710
Personal-advice task				
Appropriateness of suggestions	Basic cognitive	.393	3.987[b]	3.987[b]
	Complex cognitive	.411	0.359	2.639[b]
	Health & activity	.477	2.020	2.656[b]
	Age	.499	1.322	2.569[b]
Probable effectiveness of suggestions	Basic cognitive	.465	5.352[c]	5.353[c]
	Complex cognitive	.487	0.487	3.582[b]
	Health & activity	.508	0.688	3.002[b]
	Age	.517	0.599	2.767[a]
Unusualness of suggestions	Basic cognitive	.355	3.396[b]	3.396[c]
	Complex cognitive	.369	0.243	2.206[a]
	Health & activity	.391	0.594	1.870
	Age	.412	1.092	1.810
Number of idea units recalled	Basic cognitive	.319	2.893[a]	2.893[a]
	Complex cognitive	.333	0.233	1.887
	Health & activity	.426	2.607	2.164[a]
	Age	.434	0.384	1.977

[a] $p < .05$
[b] $p < .01$.
[c] $p < .001$.

health and activity, and age made no significant contribution. For same-feature transitions, the most powerful predictors were forward digit span, recency, and delayed free recall; for different-alternative/different-feature transitions, backward digit span was the most powerful predictor.

There was one criterion measure for the automobile-purchase task: the nonparametric correlation between the participant's rank order and the objectively derived rank order. The overall equation never achieved significance, although higher cognitive measures, health and activity, and age all made contributions that bordered on significance ($p < .10$).

There were five criterion measures for the personal-advice task: the number of suggestions, the rated appropriateness, effectiveness, and unusualness of the first three solutions offered, and the number of idea units recalled from the request for advice. The regressions are summarized in Table 18.6. For the number of suggestions, there were no significant predictors, and the equation was not significant. For the remaining criteria, the basic cognitive abilities produced significant prediction equations. Though the higher abilities and other characteristics did not significantly increase the variance accounted for, the equations remained significant throughout the analyses. The strongest predictors of both appropriateness and effectiveness were vocabulary, backward digit span, and reading span; reading span was the strongest predictor of unusualness; delayed free recall was the strongest predictor of the number of idea units recalled.

The predictive validities of the self-report measures of problem solving were also explored. The approach used was to enter all three self-report measures as predictors in a regression equation and then remove predictors successively. In addition to the criterion measures from problem solving, analyses were also carried out using the EFT, Picture Completion, and Davis Reading Test scores as criteria. The findings were not complex; simple correlation coefficients suffice to convey them. Those who rated themselves as relatively good at solving problems made less appropriate suggestions in the personal-advice task (r = –.30), but asked fewer redundant questions in the insurance-policy-choice task (r = –.34). The self-report measure of the frequency with which problems were encountered was the best predictor. Those who reported encountering more problems did better on the automobile-choice task (r = .41), the EFT (r = .44), the Picture Completion task (r = .41), and the Davis Reading Test (r = .45).

Discussion

It is important to reemphasize that the interpretation of these results is intended to generate hypotheses for further research rather than to provide conclusive tests of a priori hypotheses. The tasks were chosen to represent problems faced in everyday life, but, even so, there were numerous limitations. First, these three tasks are by no means a systematic sampling from all possible problems. Second, for any particular problem, there are many ways to reconstitute it in the laboratory and many ways that performance can be assessed. Third, even within a particular approach, the specific aspects of the scenario could well affect performance. For example, the processes involved in selecting an insurance policy may differ from those in selecting an over-the-counter headache remedy or selecting a nursing home for an aged parent, although all involve health-related choices. Fourth, the sample was not large; middle-aged adults were underrepresented; the subjects were relatively well educated. Despite these qualifications, there are several interesting results that suggest directions for further work.

Age and performance. The most striking finding was that the relations of age to performance were different for the three different problems. This pattern is in sharp contrast to virtually every standard laboratory problem-solving task reviewed earlier, for which there were clear age differences. In the insurance-policy-choice task, there was no relation. In the automobile-purchase task, there was a strong negative relation. In the personal-advice task, recall was negatively related to age, but the quality of solutions followed an inverse-U relation, with younger and older adults best.

The insurance-policy-choice task showed that younger and older adults performed similarly. Would they in all such problems? Medicare is more familiar and more important to the average older adult than to the average younger adult. What if a domain were selected that was more familiar and important to younger adults than to older adults? Alternatively, cognitive capabilities might be important. The amount of information available was small (32 pieces). If the number of policies or their features were increased, would that tax the more limited cognitive resources of older adults and produce age differences in performance? If the importance of information gathering were not emphasized by the task, as it was here, would age differences appear? For example, the individual might simply read a prose passage describing each policy. Regression techniques could be used with a single individual's ratings of policies to determine which pieces of information affected judgments. In general, the way in which information is organized and the form in which it is presented may affect differently the search strategies of individuals of different ages.

The automobile-purchase task showed clear effects of age. Here the information was presented in connected prose. Perhaps younger adults could see the underlying structure of relevant information, but the older adults could not. Would a matrix-like representation, such as that used in the insurance-policy-choice task, have prompted older adults to be more thorough and systematic? Successful performance requires that one notice and weigh a number of pieces of information, information that is embedded in other, extraneous information. The age differences on the EFT, Picture Completion task, and Davis Reading Test show that this is particularly difficult for older adults.

The relevant information in the personal-advice task, too, was buried in connected prose; yet the older adults produced the highest-quality suggestions. Perhaps when the schema is a highly familiar one, older adults are at least as likely as younger adults to activate the schema and use it to guide the extraction of information. If that is the case, asking for personal advice in areas with which older adults are unfamiliar should disrupt the pattern of superiority found here. In contrast, Denney (Chapter 19, this volume) reports finding that older adults perform less well even on problems selected as appropriate for their age group.

The older adults did recall less of the prose passage requesting the advice. Others have found poorer prose recall by older adults (Zelinski, Light, & Gilewski, 1984; Chapters 11 and 12, this volume). Yet, clearly, the older adults were not insensitive to the important information, because their suggestions were rated the highest in quality. Again, perhaps the familiar schema was extracted and guided problem solving even though specific details of the story were lost.

Could the unusual pattern of age differences found in this study simply be the result of an anomalous sample? Probably not. Measures of cognitive ability showed the declines with age that are commonly reported. It appears more likely that these problems were fundamentally different from standard laboratory problems.

Predicting problem-solving performance. Could the problems themselves be anomalous, calling on an idiosyncratic or variable set of abilities or strategies? Again, probably not. Individual differences in performance on many aspects of the problems were predictable. Measures of memory were significant predictors of the organization of search in the insurance-policy-choice task and of the quality of suggestions and recall in the personal-advice task. In unpublished studies, both Charness and Hartley found that measures of memory (particularly working memory) were significant predictors of problem-solving performance. In contrast, other problem-solving measures – the number of questions and frequency of redundant questions in insurance choice, the automobile-purchase task, and the number of suggestions in the personal-advice task – were not predicted. Hartley's unpublished study also found that the EFT score was correlated with performance on a variety of problems. Here, the EFT, together with other tests of more complex cognitive functioning, did not contribute significantly (though there was a tendency in that direction on the automobile-purchase task). Most important, personal characteristics (health, activity, age) did not contribute significantly when the contributions of cognitive abilities had already been taken into account.

These results raise a number of questions. Is it the case that the ability to pull critical, relevant information from a context of irrelevant information (measured by the EFT, the Picture Completion task, and the Davis Reading Test) is important in the type of problems conventionally studied in the laboratory, but not in many of the problems encountered in everyday life? Are the schemata of everyday problems so easy to pick out that individual differences are small and unsystematic?

Self-report measures of problem solving. The self-report measures of problem solving were reliable, but were uneven in predicting actual problem-solving performance. Only problem-solving frequency seemed promising. It may be that those who encounter more problems gain greater skill in solving them. An alternative explanation is that certain people are more likely to see a situation as a challenge – a problem to be solved – whereas others fail to see any challenge or simply respond in well-learned, stereotyped ways. If this explanation is correct, there should be a correlation between problem-solving frequency and "need for cognition" (Cacioppo & Petty, 1982), a measure of how attracted an individual is to cognitive challenges. Neither the extent to which one's self-description coincided with the characteristics attributed to good problem solvers nor the skill at problem solving attributed to oneself predicted performance. Thus, there is consensus on what makes someone a good problem solver, but that leaves us with three possibilities: (a) the consensus is wrong, or (b) it is right, but there are other, untapped characteristics that are necessary for good problem solving, or (c) such people are good at solving problems other than those investigated here. Each of these possibilities can be subjected to empirical test.

Conclusions

It has been argued that representative problems should be studied not simply because they are ecologically valid but rather because it is possible that the strategies and processes and the relations to basic abilities and personal characteristics such as age may be different from those for the domain of problems studied in the laboratory. The outcomes of this study indicate that that is a very likely possibility. The relationships of age and abilities to performance differed in nontrivial ways from those found with conventional problem-solving tasks. The study raised many questions, but it answered the principal question it was designed to address: Is it of value to study representative problems? Modeling the natural ecology of problems in the laboratory should be a fruitful exercise.

References

Anderson, J. R. (1980). *Cognitive psychology and its implications.* San Francisco: W. H. Freeman.

Anzai, Y., & Simon, H. A. (1979). The theory of learning by doing. *Psychological Review, 86,* 124–140.

Borgatta, E. F., & Corsini, R. J. (1964). *Manual for the Quick Word Test.* New York: Harcourt, Brace & World.

Botwinick, J. (1978). *Aging and behavior* (2nd ed.). New York: Springer.

Bourne, L. E. (1966). *Human conceptual behavior.* Boston: Allyn & Bacon.

Bruner, J. S., Goodnow, J. J., & Austin, G. A. (1956). *A study of thinking.* New York: Wiley.

Cacioppo, J. T., & Petty, R. E. (1982). The need for cognition. *Journal of Personality and Social Psychology, 42,* 116–131.

Card, S. K., Moran, T. P., & Newell, A. (1983). *The psychology of human–computer interaction.* Hillsdale, NJ: Lawrence Erlbaum.

Chance, J., Overcast, T., & Dollinger, S. J. (1978). Aging and cognitive regression: Contrary findings. *Journal of Psychology, 98,* 177–183.

Charlesworth, W. R. (1979). Ethology: Understanding the other half of intelligence. In M. von Cranach (Ed.), *Human ethology: Claims and limits of a new discipline.* Cambridge University Press.

Charness, N. (1979). Components of skill in bridge. *Canadian Journal of Psychology, 33,* 1–16.

Charness, N. (1981a). Aging and skilled problem solving. *Journal of Experimental Psychology: General, 110,* 21–38.

Charness, N. (1981b). Search in chess: Age and skill differences. *Journal of Experimental Psychology: Human Perception and Performance, 7,* 467–476.

Charness, N. (1981c). Visual short-term memory and aging in chess players. *Journal of Gerontology, 36,* 615–619.

Chase, W. G., & Simon, H. A. (1973). The mind's eye in chess. In W. G. Chase (Ed.), *Visual information processing.* New York: Academic Press.

Cunningham, W. R., Clayton, V., & Overton, W. (1975). Fluid and crystallized intelligence in young adulthood and old age. *Journal of Gerontology, 30,* 53–55.

Daneman, M., & Carpenter, P. A. (1980). Individual differences in working memory and reading. *Journal of Verbal Learning and Verbal Behavior, 19,* 450–466.

Denney, N. W. (1974). Classification abilities in the elderly. *Journal of Gerontology, 29,* 309–314.
Denney, N. W., & Denney, D. R. (1974). Modeling effects on the questioning strategies of the elderly. *Developmental Psychology, 10,* 458.
Denney, N. W., & Palmer, A. M. (1981). Adult age differences on traditional and practical problem-solving measures. *Journal of Gerontology, 36,* 323–328.
Dickstein, L. S. (1978). The effect of figure on syllogistic reasoning. *Memory and Cognition, 6,* 76–83.
Duncker, K. (1945). On problem solving. *Psychological Monographs, 58,* (No. 270).
Egan, D. E., & Greeno, J. G. (1974). Theory of rule induction: Knowledge acquired in concept learning, serial pattern learning, and problem solving. In L. W. Gregg (Ed.), *Knowledge and cognition* (pp. 43–104). Hillsdale, NJ: Lawrence Erlbaum.
Einhorn, H. J. (1970). Use of nonlinear, noncompensatory models as a function of task and amount of information. *Organizational Behavior and Human Performance, 6,* 1–27.
Giambra, L. M., & Arenberg, D. (1980). Problem solving, concept learning, and aging. In L. W. Poon (Ed.), *Aging in the 1980s: Selected contemporary issues in the psychology of aging* (pp. 253–259). Washington, DC: American Psychological Association.
Glass, A. L., Holyoak, K. J., & Santa, J. L. (1979). *Cognition.* Reading, MA: Addison-Wesley.
Greeno, J. G. (1974). Hobbits and orcs: Acquisition of a sequential concept. *Cognitive Psychology, 6,* 270–292.
Greeno, J. G. (1978). Natures of problem solving abilities. In W. K. Estes (Ed.), *Handbook of learning and cognitive processes* (Vol. 5). Hillsdale, NJ: Lawrence Erlbaum.
Hartley, A. A. (1981). Adult age differences in deductive reasoning processes. *Journal of Gerontology, 36,* 700–706.
Hartley, A. A., Hartley, J. T., & Johnson, S. A. (1984). The older adult as computer user. In P.E. Robinson, J. Livingston, & J. E. Birren (Eds.), *Aging and technological advances.* New York: Plenum Press.
Hartley, J. T., Harker, J. O., & Walsh, D. A. (1980). Contemporary issues and new directions in adult development of learning and memory. In L. W. Poon (Ed.), *Aging in the 1980s* (pp. 239–252). Washington, DC: American Psychological Association.
Hayslip, B., Jr., & Kennelly, K. J. (1982). Short-term memory and crystallized–fluid intelligence in adulthood. *Research on Aging, 4,* 314–332.
Hayslip, B., Jr., & Sterns, H. L. (1979). Age differences in relationships between crystallized and fluid intelligence and problem solving. *Journal of Gerontology, 34,* 404–414.
Heglin, H. (1956). Problem solving set in different age groups. *Journal of Gerontology, 11,* 310–317.
Hilgard, E. R., Irvine, R. P., & Whipple, J. E. (1953). Rote memorization, understanding, and transfer: An extension of Katona's card trick experiments. *Journal of Experimental Psychology, 46,* 288–292.
Hitch, G. (1978). The role of short-term memory in mental arithmetic. *Cognitive Psychology, 10,* 302–323.
Holtzman, T. G., Glaser, R., & Pellegrino, J. W. (1976). Process training derived from a computer simulation theory. *Memory & Cognition, 4,* 349–356.
Horn, J. L., & Cattell, R. B. (1967). Age differences in fluid and crystallized intelligence. *Acta Psychologica, 26,* 107–129.
Hornblum, J. N., & Overton, W. F. (1976). Area and volume conservation among the elderly: Assessment and training. *Developmental Psychology, 12,* 68–74.
Hoyer, W. J., Rebok, G. W., & Sved, S. M. (1979). Effects of varying irrelevant information on adult age differences in problem solving. *Journal of Gerontology, 34,* 553–560.
Hunt, E. (1974). Quote the Raven? Nevermore! In L. W. Gregg (Ed.), *Knowledge and cognition* (pp. 129–158). Hillsdale, NJ: Lawrence Erlbaum.
Hunt, E. (1978). Mechanics of verbal ability. *Psychological Review, 85,* 109–130.
Hunt, E., Frost, N., & Lunneborg, C. (1974). Individual differences in cognition: A new approach to intelligence. In G. H. Bower (Ed.), *The psychology of learning and motivation* (Vol. 7). New York: Academic Press.

Jacoby, J., Szybillo, G. J., & Busato-Schach. (1977). Information acquisition behavior in brand choice situations. *Journal of Consumer Research, 3,* 209–216.

Jeffries, R., Polson, P. G., Razran, L., & Atwood, M. E. (1977). A process model for missionaries–cannibals and other river-crossing problems. *Cognitive Psychology, 9,* 412–440.

Johnson-Laird, P. N., & Steedman, M. (1978). The psychology of syllogisms. *Cognitive Psychology, 10,* 64–99.

Kahneman, D., Slovic, P., & Tversky, A. (1982). *Judgment under uncertainty: Heuristics and biases.* Cambridge University Press.

Kanner, A. D., Coyne, J. C., Schaefer, C., & Lazarus, R. S. (1981). Comparison of two modes of stress measurement: Daily hassles and uplifts versus major life events. *Journal of Behavioral Medicine, 4,* 1–39.

Karat, J. (1982). A model of problem solving with incomplete constraint knowledge. *Cognitive Psychology, 14,* 538–559.

Katona, G. (1940). *Organizing and memorizing.* New York: Columbia University Press.

Kausler, D. H. (1982). *Experimental psychology and human aging.* New York: Wiley.

Kotovsky, K., & Simon, H. A. (1973). Empirical tests of a theory of human acquisition of concepts for sequential patterns. *Cognitive Psychology, 4,* 399–424.

Larkin, J. H., McDermott, J., Simon, D. P., & Simon, H. A. (1980). Models of competence in solving physics problems. *Cognitive Science, 4,* 317–345.

Light, L. L., Zelinski, E. M., & Moore, M. (1982). Adult age differences in reasoning from new information. *Journal of Experimental Psychology: Learning, Memory, and Cognition, 8,* 435–447.

Luchins, A. S. (1942). Mechanization in problem solving. *Psychological Monographs, 54,* (No. 248).

Lussier, D. A., & Olshavsky, R. M. (1979). Task complexity and contingent processing in brand choice. *Journal of Consumer Research, 6,* 154–165.

Maltzman, I. (1955). Thinking: From a behavioristic point of view. *Psychological Review, 62,* 275–286.

Mayer, R. E. (1982). Different problem-solving strategies for algebra, word, and equation problems. *Journal of Experimental Psychology: Learning, Memory, and Cognition, 8,* 448–462.

Mayer, R. E. (1983). *Thinking, problem solving, and cognition.* San Francisco: W. H. Freeman.

Mayzner, M. S., & Tresselt, M. E. (1966). Anagram solution times: A function of multiple-solution anagrams. *Journal of Experimental Psychology, 71,* 66–73.

Medin, D. L., & Schaffer, M. M. (1978). A context theory of classification learning. *Psychological Review, 85,* 207–238.

Meyer, J. S., & Rebok, G. W. (1985). Planning-in-action across the life span. In T. M. Shlechter & M. P. Toglia (Eds.), *New direction in cognitive science* (pp. 47–68). Norwood, NJ: Ablex.

Mikaye, N., & Norman, D. A. (1979). To ask a question, one must know enough to know what is not known. *Journal of Verbal Learning and Verbal Behavior, 18,* 357–364.

Mosher, F. A., & Hornsby, J. R. (1966). On asking questions. In J. S. Bruner, R. R. Olver, & P. M. Greenfield (Eds.), *Studies in cognitive growth.* New York: Wiley.

Mulholland, T. M., Pellegrino, J. W., & Glaser, R. (1980). Components of geometric analogy solution. *Cognitive Psychology, 12,* 252–284.

Newell, A., & Simon, H. A. (1972). *Human problem solving.* Englewood Cliffs, NJ: Prentice-Hall.

Okun, M. A. (1976). Adult age and cautiousness in decision: A review of the literature. *Journal of Gerontology, 31,* 571–576.

Papalia, D. E., & Bielby, D. (1974). Cognitive functioning in middle and old age adults: A review of research based on Piaget's theory. *Human Development, 17,* 424–443.

Payne, J. W. (1973). Alternative approaches to decision making under risk: Moments versus risk dimensions. *Psychological Bulletin, 80,* 439–453.

Payne, J. W. (1976). Task complexity and contingent processing in decision making: An information-search and protocol analysis. *Organizational Behavior and Human Performance, 16,* 366–387.

Payne, J. W. (1982). Contingent decision behavior. *Psychological Bulletin, 92,* 382–402.

Phillips, L. W., & Sternthal, B. (1977). Age differences in information processing: A perspective on the aged consumer. *Journal of Marketing Research, 14*, 444–457.

Rabbitt, P. (1977). Changes in problem solving ability in old age. In J. E. Birren & K. W. Schaie (Eds.), *Handbook of the psychology of aging* (pp. 606–625). New York: Van Nostrand Reinhold.

Raven, J. C. (1974). *Standard progressive matrices: Sets A, B, C, D, and E.* London: Lewis.

Reitman, W. R. (1965). *Cognition and thought: An information processing approach.* New York: Wiley.

Rosch, E. (1978). Principles of categorization. In E. Rosch & B. B. Lloyd (Eds.), *Cognition and categorization.* Hillsdale, NJ: Lawrence Erlbaum.

Rumelhart, D. E., & Abrahamson, A. (1973). A model for analogical reasoning. *Cognitive Psychology, 5*, 1–28.

Sacerdoti, E. (1975). The non-linear nature of plans. In *Proceedings of the Fourth International Joint Conference on Artificial Intelligence.* Tbilisi, Georgia, USSR.

Sanders, J. A., Sterns, H. L., Smith, M., & Sanders, R. E. (1975). Modification of conceptual identification performance in older adults. *Developmental Psychology, 11*, 824–829.

Scheerer, M. (1963). Problem solving. *Scientific American, 208*, 118–128.

Shortliffe, E. H. (1976). *MYCIN: Computer-based medical consultations.* New York: Elsevier.

Simon, H. A. (1975). The functional equivalence of problem solving skills. *Cognitive Psychology, 7*, 268–288.

Simon, H. A., & Gilmartin, K. (1973). A simulation of memory for chess positions. *Cognitive Psychology, 5*, 29–46.

Simon, H. A., & Kotovsky, K. (1963). Human acquisition of concepts for sequential patterns. *Psychological Review, 70, 534–546.*

Sternberg, R. J., Conway, B. E., Ketron, J. L., & Bernstein, M. (1981). People's conceptions of intelligence. *Journal of Personality and Social Psychology, 41*, 37–55.

Sternberg, R. J., & Gardner, M. K. (1983). Unities in inductive reasoning. *Journal of Experimental Psychology: General, 112*, 80–116.

Svenson, O. (1979). Process descriptions of decision making. *Organizational Behavior and Human Performance, 23*, 86–112.

Thomas, J. C. (1974). An analysis of behavior in the hobbits–orcs problem. *Cognitive Psychology, 6*, 257–269.

Trabasso, T. R., & Bower, G. H. (1968). *Attention in learning: Theory and research.* New York: Wiley.

Weisman, M. (1985, March 4). Bell's illness defied diagnosis, treatment. *Los Angeles Times.*

West, R. L., Odom, R. D., & Aschkenasy, J. R. (1978). Perceptual sensitivity and conceptual coordination in children and younger and older adults. *Human Development, 21*, 334–345.

Witkin, H. A., Oltman, P. K., Raskin, E., & Karp, S. A. (1971). *A manual for the Embedded Figures Tests.* Palo Alto, CA: Consulting Psychologists Press.

Wright, R. E. (1981). Aging, divided attention, and processing capacity. *Journal of Gerontology, 36*, 605–614.

Zelinski, E. M., Light, L. L., & Gilewski, M. J. (1984). Adult age differences in memory for prose: The question of sensitivity to passage structure. *Developmental Psychology, 20*, 1181–1192.

19 Everyday problem solving: Methodological issues, research findings, and a model

Nancy Wadsworth Denney

In recent years there has been increasing interest in the study of naturalistic, everyday problem-solving behavior in adulthood. There are many questions that could be addressed regarding the study of everyday problem solving: What kind of measures should be developed? How should these measures be developed? How should reliability and validity be established? And so forth. But the question that needs to be addressed first is *why* we should study everyday problem solving in adults, and that is the question that will be addressed first in this chapter. The rationale frequently given for studying everyday problem solving will be followed by an empirically and logically based critique of the rationale. Then the developmental research that has already been conducted with everyday problem-solving tasks will be presented, followed by presentation of a model of cognitive development that is consistent with the research findings. Then the potential of everyday problem-solving research to answer questions about nomothetic developmental functions will be called into question. Finally, the chapter closes with recommendations for further research.

The rationale for study of everyday problem solving

The recent interest in everyday problem solving has occurred as a result of developing concern over the validity of our traditional laboratory measures of problem solving when those measures are used with middle-aged and older adults. Because most traditional laboratory problem-solving tasks were developed for use with children or young adults, it is reasonable to question their relevance for middle-aged and older adults. Schaie (1978) expressed his concern about the validity of traditional intellectual measures in the following manner:

> Our analysis of external validity in the assessment of intellectual development began by stressing that psychologists in the past have attempted to search for intellectual genotypes which would display cross-situational generality in predicting behavioral consequences in specific situations. Our detailed analysis suggests that such an approach is a Sisyphean

task which should be abandoned. Instead, attention was called to the possibility of constructing alternate systems of phenotypic measurement for a basic set of major dimensions of intellect. Such measures would take into account the fact that different life stages require differential incentives (such as novelty for the young and meaningfulness for the old), and different test-taking paradigms. Moreover, we have stressed that differential combinations of intellectual genotypes may be involved in the multiplicity of criterion situations facing most individuals throughout life, particularly during adulthood and old age. The proper assessment of intellectual ontogeny therefore requires greater attention to the criterion situations within which intellectual abilities are expressed as behavioral competencies. (p. 700)

A similar view was expressed by Sinnott and Guttman (1978) with respect to performance on Piagetian tasks:

Schaie (1977–78) has recently pointed out that abilities in adulthood may be qualitatively different from those of children due to the differing experiential demands of adulthood. One of those demands is to be able to cope with the tasks of daily living in a modern, urban environment. Dealing with these demands logically may include the use of logical operations as defined by Piaget. If we wish to study intelligence as an adaptive, biological process as Piagetian theory dictates, we should now turn to the exploration of logical operations inherent in everyday, adult adaptive behavior, in all of its confusing richness. (p. 332)

The concerns expressed by Schaie, Sinnott and Guttmann, and others are all concerns about the validity of traditional measures of problem solving for use with middle-aged and older adults. There are at least three types of validity that might be questioned in this instance: predictive validity, face validity, and ecological validity.

Concerns about predictive validity

Some of the concerns that have been raised about the use of traditional problem-solving measures with middle-aged and older adults relate to their predictive validity. Traditional problem-solving measures have proved to be highly predictive of important behaviors in the everyday lives of children and young adults. For example, intelligence tests typically include measures of problem-solving ability. On the Wechsler Adult Intelligence Scale (WAIS), the Block Design, Picture Arrangement, Object Assembly, Comprehension, and possibly even Similarities subtests are measures of different aspects of problem-solving ability. Performance on such measures of problem solving predicts a variety of different types of real-life behavior in children and young adults. It predicts, among other things, academic performance (Minton & Schneider, 1980), amount of education obtained (Brody & Brody, 1976), and entry-level occupational status (Harrell & Harrell, 1945). Thus, there is some indication that traditional problem-solving measures do, in fact, measure at least a component of the ability of children and young adults to deal with the world as they are expected to deal with it. This fact should not be surprising in that many of the measures of problem solving, at least those included on intelligence tests, were selected because of their ability to discriminate between children who were and were not successful in their major task: school performance.

Although we know that many of our traditional problem-solving tasks are predictive of real-life performance for both children and young adults, we do not know if these same measures have any relevance to real-life problem-solving ability for middle-aged and older adults. Thus, many investigators have expressed concern about the predictive validity of these problem-solving measures for the adult years.

Concerns about face validity

In addition, concerns have been raised about the lack of face validity of the traditional measures of problem solving. Many of our traditional problem-solving tasks appear to be similar to at least some of the kinds of problems that children and young adults have to deal with in their everyday school settings. These same tasks do not appear to be at all similar to the kinds of problem-solving situations that most middle-aged and elderly adults deal with in their everyday work and family settings. The lack of face validity has caused a number of investigators to suggest that problems with more face validity be developed for use in research with adults.

Concerns about ecological validity

Further concerns have been expressed concerning whether or not the results of research with traditional problem-solving tasks are relevant to real-life problem-solving situations. Research on middle-aged and elderly adults' performances on traditional problem-solving tasks is responsible for some of this concern. This research indicates that performance on virtually all of the traditional laboratory problem-solving tasks that were developed for use with children and young adults decreases in a linear fashion after early adulthood. (Botwinick, 1984; Denney, 1979, 1982; Giambra & Arenberg, 1980; Kausler, 1982; Rabbitt, 1977; Salthouse, 1982). Although the vast majority of these studies have been cross-sectional in design, Arenberg's longitudinal studies also indicate an age decline in traditional problem-solving performance. As might be expected, however, the longitudinal studies show less decline, beginning at older ages, than the cross-sectional studies (Arenberg, 1982). Because cross-sectional studies tend to be biased in the direction of showing more age decline, and longitudinal studies in the direction of showing less age decline, it is not possible to know which type of study provides more accurate estimates of aging effects. However, because both types of studies indicate the same general trend, we have no alternative but to conclude that performance on traditional problem-solving tasks decreases with increasing age, whether the decline begins after early adulthood, as most of the cross-sectional studies indicate, or after middle adulthood, as Arenberg's longitudinal studies would suggest.

The finding that performance on traditional problem-solving tasks declines beginning after early adulthood has caused concern about the validity of such measures, because we assume that performance in the real world does not begin to decline after early adulthood. We do not believe that heart surgeons, historians, investment bankers, or corporate attorneys have experienced declines in their ability to do their jobs by the age of 40 or 50 years. Rather, in hiring a heart surgeon, historian, investment banker, or corporate attorney, we probably would prefer an experienced individual, because we assume that experience is tremendously important in these and other areas of real-world performance. So, whereas performance on traditional problem-solving tasks declines after early adulthood, performance on many real-world tasks appears to continue to improve at least through middle age. As a result, it is reasonable to question whether or not traditional problem-solving tasks measure abilities that are important for real-world performance.

Concerns about stability

Finally, additional concerns about the importance of traditional problem-solving tasks to the study of adult development and aging have arisen because of the results of the training research that has been conducted in the last 15 years or so. That research has demonstrated that performance on a variety of problem-solving tasks can be rather easily facilitated with very short term intervention techniques. (Botwinick, 1984; Denney, 1979, 1982; Giambra & Arenberg, 1980; Kausler, 1982.) If performance on such tasks can be so easily modified, can those tasks be measuring anything of much substance or importance? If traditional problem-solving performance is so unstable, can it predict anything?

The rationale for study of everyday problem solving: A note of caution

Caution regarding validity

One of the primary reasons for the recent interest in everyday problem-solving tasks is concern about the validity of traditional problem-solving measures. Does performance on traditional problem-solving measures predict performance in the real world? Do the traditional problem-solving tasks appear to be similar to the types of problems that adults are called on to solve in the real world? Are the findings obtained with traditional problem-solving tasks relevant to real-world problem-solving situations?

These concerns are reasonable. However, it is important that we do not conclude, without the necessary empirical evidence, that our traditional measures of practical problem solving are not predictive of important outcomes in middle and old age or that everyday problem-solving tasks are more valid for use with middle-aged and elderly adults. The fact that the more traditional measures were developed for use with either children or young adults does not mean that they are not also predictive of adult performance in real-world settings. The extent to which our traditional problem-solving tasks have predictive validity is an empirical question that should be answered.

Because performance on traditional problem-solving tasks decreases during the adult years, and performance in the real world increases at least through middle age, it is tempting to assume that what is measured by the traditional problems is not predictive of real-world performance. However, prediction is based on correlation and is therefore dependent on the relative rankings of individuals within the distributions of problem-solving performance and real-world performance, rather than on the absolute levels of performance of the individuals within either distribution. Therefore, even though performance on the traditional problems decreases with age, and performance in the real world increases with age, traditional problem-solving performance could still be highly predictive of performance on real-life problems (at least within an age group). And just as we cannot assume that traditional problem-solving tasks are not predictive of real-world performance without evidence, we also cannot assume without empirical confirmation that performance on everyday problem-solving tasks is, or will be, predictive of middle-aged and elderly adults' ability to perform in the real world. Thus, it is important to conduct research aimed at determining the relationship between performance on traditional problem-solving tasks and performance in the real world, as well as the relationship between performance on practical problem-solving tasks and real-life performance. A variety of criteria might be used for real-life performance: occupation, promotion, salary, related leadership ability, health status, psychological adjustment, marital satisfaction, life satisfaction, number of close friends, and so forth. In addition to these more general types of criteria, ratings of one's problem-solving ability by peers, family members, supervisors, or subordinates might also be used.

There is, in fact, some indication that traditional cognitive-ability tests are very useful for predicting job performance. On the basis of a meta-analysis of research on predictors of job performance, Hunter and Hunter (1984) concluded that traditional measures of cognitive ability are the best predictors available for predicting job performance:

> There have been thousands of studies assessing the validity of cognitive ability tests. Validity generalization studies have now been run for over 150 test-job combinations. . . . The results taken as a whole show far less variability in validity across jobs than had been anticipated. . . . Cognitive ability has a mean validity for training success of about .55 across all known job families. There is no job for which cognitive ability does not predict training success. Recent studies have also shown that ability tests are valid across all jobs in predicting job proficiency. (p. 80)

Hunter and Hunter found that the validity of cognitive-ability tests increased with job complexity, whereas the validity of psychomotor speed increased as job complexity decreased.

In addition, North and Ulatowska (1981) found that problem-solving ability significantly predicted competence in older adults who were living independently. In their study, competence was defined as "effectiveness in dealing with the problems and opportunities characteristic of one's environment" and was judged on the basis of an unstructured interview about various aspects of the older adults' daily lives, including their employment, hobbies, use of mass media, use of transportation, health status, and so forth. The purpose of the interview was to assess competence on the basis of how effectively the elderly adults solved problems, made decisions, planned their activities, and sought information. North and Ulatowska found that their overall competence rating was significantly related to both of the problem-solving measures that were employed in their study: the Block Design and Similarities subtests of the WAIS. North and Ulatowska also obtained measures of quality of discourse, because they believed that the ability to communicate is an essential component of competence. The measure of discourse was obtained by asking the subjects to answer a number of questions and to describe a number of situations and events. The subjects' responses were recorded and rated on the basis of relevance, clarity, and informativeness. North and Ulatowska found that both Block Design and Similarities were significantly related to all of their discourse measures, as well as to their competence measure.

In addition, Cyr and Stones (1977) found that two traditional Piagetian measures of problem-solving ability (the oscillation of a pendulum and the operations of exclusion and equilibrium in balance) also predicted behavioral competence among institutionalized elderly patients. Behavioral competence in their study was measured with the Stockton Geriatric Rating Scale (SGRS). The SGRS taps apathy, socially irritating behavior, physical disability, and communication failure.

Hultsch, Hertzog, and Dixon (1984) and Hartley (Chapter 11, this volume) have reported that traditional problem-solving measures from intelligence tests are significantly related to text recall, which could easily be construed as a test of an important real-world ability. Hultsch, Hertzog, and Dixon found that two letter-series tests (one from the kit of factor-referenced cognitive tests and the other from a primary mental-abilities test), which are tests of problem solving, loaded on a factor that predicted text memory in young and middle-aged adults, but not in older adults. Hartley, on the other hand, found that a test of abstract reasoning (Shipley Institute of Living abstract-reasoning test) predicted text memory in middle-aged and elderly adults, but not in young adults. These studies indicate that traditional problem-solving ability predicts text memory in adulthood. More research will be needed, however, before we know if the relationship increases or decreases or remains stable across age.

Finally, Willis and Schaie (in press) investigated the relationships between both fluid and crystallized measures of intellectual functioning and performance on the ETS Basic Skills Test, a test developed to assess real-life competencies, in elderly adults. They found that whereas both fluid and crystallized measures of intelligence predicted performance on the Basic Skills Test, the relationship between Basic Skills performance and fluid abilities was much stronger. Their finding is relevant because the fluid-abilities subtests are measures of problem-solving abilities. Thus, traditional measures of problem solving were highly predictive of performance on a test intended to be a measure of everyday functioning. In fact, Willis and Schaie reported that the correlations between the Basic Skills scores and the intellectual measures were on the order of those found among different intellectual subtests.

In summary, a number of studies in which a variety of measures of real-world competence were employed all indicated highly significant relationships between performance on traditional problem-solving measures and performance in either real-world settings or on problems that were intended to be realistic. These studies were presented to illustrate that it is too soon to assume that traditional measures of problem solving do not have predictive validity. Rather, the evidence to date points in the opposite direction. It appears as if traditional measures have a great deal of predictive validity. Certainly, more research on the topic is warranted, but it is clear that there is no justification, based on the empirical evidence to date, to discount the potential importance of traditional problem-solving tasks because of a presumed lack of predictive validity.

Caution regarding stability

In addition to the concerns about validity, there are also concerns about the stability of performance on traditional problem-solving tasks. The importance of the apparent instability of performance on traditional problem-solving tasks also needs to be tested empirically before it is taken too seriously. It is true that performance on traditional problem-solving tasks can be rather easily modified, but it also appears that the performances of children and young adults can be just as easily modified as those of middle-aged and older adults (Denney & Connors, 1974; Denney, Denney, & Ziobrowski, 1973; Denney, Jones, & Krigel, 1979, Denney & Turner, 1979). If the performances of children and young adults can be rather easily modified, and yet their performances still are predictive of real-world performance, then the modifiability of middle-aged and elderly adults' performances should not be a cause for alarm. Again, predictive validity should not be prejudged; it needs to be determined empirically.

An analogy will illustrate that modifiability of performance on a particular measure does not necessarily negate the importance of that measure. Both blood pressure and heart rate are easily modifiable. Yet both are measures of substantial importance – they both have a great deal of predictive validity. The same may well be true for performance on some of our traditional measures of problem-solving ability. Only empirical tests will tell.

The recent interest in everyday problem solving has grown, at least in part, out of concerns about the validity and stability of traditional measures of problem solving when those measures are used with middle-aged and elderly adults. These are reasonable concerns that need to be raised. However, it is important that we do not simply assume that traditional problem-solving measures are not valid for use with adults and/or that the modifiability of traditional problem-solving performances makes them ineffective measures for use with adults. Rather than making such assumptions, we need to test these hypotheses empirically.

Developmental research on everyday problem solving in adults

As a result of the increasing interest in everyday problem solving, a few studies of everyday problem solving have already been conducted. Many of these studies were undertaken in order to determine if the same age trends that had been found with traditional problem-solving tasks would also be obtained when the tasks were more realistic. This research will be reviewed briefly.

Problem-solving measures can be made more realistic by making either the stimuli or the task or both more realistic. Thus, problem-solving tasks can be divided into the following four classes:

1. Problems with novel stimuli and a novel task
2. Problems with novel stimuli and a realistic task
3. Problems with realistic stimuli and a novel task
4. Problems with realistic stimuli and a realistic task

The latter three types of tasks might be considered everyday problems in that they are, at least in part, more realistic than most traditional problem-solving tasks.

The everyday problem-solving tasks that have been conducted to date fall into the latter two categories: problems with realistic stimuli and a novel task, or problems with realistic stimuli and a realistic task. The results of studies with these two different types of everyday problem-solving tasks are reviewed next.

Traditional problems with realistic stimuli

Two studies of everyday or real-life problem-solving tasks were conducted in the 1950s. Bernadelli, as reported by Welford (1958), presented adults with electrical problems that were supposedly similar to those encountered in servicing radios. The subjects were given a box with six terminals on the top that were connected beneath by resistances, along with a resistance meter (ohmmeter) and a circuit diagram. The circuit diagram showed the connections between the terminals on the box, but it did not show which of the terminals pictured in the diagram corresponded to the terminals on the box. The subjects' task was to determine that correspondence. The older adults had to take more meter readings than the younger adults in order to arrive at the solution. Also, many of the meter readings that the older adults took were redundant; that is, because of their previous readings, the older adults should already have had the information that they were seeking in subsequent meter readings.

The second study was performed by Clay, as reported by Welford (1958). Clay used the same type of problem as Bernadelli, but changed the stimuli so that no electrical knowledge would be required. She presented her subjects with a box with six buttons on top. The subjects were also presented with a diagram that represented the order in which six horses finished a race. Each of the six buttons on the box was supposed to represent one of the horses, and it was the subjects' task to find out which horse was represented by each button. The subjects were supposed to solve the problem by pushing two of the buttons simultaneously, after which they would be given information about the positions of the horses that were represented by the two buttons. They were to continue pressing buttons until they had matched all the buttons with the horses. Clay's results were similar to those of Bernadelli. The older individuals made more errors, took more readings, and took more time to solve the problems.

Arenberg (1968) attempted to make a traditional concept-learning problem more realistic by using food as stimuli, rather than abstract geometric stimuli. He told his subjects that one of the foods was poisoned, and it was their task to figure out which one. Rather than telling the subjects that each stimulus either was or was not an example of the concept, the subjects were told that they either "lived" or "died" after each "meal" of three foods was presented. "Lived" indicated that the poisoned food was not included in the meal; "died" indicated that it was included. Arenberg found that older individuals could solve the poisoned-food problems more readily than they could solve traditional problems. However, older adults did not perform as well as younger adults, even with the poisoned-food problems.

Sinnott (1975) obtained similar findings with respect to Piagetian formal operational tasks. She presented her subjects with a problem that required the subject to make all possible binary combinations of items and a problem that required the subject to deal simultaneously with several proportional relationships. She used both traditional stimuli and familiar, realistic stimuli with both problems. The performances of both younger adults and older adults were facilitated by the use of the realistic stimuli, but the age differences were not eliminated by the use of familiar stimuli. In fact, if anything, the age differences were increased by the use of the realistic stimuli.

Harber and Hartley (1983) compared performance on the Raven Progressive Matrices with performance on a similar task with more realistic stimuli. Use of the realistic stimuli facilitated the performances of younger adults, but not the performances of older adults. The older adults performed less well than the younger adults on both the Raven and the task with more realistic stimuli.

What conclusions can be drawn on the basis of this research in which realistic stimuli were used with traditional problems? Although the results are not entirely consistent, these studies indicate that individuals of all ages may perform better on traditional problem-solving tasks when an attempt is made to use stimuli and feedback that are more meaningful or realistic. But the results further indicate that the use of more realistic stimuli does not eliminate the age differences that typically are found with more traditional problem-solving tasks. Rather, even with more realistic stimuli, younger adults perform at higher levels than do older adults. In fact, in some cases, the use of realistic stimuli seems to facilitate performance for younger adults more than for older adults.

Problems with realistic stimuli and a realistic task

My colleagues and I conducted a series of studies on everyday or practical problem solving. For these studies we developed sets of problems that adults might encounter in their daily lives. These problems were not traditional problems with realistic stimuli, but rather were realistic in every regard. In order to test adults' general ability to solve problems rather than their ability to deal with problems in only one or two life domains, the problem sets were developed so that they involved a diversity of types of activities from many different life domains. The problems dealt with topics as diverse as cooking, consumer issues, weather, crime, transportation, housing, work, and so forth. The following is an example of one of the problems:

> Let's say that one evening you go to the refrigerator to get something cold to drink. When you open the refrigerator, you notice that it is not cold inside, but rather, is warm. What would you do?

All of the problems presented the subjects with real-life problem situations and asked how they would deal with the situations. Their responses were judged according to the number of solutions that were given that were both safe and effective.

Three studies were conducted with such problems. In the first study (Denney & Palmer, 1981), nine problems were employed in a cross-sectional study of individuals from age 20 to 80. Performance on the problems improved from the 20-year-old group up to the 40- and 50-year-old groups and decreased thereafter.

The developmental function obtained in the first study may have occurred because the set of problems in that study may have been unintentionally biased in favor of middle-aged individuals. As a result, a second study (Denney, Pearce & Palmer, 1982) was conducted with three different sets of problems: a set of the kinds of problems that young adults might encounter in their daily lives, a set of the kinds of problems that middle-aged adults might encounter, and a set of the kinds of problems that elderly adults might encounter. The following is an example of one of the young-adult problems:

> Let's say that a young man who is living in an apartment building finds that the heater in his apartment is not working. He asks his landlord to send someone out to fix it and the landlord agrees. But, after a week of cold weather and several calls to the landlord, the heater is still not fixed. What should the young man do?

An example of one of the middle-aged-adult problems:

> Let's say that a middle-aged woman is frying chicken in her home when, all of a sudden, a grease fire breaks out on top of the stove. Flames begin to shoot up. What should she do?

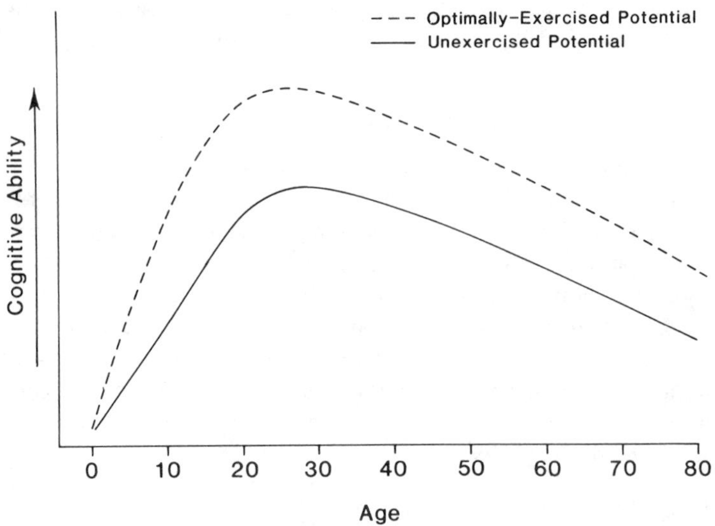

Figure 19.1. Hypothesized relationships between age and both unexercised and optimally exercised potential.

An example of one of the elderly adult problems:

Let's say that a 60-year-old man who lives alone in a large city needs to go across town for a doctor's appointment. He cannot drive because he doesn't have a car and he doesn't have any relatives who live nearby who could drive him. What should he do?

Individuals between the ages of 20 and 80 were presented with all three sets of problems. Performance on the young-adult problems decreased with increasing age, whereas performances on both the middle-aged-adult problems and the elderly adult problems increased up to middle age and decreased thereafter.

In the second study, both the young adults and the middle-aged adults performed better than any other age group on those problems that were designed specifically for them. However, the elderly adults did not perform better than the other age groups on the problems that were designed specifically for them. The elderly adults may not have performed better than the other age groups on the elderly adults' problems because we had not developed a good set of problems for them – a set of problems that adequately reflected the kinds of problems that they might encounter in their daily lives. As a result, in a third study (Denney & Pearce, in press), a number of elderly adults were recruited to help develop a new set of elderly adult problems. The elderly adults who helped develop the problems were told that we wanted them to help us develop problems that would give elderly adults the advantage. The following is an example of one of the problems that the elderly adults provided:

Let's say that a 65-year-old woman has just been widowed and now lives alone. What can she do to continue associating with people?

Individuals between the ages of 20 and 80 were presented with 10 problems that were developed in collaboration with the elderly adults. Again, just as with the elderly adult problems in the second study, performance increased from the 20-year-old group up to the 50-year-old group and declined thereafter.

What conclusions can be drawn on the basis of this series of studies of realistic problems? First, the research has demonstrated that we can determine the level of developmental function that will be obtained with practical problem-solving tasks, in large part by the types of problems we choose to employ. We can develop problems on which young adults will perform better than older adults, or we can develop problems on which middle-aged adults will perform better than either younger or older adults. This latter fact is interesting because it demonstrates that even though performance on traditional problem-solving tasks declines after early adulthood, middle-aged individuals (those in their 40s and 50s) perform better than younger individuals on at least some practical everyday problems. Thus, it appears that the additional experience that middle-aged adults have gained as a result of living longer facilitates performance on at least some types of practical problems.

Another conclusion that I have tentatively drawn is that it may not be possible to develop practical everyday problems on which older individuals will perform better than young and middle-aged adults. Middle-aged adults have performed better than elderly adults on all of the problems that I and my colleagues have developed, even on those that were developed specifically to give elderly adults the advantage. And young adults have performed just as well as elderly adults on such problems. Whereas one can easily develop a set of problems on which middle-aged adults will do better than either younger or older adults, or a set of problems on which young adults will do better than either middle-aged or older adults, it appears to be much more difficult, if not impossible, to develop a set of questions on which older individuals will do better than middle-aged or younger individuals.

The two conclusions drawn earlier (that the developmental function of performance on practical problem-solving tasks varies as a result of the types of practical problems that are employed, and that the performances of older adults are limited, in spite of the fact that they have had more real-world experience than younger adults) are consistent with my model of life-span cognitive development. That model is presented next.

A relevant model of cognitive development

In my model of life-span cognitive development (Denney, 1982, 1984), a distinction is drawn between unexercised potential and optimally exercised potential. Unexercised potential refers to how well an individual will perform if given no exercise or training on the ability in question. Optimally exercised potential refers to how well an individual will perform if given optimal exercise and/or training on the ability in question. As can be seen in Figure 19.1, the

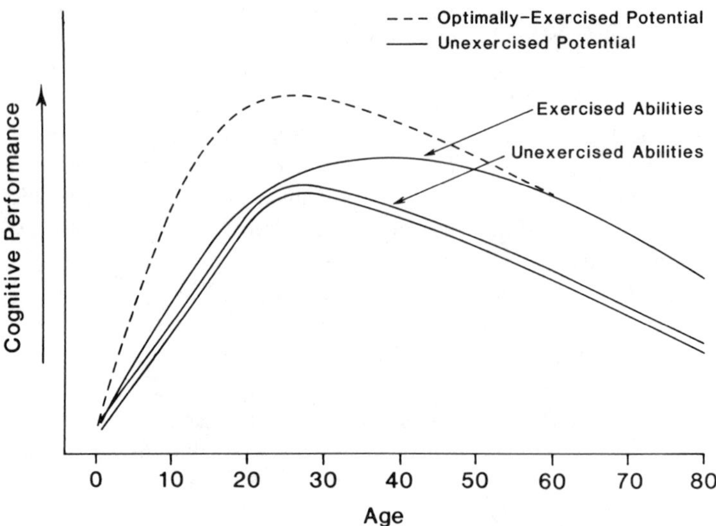

Figure 19.2. Hypothesized relationships between both exercised and unexercised abilities and levels of optimally exercised and unexercised potential.

levels of both unexercised potential and optimally exercised potential are proposed to increase up to early adulthood and decrease gradually thereafter. The region between the curves for levels of unexercised and optimally exercised potential is meant to represent the extent to which learning and experience can affect performance.

According to the model, the performance curve for abilities that are frequently exercised will fall somewhere between the curves for unexercised potential and optimally exercised potential. Just where the performance level will fall in this range will be determined by the amount and timing of the exercise and/or training experienced. Performance for abilities that are not exercised frequently, on the other hand, will tend to follow the curve for unexercised potential, because no exercise or training intervenes to direct the function away from that particular course. Two different hypothetical performance curves – one that might be obtained for frequently exercised abilities and one that might be obtained for infrequently exercised abilities – are illustrated in Figure 19.2.

This model of life-span cognitive development accounts for all of the findings obtained in the series of practical problem-solving studies reported earlier. First, the model predicts that problem-solving abilities that are not frequently exercised during the adult years will decline after the early adult years. Performance on the traditional problem-solving tasks, which is not frequently exercised, does in fact decline after early adulthood.

Second, the model predicts that problem-solving abilities that are frequently exercised during the adult years will be maximal at the age at which they are exercised most frequently. Performance on the practical problem-solving tasks

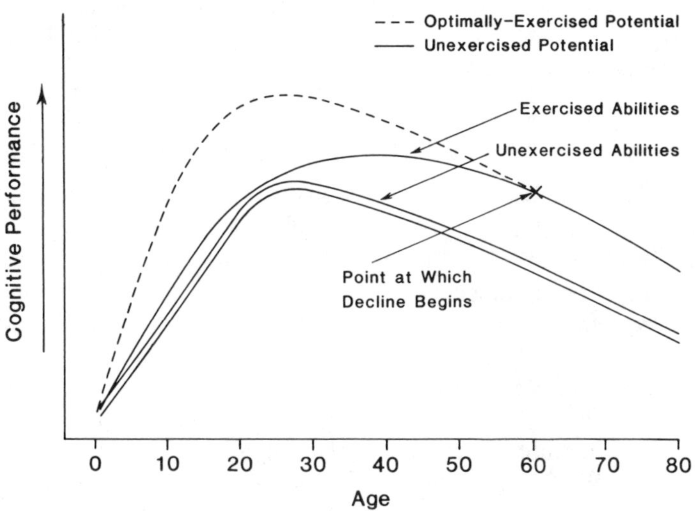

Figure 19.3. The point at which the level of optimally exercised potential falls below the level of performance of exercised abilities.

does in fact tend to be highest in those age groups that would be expected to have had the most exercise with the specific types of problems in question. That is, young adults perform better than other age groups on those problems that were developed to be similar to the ones they might encounter in their daily lives, and middle-aged adults perform better than other age groups on those problems designed for them.

Third, the model predicts that problem-solving abilities that are exercised frequently throughout the adult years will increase, or be maintained, until the age at which the level of optimally exercised potential falls below the level at which the individual has been functioning (Figure 19.3). After that age, the model predicts that performance on even highly exercised abilities will be limited. Again, as predicted, performance levels on the practical problems that were designed to be like those that elderly adults would be most likely to encounter in their daily lives were not as high for the elderly adults as for the younger age groups. Thus, it appears that the practical problem-solving performances of elderly adults are limited relative to those of younger adults, just as the model predicts.

In summary, my model of life-span cognitive development accounts for the results of research with traditional problem-solving tasks, as well as for the results of research with everyday problem-solving tasks of various kinds. According to the model, those abilities that are not exercised much during the adult years, such as those measured by traditional problem-solving tasks, should tend to decline with age, whereas those that are exercised, such as those measured by everyday problems, should be maximal at the age at which they are exercised most frequently. However, according to the model, performance during the later adult years should be somewhat limited by the age-related decline in the level of optimally exercised potential. These predictions have, so far, been supported by the results of the problem-solving research.

Everyday problem solving: What have we learned?

The research that has been conducted with everyday problem solving up to this point has answered some of the questions that instigated the initial interest in everyday problem solving. The initial interest grew out of the belief, on the part of a number of investigators, that older individuals were disadvantaged on traditional problems because the types of problems that have traditionally been used are not relevant to their everyday lives. The assumption on the part of some of those investigators was that older individuals might perform even better than younger individuals on everyday problems, because they will have had more experience with such problems as a result of living longer. This was a very reasonable hypothesis. What does the research to date tell us about its accuracy?

First, the research suggests that simply using more realistic stimuli with traditional problem-solving tasks does not eliminate, or even reduce, the age differences that are almost inevitably found on traditional problem-solving tasks. If anything, it appears that the use of more realistic stimuli may even increase the differences between younger and older adults. Thus, these studies do not support the hypothesis that older individuals may do better, relatively speaking, on everyday problems than on traditional problems.

Second, the research suggests that using problems that are realistic in both form and content results in a variety of different developmental patterns across the adult years, depending on the particular problems that are employed. Problems can be developed that will give the advantage to either young adults or middle-aged adults. These results support the hypothesis that individuals who have lived longer and therefore have had more experience do better, relatively speaking, on everyday problems, for two different reasons. First, middle-aged individuals perform better than young adults on many of the everyday-problem sets that my colleagues and I have developed. These results are in clear contrast to the results of studies of traditional problem solving, in which young adults almost inevitably perform better than middle-aged adults. Second, older adults perform as well as young adults on all of the everyday-problem sets that have been investigated, with the exception of the problems that were designed specifically to give young adults the advantage. Again, these results are in contrast to the results of studies of traditional problem solving. Both of these results suggest that the level of developmental function obtained for problem-solving ability is in fact influenced by the extent to which the various age groups have had experience with the particular problems under investigation, and on many types of practical problems, older individuals have the advantage.

Third, the research indicates that elderly adults do not perform better than younger adults on any of the sets of practical everyday problems that have been employed. This finding suggests that the performances of elderly adults on everyday problems are somewhat limited in a way that the performances of other age groups are not. This finding does not support the hypothesis that the age-related decline in performance on traditional problem-solving tasks is simply a result of the fact that the traditional problem-solving tasks are biased against elderly adults. Rather, there does appear to be an age-related decline in problem-solving ability in general, although the decline may not be apparent in everyday practical problem solving until after middle age.

In summary, the research has provided support for the initial view that older individuals may perform better on everyday problem-solving tasks than on traditional tasks. However, it has also indicated that there probably are age declines – during the later adult years – in everyday problem solving as well as in traditional problem solving. Given these findings, the research on everyday problem solving that has been conducted to date has been worthwhile. It has answered a number of questions that arose from the results of research on age differences in traditional problem-solving tasks. Next, the potential for future research on everyday problem solving is addressed.

Everyday problem solving: How much potential?

On the basis of the results of the research on everyday problem solving, I have reservations about the usefulness of research on everyday problem solving for at least certain purposes. For example, I believe that everyday problem-solving tasks have less predictive validity than do traditional tasks, in spite of the fact that the everyday problems appear to have more in common with the types of problems that individuals typically encounter in their daily lives. My reasoning is as follows: Traditional problem-solving tasks tend to measure abilities that are not typically used in daily life; rather, they tend to measure the ability to deal with novel problems. Thus, all individuals are given a more or less equal opportunity with respect to performance on traditional problem-solving tasks. With traditional problems, it tends *not* to be the case that some individuals are advantaged as a result of the types of experiences that they have had, whereas others are disadvantaged as a result of their experiential histories. With everyday problems, on the other hand, it is much more likely that some individuals will have the advantage of extensive experience in the problem domain or problem domains that are measured on a particular test, whereas others will not. So, whereas traditional problem-solving tasks may provide a good measure of one's ability to solve problems that is relatively "uncontaminated" with differential experience, everyday problem-solving tasks are less likely to be able to provide a measure that is equally "fair" to all individuals regardless of the types of experiences they have had.

I shall illustrate this point with the types of problems that I have used in my own research. One of the questions dealt with how to put out a grease fire on a stove. Why should we expect adults who do not cook and who do not know anything about chemistry and/or fires to have a particularly good answer to that question? And what does it tell us about the cognitive abilities of a Pulitzer Prize winner if he or she does not know how to answer that question correctly? All it tells us is that he or she has not had the relevant experience in the domain being measured. Another question asked what one could do if one discovered that the refrigerator was not working properly in the evening. If a brilliant mathematician does not have a good answer to that question because his or her spouse has always taken care of the repair of household appliances, what does it tell us about that individual's problem-solving abilities? Again, it tells us more about an individual's experience than about his or her ability.

Whereas traditional problems tend to measure general problem-solving *ability,* everyday problems tend to measure *ability plus experience*. Because experience is, at least to a certain extent, unrelated to ability, everyday problem-solving measures presumably will be less accurate measures of general problem-solving ability than will more traditional measures, because they include a component that is unrelated to ability. Whereas everyday problem-solving measures may predict well in the particular life domains included in the measures, their predictive ability presumably will be less impressive in domains that are not tapped by the measures. In domains that are not tapped, traditional measures should predict better because they come closer to being measures of pure ability; everyday measures, on the other hand, should predict less well because of their ability-independent component.

Let me state my argument in a different way – with the help of a computer metaphor. According to my model of life-span cognitive development, biologically determined potential and experience interact to determine performance. Let us refer to the biologically determined component of the organism as the "hardware" and to the experientially based component as the "software." According to my model, the hardware increases up to early adulthood and decreases thereafter. And experience can affect performance at any age. During childhood and early adulthood, individuals all tend to have more or less the same software because most schools tend to teach more or less the same material. As a result, for children and young adults, problem-solving tasks that are good measures of either hardware or software will be expected to be predictive of real-world performance.

After early adulthood, however, individuals do not all have the same software. One individual might have "developmental psychologist" software as well as "tennis" and "chess" software. Another might have "truck driver" and "sports trivia" software. And yet another might have "heart surgeon," "gourmet cook," and "parent" software. Thus, many measures of experience-based performance or software will not be equally applicable to, or "fair" to, all adults, because some adults will have had experience with the domains that are tapped by the measures, and others will not. With everyday problem-solving measures, an individual's score will be a function of the individual's hardware and of the match between the individual's software and the type of software tapped by the particular practical problem-solving measure. It does not seem reasonable to test individuals who have different software on the same measures of practical problem solving if those measures tap domains in which individuals have had differing amounts of experience.

Measures of practical problem solving that tap domains in which individuals differ in experience will, in my opinion, not have as much predictive validity as measures of traditional problem solving. Traditional problems tend to be novel, and as a result, everyone is given more or less equal opportunity. When individuals are tested with novel problems (problems on which they are given equal opportunity), the scores obtained should be predictive of performance in other areas, because the scores should reflect differences in ability. But when the problem-solving measures are measures of ability plus experience, the measures should then become less predictive of general real-world performance, because the scores will reflect, in part, experiential differences that are partly determined by factors other than ability.

Of course, if we study everyday practical problem solving within a domain in which all of the individuals who are being tested have specialized, then the practical problem-solving measures will have more predictive power. We might, for example, study the ability to solve electrical problems in individuals who have electrical engineering software, that is, among electrical engineers. That, of course, is currently being done under the rubric of "expertise" (Charness, Chapter 24, this volume). The study of everyday problem solving in individuals' areas of expertise seems to hold more potential in some regards than does the study of everyday problem solving. Presumably, measures of one's expertise will have more predictive validity than measures of more general everyday problem solving. In addition, it seems reasonable to try to determine nomothetic developmental functions for problem solving in individuals' areas of expertise, whereas it would be futile to try to determine the nomothetic developmental function for everyday problem solving.

My reservations about the usefulness of everyday problem solving for some purposes do not necessarily apply to other areas of everyday cognition. In other areas of everyday cognition it may be easier to develop measures on which all adults are given a more or less equal chance – measures on which adults can all be expected to have experience. In everyday-memory tasks, for example, adults might be given a list of items they were supposed to remember to buy at the grocery store. Even though adults will differ in the extent to which they frequent grocery stores, we can be fairly certain that all adults have had to remember lists of things to do in their everyday lives. We can, further, be fairly certain that all adults will be familiar with items that might be included on a hypothetical grocery list (e.g., milk, eggs, bread). Thus, both the stimuli and the task in such a test of everyday memory will be familiar to most adults. As a result, individual differences that are obtained with such measures will, in all likelihood, be better indices of ability than any measures of everyday problem solving could be. As a result, those measures should have more predictive validity than everyday problem-solving measures. So, although I have reservations about the predictive validity of everyday problem-solving measures, these concerns do not necessarily generalize to other types of everyday cognition.

In addition to my concerns about the predictive validity of everyday problem-solving measures, I also have reservations about their usefulness in determining nomothetic developmental functions. As the series of practical problem-solving studies reported in this chapter illustrates, there is no one nomothetic developmental function for everyday practical problem solving. However, even if I am correct in assuming that everyday problem-solving measures lack predictive validity and will not be useful in determining nomothetic developmental functions, that does not mean that the study of everyday problem solving will not prove to be useful for other purposes. Certainly there are reasons for studying everyday problem solving for more practical reasons. For example, if one is interested in finding ways of better protecting the elderly population from some of the fraud schemes that currently are being directed primarily at their age group, studies of everyday problem solving might be conducted to determine why older adults are more susceptible to such schemes and what can be done to reduce that susceptibility. In other words, the problem solving of elderly adults in domains that relate to such fraudulent crimes might be assessed in order to determine what things older adults typically do not do that younger, less susceptible individuals do to protect themselves from such crimes. This research might then be followed with research on how to teach older adults to better protect themselves. In addition, there are many other practical reasons for studying everyday problem solving in adults.

In summary, on the basis of the results of research on everyday problem solving, I have reservations about the predictive validity of everyday problem-solving measures and about the use of everyday problem-solving measures for determining a general nomothetic developmental function. Both of these reservations are based on the fact that performance on everyday problem-solving tasks is a result of both ability and experience. Because experience depends on many factors that are unrelated to ability, the fact that experience is an important component of everyday problem-solving performance will ensure that predictive validity is limited. And the fact that different individuals will have different amounts of experience with different types of everyday problems at different times in their lives will ensure that no one general developmental function will be obtained for all types of everyday problem-solving tasks.

Recommendations for future research

Although I do not believe that studies aimed at determining the developmental function of everyday problem solving will be useful, I do think that there are several research issues that should be addressed. The following are some recommendations for future research on everyday and traditional problem solving that I believe to be of value:

1. To what extent are both traditional and everyday problem-solving measures predictive of real-world performance and success?
2. Are the predictive validities of the two types of problem solving different at different ages?
3. What is the relationship between traditional problem-solving ability and everyday problem-solving ability? Does this relationship change with age?
4. What are the relationships between standard intelligence measures and both traditional and everyday problem-solving measures? Do traditional and everyday problems relate differently to basic cognitive abilities, such as short-term memory, spatial abilities, verbal abilities, abstract-reasoning abilities, and so forth?
5. Are the relationships between traditional and everyday problem solving and the other basic intellectual abilities different at different ages?
6. Is it possible to develop problems of a practical everyday nature that will be relevant to the life-styles of all individuals? It might be useful to focus on social problem solving. The work of Sternberg, Conway, Ketron, and Bernstein (1981) indicates that in adults' implicit theories of intelligence, social competence is one of the three main factors, in addition to problem solving and verbal ability. Further, social interaction may be one of the domains in which virtually all adults have experience. Thus, it may be a domain in which most adults actually have more or less common experience.
7. Are there age differences in social problem-solving ability?
8. How does social problem-solving ability relate to measures of traditional problem solving and everyday problem solving?
9. What are the relationships between performance on measures of expertise and measures of both traditional and everyday problem solving?
10. What are the relationships between everyday problem-solving abilities in different domains? Is there a generally positive relationship between everyday problem-solving abilities in different domains? Or are they independent?
11. In what ways do everyday problem-solving approaches change with increasing age?

Conclusion

Virtually all studies of performance on traditional problem-solving tasks indicate that performance begins to decline after early adulthood. This finding caused concern about the validity of traditional problem-solving measures when used with middle-aged and elderly adults and resulted in an interest in the use of more realistic problem-solving tasks. The little research that has been done on everyday problems suggests that there is not a single developmental function for problem-solving ability during adulthood. Rather, the age groups that have had the most experience with a particular type of problem tend to perform better than less experienced age groups. But whereas both young and middle-aged adults perform better than other age groups on problems designed specifically to give them the advantage, there appears to be a limit on performance during the later adult years. Elderly adults do not perform better than other age groups on problems designed to give them the advantage. These findings are consistent with my model of life-span cognitive development. The model suggests (a) that experience facilitates performance at all ages and (b) that there is a decrease in potential that becomes great enough during the later adult years to actually interfere with performance.

Because experience affects everyday problem-solving performance, and because different adults have different types of experience, everyday problem-solving measures will be limited in at least two respects. First, everyday problem-solving measures probably will not have as much predictive validity as traditional problem-solving measures. Second, it will not be possible to establish a general nomothetic developmental function for everyday problem solving.

References

Arenberg, D. (1968). Concept problem solving in young and old adults. *Journal of Gerontology, 23,* 279–282.

Arenberg, D. (1982). Changes with age in problem solving. In F. I. M. Craik & S. Trehub (Eds.), *Aging and cognitive processes.* New York: Plenum Press.

Botwinick, J. (1984). Problem solving: Forming concepts. In J. Botwinick (Ed.), *Aging and behavior.* New York: Springer.

Brody, E. B., & Brody, N. (1976). *Intelligence: Nature, determinants, and consequences.* New York: Academic Press.

Cyr, J., & Stones, M. J. (1977). Performance on cognitive tasks in predicting the behavioral competences in the institutionalized elderly. *Experimental Aging Research, 3,* 253–264.

Denney, N. W. (1979). Problem solving in later adulthood. In P. B. Baltes & O. G. Brim (Eds.), *Life-span development and behavior* (Vol. 2). New York: Academic Press.

Denney, N. W. (1982). Cognitive change. In B. B. Wolman & G. Stricker (Eds.), *Handbook of developmental psychology.* Englewood Cliffs, NJ: Prentice-Hall.

Denney, N. W. (1984). A model of cognitive development across the life span. *Developmental Review, 4,* 171–191.

Denney, N. W., & Connors, G. J. (1974). Altering the questioning strategies of preschool children. *Child Development, 45,* 1108–1112.

Denney, N. W., Denney, D. R., & Ziobrowski, M. (1973). Alterations in the information-processing strategies of young children following observation of adult models. *Developmental Psychology, 8,* 202–208.

Denney, N. W., Jones, F. W., & Krigel, S. H. (1979). Modifying the questioning strategies of young children and elderly adults. *Human Development, 22,* 23–36.

Denney, N. W., & Palmer, A. M. (1981). Adult age differences on traditional and practical problem-solving measures. *Journal of Gerontology, 36,* 323–328.

Denney, N. W., & Pearce, K. A. (in press). A developmental study of practical problem solving in adults.

Denney, N. W., Pearce, K. A., & Palmer, A. M. (1982). A developmental study of adults' performance on traditional and practical problem-solving tasks. *Experimental Aging Research, 8,* 115–118.

Denney, N. W., & Turner, M. C. (1979). Facilitating cognitive performance in children: A comparison of strategy modeling and strategy modeling with overt self-verbalization. *Journal of Experimental Child Psychology, 28,* 119–131.

Giambra, L. M., & Arenberg, D. (1980). Problem solving, concept learning, and aging. In L. W. Poon (Ed.), *Aging in the 80s: Psychological issues,* (pp. 253–259). Washington, DC: American Psychological Association.

Harber, K. D., & Hartley, A. A. (1983). Meaningfulness and problem solving performance in younger and older adults. *Experimental Aging Research, 9,* 93–95.

Harrell, T. W., & Harrell, M. S. (1945). Army General Classification Test scores for civilian occupations. *Educational and Psychological Measurement, 5,* 229–239.

Hultsch, D., Hertzog, C., & Dixon, R. (1984). Text recall in adulthood: The role of intellectual abilities. *Developmental Psychology, 20,* 1193–1209.

Hunter, J. E., & Hunter, R. F. (1984). Validity and the utility of alternative predictors of job performance. *Psychological Bulletin, 96,* 72–89.

Kausler, D. H. (1982). Thinking. In D. H. Kausler (Ed.), *Experimental aging and human behavior.* New York: Wiley.

Minton, H. L., & Schneider, F. W. (1980). *Differential psychology.* Monterey, CA: Brooks/Cole.

North, A. J., & Ulatowska, H. K. (1981). Competence in independently living older adults: Assessment and correlates. *Journal of Gerontology, 36,* 576–582.

Rabbitt, P. (1977). Changes in problem solving ability in old age. In J. E. Birren & K. W. Schaie (Eds.), *Handbook of the psychology of aging* (pp. 606–625). New York: Van Nostrand Reinhold.

Salthouse, T. A. (1982). Decision making and problem solving. In T. A. Salthouse (Ed.), *Adult cognition* (pp. 83–102). New York: Springer.

Schaie, K. W. (1978). External validity in the assessment of intellectual development in adulthood. *Journal of Gerontology, 33,* 695–701.

Sinnott, J. D. (1975). Everyday thinking and Piagetian operativity in adults. *Human Development, 18,* 430–443.

Sinnott, J. D., & Guttmann, D. (1978). Piagetian logical abilities and older adults' abilities to solve everyday problems. *Human Development, 21,* 327–333.

Sternberg, R. J., Conway, B. E., Ketron, J. L., & Bernstein, M. (1981). People's conceptions of intelligence. *Journal of Personality and Social Psychology, 41,* 37–55.

Welford, A. T. (1958). *Aging and human skill.* London: Oxford University Press.

Willis, S. L., & Schaie, K. W. (1986). Practical intelligence in later adulthood. In R. J. Sternberg & R. K. Wagner (Eds.), *Practical intelligence: Origins of competence in the everyday world* (pp. 236–268). Cambridge University Press.

20 Prospective/intentional memory and aging: Memory as adaptive action

Jan D. Sinnott

Something very complex and at the same time very common happened to all the authors of the chapters in this book. All of them managed to arrive at the Talland memorial conference. A number of things could have stood in the way of that arrival, and if they had, the participants would never have convened to produce these chapters. One of those things is a sort of memory. To get the flavor of this sort of memory, imagine that you are going on a trip. Think for a moment about some of the many memory-related things you need to do to accomplish that. You need to remember to plan your trip, or to get someone to do that. You need to prepare your house and spouse and children and cats and office for your departure. You need to remember to wash your socks and to bring those clean socks in a well-packed suitcase. And you need to remember when and how to return home again.

As you scan, for a moment, what you would need to remember, you may notice that much of it falls into two categories: things you remember to *do* ("memory for planned action"), and things you remember because you need them in order to do the things you plan to do. An example of the former is "get on the plane"; an example of the latter is "remember the way to the airport." These two sets of memories are prospective/intentional memories and will be discussed in this chapter. These types of memories may be of major interest in assessment of adults' optimum everyday memory capacities. These memories may reflect an underlying action-oriented function for memory, one that is adaptive in a world where there is some stability and where taking action is often useful (Sinnott, Chapter 5, this volume).

In spite of the complexity of the topic and the frequency with which this behavior occurs, this will be a short discussion. It is short because there has been

The support of David Arenberg, chief of the Cognition Section, Gerontology Research Center, National Institute on Aging (NIA) is gratefully acknowledged. This work was partly funded by an NIA Postdoctoral Fellowship to the author and by a grant from Towson State University. The assistance of Robin Armstrong, Judy Friz, Sandra Kafka, Lena Phillips, Judy Plotz, and Susan Robinson, and of participants in the Baltimore Longitudinal Study of Aging, is appreciated.

so little work in this area. It is included because this area of study is potentially important for the study of memory because it permits the experimenter to directly address and manipulate the factors of motivation and intention, while conceptualizing the subject as an adaptive system.

This chapter explores several topics. Why study prospective/intentional memory at all? What data – especially age-related data – on prospective memory performance, either in the laboratory or life, exist? What are the main issues and methodological questions?

Why study prospective/intentional memory?

In this section it is argued that prospective/intentional memory should be studied for several reasons: Little is known about it; such memories are highly motivated and salient, allowing a manipulation of that factor; they are adaptive; they have interpersonal implications.

Prospective memory is memory for planned action (Meacham, 1982). Intentional memory (Sinnott, 1986b) is memory for whatever lets one accomplish one's plan. Prospective/intentional memory may be compared with retrospective memory (i.e., memory for past events). Prospective/intentional memory involves some retrospective elements, because planning the action did occur in the past. But prospective/intentional memory includes more than memory for just any past events, because it includes memory for events that will continue through time and that are personally motivating and relevant to the life of the rememberer.

As Baddeley and Wilkins (1984) point out, the dichotomy between prospective/intentional memory and retrospective memory is somewhat artificial. Much of prospective/intentional memory involves retrospective remembering. In the study by Poon and Schaffer (1982), when respondents remembered to telephone, they also drew on their memories of how to telephone and of the manner in which they had been asked to do so in that experiment. Although research to examine the question has not yet been carried out, it seems conceptually reasonable that both prospective/intentional memory and retrospective memory probably draw on similar processes. There may be episodic and semantic prospective/intentional memory, for example. It may be that retrospective memories might never be stored if they were not, at the point of storage, considered prospective/intentional, or "needed again." But other dichotomies in memory research (e.g., episodic/semantic) are also weak. It simply makes sense, as Baddeley and Wilkins (1984) note, to use the prospective/intentional label to draw attention to an area of research that has been neglected in the past and that is important in everyday functioning. To make a generalization, it seems that the more prospective/intentional an item is, the less investigators have studied it, and the more important it is perceived by subjects to be for everyday functioning.

One more reason to study prospective/intentional everyday memory is this: It probably is a factor in everyday problem solving. When individuals see a problem, interpret that problem as a real-life or everyday problem (as opposed to

Table 20.1. *Summary of major prospective memory studies*

Study	Subjects	Behavior measured	Major findings	Major issues raised and factors discussed
Baddeley & Wilkins (1984)[a]	Theoretical paper			Three way categorization of memory tasks: prospective, retrospective; short term, long-term; episodic, semantic
Ceci & Bronfenbrenner (1985)	10- and 14-year-old children	Remembering to monitor time	Strategic time monitoring less frequent in lab than at home; strategies used were more complex at home; roles influenced strategy use	Life may make a better lab than the lab itself
Drew (1940)	Pilots	Monitoring simulated gauges, fuel indicators (task considered analogue of demands during flight)	Omissions few at first, many later	Task analysis
Harris (1980)	Women ($\bar{X}$ age 47)	Memory aids used to recall birthdays, anniversaries	Memory aids like calendars were habitually used	Roles may influence memory strategies
Harris (1984)[a]	Theoretical & review paper			Habitual vs. episodic prospective memory; types of monitoring prospective vs. retrospective
Harris & Wilkins (1982)	Adults	Remembering to press a button (analogue of pill taking)	Subjects used a test–wait–test–exit loop to monitor	Cost–benefit factors in processing during monitoring; critical period's shape & duration
Kreutzer, Leonard, & Flavell (1975)	Children, grades K–5	Awareness of techniques for remembering to bring ice skates	Children were aware of memory aids they used to improve prospective memory	Metamemory questions may apply to prospective memory too

Levy (1977)	Mothers of children in behavior therapy	Remembering to telephone for information on procedures at next stage of treatment	Commitment did not reliably increase compliance	Compliance vs. simple memory
Levy & Clark (1980)	Hospital outpatients	Remembering to make clinic appointments	Commitment did not reliably increase compliance	Compliance vs. simple memory
Levy & Loftus (1984)[a]	Review of studies on compliance with instructions			
Levy, Yamashita, & Pow (1979)	Adults getting flu shots	Remembering to record symptoms for 2 days after shot	Commitment did not reliably increase compliance	Compliance vs. simple memory
Loftus (1971)	Adults	Remembering to do one task *after* another	Interval is important	Same models useful for prospective and other memory
Meacham (1982)[a]	Theoretical paper on prospective memory			Prospective memory considered in context of activities, actions, operations, as described by Soviet developmental psychologists; prospective vs. retrospective
Meacham & Colombo (1980)	Children, ages 5–7	Remembering to remind experimenter to get their toy from box	Strategies change with age	
Meacham & Dumitru (1976)	Children, ages 5–7	Remembering to enter their pictures in a contest	Type of cue less important; age more important	
Meacham & Kushner (1980)	Undergraduates	Memory of behavior and memory in prospective situations	Anxiety leads to remembering prospective actions, but not performing them; external retrieval cues help	Motivational components in good performance
Meacham & Leiman (1982)	College students	Remembering to mail postcards	External retrieval cues assist episodic prospective remembering	Kinds of prospective memory; habitual vs. episodic distinction; external retrieval cues used to convert episodic into habitual task?

Table 20.1 *(cont.)*

Study	Subjects	Behavior measured	Major findings	Major issues raised and factors discussed
Meacham & Singer (1977)	College students	Remembering to mail postcards	Regularity of demand and incentive had no effect	Compliance vs. memory
Morris (1979)				
Moscovitch (1982)	College students; graduates, ages 65–75	Remembering to telephone	Old outperformed young	Old rely on external cues more? Old more motivated?
Orne (1970)	Adults	Remembering to send postcards	Payment *in advance* significantly influenced return rate, but amount of payment did not	
Pajurkova & Wilkins (1983)	Normal adults and epileptic adults	Remembering to change pencils during lab task	Left-hippocampal excisions related to forgetting	Physiological correlates
Poon & Schaffer (1982)	Young adults ($\bar{X}$ age 25 years); old adults ($\bar{X}$ age 73 years)	Remembering to telephone	Motivation determined performance; performance not always due to memory	
Reason (1979)	Adults	Keeping a diary of planned actions not taken	Failures can be categorized four ways	Theoretical considerations behind *not* acting as planned, including overautomatization
Sinnott (1984c, 1986b)	Young and old adults	Remembering incidental and prospective items that were part of experiences as a research subject; remembering to follow set of three instructions after test	Prospective items not influenced by age and time, whereas incidental items were influenced	Motivation and contextual relevance; memory as adaptive action; effortfulness
Welford (1958)	Adults	Remembering to press a key during a lab task	Increasing forgetting with age	Utility of memory aids; vigilance demands

West (1984)	Young, middle-aged, old adults	Remembering to complete diary and telephone; remembering to telephone and mail a postcard with a certain message; remembering location of folder and appointment	Prospective memory is large part of everyday memory activity; external mnemonics most useful; no major age effects	Contrast prospective, retrospective memory; motivational components; penalty for failure
Wilkins (1976)	Adults	Remembering to send postcards	Length of interval did not influence retention	Compliance vs. simply remembering; short-term vs. long-term tasks
Wilkins & Baddeley (1978)	Women aged 35–49	Remembering to operate a printout clock four times a day (task considered an analogue of pill-taking)	Success inversely related to free-recall scores	Methods of cuing recall; failure to report failures of recall leads to bias

[a]Theoretical or review paper.

abstract, unrealistic), and think aloud on their way to solution, they seem to pay attention to storing problem elements they think they will need later (Sinnott, 1986a). "I've got to remember to . . . " is a familiar phrase, as is "Taking into account that you'll eventually have to. . . . " Actually, "backward" processing (solving from the *last* move back to earlier ones) seems impossible without the use of a form of prospective memory. Certain types of "inquiring systems" (Singer's, for example) *demand* intentional/prospective controls over processing (Churchman, 1971). So task analysis suggests that learning about prospective/intentional memory will aid in understanding everyday problem solving, as well as problem solving of all kinds.

It is argued that prospective/intentional memory should be studied because it has not been explored in memory literature and because it can be distinguished from retrospective memory, which has been investigated. Prospective/intentional memory study permits manipulation of motivation. Such memory abilities are certain to be adaptive for the functioning of the organism, and because they involve interpersonal relations in both goal setting and reinforcements, they permit analyses of a social component in cognition.

What are the major findings so far?

In this section, the relatively small number of available studies is reviewed. The focus is on the stimulus materials used, on studies done with older respondents, and on the author's own recent research. Four studies will be discussed in detail. The studies are summarized in Table 20.1 in terms of subjects, behavior measured, results, and issues raised.

There have been studies of prospective/intentional memory, but usually they have used young subjects and somewhat artificial situations, such as remembering to mail postcards. (Mailing postcards is, of course, an everyday task. What is somewhat artificial is that subjects are mailing them to someone they do not know simply because they were told to do so.) They also have been based on Meacham's strict definition of *prospective* memory as "remembering to act." Among 25 studies, in only 4 studies were older adults tested as subjects. The 21 studies of other-than-old individuals focused on (in order of frequency) remembering to send postcards or call, monitoring (although this was present in all studies, it was the salient feature in certain studies), metacognitive awareness of prospective/intentional memory, diary studies, and aids to prospective/intentional memory. Some studies addressed more than one area. Major findings (Table 20.1) were impossible to categorize or summarize, because the studies did not build on each other so much as on the other memory-related interests of the authors.

Four studies included older respondents and will be discussed in detail, in this order: Poon and Schaffer (1982); Moscovitch (1982); West (1984); Sinnott (1984c, 1986b). Poon and Schaffer (1982), in one such study with older respondents, asked young (mean age 25.3 years) and old (mean age 73.2 years) adults to remember to telephone at certain times over a 3-week period. The elderly remembered more calls than did the young, called more closely to target times, and were more consistent over the 3-week period than were the young. Results were similar for other studies with older adults, such as those reported by West (1984) and by Sinnott (1984c, 1986b). This suggests that prospective/intentional memory and goal-related memory may be of major interest in assessing adults' optimum everyday memory capabilities. Such tasks may reflect an underlying action-oriented adaptive function for memory. Performance might also reflect a compensatory focusing of older adults' skills on salient, context-embedded events. In another study, Moscovitch (1982) requested college students and older college graduates (ages 65–75) to remember to make telelphone calls. Once again the old outperformed the young. In a third study (West, 1984) young, middle-aged, and old adults were to remember to complete a diary, to telephone, to mail a card with a certain message, and to be able to locate a folder and keep an appointment. Results indicated that prospective/intentional memory was a large part of everyday memory activity and that external mnemonics (such as notes) were useful in cuing recall. Age decrements were not generally found.

Finally, Sinnot (1984c, 1986b), in a longitudinal study, asked 79 older and younger adults (ages 23–93) to recall or recognize information that was incidental or prospective/intentional in nature and that should have been acquired by subjects in the course of 2 days of activities as a research volunteer in the Baltimore Longitudinal Study of Aging (BLSA). For example, subjects were asked to return to a certain room; they were asked to remember how they would get to the cafeteria that day for dinner. All respondents to date (but one) have performed the requested prospective/intentional tasks. Memory for prospective/intentional items was not influenced by age or passage of time (18 months), whereas memory for incidental items was influenced. The results suggested that context and salience are important factors in everyday aging memory performance over time. The study just mentioned is part of a larger everyday-memory investigation that also examines parameters of spatial and salient items (but not prospective/intentional items) that are everyday in nature. This study is linked with others on everyday problem solving and studies of laboratory-tested memory so that a more complex picture of memory processes can be obtained.

In reviewing the available prospective/intentional memory studies, it was found that most studies used relatively artificial situations and young respondents. Studies of older respondents resulted in the old at least matching the young in performance.

Issues and methodological questions

Numerous issues have been raised by those doing research in prospective/intentional memory. Some focus on methodology, others on general theoretical issues or issues concerning the philosophy of science. In this section, methodology is addressed, with a focus on tasks, compliance, motivation, individual differences, cues, failure, and definitions.

Methodology

The study of prospective/intentional memory is still so new that most methodological approaches are not satisfactory or standardized. Some strategies, however, are more widely used than others. One frequently used strategy (Levy, 1977; Meacham & Singer, 1977; Meacham & Leiman, 1982; Moscovitch, 1982; Orne, 1970; Poon & Schaffer, 1982; West, 1984; Wilkins, 1976) is to ask subjects to return postcards or to make calls, and a number of variations on those themes have been pursued (Table 20.1). Investigators are still exploring the utility of various forms of those postcard tasks and barely beginning the development of others. Most of the investigators in this area are sensitive to contextual relativism in their studies and know that performance is likely to vary from context to context. It is therefore probable that several of the methods will be perfected and will cover a wider number of situations and contexts.

The potential confounding of compliance and prospective/intentional memory in most approaches has been noted (Levy & Loftus, 1984). When an individual *remembers* to mail his or her postcard, that individual must also be willing to actually *do* so for researchers to record that event as an instance of prospective/intentional memory, in most studies. Some items on Sinnott's scale are exceptions to this rule. Yet the perversity of human research participants is such that many may remember but *refuse* to act, for their own good reasons. If asked to report failures to recall, they fail to do that (Wilkins & Baddeley, 1978). So discriminating between remembering and compliance is extremely difficult and may bias results. However, noncompliance, in a sense, might influence any memory study, not only prospective-intentional studies. Respondents may never tell us all they know when we ask them to recall. As the work of Harris (1980) suggests, even social roles may be factors in whether or not a respondent bothers to struggle to find ways to respond appropriately. The compliance issue, then, reduces itself to a motivation issue.

Experimenters need to get a better grasp on what motivates respondents to do their best, and study of prospective/intentional memory may help reach this goal. Experimenters who wish to generalize from their findings also need to know how motivated the respondents are to do well in various situations in real life. Experimenters are highly motivated persons and tend to favor that stance as adaptive, but there is nothing ignoble about those larger numbers of humanity who generally meander through life propelled by a much lower motivation to do anything. If these latter are the majority, and yet studies are peopled by the others, that is, the highly motivated, then results will be ungeneralizable anyhow! Now, because one argument for testing prospective/intentional memory is that motivation to do those tasks is high and performance is therefore "optimal" (Sinnott, 1984c,

1986b), a dilemma exists. Perhaps generalization from apparent prospective/intentional ability to other kinds of memory ability is invalid. But this problem is easily resolved. Everyday-memory test batteries (and lab test batteries) can be engineered to capture many points on the continuum of motivation so that performance under many "normal" motivation levels can be measured. This will capture the range and context of individuals' varying abilities and performance, insofar as they choose to disclose. One way to do this is to vary the degree of prospective/intentional involvement of the task systematically, while also varying the familiarity or "everydayness" of the task.

Using these tasks, information can also be obtained on the potential variety of *processes* a person might resort to in various contexts, under various levels of motivation and in different states of physical and mental decline. This is possible if investigators do what has been recommended before (Giambra & Arenberg, 1980): intensive study and model building for *individuals* (Hartley, Chapter 18, this volume). Although obviously there is a need to know how "most people" (the mythical "average persons") behave on any task, there is no reason other than lack of awareness to adhere slavishly to either nomothetic or idiographic analyses alone. The real solution to the dilemma involving compliance, motivation, and range of performance is partly based on better control and largely based on expanded ranges of tasks, contexts, and analytic approaches. It is important to keep in mind that a complexity of physical and psychological systems operates here. One can foresee a time when a model of a respondent's performance (on a physical and psychological level) will specify conpensatory strategies, strengths, and weaknesses in cognitive performance over a variety of tasks so that targeted interventions can maintain near-optimal performance until death.

Better studies would also result from extentions and refinements of some of the approaches seen in Table 20.1. Further work on cues, especially differential age/context aids to prospective/intentional memory, would help. There has been a suggestion that the old make good use of external cues (Moskovitch, 1982). This knowledge can be useful in interventions, as can additional knowledge of metamemory. Task analysis of any sort would also be a useful step forward. Further exploration of reasons for memory failure (seldom attempted in most of this research) could be a major source of knowledge for us here, as it was for Piaget in the early phases of his studies. Further understanding of some systems elements (e.g., cost–benefit, critical periods, physiological parameters) influencing the monitoring that leads to a successful prospective/intentional response would be useful, because monitoring should of necessity be a part of any prospective/intentional memory operations. These are very general suggestions, but more specific recommendations seem premature when so little has been done.

Some final methodological questions revolve around the definition of prospective/intentional memory, the differences between it and retrospective memory, the various types of prospective/intentional memory that might be teased out of the general concept, and the overlap with established models of nonprospective memory. Much has been made of these questions and definitional distinctions (see the studies cited in Table 20.1). A higher-level question may be to what degree is it useful in a given case to separate and define and label, rather than to describe the ongoing processes. Investigators with a systems-theory bias (Sinnott, Chapter 5, this volume) usually are most concerned with examination of process and its place in the nested arenas of processes. For them, labeling is only "more or less" useful, because anything out there in real life is only "more or less" an exemplar of some concept. The only exceptions to such probabilistic conceptualizations are abstract systems with severe constraints. The experimental results of these severe-constraint studies may generalize only to the information-processing behavior of people who frame the world in a black-and-white manner. So labeling a memory study as "prospective" or "retrospective" suggests to the systems thinker that the former is *relatively* more focused on memory in service of doing something in the future, whereas the latter is *relatively* more focused on memory in service of other goals, all goals being somehow adaptive at some system level. As Meacham (1982) says, memory must be *from* the past, but not necessarily *about* the past. Many of the same processes (e.g., short-term, long-term, episodic, semantic) may be used in prospective/intentional memory.

Differentiating memory as prospective/intentional or retrospective serves a purpose only when one expects to argue that different systems are served, different compensations occur, parameters of functioning differ, individuals' styles differ, or any process-related element with adaptive implications varies between the two. Are different processes involved in prospective/intentional versus retrospective memory? Meacham (1982) addresses this, as does Harris (1984). The answer seems to be yes. Although many theorists appear to ignore the attention, monitoring, metamemory, and motivation components of memory, Meacham gives them a role in prospective memory and then even creates analogues for them in retrospective memory. When Harris discusses "remembering what to recall," he addresses the monitoring function that appears so frequently in Table 20.1 (Welford, 1958), but not in most memory studies. The involvement of attention, monitoring, and metamemory processes, as well as of motivation, makes prospective/intentional memory different. Doing prospective/intentional memory studies permits easier analyses and control of the monitoring and motivational processes within ongoing cognitive processes. This permits broadening of analyses and linking emotion and intention to cognition. In addition to this, prospective/intentional memory studies offer a controllable way to link the personal-psychological-cognitive system to the social-interpersonal system. Most of the studies in Table 20.1 demanded responses that would link one individual with another, or with a group, or with a role, to avoid social punishments. From a systems perspective (Sinnott, Chapter 5, this volume), prospective/intentional studies are worth doing because they show the adaptive information flow between the bounded person system and other bounded person or social or physical systems. For example, failure to act as planned (to come home on time for dinner) often leads to feedback from the social system (family is angry) that modifies further attempts at remembering. The social "memory" (dinner is ritually at 6 p.m.) communicates to the individual memory, which then modifies person behavior, or acts with others to modify the social rituals. This means that memory can be studied in social context. Such complex cognitive processes can therefore be analyzed. Right now, some investigators in this area concentrate on studying memory for *doing*, and others study memory for *planning to do*, but seem aware of the artificial fractionalization and the overriding goal. So, study of prospective/intentional memory serves a special set of purposes.

Issues

On a theoretical level, the study of prospective/intentional memory demands that we address the following issues: the dialectic between phenomenological science and objective science; consciousness, awareness, attention, and vigilance; the extent to which persons construct their known reality; embeddedness (of memory in other cognitive processes, and of cognitive systems in other systems). They are addressed in this section. These issues will bring to mind some of the theoretical and other chapters in this book (Chapters 5, 7, and 23).

Students of the history of psychology will be aware that psychology is once again, after a long hiatus, putting subjectivity and the person back into objective studies. Psychology is not alone in this. The "new physics" (relativity theory, quantum theory, etc.) honors a sophisticated subjectivity in physical universal laws (Einstein, 1961; Wolf, 1981) such that the knower or measurer of reality is, through action (Ilyenkov, 1977; Monod, 1971), the partial creator of reality over time (Hofstadter, 1979; Sinnott, 1981, 1984a, 1984b). Neo-Piagetians know this stage as *post*-formal thought (Commons, Richards, & Armon, 1984). Destiny and truth are created concurrent with events. What the actor feels, believes, and then does partly determines what "is," *within* the limits of the other realities already out there on the stage, and *within* the limits of adaptivity and survival (one cannot create just anything). Perhaps behavior exists largely "in relation to" important others. Perhaps by those interactions, within the limits that the significant other allows, the individual constructs or distorts identities and personalities (Kelly, 1955). Prospective/intentional memory studies suggest that the goal of "doing something" is a goal only if it is a goal in the mind of the subject and that it will be performed only if the subject is conscious of it as a goal at some level. Thus, the phenomenological is necessarily made part of the objective, and vice versa, within the memory task itself.

Notice, then, that consciousness is addressed here, and with it attention, vigilance, and states of awareness. Only to the degree a respondent is conscious of something to do *as* something to do can that respondent demonstrate prospective/intentional memory. Only when the respondent is monitoring the baking time of the cupcakes, attending to them, can he or she remember to take them, on time, from the oven. Sometimes, in one state of awareness, the task to be done will be forgotten: With a bridge between states of awareness, another state may be reached that does give access to a memory of the task to be done. A process like

Monitor/control processes

Automatically process incoming information and behavior

Shift attention

Permit input

Decide that to do *X* is important

Attend to passage of time

Seek input

Evaluate

Decide time to act

Decide *to* act

Interrupt program of habitual action

Be aware of extent of *need* to monitor

Categorize as "a goal" or as "useful information in light of a plan"

Lower-level processes

Input information concerning planned action and means to planned action

Recapture state at which plan reaches consciousness

Recall goal and needed mediating information

Actually monitor time, date, etc.

Act

Figure 20.1. Monitor and lower-level processes during prospective memory.

that in Figure 20.1 may be operating during prospective/intentional memory. A look at the terms Ceci and Howe (1982) use for conscious attentional processing could alert readers that this is so: planfulness; strategic processes; purpose; intention; expectation; pertinence. When Hilgard (1980) distinguishes between active and passive consciousness, he draws attention to the former's involving planfulness and action to reach a goal. Reason (1979) attends to the difficulties for prospective/intentional memory when automatic processes are so strong that they lead to acting "not as (*consciously*) planned." Conscious attentional processing seems to be involved in prospective/intentional memory.

In Figure 20.1, a monitor level can be seen to control attentional shifts, decision making, and input of information, in addition to permitting interruption of automatic processes that need interrupting for the planned activity to be done. Consciousness must shift from active to passive and back again. Attention must shift from focused to diffuse and back, and the individual must orchestrate this while carrying on with other tasks. Can prospective/intentional memory be a vehicle for exploring everyday attention, consciousness, and monitoring processes in information-processing models? It would seem so. What are the limits of prospective memory ability, or of the attention, consciousness, and monitoring needed for that memory to function? These data are not yet available.

Perhaps these very necessary prospective/intentional memory skills can even be improved. This might involve training in attention, improvements in monitoring, increasing one's awareness of good and poor processing by focusing on metamemory, training in "slipping" between levels of processing, or changing the balance between active and passive. It might involve greater awareness that a portion of reality is "out there" *and* is co-created, made more important, by those knowing it when it is made the focus of a plan. Clinicians use these shifts in focus to help bring about the changes desired by clients. They could be used simply to improve memory skill and to compensate for losses in aging.

The last entry in the monitor/control part of Figure 20.1 relates to categorizing something as a "goal" or as "useful information in light of a plan." The last function has considerable bearing on problem solving, especially that area of problem-solving study comparing solutions to well-structured versus ill-structured problems. Many articles (Sinnott, 1984a; Sweller, 1983; Sweller & Levine, 1982) and books (Churchman, 1971) have addressed this area. A model of processes used during planning was described by Hayes-Roth and Hayes-Roth (1979). Prospective/intentional memory would seem to relate to problems being conceptualized as well or ill structured. If one sees a problem as *well* structured – having a clear goal (or plan) – one needs simpler processes (Figure 20.1) to monitor, evaluate, and act; if one sees a problem as *ill* structured – not having a clear goal (or plan) – one needs additional processes to evaluate and categorize. This seems to imply either that the judgment about the nature of the problem influences the prospective-intentional memory processes used or that the reverse could be true. Having the memory capacity or the monitors or the "processes" could determine whether one can make the effort of seeing the problem as ill structured, or *must* see the problem as well structured. With few mental resources, planned actions *must*, perhaps, be seen as clear and simple; with greater resources, they might be given the benefits of exploration, hypothesizing, and alteration.

This brings us back to the problem of memory and aging. When prospective/intentional tasks are clear, older respondents do as well as or better than the young and continue to remember well even over time. If motivation and salience are the only key factors behind this optimistic finding, creation of and testing with *ill*-structured prospective memory tasks should lead to the same results: no age difference. If, however, T. A. Salthouse (private communication) is correct and older adults have more trouble processing and monitoring simultaneously, or if resources are more important than motivation/salience, then older adults should show declines on ill-structured prospective/intentional memory tasks. If these models of everyday problem solving and Figure 20.1 are reasonable, prospective memory ability should predict certain elements of problem-solving style and success for older adults, as well as, to some extent, attentional processes and one's propensity to view the world as "black and white" rather than relativistic.

Relation to the systems approach

One last issue is the relationship between prospective/intentional memory aging studies and two other theories: action theory and general systems theory (GST) (Sinnott, Chapter 5, this volume). That is the focus of this last section.

Prospective/intentional memory is a useful memory category in view of several theoretical views mentioned in this book. A researcher's model of memory processes seems to influence and limit research results by limiting the questions posed by the memory researcher. The earlier associative model was based on a mechanistic metamodel and led to an irreversible-decrement view of aging, with biological antecedents. The next approach historically was the information-processing approach, based on an organismic metamodel and leading to a view of age-related decrement balanced by an individual's compensation. Lately, a contextual approach, suggesting that what is relevant in a context is what is remembered, has projected a nondecremental view of aging, depending on the context of the situation (Hultsch, 1977). The contextual view has similarities to a living-systems metamodel (Miller, 1978) in that what is remembered at any age is a function of all intraorganismic and extraorganismic system parameters. The contextual view would suggest that we ask whether or not there is a decrement at all for those memories that are salient in a given context, as prospective/intentional memories are.

Bruce's adaptation theory, Rubin's regularity and control approach, and my systems approach can be discussed in terms of prospective/intentional memory. Action theory (Chapman, 1984), a view probably not as well known here as in Europe, also fits well with a prospective/intentional view of memory. Action theory is a family of theories [see Chapman (1984) and that entire issue of *Human Development]*. Action theorists are committed to the ideas that a person's intentions influence behavior, that observer and observed share some meaning system, if they can interact at all, and that thought is internalized action that has an overall social/interpersonal adaptive function. The theory has further intersubjective implications: the agent's understanding and the observer's understanding of the agent's behavior are partly *derived* from membership in a community.

These three (prospective/intentional memory, action theory, GST) overlap and offer many intriguing questions. GST suggests that person systems are nested in social systems; so does action theory, and so does prospective/intentional memory theory, because its impetus and consequences are very social in nature. Action theory suggests that the ability to be reflective and intentional does develop over time. So prospective/intentional memory may grow along with the conscious or subconscious awareness of the potential ill-structured nature of the human system and problems of life. It may be related to awareness that individuals co-create their own multisystem reality and ultimately need to make adaptive *choices* of action (or Truth) in a "new physics" world where many values can satisfy the equation of life. Prospective/intentional memory may help persons survive in such a world, even if they are not yet conscious of it. But if they *are* conscious of it, they could be simultaneously the audience and the conductors of this symphony of cognitive and emotional processes. As prospective/intentional memory is studied, information about other complex cognitive processes promises to be uncovered.

Methodological development in this area is in its infancy. Compliance frequently is confounded with memory. The full range of motivational and individual differences needs to be explored, as should cuing and reasons for failure. It is suggested that consciousness, attention, complex cognitive processes, vigilance and states of awareness, systems approaches to behavior, and monitoring should be studied and easily might be studied within this memory paradigm.

Conclusion

This chapter reviews work on prospective/intentional memory, addressing several issues: reasons for studying prospective/intentional memory; data (especially age-related data) that already exist; the main issues and methodological questions. It is argued that prospective/intentional memory should be studied because it is a relatively unexplored area and because it has some features that make it different from retrospective memory. Prospective/intentional memory, by definition, is highly motivated, permitting paired experiments with varying motivational involvement. Prospective/intentional memory seems adaptive for the organism, and because it often involves social reinforcers, it permits inclusion of an interpersonal component. In reviewing the available studies, I found that most relied on tasks such as returning postcards, and most tested young respondents. Studies including older respondents resulted in the old matching or bettering the performance of the young. Methodological developments are necessary because this area is in its infancy. Compliance could be a confound for memory performance here. The full range of motivational, individual, and context influences on performance needs to be addressed, as do potential intervention strategies and reasons for failure. It is suggested that consciousness, vigilance, complex cognitive processes, systems approaches to human behavior, and monitoring functions might be studied within the prospective/intentional memory paradigm.

References

Baddeley, A. D., & Wilkins, A. (1984). Taking memory out of the laboratory. In J. E. Harris & P. E. Morris (Eds.), *Everyday memory, actions, and absentmindedness* (pp. 1–17). New York: Academic Press.

Ceci, S. J., & Bronfenbrenner, U. (1985). "Don't forget to take the cupcakes out of the oven": Prospective memory, strategic time monitoring, and context. *Child Development, 56.*

Ceci, S. J., & Howe, M. J. A. (1982). Metamemory and effects of intending, attending, and intending to attend. In G. Underwood (Ed.), *Aspects of consciousness. Vol. 3: Awareness and self awareness* (pp. 147–164). New York: Academic Press.

Chapman, M. (1984). Action, intention, and intersubjectivity. *Human Development, 27,* 139–144.

Churchman, C. (1971). *The design of inquiring systems: Basic concepts of systems and organizations.* New York: Basic Books.

Commons, M. L., Richards, F. A., & Armon, C. (1984). *Beyond formal operations: Late adolescent and adult cognitive development.* New York: Praeger.

Drew, G. C. (1940). An experimental study of mental fatigue (British Air Ministry, Flying Personnel Research Committee Paper No. 277); reprinted in Harris (1984).

Einstein, A. (1961). *The ABC's of relativity.* New York: Mentor.

Giambra, L., & Arenberg, D. (1980). Problem solving, concept learning, and aging. In L. Poon (Ed.), *Aging in the 1980s: Psychological issues* (pp. 253–259). Washington, DC: American Psychological Association.

Harris, J. E. (1980). Memory aids people use: Two interview studies. *Memory and Cognition, 8,* 31–38.

Harris, J. E. (1984). Remembering to do things: A forgotten topic. In J. E. Harris & P. E. Morris (Eds.), *Everyday memory, actions, and absentmindedness* (pp. 71–92). New York: Academic Press.

Harris, J. E., & Wilkins, A. J. (1982). Remembering to do things: A theoretical framework and an illustrative experiment. *Human Learning, 1,* 123–136.

Hayes-Roth, B., & Hayes-Roth, F. (1979). A cognitive model of planning. *Cognitive Science, 3,* 275–310.

Hilgard, E. R. (1980). Consciousness in contemporary psychology. *Annual Review of Psychology, 31,* 1–26.

Hofstadter, D. (1979). *Gödel, Escher, & Bach: An eternal golden braid.* New York: Random House.

Hultsch, D. (1977). Changing perspectives on basic research in adult learning and memory. *Educational Psychology, 2,* 367–382.

Ilyenkov, E. V. (1977). *Dialectical logic.* Moscow: Progress Publishers.

Kelly, G. A. (1955). *The psychology of personal constructs.* New York: Norton.

Kreutzer, M. A., Leonard, C., & Flavell, J. H. (1975). An interview study of childrens' knowledge about memory. *Monographs of the Society for Research in Child Development, 40* (1, Serial No. 159).

Levy, R. L. (1977). Relationship of an overt commitment to task compliance in behavior therapy. *Journal of Behavior Therapy and Experimental Psychiatry, 8,* 25–29.

Levy, R. L., & Clark, H. (1980). The use of an overt commitment to enhance compliance: A cautionary note. *Journal of Behavior Therapy and Experimental Psychiatry, 11,* 105–107.

Levy, R. L., & Loftus, G. R. (1984). Compliance and memory. In J. E. Harris & P. E. Morris (Eds.), *Everyday memory, actions, and absentmindedness* (pp. 92-112). New York: Academic Press.

Levy, R. L., Yamashita, D., & Pow, G. (1979). The relationship of an overt commitment to the frequency and speed of compliance with symptom reporting. *Medical Care, 17,* 281–284.

Loftus, E. F. (1971). Memory for intentions. *Psychonomic Science, 23,* 215–316.

Meacham, J. A. (1982). A note on remembering to execute planned actions. *Journal of Applied Developmental Psychology, 3,* 121–133.

Meacham, J. A., & Colombo, J. A. (1980). External retrieval cues facilitating prospective remembering in children. *Journal of Educational Research, 73,* 299–301.

Meacham, J. A., & Dumitru, J. (1976). Prospective remembering and external retrieval cues. *JSAS Catalog of Selected Documents in Psychology,* 6(65, Ms. No. 1284).

Meacham, J. A., & Kushner, S. (1980). Anxiety, prospective remembering, and performance of planned actions. *Journal of General Psychology, 103,* 203–209.

Meacham, J. A., & Leiman, B. (1982). Remembering to perform future actions. In U. Neisser (Ed.), *Memory observed: Remembering in natural contexts* (pp. 327–336). San Francisco: W. H. Freeman.

Meacham, J. A., & Singer, J. (1977). Incentive in prospective remembering. *Journal of Psychology, 97,* 191–197.

Miller, J. (1978). *Living systems.* New York: McGraw-Hill.

Monod, J. (1971). *Chance and necessity.* New York: Knopf.

Morris, P. E. (1979). Strategies for learning and recall. In M. M. Gruneberg & P. E. Morris (Eds.), *Applied problems in learning and memory* (pp. 25–58). New York: Academic Press.

Moskovitch, M. (1982). A neuropsychological approach to memory and perception in normal and pathological aging. In F. I. M. Craik & S. Trehub (Eds.), *Aging and cognitive processes* (pp. 55–78). New York: Plenum.

Orne, M. T. (1970). Hypnosis, motivation, and the ecological validity of the psychological experiment. In W. J. Arnold & M. M. Page (Eds.), *Nebraska symposium on motivation* (Vol. 18, pp. 187–266). Lincoln: University of Nebraska Press.

Pajurkova, E. M., & Wilkins, A. J. (1983). *Prospective remembering in patients with unilateral temporal or frontal lobectomies.* Paper presented at a European conference of the International Neuropsychological Society, Lisbon.

Poon, L. W., & Schaffer, G. (1982). *Prospective memory in young and elderly adults.* Paper presented to the American Psychological Association, Washington, DC.

Reason, J. (1979). Actions not as planned: The price of automatization. In G. Underwood & R. Stevens (Eds.), *Aspects of consciousness: Vol. 1, Psychological issues* (pp. 67–90). New York: Academic Press.

Sinnot, J. D. (1981) The theory of relativity: A meta-theory for development? *Human Development, 24,* 293–311.

Sinnott, J. D. (1984a). *A model for the solution of illstructured problems: Implications for everyday and abstract problem solving.* Paper presented to the Gerontological Society, San Antonio, TX.

Sinnott, J. D. (1984b). Postformal reasoning: The relativistic stage. In M. Commons, F. Richards, & C. Armon (Eds.), *Beyond formal operations* (pp. 288–315). New York: Praeger.

Sinnott, J. D. (1984c). *Prospective/intentional and incidental everyday memory: Effects of age and passage of time.* Paper presented to the American Psychological Association, Toronto.

Sinnott, J. D. (1985). *General systems theory: A rationale for the study of everyday memory.* Presentation at Talland Conference, Cape Cod.

Sinnott, J. D. (1986a). Lifespan relativistic postformal thought: Methodology and data from everyday problem solving studies. In M. Commons, J. Sinnott, F. Richards, & C. Armon (Eds.), *Beyond formal operations. II: Comparisons and applications of adolescent and adult developmental models.* New York: Praeger.

Sinnott, J. D. (1986b). Prospective/intentional and incidental everyday memory: Effects of age and passage of time. *Psychology and Aging, 2,* 110–116.

Sweller, J. (1983). Control mechanisms in problem solving. *Memory and Cognition, 11,* 32–40.

Sweller, J., & Levine, M. (1982). The effects of goal specificity on means–end analysis and learning. *Memory and Cognition, 8,* 463–474.

Welford, A. T. (1958). *Aging and human skill.* London: Oxford University Press.

West, R. L. (1984). *An analysis of prospective everyday memory.* Paper presented to the American Psychological Association, Toronto.

Wilkins, A. J. (1976). *A failure to demonstrate the effects of "retention interval" in prospective memory.* Unpublished manuscript.

Wilkins, A. J., & Baddeley, A. D. (1978). Remembering to recall in everyday life: An approach to absent-mindedness. In M. M. Gruneberg, P. E. Morris, & R. N. Sykes (Eds.), *Practical aspects of memory* (pp. 27–34). New York: Academic Press.

Wolf, F. A. (1981). *Taking the quantum leap.* New York: Harper & Row.

Part IIB

Concomitant influences

21 Motivation and aging

Lawrence C. Perlmuter and Richard A. Monty

This literature review will examine the effects of motivation on mental activity in the aged. It will show that motivation significantly affects performance on a variety of tasks, but does not eliminate age-related cognitive deficits. The findings demonstrate that failure to consider the influence of motivation on performance in the aged can lead to an exaggeration of the magnitude of the deleterious effects of aging on cognitive functioning, and an increase in motivation can improve memory functioning in aged individuals, including those who are experiencing memory problems.

Statement of the problem

Historically, one of the major foci of experimental psychology was on variables associated with the phenomenon of learning. Because learning was differentiated from performance, an attempt was made to identify variables that affected performance versus those that affected learning. Specifically, it was recognized (Hull, 1943) that learning, defined as a relatively permanent change in behavioral potential, needed to be distinguished from performance, defined as the measurable expression of that which an organism had learned. Moreover, performance was not considered to be isomorphic with learning; rather, learning set an upper bound on performance. An organism could not display (perform) more than it had learned. On the other hand, an organism could and in most cases did perform at a lower level than that attained by learning.

Motivation was considered to be one of the primary variables that affected performance. Learning or, more precisely, habit strength [acquired stimulus–response (S–R) associations] entered into a multiplicative relationship with motivation or drive such that the levels of performance in a given organism at two

The preparation of this chapter was supported by grants from the National Institute on Aging (AG02300), the U.S. Army Human Engineering Laboratory, and the Veterans Administration Medical Services. Special thanks go to Kathleen Flannery for her helpful suggestions and to Janice Yates and Patti Russo for their assistance.

slightly different times likely would be measurably different. Thus, learning is the relatively permanent variable in the equation, whereas motivation is the relatively more labile variable, reflecting the immediate and changing needs of the organism.

There are several important, albeit subtle, features associated with the Hullian conception of behavior. First, in this system, motivation has no independent existence. It is strictly a conceptual term, defined operationally by antecedent conditions that can be experimenter-controlled. A variety of antecedent conditions have been shown to affect motivation, including anxiety, fear, and any number of physical or social needs. In short, any change that alters homeostasis may alter motivation. Second, motivation is a blind energizer of all habits. Third, as a conceptual term in a mechanistic system of behavior, motivation cannot be controlled by self-directed desires or wishes of the individual. Rather, it is a reflection of the needs or lacks within the internal or external environment of the individual. Because motivation is conditionable, such needs or lacks can be affected by learning.

The orientation of this chapter is generally compatible with the first and second features stated earlier. However, our conception will directly challenge the third feature and will attempt to show that the organism is capable of self-directed decision-making behaviors and that these, in turn, can augment motivation and improve performance significantly.

Although most contemporary laboratory-based theories that focus on age-related changes in performance have rejected Hullian-like theoretical formalism, they have also minimized the distinction between learning and performance and thus have found little justification for the motivation construct (Okun, 1980). In addition, the popularity of learning and memory models derived from computer "boxologies" may have further diminished any explicit theoretical concern with motivation. Because computers have all of their personal needs permanently satisfied a priori, provisions for a motivation concept in such models could be considered specious.

The failure to distinguish between learning and performance may be a significant problem for theorists investigating age-related changes in cognition. If it is assumed that age-related performance deficits isomorphically reflect corresponding declines in learning, ability, or competence, such conclusions may result in serious overestimation of the degree to which cognition changes with age. Moreover, if, as Prohaska, Parham, and Teitelman (1984) have shown, cognitive tests are more anxiety-provoking or even more demotivating to aged subjects than to young subjects, then age-related cognitive deficits may be overstated. Further, motivation levels may decrease with age. There is evidence that one recognized antecedent of motivation, namely, perceived control, may decline with increasing age, as well as with elevations in depression (Perlmuter, Monty, & Chan, 1986; Weisz, 1983). Finally, there is evidence (Berlyne, 1967; Kleinsmith & Kaplan, 1963) that motivation can affect many of the putative cognitive processes (e.g., consolidation, retrieval) that underlie performance on many of the tests that are used to assess age-related changes in performance.

Purpose of this chapter

Our approach to the study of motivation is guided by two objectives: concern with ecological validity and with minimizing reliance on self-report measures. We shall briefly review the effects of incentive motivation on performance in the aged. This review will show that motivational variables do not have a simple input-output effect on performance. Presumably, the effects of motivation on performance are conditioned in part by the nature of the task. This will be illustrated by an examination of the effects of incentives or rewards on performance in the aged. After that we shall examine another source of motivation, one that derives from allowing individuals to control some aspect of their environment.

Although theorizing about motivation has not been the exclusive domain of Hull, many of the competing theories share an important kinship with the Hullian approach. To review more thoroughly other approaches to motivation, the reader is invited to consult Elias and Elias (1977), McClelland (1985), and Nicholls (1979).

Up to this point, we have sought to justify the importance of motivation for a more complete understanding of behavior. We have described, in capsule form, some of the ways by which ignorance of motivation can lead not only to an overestimation of age-related changes in cognition but also to a confounding of the assessment of cognition because of uncontrolled differences between young and aged subjects. These contentions are not to suggest that learning and motivation are two distinct and independent noninteracting processes. Unfortunately, the situation is more complicated than that. Motivation is neither a chimera nor a process that can be wished away. Rather, as will be seen below, its effects on performance can be systematically manipulated and evaluated.

Antecedents of motivation

Rewards and incentives have traditionally been considered to affect motivation. The relationship between reward magnitude and motivation, however, cannot always be intuited. We shall examine the effects of reward on performance in a learning situation. We shall also examine other less traditional sources of motivation, namely, the effects of choice and control on motivation. When individuals are enabled to personalize a task, either by learning materials that they themselves have generated or by making certain choices over the task, it is likely that motivation will increase. These issues will be examined in young and aged learners. The relationship of motivation to performance has both theoretical significance and practical significance in understanding how performance changes with advancing age and how such changes can be remediated.

Effects of rewards on performance

The experimental literature has shown that motivational levels can be altered in a variety of ways. One of these is by the use of extrinsic rewards (e.g., money for good performance), and another is by manipulating intrinsic factors, such as making a task more interesting, relevant, or personalized. If an age-related decrement in performance is merely the result of low motivation, rewards should enhance performance relative to a no-reward group of young subjects. In describing such a hypothetical study, it must be stated at the outset that it is neither our assumption nor our purpose to explain away age-related decrements as mere reflections of lowered motivation. Rather, our purpose is to show that motivation, if effectively manipulated, is an important variable that influences performance in young and aged subjects and should not be ignored as a potential source of variance in the investigation of performance across the life span.

In one such study, Grant, Storandt, and Botwinick (1978) rewarded subjects monetarily for showing improvement on a digit-symbol task relative to a previously established no-reward level. Rewards improved performance very slightly and thus clearly failed to eliminate differences between young and aged subjects.

Hartley and Walsh (1980) employed a single-trial free-recall task in which subjects received either 0, 5, or 50 cents for correct recall. Although reward did improve performance for young and old, these effects were apparent only during the first minute of the 3-min report period, and the greatest effect was observed for the 5-cent reward. More important, age did not interact with incentive, thus leading the authors to conclude that age-related deficits in performance were not attributable to motivational factors.

The overall results of that experiment lead one to question that it provided an adequate test of the motivation hypothesis. First, because primary memory was not expected to vary for the two age groups, it is curious that the largest age effects were seen in recall within the initial 15 sec of the 3-min report period. When recall was examined after 30 sec, young and aged performed similarly. Despite these somewhat atypical findings, Hartley and Walsh (1980) stated that "motivational factors, such as task involvement contribute little to age-related differences in memory performance across the life span" (p. 905), and they went on to conclude that "motivational *differences* are not an *important [sic]* factor in the causal equation which provides large age-related differences in performance on laboratory memory tasks."

Manipulation of incentives may fail to provide an effective test of the relationship between motivation and performance. An increase in reward magnitude may not ineluctably enhance motivation in rats or humans; see Kruglanski (1975) and Lepper and Greene (1978) for a discussion of these matters. Moreover, such manipulations can reduce intrinsic motivation associated with task performance. This latter relationship can be understood if the individual is viewed as an active rather than a passive participant in a learning situation, because the attributions that are made in response to a reward are likely to mediate its effects on behavior.

Consistent with the notion of the active organism are the data to be discussed in a subsequent section of this chapter that will show how motivation can be augmented by increasing the individual's level of engagement in the task, even in the absence of extrinsic rewards.

Previous research has shown that monetary incentives are limited in their beneficial effects on behavior (Nelson, 1976). Because Hartley and Walsh (1980) discussed Nelson's findings, it is not clear why they expected that monetary rewards would be effective in aged subjects. More direct evidence for the effects of motivation needs to be made available before concluding that motivation does or does not reduce the gap in performance between young and aged subjects.

Adapting the task to the learner

A study by Wittels (1972) examined the hypothesis that age-related declines in performance may be secondary to the fact that laboratory stimuli often are generation-bound (age-bound) and thus may differ in meaningfulness for different age groups. Wittels attempted to control for possible intergenerational differences by controlling the meaningfulness of the response words to be learned by young and old subjects on a paired-associates task. The experimental conditions relevant to the present discussion are those in which subjects were instructed to generate a set of 10 response words to each stimulus. The fifth word in each set served as the response to the respective stimuli in a subsequent paired-associate task. Presumably, such a procedure allowed subjects an opportunity to learn their own words, thus minimizing task-related intergenerational bias between young and old. The opportunity to learn self-generated words had no beneficial effects on error scores or trials to criterion in either young or aged subjects. In other words, there was no evidence to support the hypothesis that age differences in learning are mitigated by using materials that are designed to eliminate intergenerational bias.

Slamecka and Graf (1978) utilized a procedure similar to that of Wittels, with one major exception. Each subject was presented with a stimulus word and was required to generate a *single* response word to it. A comparison group simply read the identical S–R pairs. Cued recall was higher in the "generate" condition than in the "read" condition, a result that is discrepant with that of Wittels. Apparently, the generation procedure is effective for the first or initially generated response. Thus, Wittels's procedure may have been ineffective in adequately personalizing the task, because her subjects learned not the first response but rather the fifth response in the set of 10 responses.

A recent study (McFarland, Warren, & Crockard, 1985) with aged learners replicated the procedure and results of Slamecka and Graf, thus providing additional support for the conclusion that performance can be improved in the aged by increasing the subjects' active participation in the learning task. It is also likely that the generation procedure personalizes the task and in turn increases motivation.

Personalization of tasks

Allowing subjects to make choices relevant to the specific task may provide an effective procedure for personalizing a task. Presumably, as the task becomes more personalized, the subject's involvement in the task increases, and this in turn may increase motivation. The rationale for this approach to motivation is based on the assumption that the personalization of a task implicitly increases its resemblance to relatively pleasant tasks that individuals may perform routinely. For example, when offered a choice of materials to be learned in the laboratory, this procedure may, to some extent, resemble the opportunity for choice and control that individuals enjoy and appreciate in more positive settings, such as ordering from a restaurant menu. To some extent, the laboratory procedure and the restaurant experience are in some sense self-initiated and self-directed. As individuals come to perceive the self-directed features of their behavior, there should be an accompanying increase in the perception of control.

It is assumed that when an individual is able to make a conscious and meaningful choice, there is an increment in the perception of control over the environment that, as will be seen later, has motivational properties that facilitate performance. However, not all choices are conscious and meaningful, and thus not all choices increase motivation (Savage, Perlmuter, & Monty, 1979). Moreover, especially when the performances of young and aged are compared, an abundance of research shows that certain environments in which the infirm or the aged may be living serve to diminish opportunities for choice, thereby attenuating motivation and the perception of control (Langer & Rodin, 1976). Parenthetically, it has been observed that mere beliefs about control can enhance morale in the institutionalized aged (Sellers, 1986) and that very simple adjustments within these environments may be sufficient to enhance control; morbidity decreases, and life itself may be prolonged (Langer, 1979).

A reading of Hartley and Walsh's study (1980) and Wittels's study (1972) provides little justification for continuing to investigate the possible contribution of motivation to age-related declines in performance. However, we believe that the study of motivation should not be put to rest based on these moot findings. Throughout much of the remainder of this chapter we shall examine performance on tasks that have been personalized, and we shall attempt to show that such procedures do heighten motivation and enhance performance in young and aged learners.

In a paired-associate experiment, aged subjects were presented with an opportunity to choose words to be learned in response to the stimulus words (Fleming & Lopez, 1981). In the "choice" condition, each stimulus word was accompanied by three response words, and subjects selected one of these to be learned. In the "force" condition, subjects were assigned response words to be learned. Subjects who chose learned significantly more S–R pairs across the six trials than did the force subjects (Figure 21.1). Fleming and Lopez attributed these findings to an increased perception of control over the task as a consequence of choice. Pre-

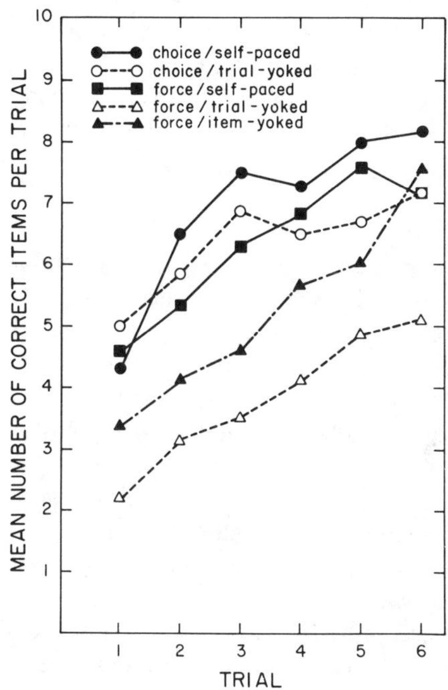

Figure 21.1. Mean number of correct items per trial for choice and force groups. (Adapted from Fleming & Lopez, 1981; copyright Beech Hill Enterprises, Inc., 1981.)

sumably, an increase in the perception of control enhanced motivation, which in turn was reflected in significant improvement in performance.

The study by Fleming and Lopez (1981) provides important methodological and theoretical contributions to an understanding of the effect of motivation on performance. However, manipulation of a motivational variable does not guarantee that it will measurably affect performance. In Wittels's study (1972) and in that of Fleming and Lopez, when subjects learned their own personally selected words, this manipulation was effective only if subjects were provided with an opportunity to make direct or concise choices. Wittels's procedure requiring successive decisions may have attenuated the salience of perceived control. Consistent with this explanation, McFarland and associates (1985) found positive effects following a single decision. Moreover, previous research had shown that the act of choosing per se was not sufficient to increase the perception of control (Monty, Geller, Savage, & Perlmuter, 1979). In order for choice to enhance performance, the alternatives (word pairs) from which the selections are made must be similar. A choice between a word of high meaningfulness (e.g., river) and a word of low meaningfulness (e.g., zobel) results in nearly unanimous selection of the word "river," but more important, it fails to provide the subject with a meaningful or autonomous opportunity for choice. Hence, such restricted choices do not benefit performance.

When motivational effects are evaluated in either young or aged subjects, ample consideration is required to assure that motivation has been manipulated effectively. Although the conditions that will foster an increase in motivation may sometimes be elusive, once it has been manipulated effectively, its consequences are sufficiently robust to improve performance even on a task such as paired-associate learning that by most aesthetic or ecological-validity criteria would not rank high.

Because Fleming and Lopez (1981) did not examine the effects of choice developmentally, it was not possible to determine the extent to which choice was effective in minimizing age-related declines in performance. Currently, we are aware of no studies that have addressed this important issue. However, the results from a recent paired-associate learning experiment showed that when young and aged subjects learned materials of their own choosing, age-related decrements persisted (Perlmuter et al., 1986). The authors did not include data for subjects who were denied an opportunity to choose. Hence, it cannot be determined to what extent motivation per se might have diminished the performance gap between young and old. Such an evaluation would require a complete factorial design (age and choice), with one of the major tests involving a comparison between aged subjects who learned words of their own choosing and young subjects who learned either identical or comparable words in the absence of choice. This comparison would determine the extent to which age-related performance deficits can be eliminated by enhancing motivation. Other analyses might involve comparisons between young and aged subjects that would index the extent to which motivation is effective within age groupings. Despite the absence of this information, there are self-report data from their experiment that bear on this question. That is, even when provided with an opportunity for choice, aged subjects reported significantly lower levels of choice or of freedom to choose than did young subjects. Thus, extrapolating from the self-report data, it may be surmised that the opportunity for choice will be expected to diminish, but not eliminate, age-related performance decrements.

The motivational effects of choice have been observed even for subjects who have sought clinical assistance for problems of memory. In a paired-associate study by Perlmuter and Smith (1979), subjects ranged in age from 60 to 75 years. Each of the 12 stimulus words was accompanied by five potential response words, and subjects were permitted to choose one response word within a 10-sec period. A matched group of force subjects was exposed to the identical materials, but was required to learn one response based on a choice-force yoking procedure. The results (top panel of Figure 21.2) essentially replicated those of Fleming and Lopez (1981) and showed that the choice subjects learned significantly more words than did the force subjects, and they tended ($p > .05$) (bottom panel of Figure 21.2) to make fewer errors of intrusion (misplaced responses) than did the force subjects. In fact, the percentage of correct responses and the percentage of intrusions in the force condition were similar. Thus, the opportunity to choose affects motivation in aged subjects, even those seeking assistance for problems with everyday memory.

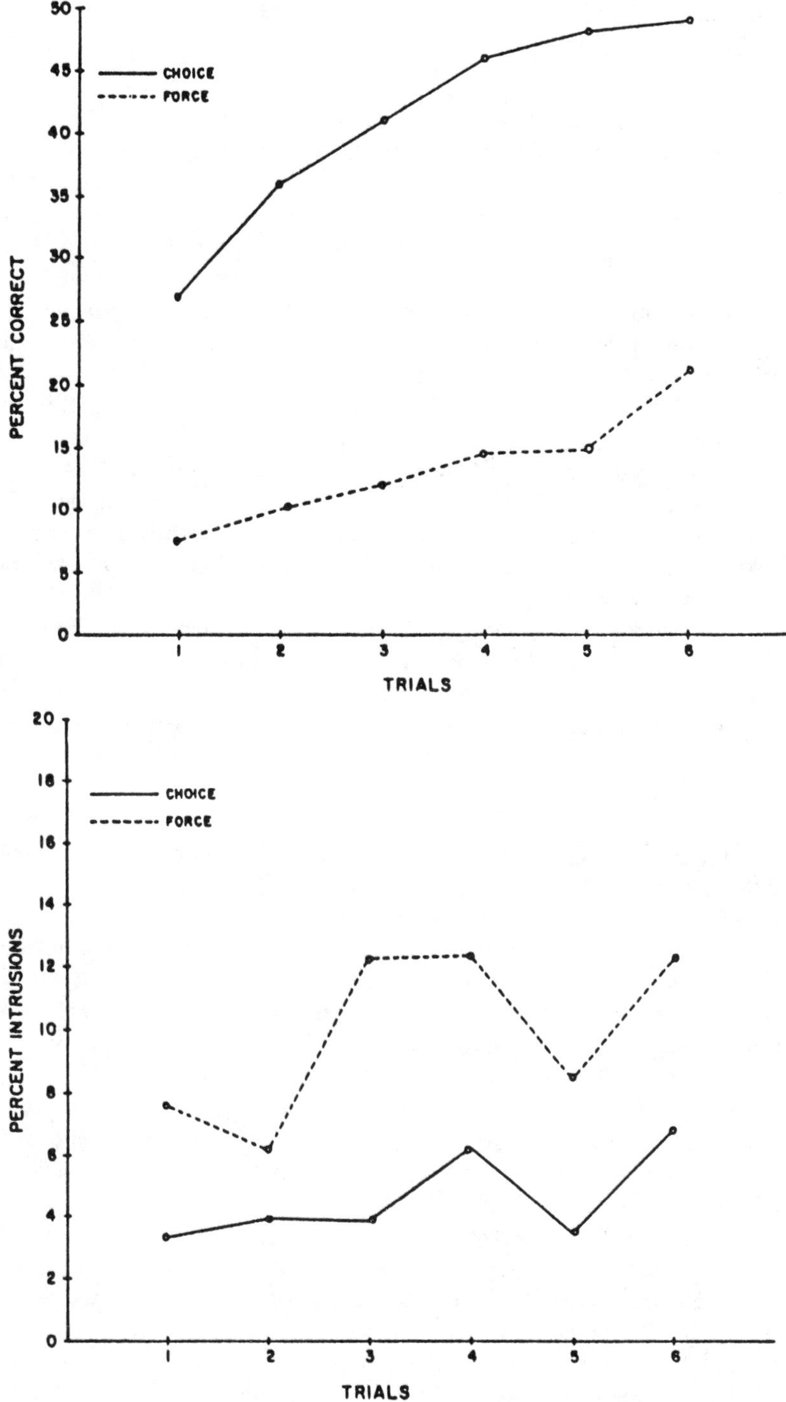

Figure 21.2. Mean percentage correct and mean percentage intrusions for choice and force groups. (Adapted from Perlmuter & Smith, 1979.)

Generalized effects of choice

To this point, the results show that providing subjects with an opportunity to choose can have beneficial effects on performance. One possible explanation for these results is that in the choice condition, performance improved as a result of the learning of self-selected words that may have had idiosyncratic associations – an advantage denied to the force subjects. A second and more plausible explanation for the effects of choice is that when an individual is provided with an opportunity to make choices, there is an increase in the perception of control that in turn affects motivation. We shall examine these alternative hypotheses.

To test the robustness of these competing hypotheses, we initially employed a paradigm that bore little resemblance to the paired-associate paradigm from which they were derived. A reading-comprehension study with 7–8-year-old subjects was conducted by White, as reported by Perlmuter and Monty (1977). Subjects were informed that they would be reading a series of short stories and would have to answer questions about these. In the Early Choice condition, subjects were presented with informative titles describing each of three stories and asked to choose one of these for subsequent reading and testing. They were next presented with three other titles, but in this instance were informed of the story that they would be required to read (i.e., in the absence of choice). This latter procedure occurred twice more. The first story that subjects read and answered questions about was drawn from the final series and was one over which no choice had been permitted.

A second group of subjects (Force group) was exposed to a set of three titles as was the previously described group, but the Force group was assigned one of these. This procedure was repeated again and again until four stories had been assigned. This group was then tested on one story from the final assignment.

When performances for these two groups were compared on the initial test, the Early Choice group answered significantly more questions correctly than did the Force group. Both groups read the identical (assigned) story on this test. Of central importance in this comparison is that both groups were performing a task over which they had no choice. What distinguished these groups is that the Early Choice group had been permitted to make a choice at the start of the task, and on this basis they may have developed a perception of control that increased motivation and in turn generalized to portions of the task over which no choice was permitted. In this way, the explanatory role of idiosyncratic factors was eliminated.

The motivational effects of choice were similarly evaluated in a paired-associate task with college-age subjects (Monty, Rosenberger, & Perlmuter, 1973). Subjects were presented with a series of 12 stimulus words, each accompanied by five potential response words. The Early Choice group selected responses to the first three stimulus words, and the Late Choice group selected responses to the final three response words. For both groups, the majority of S–R pairs were experimenter-selected. A 100% Choice group selected response words

Table 21.1. *Mean number of correct responses on the first trial of a 12-item S–R pair test (N = 20 in each group)*

Group	Mean number correct
100% Choice	4.80
Early Choice	4.75
Late Choice	2.90
Force	3.40

Source: Adapted from Monty et al. (1973).

to each of the stimuli, and a Force group selected response words to none of the stimuli. The Early Choice group and the 100% Choice group performed similarly. More important, these groups learned significantly more words across trials than did either the Late Choice or Force group, and the latter two groups did not differ from each other (Table 21.1).

It is apparent that choice enhances performance even when limited to a selection of only 25% of the materials. Apparently, choice must occur early in the task in order to enable the subject to perceive control. Choice in the concluding segment of the task failed to establish such a perception of control. Thus, the effects of choice were generalizable within the same overall task. But are they motivational, and do they affect performance on tasks other than the choice?

To attempt to answer these questions, one group of subjects (Choice) was permitted to choose response words to be learned on a paired-associate task, and another group (Force) was exposed to these materials and assigned response words (Perlmuter, Scharff, Karsh, & Monty, 1980). The paired-associate task used an anticipation procedure in which the stimulus was presented on a screen, and the subject anticipated the appropriate response word, as was done in the previously described experiment (Monty et al., 1973). The next slide to appear in the series contained the S–R pair.

The novel feature of the procedure involved the introduction of an unanticipated reaction-time task concurrent with the start of the paired-associate task. Following the conclusion of the choice/force procedure, subjects were instructed to hold an index finger on a key and to lift it and strike a second key as soon as possible each time a tone was sounded. The tone was sounded without warning, and this occurred only during the presentation of the S–R pair, thus not competing with the vocalization of the anticipated response word.

As expected, Choice subjects learned their S–R pairs significantly better than did Force subjects. Of more importance, reaction times were significantly faster for Choice subjects than for Force subjects, an outcome consistent with a motivational interpretation of choice (Figure 21.3).

A second experiment with college-age participants, comparable to the first, was conducted in order to evaluate performance on the reaction-time task inde-

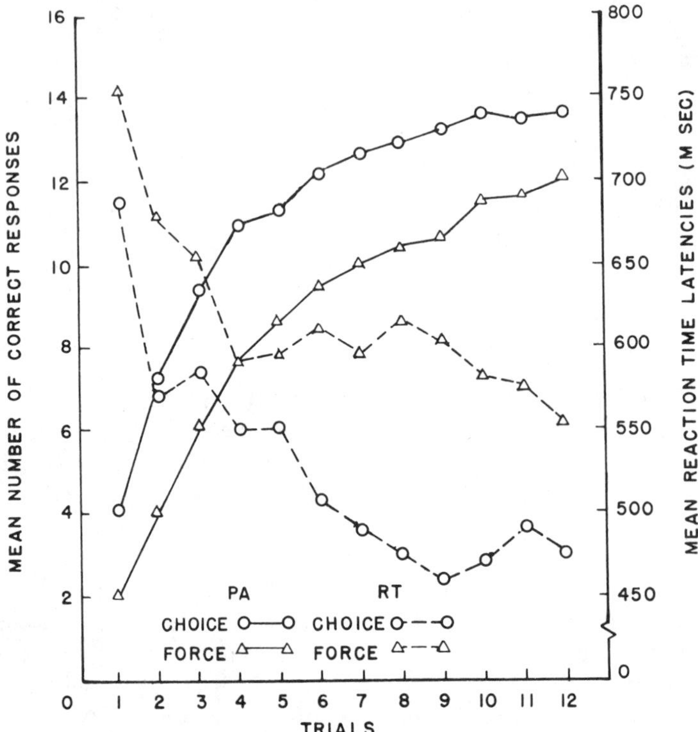

Figure 21.3. Mean number of correct responses on the paired-associate task (left ordinate) and mean reaction-time latencies (right ordinate) for the choice and force groups. (Adapted from Perlmuter et al., 1980; copyright Plenum Publishing Corporation, 1980.)

pendent of paired-associate learning. As described in the previous experiment, one group chose their response words, but words for a second group were assigned. On completion of the choice/force procedure, both groups were informed that prior to learning the S–R pairs, a reaction-time task was to be performed. The Choice subjects reacted significantly faster than did the Force subjects (Figure 21.4), a result similar to that reported previously.

These findings indicated that the effects of choice generalized to an (unanticipated) task over which no choice had been permitted. More important, they showed that the opportunity to make choices energized behavior and resulted in increased speed of behavior. Such findings are in harmony with a generalized-motivation hypothesis (Hull, 1943). Obviously, the idiosyncratic hypothesis is mute with respect to the effects of choice on reaction time.

Effects of choice on memory performance in the aged

There is some evidence (Kausler & Kleim, 1978) that the aged may be relatively more susceptible to interference from background cues than are the

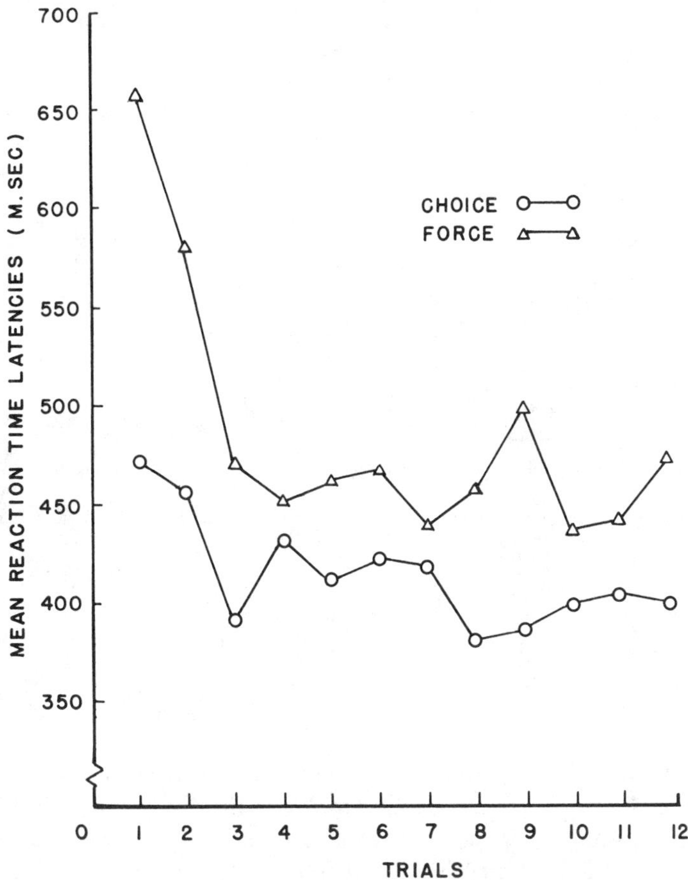

Figure 21.4. Mean reaction-time latencies for the choice and froce groups. (Adapted from Perlmuter et al., 1980; copyright Plenum Publishing Corporation, 1980.)

young. Perlmuter and associates (unpublished data) adapted a paradigm used by Kausler and Kleim to determine if choice would attenuate background interference. Background cues consisted of words that were presented along with to-be-learned target words. No instructions were provided to the subjects about the specific role of the background words. Aged subjects were presented with a page of 24 lines of words. Half of the lines contained two words, and the remainder contained four. The short and long lines were randomly positioned on the page. The words were composed of five letters and were of moderate meaningfulness levels. On half of the lines, subjects selected a target to be learned, and on the remainder, targets were assigned. Thus, subjects chose six targets (one from each of the two-word lines) and then six more targets (one from each of the four-word lines). The remaining 12 target words to be learned were assigned by the experimenter.

Table 21.2. *Mean number of correct discriminations as a function of condition and number of words*

	Words per line	
Condition	2	4
Choice	5.33	5.33
Force	3.67	4.42

Table 21.3. *Mean proportion correct: recognition test*

	Choice condition		Force condition	
Words per line	Target	Background	Target	Background
2	.79	.64	.81	.46
4	.94	.46	.65	.30

Following the choice/force procedure, there was a 15-min break. Next, a discrimination test was presented in which the lines were haphazardly rearranged on the page, and the positions of the words within the lines were also reordered. The results, shown in Table 21.2, indicated that discrimination performance was significantly higher on choice lines than on force lines. With corrections for guessing, no effects of line length were observed.

A free-recall task was presented next, and again significantly more targets from choice lines than from force lines were recalled. There was a tendency for higher recall on four-word choice lines than on two-word choice lines, whereas on the force lines this effect was not seen; however, the interaction was not significant.

In a second experiment with aged subjects, the procedure was nearly identical with that just described. The novel feature of this experiment was the unanticipated introduction of a recognition task in which the 72 old words (target and background) were presented along with an equal number of new distractors. The words on the recognition test were presented individually. Table 21.3 presents a breakdown of the significant interaction of Choice/Force × Target/Background × Words Per Line. The effect of choice on target learning was limited to long lines (four words per line), but more important, choice significantly facilitated background recognition. Further, it appears that the adverse effects of the number of background words on targets are limited to the force lines.

Thus, the within-subject manipulation of the choice variable indicated that its effects were specific to the lines on which choice occurred. This is not to gainsay the possibility that there may have been some generalized effects of choice as well. However, the most important aspect of these results is in showing that choice enabled subjects to extract more information from the task than did the force condition, because both background and target recognitions were significantly benefited by choice. Presumably, choice improves performance by providing an increase in processing resources (via motivation), thereby enabling subjects to learn intentional as well as incidental cues more effectively. Such an outcome is of theoretical as well as practical importance, because it has been found (Farkas & Hoyer, 1980) that the aged often are more susceptible to the adverse effects of background or contextual cues.

In summary, although these experiments were not designed to show the extent to which the effects of choice and perceived control would change with advancing age, they do show that choice can be effective through eight decades of life. Presumably, choice increases the perception of control, and this in turn enhances motivation. Such effects have been observed with a variety of experimental paradigms ranging from simple reaction time to reading comprehension. Moreover, this procedure was effective even for aged subjects who presented with memory problems.

The effects of choice are labile and robust. That is, once the perception of control has been established, its effects generalize across portions of tasks and even to new tasks. On the other hand, the perception of control cannot be established by fiat. Whereas choice that is permitted at the inception of a task significantly improves performance on portions of a task over which no choice had been permitted, choice that is limited to the concluding portion of the task appears to have little, if any, beneficial effect on performance.

Enhancing perceived control in natural settings

Routine behaviors can be exploited to enhance the perception of control (Perlmuter & Langer, 1982). Once an individual has consented to perform a laboratory task (e.g., paired-associate learning), it is relatively easy to provide an opportunity for choice. Although the laboratory task presents an unfamiliar paradigm to the naive subject, the opportunity for choice has meaningful features that render it a potentially effective intervention for manipulating motivation.

Extrapolation of the effects of perceived control to the everyday world is hindered by the subjective nature of control. Moreover, to inform individuals that they have been granted control over some routinely performed behavior (e.g., selecting an item of clothing), as if by fiat, fails to constitute an effective transfer of control. The arbitrary award of control by a benevolent agent underlines its provisional nature. On the other hand, individuals may come to perceive control primarily through feedback intrinsic to their own behavior (Chan, Karbowski, Monty, & Perlmuter, 1986). That is, individuals may be vigilant to their behavior and may derive an increased perception of control from it to the extent that the behavior is perceived to have controlling features. The preliminary results of an experiment that encourages individuals to monitor their own behavior will be examined.

Attention to routine behavior and perceived control

Repeatedly performed behaviors often grow automatic (Kimble & Perlmuter, 1970) or mindless (Langer, 1975). Thus, even though an individual apparently elects or chooses to perform a particular behavior, there is no guarantee that such a chosen action will inevitably be performed in a mindful or intentional fashion. A number of actions, many of which are performed daily, appear to be self-initiated, but are nevertheless performed without the sense of a willful choice. Moreover, even overt decisions appear to grow automatic. Examples of mindlessly chosen decision sequences include the following: tying one's left or right shoelace first; shaving the left or right side of the face first; brushing upper teeth or lower teeth first.

Presumably, it is likely that a chosen behavior increases the perception of control or a sense of competence, in White's terminology (1959), only when such an act is performed as a willful and chosen act. Thus, an attempt was made to "deautomatize" certain daily routine behaviors in order to determine if such an intervention would enable the individual to gain a restored perception of control over actions that most recently had been performed automatically (Perlmuter & Langer, 1982).

Aged subjects were recruited from a day-treatment program. One group was asked to monitor one behavior each day for 2 weeks. Specifically, they were asked to respond to the following questions: What was your first beverage of the day? How much did you drink? Did you enjoy it? A second group was asked to monitor a different behavior on each of 7 days and then to repeat the cycle in week 2. For example: What snack did you choose in the evening? How much did you consume? Did you enjoy it? On another day, the questions were these: What was your first beverage of the day? How much did you drink? Did you enjoy it? And so forth. The third group was asked the same questions as those used in the second group, but in a critically different way. For example: What was your first beverage of the day? What other beverages might you have chosen but did not? They were then asked to list three nonchosen alternatives.

Following completion of the 2 weeks of monitoring, all subjects were presented with a series of eight questions about the amount of control they had over their lives, whether or not they would be willing to participate in future research, and so forth. The questions were answerable with a four-category qualitative scale, ranging from "a little" to "a lot." Owing to the small sample sizes, no statistical treatments were carried out, but the results were very consistent and showed that on each of the questions, the third group had higher (more positive) scores than did the second group, which in turn had more positive scores than did the first group.

These results were consistent with our predictions. That is, when subjects repeatedly monitored the same behavior each day, initially this activity may have appeared novel and attention-demanding. However, within the 2-week period of the study, repetition may have facilitated automaticity. To informally assess the subjects' perceptions of these tasks, we interviewed them following the completion of the study. Subjects in the "repeat" monitoring condition indicated that they grew bored with the task. It may be conjectured that what was boring was not the task but rather the fact that without exception the first beverage of the day for any one subject did not change during the 2-week period. Orange juice drinkers drank it daily; water consumers, the same. The participants had, through automaticity, relinquished the opportunity for choice and hence control.

By comparison, for the "varied" monitoring group, their choices may have become more salient during the course of the study, because they monitored a different selection each day. The "rejection" group was, as expected, the one for whom choice became most salient, because on each day these individuals not only monitored that which was chosen but also were forced to consider alternatives that presumably had not been considered recently or that they had implicitly rejected.

The process of rejection may be more important than selection in constituting an autonomous choice. When presented with qualitatively dissimilar alternatives, the benefits of choice are nil (Monty et al., 1979). For example, in choosing between a sterling pen and a gold-plated pen, a subject may select the latter. In another scenario with a wooden pencil and a gold-plated pen, the latter is likely to be chosen. The motivational consequences to the chooser of these selections will be markedly different, despite the selection of the identical object in each scenario. Apparently, the motivating effects of a choice are more affected by certain features of the rejected alternative than by that which has been selected. In other words, for choice to be motivating, the rejection process apparently must receive consideration. In the monitoring experiment, the rejection condition actively confronted the subjects with alternatives to that which had been chosen, leading to the highest perception of control. Behavioral monitoring, when effective, transforms choice from an automatic to a mindful behavior, from which subjects can learn that they have control.

The clinical potential of these techniques is now being evaluated with aged subjects who have problems with memory. Participants performing such exercises indicate that they have become increasingly aware of their environment. In some cases they even report pleasant surprise at discovering cues in their environment that they had not observed previously.

Changes in self-narrative description with age

In this study (Perlmuter & Langer, unpublished data), a group of community-dwelling aged subjects living in a semirural college town were examined along with college-age subjects. The subject's task was to report, in as great detail as possible, everything about four different time periods: today, yesterday, the last Fourth of July, and a week from Sunday. Subjects spoke about their activities within these time periods, and their speech was recorded by a tape recorder that was placed out of view. All subjects were told that their speech was being recorded and completed an informed-consent form explicitly describing the procedure. As subjects completed each of their reports, the experimenter prompted them for more information.

The reports were examined for a number of characteristics (e.g., amount of detail, references to time, use of the personal pronoun "I"). Elderly subjects, relative to the young, provided significantly less detail in recounting the last Fourth of July and today's activities. With respect to yesterday and the future, no differences were found between age groups.

The elderly used the pronoun "I" significantly more frequently than did the young with respect to today, but for other time periods there were no differences between groups. More important, for the aged, the frequency of "I" declined significantly when the future period was compared with the present. No comparable change was found for the young. At this point, we can only conjecture that for the aged, the decline in the use of "I" may reflect a lesser sense of personal control or involvement in the future. The next study to be described examined how forced usage of the personal pronoun affected perceptions of the future.

Aged subjects participating in a day-treatment program read a short story detailing plausible activities that might be engaged in at the start of an ordinary day. Prior to reading the page, all subjects personalized it by completing a blank that made it appear as if the story were about themselves. As they read through the story, they came upon an intermittent number of blanks. The blanks preceded simple action verbs; when filled in by the subject, the result was a completed sentence such as "I drank the orange juice" or "He/She drank the orange juice." One group was instructed to write "I" in the blank spaces, whereas for another group, the blanks were to be completed by "He" or"She," depending on the subject's gender. There were 13 blanks.

Following this exercise, all subjects received an unanticipated recognition test in which key words from the story were presented, along with an equal number of filler words [e.g., orange juice (old) or cranberry juice (new)]. Unfortunately, recognition performance was uniformly high, and the I versus He/She manipulation could not be assessed.

Following the recognition task, subjects responded to a series of questions, one of which related to their willingness to participate in future experiments. Another question dealt with their willingness to lead a discussion group concerned with problems of the aged. The remainder of the questions were oriented toward past or present personal issues, such as perceived health, control, and so forth. All questions were answerable by a four-category qualitative scale. The results indicated that on all questions dealing with the past or present, the two groups performed similarly. This lack of a difference is important in interpreting the significant differences that were found for the future-oriented questions. That is, the I versus He/She manipulation did not indiscriminately increase optimism about events over which no control was possible, such as past events or current health status. Rather, this manipulation may have selectively increased optimism and hope for the future. On the question related to possible leadership of a to-be-formed senior-citizen group, there was signficantly more positiveness in the "I" condition than in the "He/She" condition. Similarly, in response to a question about willingness to participate in a to-be-scheduled psychology experiment, the "I" condition was significantly more positive.

Apparently, older subjects are likely to be somewhat less optimistic about participation in and control over future events. Simple and direct manipulations, as described earlier, appear to reverse these tendencies.

In summary, behaviors appear to grow automatic with repetition. For aged individuals, dwelling in staid environments, a large number of behaviors, perhaps the majority, may be considered automatic. Although automatically performed behaviors are likely to be performed effectively, proficiently, and with an economy of energy and attention, at the same time automaticity deprives the individual of a sense of control and competence that can be derived from behavior.

Apparently, the perception of control can be increased by requiring subjects to monitor even one routine behavior each day. Monitoring may interfere with automaticity. The most effective monitoring procedure is one that informs the subject of the availability of alternatives or choices. When behaviors are transformed into intentional actions, individuals have an opportunity to derive a sense of competence and control from performance.

Conclusions

Although it is acknowledged that performance derives from the combination of ability and motivation, relatively little attention has been devoted to quantifying the relative contribution of each of these factors to age-related changes in performance. Aged individuals may approach cognitive tasks with less motivation than young subjects. Moreover, to old subjects, such tasks may be anxiety-provoking and even demotivating.

Most textbooks and theories of cognitive aging have ignored the construct of motivation for a variety of reasons. The popularity of computer-driven metaphors for cognitive processes, the intangible quality of motivation, and the fact that, historically, motivation in adults was studied by manipulating rewards and was found to have little effect on cognitive performance – all these factors contributed to its current moribund state.

An alternative to the extrinsic (via rewards) approach to motivation is one in which the perception of control is enhanced by allowing individuals to make choices or to perceive choices in the performance of their routine behaviors. Effecting a change in individuals' beliefs about the perception of control is motivating to young and old. It is not known, however, to what extent motivation changes with age nor to what extent age-related changes in cognitive performance are the consequences of changes in motivation versus ability. Work is under way to answer these questions.

In this chapter we have shown that the perception of control can be increased even under sterile laboratory conditions, and its effects on performance can be thoroughly quantified. Moreover, similiar manipulations can be used to increase the perception of control and motivation in natural settings as well. Whether the purpose is to chart age-related changes in cognitive performance or to improve the quality of life in the aged, it is difficult to accomplish either of these objectives without attention to motivation.

References

Berlyne, D. E. (1967). Arousal and reinforcement. In D. Levine (Ed.), *Nebraska symposium on motivation.* Lincoln: University of Nebraska Press.

Chan, F., Karbowski, J., Monty, R. A., & Perlmuter, L. C. (1986). Performance as a source of perceived control. *Motivation and Emotion, 10,* 59–70.

Elias, M. F., & Elias, P. K. (1977). Motivation and activity. In J. E. Birren & K. W. Schaie (Eds.), *Handbook of the psychology of aging* (pp. 357–383). New York: Van Nostrand Reinhold.

Farkas, M. S., & Hoyer, W. J. (1980). Processing consequences of perceptual grouping in selective attention. *Journal of Gerontology, 35,* 207–216.

Fleming, C. C., & Lopez, M. A. (1981). The effects of perceived control on the paired-associate learning of elderly persons. *Experimental Aging Research, 1,* 71–77.

Grant, E. A., Storandt, M., & Botwinick, J. (1978). Incentive and practice in the psychomotor performance of the elderly. *Journal of Gerontology, 33,* 413–415.

Hartley, J. T., & Walsh, D. A. (1980). The effect of monetary incentive on amount and rate of free recall in older and younger adults. *Journal of Gerontology, 35,* 899–905.

Hull, C. L. (1943). *Principles of behavior.* New York: Appleton-Century-Crofts.

Kausler, D. H., & Kleim, D. M. (1978). Age differences in processing relevant versus irrelevant stimuli in multiple-item recognition learning. *Journal of Gerontology, 33,* 87–93.

Kimble, G. A., & Perlmuter, L. C. (1970). The problem of volition. *Psychological Review, 77,* 361–384.

Kleinsmith, L. J., & Kaplan, S. (1963). Paired-associate learning as a function of arousal and interpolated interval. *Journal of Experimental Psychology, 65,* 190–193.

Kruglanski, A. W. (1975). The endogenous–exogenous partition in attribution theory. *Psychological Review, 82,* 387–406.

Langer, E. J. (1975). The illusion of control. *Journal of Personality and Social Psychology, 32,* 311–328.

Langer, E. J. (1979). The illusion of incompetence. In L. C. Perlmuter & R. A. Monty (Eds.), *Choice and perceived control* (pp. 301–314). Hillsdale, NJ: Lawrence Erlbaum.

Langer, E. J., & Rodin, J. (1976). The effects of choice and enhanced personal responsibility for the aged: A field experiment in an institutional setting. *Journal of Personality and Social Psychology, 34,* 191–198.

Lepper, M. R., & Greene, D. (1978). Overjustification research and beyond: Toward a means–end analysis of intrinsic and extrinsic motivation. In M. R. Lepper and D. Greene (Eds.), *The hidden costs of reward: New perspectives on the psychology of human motivation.* Hillsdale, NJ: Lawrence Erlbaum.

McClelland, D. C. (1985). How motives, skills and values determine what people do. *American Psychologist, 40,* 812–825.

McFarland, C. E., Warren, L. R., & Crockard, J. (1985). Memory for self-generated stimuli in young and old adults. *Journal of Gerontology, 40,* 205–207.

Monty, R. A., Geller, E. S., Savage, R. E., & Perlmuter, L. C. (1979). The freedom to choose is not always so choice. *Journal of Experimental Psychology: Human Learning and Memory, 5,* 170–178.

Monty, R. A., Rosenberger, M. A., & Perlmuter, L. C. (1973). Amount and locus of choice as sources of motivation in paired-associate learning. *Journal of Experimental Psychology, 97,* 16–21.

Nelson, T. O. (1976). Reinforcement and human memory. In W. K. Estes (Ed.), *Handbook of learning and cognitive processes* (Vol. 3). Hillsdale, NJ: Lawrence Erlbaum.

Nicholls, J. G. (1979). Quality and equality in intellectual development: The role of motivation in education. *American Psychologist, 34,* 1071–1084.

Okun, M. A. (1980). The role of noncognitive factors in the cognitive performance of older adults. *Contemporary Educational Psychology, 5,* 321–345.

Perlmuter, L. C., & Langer, E. J. (1982). The effects of behavioral monitoring on the perception of control. *Clinical Gerontologist, 1,* 37–43.

Perlmuter, L. C., & Monty, R. A. (1977). The importance of perceived control: Fact or fantasy? *American Scientist, 65,* 759–765.

Perlmuter, L. C., Monty, R. A., & Chan, F. (1986). Learning, choice, and control. In M. M. Baltes & P. B. Baltes (Eds.), *Aging and control.* Hillsdale, NJ: Lawrence Erlbaum.

Perlmuter, L. C., Scharff, K., Karsh, R., & Monty, R. A. (1980). Perceived control: A generalized state of motivation. *Motivation and Emotion, 4,* 35–45.

Perlmuter, L. C., & Smith, P. (1979). *The effects of choice and control on paired-associate learning in the aged.* Presented at a meeting of the New England Psychological Association.

Prohaska, T. R., Parham, I. A., & Teitelman, J. (1984). Age differences in attributions to causality: Implications for intellectual assessment. *Experimental Aging Research, 10,* 111–117.

Savage, R. E., Perlmuter, L. C., & Monty, R. A. (1979). Effect of reduction in the amount of choice and the perception of control on learning. In L. C. Perlmuter & R. A. Monty (Eds.), *Choice and perceived control* (pp. 91–106). Hillsdale, NJ: Lawrence Erlbaum.

Sellers, J. B. (1986). *The influence of a confidant on the morale of institutionalized elderly women.* Unpublished doctoral dissertation, Boston University School of Nursing.

Slamecka, N. J., & Graf, P. (1978). The generation effect: Delineation of a phenomenon. *Journal of Experimental Psychology: Human Learning and Memory, 4,* 592–604.

Weisz, J. R. (1983). Can I control it? The pursuit of veridical answers across the life span. In P. B. Baltes & O. G. Brim (Eds.), *Life-span development and behavior.* New York: Academic Press.

White, R. W. (1959). Motivation reconsidered: The concept of competence. *Psychological Review, 66,* 297–333.

Wittels, I. (1972). Age and stimulus meaningfulness in paired-associate learning. *Journal of Gerontology, 27,* 372–375.

22 Questionnaire research on metamemory and aging: Issues of structure and function

Roger A. Dixon

The title of this chapter is so commodious that it may be useful to begin by tidying up the domain of interest. First, there are two chapters in this section devoted to metamemory and aging; the other is Chapter 23 by John Cavanaugh. The field has been divided in a convenient way, and perhaps a theoretically and methodologically meaningful way. Specifically, Cavanaugh presents a discussion of the literature on metamemory and aging, where "metamemory" is operationally defined with any of multiple experimental (often on-line laboratory) tasks. I, on the other hand, have been charged with introducing the topic in a general (and certainly all too brief) manner and focusing attention on the metamemory and aging literature, where "metamemory" is indicated by verbal-report data (especially questionnaire data).

There is one further delineation in my topic I should note. Within the realm of verbal-report memory data, there are several domains, each of which is at least indirectly relevant to the issue at hand, but only one of which is immediately pertinent. These topics are summarized in Table 22.1. With the additional criterion of the consideration of developmental (especially aging) questions, this delineation follows closely that of Herrmann (1984). For the most part, I shall not address topic 1 (semantic-memory questionnaires), even those in which developmental (or aging) issues are paramount (Botwinick & Storandt, 1980; Erber, 1981; Perlmutter, Metzger, Miller, & Nezworski, 1980; Poon, Fozard, Paulshock, & Thomas, 1979; Riegel, 1973), and even though there is clear evidence that these techniques, which are verifiable against established facts, can represent valid ways of investigating memory (Herrmann, 1984). Also, I shall not discuss topic 2 (episodic-memory questionnaires), even though such research with older adults is of considerable theoretical importance, and despite such more global pertinent problems as verification of accuracy (Erber, 1981; Franklin & Holding, 1977; Robinson, 1976; Rubin, 1982; Waldfogel, 1948). Likewise, topic 3 (those metamemory questionnaires that were not designed explicitly for, or have not

The author appreciates the helpful comments of Deborah Burke, Christopher Hertzog, David Hultsch, and Timothy Salthouse on an earlier version of this chapter.

Table 22.1. *Examples of verbal-report data used in memory research*

Topic 1. Semantic-memory questionnaires: Those questionnaires that were designed to address the recognition or recall of general information, knowledge, or events

Topic 2. Episodic-memory questionnaires: Those questionnaires that were designed to address the representation of specific individual experiences

Topic 3. "Adevelopmental" metamemory questionnaires: Those metamemory questionnaires that were not designed for, or have not been applied to, life-span developmental questions

Topic 4. "Developmental" metamemory questionnaires: Those metamemory questionnaires that were designed for, or have been applied to, life-span developmental questions

Table 22.2. *Some examples of metamemory questionnaires that were designed for, or have been applied to, life-span developmental issues*

Questionnaire	Documentation
1. Memory Questionnaire (MQ)	Perlmutter (1978)
2. Memory Functioning Questionnaire (MFQ)	Gilewski et al. (1983); Zelinski et al. (1980)
3. Subjective Memory Questionnaire (SMQ)	Bennett-Levy & Powell (1980)
4. Short Inventory of Memory Experiences (SIME)	Chaffin & Herrmann (1983); Herrmann (1984)
5. Metamemory in Adulthood (MIA)	Dixon & Hultsch (1983a, 1983b, 1984); Hertzog, et al. (1985)

been applied to, aging issues) will not be discussed (Herrmann, 1982, 1984). Rather, the focus of this chapter is on topic 4: programmatic, published research associated with those metamemory questionnaires that were designed for, or have been applied to, life-span developmental questions.

As can be seen in Table 22.2, some examples of "eligible" research programs or reports include (1) the Memory Questionnaire of Perlmutter (1978), (2) the Memory Functioning Questionnaire of Zelinski, Gilewski, and colleagues (Gilewski, Zelinski, Schaie, & Thompson, 1983; Zelinski, Gilewski, & Thompson, 1980), (3) the Subjective Memory Questionnaire (Bennett-Levy & Powell, 1980), (4) the Short Inventory of Memory Experiences (Chaffin & Herrmann, 1983), and (5) the Metamemory in Adulthood (MIA) questionnaire (Dixon & Hultsch, 1983a, 1983b, 1984; Hertzog, Dixon, Schulenberg, & Hultsch, 1985b). Certainly there are other published studies that have employed interviews, questionnaires, or a restricted set of questions and have reported results on a sample including older adults (Harris, 1980; Hulicka, 1982; Riege, 1982; Sunderland, Harris, & Baddeley, 1984; Weinstein, Duffy, Underwood, MacDonald, & Gott, 1981; West, Boatwright, & Schleser, 1984; Williams, Denney, & Schadler, 1983;

Zarit, 1982; Zarit, Cole, & Guider, 1981). Some of these will be mentioned throughout this chapter. Nevertheless, the five questionnaires identified in Table 22.2 will constitute the most general domain of interest. Because of space limitations, however, I shall later use the MIA as the principal example. One final introductory note: A recent review of questionnaires applicable to the assessment of memory complaints in older adults (Gilewski & Zelinski, 1983) considers a similar sample of questionnaires from a complementary viewpoint.

Metamemory and life-span cognitive development

A definition and representation

In recent years, cognitive psychologists have focused increasing attention on putative "higher" mental processes. In an effort to describe the evolving complexities of human mental functioning, multifaceted and occasionally hierarchical models of cognition have been proffered. However, although employing such terms as "metacognition" (Brown, 1978; Brown, Bransford, Ferrara, & Campione, 1983) and "metamemory" (Cavanaugh & Perlmutter, 1982; Flavell, 1971; Flavell & Wellman, 1977), most experimental and psychometric psychologists have avoided the lure of reification. As a result, such terms – the core definitions of which are widely accepted and quoted – have spawned multiple (and sometimes mutually exclusive) operational definitions. Of course, one may argue that the fact of numerous operational definitions for a set of related constructs may be taken as nominal (but convergent) evidence for the relative autonomy of the set. Recent reviews suggest, however, that the questions (1) whether or not metacognition and metamemory sufficiently diverge from one another to be independently measurable and useful, and (2) whether or not as a class they sufficiently diverge from other well-defined and measurable classes of cognitive or affective behavior, are, for lack of appropriate data, not yet answerable (Brown et al., 1983; Cavanaugh & Perlmutter, 1982; Dixon & Hertzog, 1985).

More complete discussions of these definitional, conceptual, and empirical issues are available elsewhere. The working definition of metamemory adopted for present purposes follows closely the core properties identified in much of the literature (Brown, 1975; Cavanaugh & Perlmutter, 1982; Flavell, 1971; Flavell & Wellman, 1977). Thus, "metamemory" is a term representing one's knowledge, perceptions, and beliefs about the functioning, development, and capacities of (1) one's own memory and (2) the human memory system. It includes knowledge, perceptions, and beliefs about the demand characteristics of particular tasks or situations, the availability and employability of relevant strategies and aids, and other memory-relevant characteristics of the persons themselves. Several observers have commented conceptually on such additional characteristics of metamemory phenomena as their potential practical or functional value (Angell, 1908; Brown, 1975, 1979; Dixon & Hertzog, 1985; James, 1890) and the personological, affective, or social factors possibly active in both laboratory and everyday-

Table 22.3. *Major assumptions of metamemory research activity*

1. *Assumption of discriminant validity:* Metamemory is distinguishable from social intelligence, crystallized intelligence, other domains of self-knowledge and other knowledge, world knowledge, self-esteem, achievement motivation, metacognition, other "metas."
2. *Assumption of convergent validity:* Multiple operational definitions, factors, aspects, and domains converge in a coherent construct.
3. *Assumption of Predictive Validity:*
   - 3A. *Causality:* There is a predictive, if not causal, relationship between knowledge about memory and behavior in memory-demanding situations.
   - 3B. *Bidirectionality:* There is a dynamic bidirectional relationship between memory knowledge and memory performance.
   - 3C. *Ecological relevance:* Metamemory (broadly conceived) contributes to cognitive efficiency in everyday life.

memory situations (Baddeley, 1981a; Bower, 1981; Dewey, 1908; Hultsch & Pentz, 1980; Martin & Jones, 1984; Zarit, 1982). These additional characteristics may be particularly important when the focus of research is on understanding apparent age-related declines in memory performance in late life (Dixon & Hertzog, 1985; Dixon & Hultsch, 1983b; Hultsch, 1984; Zelinski et al., 1980).

Assumptions

The major (and generally unexpressed) assumptions of metamemory research activity are presented in Table 22.3. These assumptions appear to have been lurking behind most metamemory research activity, inadequately articulated conceptually and insufficiently tested empirically. The first assumption, which I call the assumption of discriminant validity, is simply that, as a construct, metamemory is distinguishable (both empirically and conceptually) from other related constructs, such as crystallized intelligence, social intelligence, other domains of self-knowledge and other knowledge, world knowledge, self-esteem, and achievement motivation, as well as metacognition and other "metas." The second assumption, which I call the assumption of convergent validity, is that the plethora of operational definitions of the construct – which seemingly represent multiple dimensions, factors, aspects, and domains – converges conceptually and empirically (i.e., relatively high correlations among different measures of the same construct) in a consistent, coherent construct.

The third major assumption, which I call the assumption of predictive validity, is composed of at least three related subsets. First, the assumption that has received the most empirical investigation is the assumption of a predictive relationship, or causality; that is, there is believed to be a causal relationship between knowledge and perceptions of memory, on the one hand, and remembering behavior and performance in memory-demanding situations, on the other. Indeed, this is the primary variety of validity information available in the metamemory literature. Parenthetically, one can understand why this is such a crucial consideration in metamemory research; in the absence of a demonstrable relationship between metamemory and memory, then the overall usefulness of the metamemory construct may become suspect (Chi, 1985; Schneider, in press). The second subset under the assumption of predictive validity is rather more subtle and has been less thoroughly investigated. This is the assumption that there is a dynamic, bidirectional relationship between memory knowledge, perceptions, and beliefs, on the one hand, and memory performance or behaviors, on the other. That is, from an intraindividual perspective (even, writ large, a life-course perspective), one's knowledge, perceptions, and beliefs about memory not only influence memory performance but also are shaped by a succession of memory experiences. A third subset under this assumption of predictive validity is implicit perhaps in only *some* treatments of the construct. That is, metamemory (and related phenomena such as mnemonics and memory aids) is a useful cognitive process not only because it may predict performances on laboratory tasks but also because it may contribute to cognitive efficiency in everyday life, and it may be one source of cognitive compensation. One underlying, as yet unmentioned, corollary of assumption 3 is related to aging research; that is, knowledge, perception, and beliefs about memory may be important contributors to the frequently observed age-related decrements in performance on laboratory memory tasks (Hertzog, Dixon, & Hultsch, 1985a; Hultsch, 1984).

It is a rare research program that contains information pertaining to all three assumptions, but most research is addressed to at least one of the three (usually assumption 3A). As several reviewers have noted, for most methodologies even this assumption is not often supported convincingly in both the childhood and adult literatures (Cavanaugh & Perlmutter, 1982; Schneider, in press). As we shall see later, some questionnaire research is beginning to address a larger subset of these assumptions.

Representation

One interpretation of life-span cognitive and intellectual development may be heuristically useful as applied to the domain of metamemory. As can be seen in Table 22.4, recent reviews of a wide range of literature have advanced four abstractions designed to characterize cognitive and intellectual development throughout adulthood (Baltes & Willis, 1979; Dixon, Kramer, & Baltes, 1985; Willis & Baltes, 1980). These four abstractions are (1) *multidimensionality,* or the notion that many mental constructs are composed of multiple abilities or dimensions, each with potentially distinct structural and functional properties, (2) *multidirectionality,* which signifies that there may be multiple distinct change patterns associated with these abilities, (3) *interindividual variability,* a conception reflecting the substantial interindividual differences often observed in the life-course change patterns of a given mental phenomenon, and (4) *intraindividual*

Table 22.4. *Four abstractions from the literature on life-span cognitive and intellectual development*

Abstraction	Significance
1. Multidimensionality	Many mental constructs are composed of multiple abilities or dimensions.
2. Multidirectionality	There may be multiple distinct change patterns associated with these abilities or dimensions.
3. Interindividual variability	There are substantial interindividual differences often observed in the life-course change patterns of a given phenomenon.
4. Intraindividual plasticity	In principle, some individual behavioral patterns are modifiable.

Source: Willis & Baltes (1980).

plasticity, which indicates that, in principle, some individual behavioral patterns are modifiable (e.g., through effort, training, or practice).

In subsequent sections it will be seen that these four abstractions may be applied usefully to life-span metamemory development. Indeed, as described in later sections, the work in which I am currently involved – with Christopher Hertzog and David Hultsch – is moving in the direction of investigating the applicability of all four. That is, we shall gather information pertaining to the representativeness of each of the four abstractions. Because of its inherent potential to represent a multidimensional structure, questionnaire research is one means by which all of these abstractions may be "tested." Let us turn now to a closer consideration of questionnaires as a research tool and their applications to metamemory and aging.

Questionnaire research on metamemory and aging

General issues

Questionnaire research activity (using subjective verbal reports as data) is garnished with a host of theoretical, methodological, and empirical reservations (Baddeley, 1981b; Ericssen & Simon, 1980; Nisbett & Wilson, 1977). Illustrative issues include (1) the conceptual status of introspection, (2) the plausibility of introspection regarding one's own cognitive processes, (3) the potential accuracy of such introspection, (4) the verisimilitude of subsequent reports, (5) the generality versus specificity of the content of questions or items, (6) whether the instruments are tests (e.g., memory questionnaires) or opinion surveys (e.g., some metamemory questionnaires), (7) a certain lack of experimental control, (8) the issue of "the memory introspection paradox" (that those people who experience memory failures are also those people who are likely to forget such events), (9) problems of reliability, and (10) problems of predictive and construct validity (Brown et al., 1983; Herrmann, 1982, 1984; Morris, 1984).

Table 22.5. *Some possible reasons for the dilution of observed metamemory–memory relationships*

1.	Both metamemory and memory phenomena may be distributed into multiple dimensions.
2.	The obtained correlation is limited by the reliability with which each indicator can be measured.
3.	There may be, across occasions, considerable intraindividual variability in memory beliefs and perceptions (i.e., they may be more state-like than trait-like).

Sources: Dixon & Hertzog (1985); Herrmann (1982).

On the other hand, there are several conceptual and methodological reasons for using verbal-report data on memory and metamemory: (1) They may serve as an efficient simulation or approximation of some everyday-memory phenomena, (2) they may allow for a more adequate simultaneous representation of the range of metamemory phenomena, (3) because they may participate in the psychometric tradition, they may provide a natural means of representing the apparent multidimensional nature of the phenomena, (4) for this reason they may promote theoretical work with respect to the multidimensional character of the content domain, (5) they may promote theoretical work on the relationship between specific aspects or dimensions of both metamemory and memory performance, and (6) they may provide one means of articulating and studying the linkages among social, affective, and cognitive processes. Like any method, it can be abused or used uncritically or inappropriately. When the credentials of a given questionnaire are strong – when there is a well-delineated content domain and when there are known, as well as acceptable, psychometric properties – it may be applied prudently, but confidently, in empirical research.

As several reviewers have pointed out, however, the validity evidence accruing to some metamemory questionnaires has not been of the sort to inspire a great deal of confidence (Herrmann, 1982, 1984). That is, despite the recent proliferation of metamemory questionnaires used in aging research, the evidence pertaining to even the predictive validity of such questionnaires (the metamemory–memory performance relationship) is generally inconclusive, and where conclusive, it is very often weak.

In aging research, obtained metamemory–memory correlations may be diluted for several methodologically or conceptually coherent reasons (Herrmann, 1982). As seen in Table 22.5, these reasons, taken together, are closely related to the interpretation of metamemory development in terms of the four abstractions (multidimensionality, multidirectionality, interindividual variability, intraindividual plasticity) described earlier. Specifically, some of these possible reasons are as follows. First, both memory and metamemory phenomena may not be unitary processes, and thus there is no theoretical reason to expect necessarily high correlations among all (or even most of) the multiple dimensions or the various general and specific aptitudes. Therefore, failure to consider carefully which dimensions of metamemory might be related to which dimensions of memory, and then failure to measure the appropriate dimensions, could lead to small validity coefficients (Dixon & Hertzog, 1985; Herrmann, 1982; Herrmann & Neisser, 1978; Hertzog et al., 1985b; Sehulster, 1981b).

Second, the reliability with which each variable (in the metamemory and memory domains) can be measured limits the correlation between the two variables. In the present case, a metamemory instrument with low (or unknown) reliability may not be correlated highly with even a reliably measured memory variable.

Third, there may be, across occasions, considerable intraindividual variability in memory knowledge, beliefs, and perceptions; that is, metamemory may be more state-like than trait-like. That self-reports are intraindividually inconsistent does not necessarily imply that the "error" variance is unwieldy or uninteresting. If coherent patterns can be recovered from this intraindividual variability – if such variability may be linked, for example, to variability in other labile aspects of the individual (viz., mood states such as anxiety and fatigue, "energy levels," self-efficacy, motivation, health) – then the observed variability is potentially interpretable and psychologically meaningful (Dixon & Hertzog, 1985; Hertzog et al., 1985a; Nesselroade, 1983). That is, self-perceptions regarding memory may be important antecedents of shifts in memory performance over time.

Each of these possible reasons for dilution of obtained metamemory–memory correlations can be addressed in questionnaire research. Overall, these four reasons point to multiple potential causes of individual differences in memory performance, causes that are associated with, but distinguishable from, memory knowledge. These influences, such as situation-specific memory experiences or subjective beliefs about one's own memory efficacy, may either operate independent of veridical memory knowledge or mediate its relationship to strategy use. I shall return to this validity question later when I summarize the initial results of our research program. Before that, however, I would like to turn attention to a brief comparison of some of the adult age-related results from different laboratories.

Survey of principal research

As indicated earlier, several metamemory questionnaires have been developed for, or applied to, issues of cognitive aging. These instruments range from interviews on the use of memory aids (Harris, 1980), memory strategies (Weinstein et al., 1981), and memory complaints (Gilewski & Zelinski, 1983; Zarit et al., 1981) to a set of questions concerning perceptions of memory abilities and memory aging (Williams et al., 1983). In the latter study, for example, Williams and associates found that older adults indicated that they perceived memory abilities to decline with advancing age, but not in all individuals (i.e., there is perceived interindividual variability). Prominent among the reasons given for this decline were such noncognitive influences as poor health, lack of concentration or effort, and lack of use or practice. The subjects also indicated that the activity level, the perceived importance of the information, personal expectations

Table 22.6A. *Comparison of selected age-related results from metamemory questionnaire research*

Aspect of metamemory	Study	Age differences or indication of age changes
Perceived memory abilities or capacities		
Perception of memory abilities (SMQ)	Bennett-Levy & Powell (1980)	Positive (O > Y)
Reported memory abilities (SIME)	Chaffin & Herrmann (1983)	Mixed (positive, equivalent, and negative)
Rating of memory capacity (MIA)	Dixon & Hultsch (1983b)	Negative (Y > O)
General rating of memory (MFQ)	Gilewski et al. (1983)	Negative (Y > O)
Reported use of memory strategies		
Reported use of mnemonics and strategies (MIA)	Dixon & Hultsch (1983a)	Equivalent
Reported use of mnemonics (MFQ)	Gilewski et al. (1983)	Equivalent
Reported use of memory strategies (MQ)	Perlmutter (1978)	Equivalent
Reported use of memory strategies	Weinstein et al. (1981)	Negative (Y > O)

for performance, and, to some extent, anxiety or nervousness can influence memory performance. Several of the influences identified by the older adults in that study are, as we shall see, of direct theoretical relevance to other programs of questionnaire research.

In Tables 22.6A, 22.6B, and 22.6C, some of the adult age-related results of metamemory questionnaire research can be seen. (In these tables, I use the expression "positive age differences" to refer to those cases where older adults perform better than younger adults, and "negative age differences" to indicate the reverse.) It should be noted that this comparison involves aspects of metamemory measured differently across studies (e.g., by single items, subscales, or global scores). Overall, for most aspects of metamemory, negative age differences (e.g., in perception of memory abilities) or indications of negative age changes (e.g., in expectation of memory decline) were found. Across studies and within constructs, however, there was some discrepancy. For example, although Weinstein and associates (1981) reported a negative age effect for reported use of memory strategies, on similar measures Perlmutter (1980), Gilewski and associates (1983), and Dixon and Hultsch (1983b) reported no age differences. Similarly, a mixed pattern of results appeared for indicators of perceived memory abilities or capacities. Although Bennett-Levy and Powell (1980) reported a positive age effect for their indicator, and Chaffin and Herrmann

Table 22.6B. *Further comparison of selected age-related results from metamemory questionnaire research*

Aspect of metamemory	Study	Age differences or indication of age changes
Perception of decline in memory abilities		
Rating of memory decline (MIA)	Dixon & Hultsch (1983b)	Negative (O > Y)
Retrospective rating of memory decline (MFQ)	Gilewski et al. (1983)	Negative (O > Y)
Expectation of memory decline (MQ)	Perlmutter (1978)	Negative (O > Y)
Perception of decline in memory abilities	Williams et al. (1983)	Negative (O > Y)
Reports of memory problems		
Frequency of memory problems (MFQ)	Gilewski et al. (1983)	Negative (O > Y)
Reported number of memory problems (MQ)	Perlmutter (1978)	Negative (O > Y)
Reported frequency of memory failures	Sunderland et al. (1984)	Positive (Y > O)

(1983) found a mixed pattern of results (including positive, equivalent, and negative age differences for their multiple indicators), Dixon and Hultsch (1983b), Gilewski and associates (1983), and Zelinski and associates (1980) found negative age difference for their indicators of rating of memory or memory capacity.

Table 22.6B shows four studies that included indicators of the perception of decline in memory abilities (Dixon & Hultsch, 1983b; Gilewski et al., 1983; Perlmutter, 1978; Williams et al., 1983). All reported that older adults, more than younger adults, perceived memory abilities to decline. Two studies (Gilewski et al. 1983; Perlmutter, 1978) found negative age differences for reports of memory problems, but Sunderland and associates (1984), with a slightly different focus, found that younger adults reported more frequent memory failures than did older adults. As can be seen in Table 22.6C, two studies developed measures of general knowledge of memory processes, with Perlmutter (1978) reporting no age differences and Dixon and Hultsch (1983b) reporting negative age differences. Studies investigating memory complaints have been reviewed by Gilewski and Zelinski (1983).

Obviously, some of the discrepancies described roughly in these three tables may be due to differences in samples or measures. In addition, the studies surveyed were rather uneven in reported reliability and validity. Whereas some provided little or no reliability information, others provided little or no validity information. At least two of the metamemory questionnaires, the MFQ (Gilewski et al., 1983) and the MIA (Dixon & Hultsch, 1983a, 1983b, 1984; Dixon, Hertzog, Schulenberg, & Hultsch, 1985b; Hertzog et al., 1985b), have known (and generally acceptable) psychometric properties. A range of evidence for reliability and validity has been accumulated for both instruments (Gilewski & Zelinski, 1983). In addition, both instruments were designed explicitly for work with adult development and aging, with an identifiable concern for ecologically relevant

Table 22.6C. *Further comparison of selected age-related results from metamemory questionnaire research*

Aspect of metamemory	Study	Age differences or indication of age changes
General knowledge of memory processes		
Knowledge of basic memory processes (MIA)	Dixon & Hultsch (1983b)	Negative (Y > O)
Memory knowledge (MQ)	Perlmutter (1978)	Equivalent
Assorted aspects		
Rating of influence of anxiety on memory (MIA)	Dixon & Hultsch (1983b)	Equivalent
Perceived importance of good memory (MIA)	Dixon & Hultsch (1983b)	Equivalent
Perceived personal control over memory (MIA)	Dixon & Hultsch (1983b)	Negative (Y > O)
Rating of recall of past events (MFQ)	Gilewski et al. (1983)	Negative (Y > O)
Rating of seriousness of memory problems (MFQ)	Gilewski et al. (1983)	Negative (Y > O)
Everyday memory demands (MQ)	Perlmutter (1978)	Equivalent

constituent metamemory behaviors and a range of laboratory and presumably ecologically valid memory tasks for validation work. Although the content domains tapped by these two instruments are similar, they are rather different in focus. Whereas the MFQ focuses on multiple aspects of one's perception of memory ability in everyday situations, the MIA attends to a subset of this domain and, in addition, various aspects of memory-related knowledge, personal beliefs, and affect (whether or not they are veridical). As one illustration, I shall turn now to a closer examination of one of these instruments and the accompanying evidence for the relationship between metamemory and memory performance throughout adulthood.

The Metamemory in Adulthood (MIA) questionnaire

As mentioned earlier, the principal issues for research using verbal-report data (especially questionnaire data) to examine metamemory development in adulthood are as follows: (1) the content domain of the construct, especially its constitution and scope, (2) the reliability of the instrument and constituent subscales, including internal consistency and repeatability, and (3) the associated validity, especially empirical (concurrent and predictive) and construct (convergent and discriminant) validity. The continuing work with the MIA is addressed to these issues.

Eight initial dimensions

Our first efforts were directed at "enriching" the construct of metamemory; that is, we examined multiple memory, metamemory, metacognition, and

Table 22.7. *The eight dimensions of the MIA instrument*

Dimension	Description	Sample item
1. Strategy	Knowledge of one's remembering abilities such that performance in given instances is potentially improved; reported use of mnemonics, strategies, and memory aids (+ = high use)	Do you write appointments on a calendar to help you remember them?
2. Task	Knowledge of basic memory processes, especially as evidenced by how most people perform (+ = high knowledge)	For most people, facts that are interesting are easier to remember than facts that are not.
3. Capacity	Perception of memory capacities as evidenced by predictive report of performance on given tasks (+ = high capacity)	I am good at remembering names.
4. Change	Perception of memory abilities as generally stable or subject to long-term decline (+ = stability)	The older I get, the harder it is to remember things clearly.
5. Activity	Regularity with which respondent seeks and engages in activities that might support cognitive performance (+ = high regularity)	How often do you read newspapers?
6. Anxiety	Rating of influence of anxiety and stress on performance (+ = high anxiety)	I do not get flustered when I am put on the spot to remember new things.
7. Achievement	Perceived importance of having a good memory and performing well on memory tasks (+ = high achievement)	It is important that I am very accurate when remembering names of people.
8. Locus	Perceived personal control over remembering abilities (+ = internality)	It's up to me to keep my remembering abilities from deteriorating.

Sources: Dixon & Hultsch (1983b, 1984).

perception-of-self and cognition interviews and questionnaires. From these we initially abstracted eight theoretically meaningful dimensions, began operationalizing them in the form of a pool of 206 items, and established content validity. All items were designed to reflect everyday, ecologically relevant activities, behaviors, or conditions. These dimensions are summarized in Table 22.7.

Use of memory strategies (Strategy). This category refers to the use of memory strategies of various types. The basic question is this: Does the respondent (know and) use information about his/her general remembering abilities that is designed to assist or improve performance in given instances? Although what a person both knows and does about strategies is of interest, the focus here is on the *use* of strategies, mnemonics, and memory aids. That is, a high score will come from reported frequent use of memory aids. Examples would include activities such as writing reminder notes, repeating to oneself the information to be remembered, and making mental associations of one item with another.

Knowledge of memory tasks and processes (Task). This category refers more to fundamental knowledge of memory processes than to reported use. It is task-oriented (i.e., relating more to knowledge of task/process differences than to person differences). The expected source of variance lies in the task and task characteristics. The basic question is this: Does the respondent have an understanding of basic memory processes, especially as evidenced by knowledge of how most people would perform? Examples would include the knowledge that most people find it easier to remember short lists than long lists, and important things than unimportant things. A high score here is indicative of a high level of understanding of general memory processes.

Perception of own memory capacities (Capacity). This category refers to the respondent's predictive report regarding recall performance in designated situations. The respondent's remembering ability (of, for example, names, places, dates) or perception of that ability is of critical interest. The basic question is this: How does the individual perceive his/her performance on given memory tasks, and what does the individual perceive about his/her competence in memory activities? Examples would include perception skill at remembering names, where one parked the car, and birthdates. A high score is indicative of a high level of reported memory capacity.

Perception of change (Change). This category focuses on the perceived developmental process of remembering capacities for the individual and for others in general. The basic question is this: Does the respondent perceive his/her everyday remembering abilities as subject to change, and if so, in what direction (better or worse) is that change? Examples would include the perception that memory generally gets better or worse with age, or that the respondent's memory is getting better or worse with age. It was decided that a positive perception of memory adaptability and functioning would be assigned a higher score than a negative view.

Activities supportive of memory (Activity). The basic question is this: Does the respondent *regularly* engage in activities that might support cognitive skill in general and remembering skill in particular? Activities that might be considered supportive of memory skill are those of a "mental" or social variety in which thinking and remembering processes are exercised in the course of the activity. Examples would include activities such as reading, watching television, attending social gatherings, traveling, and solving problems. A high score results from a reported high level of cognitively supportive activities.

Memory and state anxiety (Anxiety). This refers both to (1) ratings of the influence of the respondent's emotional state (considered in terms of a continuum from equanimity-calmness to agitation-anxiety) on performance on cognitive tasks and (2) ratings of the influence of being presented with a cognitive task on the respondent's emotional state. Examples would involve knowledge that general cognitive demands or particular cognitive tasks may result in heightened levels of emotional tension or anxiety, or knowledge that the individual finds it difficult to perform cognitive tasks when anxious. A high score indicates a high level of anxiety associated with performance.

Memory and achievement motivation (Achievement). The basic questions are these: How important is it to the respondent to have a good memory and to do well on memory tasks, and how hard does he/she work on remembering and related activities? Examples would include statements reflecting the value and importance of memory functioning and positive responses to statements that indicate a desire, willingness, or attempt to improve or perfect remembering skills. A high score here indicates a high level of motivation to achieve in memory.

Personal control in memory abilities (Locus). This refers to the respondent's perceived sense of control over remembering skills. The basic question is this: Does the respondent believe that he/she has control over his/her remembering abilities or, alternatively, that his/her remembering abilities are largely determined by factors outside of his/her control (e.g., age, inheritance, health)? Examples would include statements indicating that memory depends largely on hard work, practice, and determination, or, conversely, that it depends largely on health, other person's activities, age, or other factors outside the respondent's control. A high score here is associated with a personal (or internal) sense of control.

This instrument was administered sequentially to, at first, three independent samples of community-dwelling adults, ranging in age from 18 to 84 years [see Dixon & Hultsch (1983b) for further sample information], and then to three more similar independent samples (Hertzog et al., 1985b). On the basis of Cronbach's α, item-to-total-subscale correlations, item-to-other-subscale correlations, and factor analyses [iterative principal axis, with oblique (promax) rotation], successive item selections occurred until a 120-item instrument, with acceptable psychometric properties, was completed. Some psychometric features of this instrument are described in Table 22.8. Six of the subscales (Strategy, Task, Change, Anxiety, Achievement, and Locus) appeared to be acceptably reliable and factorially valid. The Capacity subscale was internally consistent, but was highly correlated with the Change subscale. The Activity subscale behaved consistently across samples, but with more modest psychometric properties. Because, further, this subscale is addressed to reported frequency of cognitively supportive activities (not to knowledge, perceptions, or beliefs about memory), it is perhaps best to exclude it from the present representation of the construct of metamemory. It should not, however, be excluded in principle from consideration in the prediction of ecological memory performance in adulthood. Notably, it represents one of the three features of metamemory identified initially by Flavell (1971).

As may be apparent from the earlier tables, much of the conceptual space of this metamemory construct has been tapped in other research projects, most notably those of Gilewski and associates (1983), Zelinski and associates (1980), and

Table 22.8. *Summary of internal consistency (Cronbach's α) and item factor loadings for eight MIA subscales*

Subscale	Range of α across 3 samples	Factor loadings across 3 samples
Strategy (21)	.78 to .90	.32 to .75
Task (15)	.74 to .87	.34 to .76
Capacity (20)	.74 to .90	.30 to .67
Change (19)	.82 to .92	.38 to .83
Activity (16)	.28 to .76	.32 to .55
Anxiety (14)	.78 to .87	.33 to .73
Achievement (14)	.61 to .84	.30 to .64
Locus (11)	.71 to .80	.31 to .67

Table 22.9. *MIA subscales similar to, or represented in, other metamemory questionnaires or associated research*

Other questionnaires	MIA dimensions							
	STRAT	TASK	CAP	CHANGE	ACT	ANX	ACH	LOCUS
SMQ: Bennett-Levy & Powell (1980)			X					
SIME: Chaffin & Herrmann (1983)			X					
MFQ: Gilewski et al. (1983)	X		X	X	Y		Y	
MQ: Perlmutter (1978)	X	X		X				
Weinstein et al. (1981)	X							
Williams et al. (1983)				X	Z			Z

Note: X = close correspondence; Y = contains items similar to those in these subscales; Z = Additional questions or responses addressed these issues.

Perlmutter (1978). This overlap is depicted in Table 22.9. One interesting aspect of the MIA is its multiple measures (subscales) of three potentially salient "sub-constructs" of metamemory. Elsewhere (Dixon et al., 1985b; Hertzog et al., 1985b) we have tentatively identified these subconstructs as Memory Knowledge (composed of Task, Strategy, and perhaps Locus), Memory Self-efficacy (composed of Capacity, Change, Achievement, and perhaps Locus), and Memory-related Affect (composed of Anxiety, Achievement, and perhaps Locus). This latter "subconstruct" is generally unrepresented in other instruments. We are currently engaged in testing this hypothesis in higher-order factor analyses on the covariance matrices of six samples of young, middle-age, and old adults.

Table 22.10. *Summary of mean age differences and prediction of text-recall performance for eight MIA subscales across three samples of adults*

Subscale	Age differences	Cross-sample recall-prediction pattern
Strategy	n.s.	Young, middle-age
Task	Young > old (samples 1, 3)	Young, middle-age, old
Capacity	Young > old (samples 1, 2, 3)	Young, middle-age
Change	Young > old (samples 1, 2, 3)	Young
Activity	n.s.	—
Anxiety	n.s.	—
Achievement	n.s.	Middle-age, old
Locus	Young > old (samples 1, 2, 3)	Old
Total scale	Young > old (samples 1, 2, 3)	Young and old

Source: Dixon & Hultsch (1983a).

In one of these recent studies (Dixon et al., 1985b), the hypothesis that these subconstructs were derivable empirically from the seven subscales (minus Activity) was tested on a sample of 146 young (ages 21–39), 86 middle-aged (ages 39–58), and 146 old (ages 60–74) community-dwelling adults. The results of an exploratory factor analysis (EFAP II) and an age-comparative procedure (using LISREL VI) indicated that it was indeed plausible to model the three hypothesized higher-order factors. However, whereas Memory Knowledge and Memory-related Affect had an isomorphic structure across age groups, Memory-related Self-efficacy appeared to have an age-related variation in structure. These initial results are presently being compared with those emerging from identical analyses on a separate sample (Hertzog et al., 1985b).

Issues of validity

As was suggested earlier, the predictive-validity question is important: Do these multiple subscales, or hypothesized subconstructs, predict memory performance? Several reviews and studies have addressed this issue (Gilewski et al., 1983; Herrmann, 1984; Morris, 1984; Perlmutter, 1978; Salthouse & Kausler, 1985; Zelinski et al., 1980). Our own initial efforts were directed at cross-sample validation of age-related prediction patterns for memory for text (Dixon & Hultsch, 1983a). These results are summarized in Table 22.10 (columns 1 and 3). The most important finding is not that there are certain consistent linkages among at least six of the MIA subscales and memory for text performance across three independent samples but that these linkages are somewhat different for each age group. For younger adults, reported use of memory strategies and physical reminders (Strategy), as well as perception of own memory abilities (Capacity) and

Table 22.11. *Summary of age-related correlations between MIA subscales and ability measures*

Strategy is related to:
Induction in Y
Verbal Comprehension in MA and O
Backward Span and Word Memory in all
Figures of Speech in O

Task is related to:
Verbal Comprehension in all
Backward Span in all
Forward Span in O
Word Memory and Figures of Speech in Y and O

Capacity is related to:
Verbal Comprehension, Backward Span, Object Number, Figures of Speech, Theme Test in O (inversely)

Activity is related to:
Verbal Comprehension in MA and O
Induction, Word Memory, Figures of Speech in O

Anxiety is related to:
Forward Span in Y and O (inversely)

Note: Range of magnitude of correlations = .25 to .53; Y = young; MA = middle-aged; O = old.
Source: Dixon et al. (1985a, 1985b).

what is known about general memory processes (Task), best predicts memory performance. For middle-aged adults, reported use of strategies and reminders (Strategy), general memory knowledge (Task), perception of own abilities (Capacity), and level of motivation to achieve in memory performance (Achievement) predict memory for text performance. For older adults, general memory knowledge (Task), level of motivation to achieve in memory performance (Achievement), and sense of personal control of memory functioning (Locus) best predict memory performance.

In general, whereas the memory for text performance of younger adults is associated primarily with the "knowledge" (Task, Strategy) and "self-efficacy" (Capacity) dimensions of the MIA, the performance of older adults is predicted by a "knowledge" dimension (Task) and by an "affect" dimension (Achievement, Locus). Referring to our earlier discussion of possible reasons for low obtained metamemory–memory relationships, one may speculate that this apparent shift in prediction patterns across the adult years is not capturable with operational definitions that do not include (or distinguish among) memory knowledge, memory-related self-efficacy, and memory-related affect.

A second form of the predictive-validity issue emerges. Does the MIA predict performance also on laboratory cognitive and memory tasks? The initial evidence for this is summarized in Table 22.11. Performance on a wide range of ability measures – including two indicators each of Verbal Comprehension (Vocabulary 1, Advanced Vocabulary), Induction (Letter Sets, Letter Series), Span (Forward,

Backward), Associative Memory (Object Number Test, Memory for Words), Associational Fluency (Controlled Associations, Figures of Speech), and Ideational Fluency (Topics Test, Theme Test) (Ekstrom, French, Harman, & Derman, 1976) – was correlated with performance on the MIA (Dixon et al., 1985). The sample included three adult age groups: young ($\bar{X}$ = 32.0; n = 50), middle age ($\bar{X}$ = 49.5; n = 50), and old ($\bar{X}$ = 68.9; n = 50).

As can be seen in the table, Task is related to the Verbal Comprehension indicators across the three age groups. Strategy is related to Verbal Comprehension for middle-age and older adults, whereas for young adults it is related to the Induction indicators. There are multiple examples of significant correlations across the three age groups for these two subscales. For Capacity, however, a typical indicator of metamemory, the bulk of significant correlations was for the old adults, and these were negative. That is, for older adults, the higher the rating of self-efficacy (Capacity), the lower the performance on 6 of 12 laboratory cognitive tasks. Overall, the two indicators of memory knowledge (Strategy and Task) were related to several indicators, especially Verbal Comprehension, Induction (for the young), Backward Span, Word Memory, and Figures of Speech (for the old). This suggests that self-ratings of ability may not be as closely related to typical laboratory tasks as is general knowledge. In contrast to the memory for text results, there is no evidence here that the affect subscales predicted performance on laboratory tasks for any of the age groups. (Of course, a complete sampling of laboratory memory tasks is in order.) All of this, again, suggests the specificity of prediction patterns among the multiple dimensions of metamemory and the multiple dimensions of memory performance (Chaffin & Herrmann, 1983; Sunderland et al., 1984; Zelinski et al., 1980).

Conclusion: Avenues for future research

This review of the applicability of questionnaire research to the investigation of metamemory in adulthood has indicated that there may be (1) a heterogeneous content domain (i.e., there may be multiple dimensions of metamemory in adulthood), (2) differential predictive relationships among memory tasks and these multiple dimensions, and (3) some greater influence of affective metamemory dimensions on memory for text performance in older adults. These findings buttress the three issues raised earlier regarding the modest magnitude of metamemory–memory correlations in adult samples. In particular, they suggest the need to identify short-term change and variability in subjective dimensions of metamemory.

One conclusion is that a thorough understanding of the relationship between metamemory and memory performance requires further investigation of intraindividual variation. As has been indicated elsewhere (Dixon & Hertzog, 1985; Hertzog et al., 1985a; Hultsch, 1984), both cognitive performance measures and metamemory measures have been assumed to provide a valid indication of abilities. Thus, the assumption is that these abilities are stable over the adult life span, except for age-related (generally decremental) change. Inextricably interwoven with this assumption is the position that the observed cognitive performance is more trait-like than state-like, that there is relatively little intraindividual fluctuation associated with corresponding changes in labile characteristics of individuals, such as interest patterns, motivations, mood states, health, alcohol or drug intoxication, sleep loss, familiarity, and perceptions of self-efficacy in situations demanding cognitive skills.

Therefore, some current work proceeds from a recognition that ontogenetic change in underlying mental processes may be but one contributing factor to age-correlated changes in complex cognitive behaviors (Dixon & Hertzog, 1985; Hertzog et al., 1985a; Hultsch, 1984). From this perspective, it is suggested that (1) single-session memory-assessment procedures may not necessarily provide a valid indication of underlying "traits," (2) multiple-session memory-assessment procedures may uncover fluctuations in cognitive performance of older adults that are associated with lability in physiological and psychological states, (3) these fluctuations are conceptually distinct from age change per se, and (4) perceptions of self-efficacy in cognitive situations may have a substantial impact on the cognitive performance of older adults (and vice versa) (Hertzog et al., 1985a). It is possible, as well, that these suggestions may apply as much to memory as to metamemory (Dixon & Hertzog, 1985; Hertzog et al., 1985a; Hultsch, 1984). That is, evidence that fluctuations in memory performance were predicted by contemporaneous fluctuations in affective states or perceptions of cognitive competence might suggest that a major component of variance in the cognitive performance of older adults may be somewhat indirectly related to "natural" or single-session assessments of memory skills. Thus, important components may be perceptions, beliefs, attitudes, and expectations regarding performance in situations demanding cognitive skills (Hertzog et al., 1985a).

Several specific issues have been outlined for further study (Hertzog et al., 1985a): (1) examination of the convergent factorial validity of multiple measures of metamemory; (2) determination of the divergence of dimensions of metamemory from more general constructs of self-perception, personality, and affect; (3) delineation of intraindividual fluctuation in perceptions of memory-related self-efficacy and affect. Of particular concern is the question whether or not fluctuations in these dimensions covary with perceived memory failures in older adults and, if so, whether or not these shifting perceptions influence memory performance. As answers to these questions become available, our understanding of the complexities involved in metamemory development across adulthood, memory development across adulthood, and metamemory–memory performance relationships across adulthood should become further refined.

References

Angell, J. R. (1908). *Psychology: An introduction to the structure and function of human consciousness* (4th ed.). New York: Henry Holt.

Baddeley, A. D. (1981a). Cognitive psychology and psychometric theory. In M. P. Friedman, J. P. Das, & N. O'Connor (Eds.), *Intelligence and learning* (pp. 479–486). New York: Plenum Press.

Baddeley, A. (1981b). The cognitive psychology of everyday life. *British Journal of Psychology, 72,* 257–269.

Baltes, P. B., & Willis, S. L. (1979). The critical importance of appropriate methodology in the study of aging: The sample case of psychometric intelligence. In F. Hoffmeister & C. Müller (Eds.), *Brain function in old age* (pp. 164–187). Heidelberg: Springer.

Bennett-Levy, J., & Powell, G. E. (1980). The Subjective Memory Questionnaire (SMQ). An investigation into the self-reporting of 'real life' memory skills. *British Journal of Social and Clinical Psychology, 19,* 177–188.

Botwinick, J., & Storandt, M. (1980). Recall and recognition of old information in relation to age and sex. *Journal of Gerontology, 35,* 70–76.

Bower, G. H. (1981). Mood and memory. *American Psychologist, 36,* 129–148.

Brown, A. L. (1975). The development of memory: Knowing, knowing about knowing, and knowing how to know. In H. W. Reese (Ed.), *Advances in child development and behavior* (Vol. 10). New York: Academic Press.

Brown, A. L. (1978). Knowing when, where, and how to remember: A problem of metacognition. In R. Glaser (Ed.), *Advances in instructional psychology.* Hillsdale, NJ: Lawrence Erlbaum.

Brown, A. L. (1979). Theories of memory and the problems of development: Activity, growth, and knowledge. In L. S. Cermak & F. I. M. Craik (Eds.), *Levels of processing in human memory.* Hillsdale, NJ: Lawrence Erlbaum.

Brown, A. L., Bransford, J. D., Ferrara, R. A., & Campione, J. C. (1983). Learning, remembering, and understanding. In J. H. Flavell & E. M. Markman (Eds.), *Handbook of child psychology. Vol. 3: Cognitive development* (pp. 77–166). New York: Wiley.

Cavanaugh, J. C., & Perlmutter, M. (1982). Metamemory: A critical examination. *Child Development, 53,* 11–28.

Chaffin, R., & Herrmann, D. J. (1983). Self reports of memory abilities by old and young adults. *Human Learning, 2,* 17–28.

Chi, M. T. H. (1985). Changing conceptions of sources of memory development. *Human Development, 28,* 50–56.

Dewey, J. (1908). What does pragmatism mean by practical? *Journal of Philosophy, Psychology and Scientific Methods, 5,* 85–99.

Dixon, R. A., & Hertzog, C. (1985). A functional approach to memory and metamemory development in adulthood. In F. E. Weinert & M. Perlmutter (Eds.), *Memory development across the life span: Universal changes and individual differences.* Hillsdale, NJ: Lawrence Erlbaum.

Dixon, R. A., Hertzog, C., & Hultsch, D. F. (1985a). *The multiple relationships between metamemory and cognitive abilities in adulthood.* Unpublished manuscript, Max Planck Institute for Human Development and Education, Berlin, West Germany.

Dixon, R. A., Hertzog, C., Schulenberg, J., & Hultsch, D. F. (1985b). *Adult age differences in the second-order factor structure of metamemory.* Paper presented at the eighth biennial meeting of the International Society for the Study of Behavioral Development, Tours, France.

Dixon, R. A., & Hultsch, D. F. (1983a). Metamemory and memory for text relationships in adulthood: A cross-validation study. *Journal of Gerontology, 38,* 689–694.

Dixon, R. A., & Hultsch, D. F. (1983b). Structure and development of metamemory in adulthood. *Journal of Gerontology, 38,* 682–688.

Dixon, R. A., & Hultsch, D. F. (1984). The Metamemory in Adulthood (MIA) instrument. *Psychological Documents, 14,* 3.

Dixon, R. A., Kramer, D. A., & Baltes, P. B. (1985). Intelligence: A life-span developmental perspective. In B. B. Wolman (Ed.), *Handbook of intelligence: Theories, measurements, and applications.* New York: Wiley.

Ekstrom, R. B., French, J. W., Harman, H. H., & Derman, D. (1976). *Manual for kit of factor-referenced cognitive tests.* Princeton, NJ: Educational Testing Service.

Erber, J. T. (1981). Remote memory and age: A review. *Experimental Aging Research, 7,* 189–199.

Ericsson, K. A., & Simon, H. A. (1980). Verbal reports as data. *Psychological Review, 87,* 215–251.

Flavell, J. H. (1971). First discussant's comments: What is memory development the development of? *Human Development, 14,* 272–278.

Flavell, J. H., & Wellman, H. M. (1977). Metamemory. In R. V. Kail, Jr., & J. W. Hagen (Eds.), *Perspectives on the development of memory and cognition.* Hillsdale, NJ: Lawrence Erlbaum.

Franklin, J. C., & Holding, D. H. (1977). Personal memories at different ages. *Quarterly Journal of Experimental Psychology, 29,* 527–532.

Gilewski, M. J., & Zelinski, E. M. (1983). *Assessment of memory complaints in the community-dwelling elderly.* Paper presented at the second George A. Talland Memorial Conference, Boston, MA.

Gilewski, M. J., Zelinski, E. M., Schaie, K. W., & Thompson, L. W. (1983). *Abbreviating the Metamemory Questionnaire: Factor structure and norms for adults.* Paper presented at the annual meeting of the American Psychological Association, Anaheim, CA.

Harris, J. E. (1980). Memory aids people use: Two interview studies. *Memory & Cognition, 8,* 31–38.

Herrmann, D. J. (1982). Know thy memory: The use of questionnaires to assess and study memory. *Psychological Bulletin, 92,* 434–452.

Herrmann, D. J. (1984). Questionnaires about memory. In J. E. Harris & P. E. Morris (Eds.), *Everyday memory, actions and absentmindedness* (pp. 133–154). London: Academic Press.

Herrmann, D. J., & Neisser, U. (1978). An inventory of everyday memory experiences. In M. M. Gruneberg, P. E. Morris, & R. N. Sykes (Eds.), *Practical aspects of memory* (pp. 35–51). London: Academic Press.

Hertzog, C., Dixon, R. A., & Hultsch, D. F. (1985a). *Assessment of short term change and fluctuation in memory and metamemory in adulthood.* Unpublished manuscript, College of Human Development, Pennsylvania State University, University Park. PA.

Hertzog, C., Dixon, R. A., Schulenberg, J., & Hultsch, D. F. (1985b). *Adult age differences in the factor structure of metamemory.* Paper presented at the 93rd annual meeting of the American Psychological Association, Los Angeles, CA.

Hulicka, I. M. (1982). Memory functioning in late adulthood. In F. I. M. Craik & S. Trehub (Eds.), *Aging and cognitive processes (pp. 331–351).* New York: Plenum Press.

Hultsch, D. F. (1984). *Memory perceptions and memory performance in adulthood and aging.* Paper presented to the Canadian Association on Gerontology, Vancouver, BC.

Hultsch, D. F., & Pentz, C. A. (1980). Encoding, storage, and retrieval in adult memory: The role of model assumptions. In L. W. Poon, J. L. Fozard, L. S. Cermak, D. Arenberg, & L. W. Thompson (Eds.), *New directions in memory and aging: Proceedings of the George A. Talland memorial conference* (pp. 73–94). Hillsdale, NJ: Lawrence Erlbaum.

James, W. (1980). *The principles of psychology* (Vol. 1). New York: Dover.

Martin, M., & Jones, G. V. (1984). Cognitive failures in everyday life. In J. E. Harris & P. E. Morris (Eds.), *Everyday memory, actions and absentmindedness.* London: Academic Press.

Morris, P. E. (1984). The validity of subjective reports on memory. In J. E. Harris & P. E. Morris (Eds.), *Everyday memory, actions and absentmindedness* (pp. 153–172). London: Academic Press.

Nesselroade, J. R. (1983). *Some implications of the trait–state distinction for the study of adult development and aging: "Still labile after all these years."* Paper presented at the 91st annual meeting of the American Psychological Association, Anaheim, CA.

Nisbett, R. E., & Wilson, T. D. (1977). Telling more than we can know: Verbal reports on mental processes. *Psychological Reivew, 84,* 231–259.

Perlmutter, M. (1978). What is memory aging the aging of? *Developmental Psychology, 14,* 330–345.

Perlmutter, M., Metzger, R., Miller, K., & Nezworski, T. (1980). Memory of historical events. *Experimental Aging Research, 6,* 46–60.

Poon, L. W., Fozard, J. L., Paulshock, D. L., & Thomas, J. C. (1979). A questionnaire assessment of age differences in retention of recent and remote events. *Experimental Aging Research, 5,* 401–411.

Riege, W. H. (1982). Self-report and tests of memory aging. *Clinical Gerontologist, 1,* 23–36.

Riegel, K. F. (1973). The recall of historical events. *Behavioral Science, 18,* 354–363.

Robinson, J. A. (1976). Sampling autobiographical memory. *Cognitive Psychology, 8,* 578–595.

Rubin, D. C. (1982). On the retention function for autobiographical memory. *Journal of Verbal Learning and Verbal Behavior, 21,* 21–38.

Salthouse, T. A., & Kausler, D. H. (1985). Memory methodology in maturity. In C. J. Brainerd & M. Pressley (Eds.), *Basic processes in memory development.* New York: Springer.

Schneider, W. (in press). Developmental trends in the metamemory–memory behavior relationship: An integrative review. In D. L. Forrest-Pressley, G. E. MacKinnon, & T. G. Waller (Eds.), *Cognition, metacognition and performance.* New York: Academic Press.

Sehulster, J. R. (1981a). Phenomenological correlates of a self theory of memory. *American Journal of Psychology, 94,* 527–537.

Sehulster, J. R. (1981b). Structure and pragmatics of a self-theory of memory. *Memory & Cognition, 9,* 263–276.

Sehulster, J. R. (1982). Phenomenological correlates of a self theory of memory, II: Dimensions of memory experience. *American Journal of Psychology, 95,* 441–454.

Sunderland, A., Harris, J. E., & Baddeley, A. P. (1984). Assessing everyday memory after severe head injury. In J. E. Harris & P. E. Morris (Eds.), *Everyday memory, actions and absent-mindedness* (pp. 191–206). London: Academic Press.

Waldfogel, S. (1948). The frequency and affective character of childhood memories. *Psychological Monographs, 62*(4, Whole No. 291).

Weinstein, C. E., Duffy, M., Underwood, V. L., MacDonald, J., & Gott, S. P. (1981). Memory strategies reported by older adults for experimental and everyday learning tasks. *Educational Gerontology, 7,* 205–213.

West, R. L., Boatwright, L. K., & Schleser, R. (1984). The link between memory performance, self-assessment, and affective status. *Experimental Aging Research, 10,* 197–200.

Williams, S. A., Denney, N. W., & Schadler, M. (1983). Elderly adults' perception of their own cognitive development during the adult years. *International Journal of Aging and Human Development, 16,* 147–158.

Willis, S. L., & Baltes, P. B. (1980). Intelligence in adulthood and aging: Contemporary issues. In L. W. Poon (Ed.), *Aging in the 1980s: Psychological issues* (pp. 260–272). Washington, DC: American Psychological Association.

Zarit, S. H. (1982). Affective correlates of self-reports about memory of older people. *International Journal of Behavioral Geriatrics, 1,* 25–34.

Zarit, S. H., Cole, K. D., & Guider, R. L. (1981). Memory training strategies and subjective complaints of memory in the aged. *Gerontologist, 21,* 158–164.

Zelinski, E. M., Gilewski, M. J., & Thompson, L. W. (1980). Do laboratory tests relate to self-assessment of memory ability in the young and old? In L. W. Poon, J. L. Fozard, L. S. Cermak, D. Arenberg, & L. W. Thompson (Eds.), *New directions in memory and aging: Proceedings of the George A. Talland memorial conference* (pp. 519–544). Hillsdale, NJ: Lawrence Erlbaum.

23 The importance of awareness in memory aging

John C. Cavanaugh

It's seven o'clock. The incessant chirping of the alarm rudely jolts you out of blissful slumber. In a seemingly reflex reaction, you grope around and silence the offender. Lying in the comfort of your bed, dreading the shock of cold floors, you begin to think. Even in your semiconscious state, you start remembering what the new day has in store: three committee meetings, class, several errands to run, a paper to write, a dentist appointment, and a very special dinner date. With a solemn promise to yourself that you won't (meaning can't) forget any of them, you finally get up and charge into the safety of a nice hot shower. During the day, you check the clock from time to time, talk to yourself about when the next appointment is, look at your calendar, and so on.

Embedded in these typical, everyday activities is a very intriguing notion: that we are aware that we need to remember things, that we tell ourselves to remember, and that we periodically check to see how we are doing. That awareness and memory are inextricably linked (Tulving, 1985) is obvious in everyday life. Unfortunately, it seems that memory researchers have been reluctant to recognize that fact (Hilgard, 1980; Miller, 1980; Neisser, 1979; Tulving, 1985). The goal of this chapter is to address this lack of concern, because the role of awareness in memory provides insights into memory development across adulthood.[1]

I could not have prepared this chapter without the help of many people. To all of my colleagues I owe a debt of gratitude for many fruitful discussions over the years at conferences, over the phone, and through the mails. Special thanks go to Cameron, Deirdre, Jan, Lennie, and Chris; they all kept me going through the tough times. You all helped shape the good points. The mistakes, of course, are all mine.

[1]Before presenting the framework I shall use throughout the remainder of this chapter, a few words about the use of the terms "consciousness" and "awareness" are in order. In some psychological writings on the topic, the terms "consciousness" and "awareness" have closely related, but not identical, meanings. For example, "consciousness" may refer to an ability of people to engage in self-reflective thinking, whereas "awareness" may refer to the subjective, phenomenally experienced outcome of self-reflective thinking in a specific situation. Stated somewhat differently, consciousness is what enables us to be

Three questions need to be considered in order for this goal to be met: (1) What are we aware of? (2) What is the experience of memory awareness like? (3) How does memory awareness change with age? This chapter will explore some answers to these questions from perspectives that differ from those that others have taken (Camp, Chapter 25, this volume; Dixon, Chapter 22, this volume). First, alternative approaches to defining what is meant by "awareness of memory" will be discussed. Second, different ways of operationalizing awareness will be described, along with a brief summary of the research examining age differences in these abilities. Finally, a framework that could serve as a guide to future research efforts will be presented. Thus, over the course of the chapter we shall see what kinds of things might be going on when we are aware of memory, why such an interesting and important topic has so many problems, how awareness fares with increasing age, and where such kinds of thinking might fit in the overall cognitive system.

Conceptual background and definitional issues

Interest in what people know about or are aware of concerning memory is an old topic in both philosophy and psychology (Cavanaugh & Perlmutter, 1982). Psychologists have dabbled with the topic for over 80 years, studying everything from reports of children's awareness of problem-solving strategies (Binet, 1903) to computer simulation of self-monitoring systems (Bobrow & Collins, 1975). Over the last few decades, what work that has been done on memory awareness has focused on the experience of awareness that one knows something (the feeling-of-knowing phenomenon), the self-awareness of monitoring or keeping track (executive processes), and the knowledge that certain persons or task factors make a memory task easier or harder (metamemory).

Contents and nature of memory awareness

The literatures that address what we are aware of concerning memory are largely empirical rather than theoretical. By far, the most extensive is that on metamemory. By now, it has become clear that each one of us has an extensive knowledge base about the many factors that influence memory (see Dixon, Chapter 22, this volume, for an extensive review). But there are few theories or models of how being aware of these different aspects of memory affects ongoing processing. Work in this area is progressing, and a model will be presented later.

The second literature that describes what we are aware of forms the crux of this chapter. It is when we monitor our memory processing that we become aware

aware of things. This distinction, however, tends to be somewhat arbitrary and difficult to maintain in practice. Consequently, throughout the remainder of this chapter, "awareness" and "consciousness" will be used interchangeably.

of what we are doing. Predicting how well we are going to do on a task is one example that has received considerable attention over the years. This literature will be considered in later sections.

In contrast to the empirical bases for what we know concerning the kinds of things people are aware of, most of what we know about the *nature* of awareness comes from philosophical considerations of it (Mandler, 1975; Natsoulas, 1981; Underwood, 1982). Although such a perspective is important, it is primarily theoretical, with little empirically derived supporting evidence. In the area of memory, the situation is particularly bad. At present, we have at best only a few rudimentary fragments of information about the nature of memory awareness. We know very little about what it feels like to be aware. We have no idea whether or not we have control over becoming aware. We do not know whether or not becoming aware is associated with particular emotions. We do not know why we are aware in some memory situations and not others. We do not know whether or not or how awareness changes with age. As a first step in addressing these gaps, the rest of this chapter presents some ideas about what the nature of awareness might be and what we might learn by looking at its development across adulthood.

As a way to start, I propose that memory awareness be viewed as being composed of three fundamentally different categories (Klatzky, 1984): *systemic awareness, epistemic awareness,* and *on-line awareness.* The boundaries among them are not sharp, and the definitions are not yet refined, but they provide a first approximation. The distinctions, as will become clear, are based on criteria that are more empirically than theoretically derived at present. In particular, the three subtypes are derived from different forms of verbal-report data, such as surveys, on-line measures, and interviews, which in turn are based on different operational definitions of awareness. Even without a strong theoretical basis, however, these three categories serve to highlight key differences in memory awareness that have important developmental implications. For example, it may be the case that certain kinds of awareness show normative change with age and others do not. Such a differential pattern of change could shed a new light on the literature on memory aging as a whole. More important, though, is that focusing attention on categories of memory awareness forces us to consider the person doing the processing to a far greater extent than has been typical. It will also bring the study of memory out of the days when it was examined as if we were studying computer hardware to a point that will allow researchers to take a more subjective and holistic perspective. [An excellent discussion of the advantages of this research perspective is given by Lincoln & Guba (1985).] The differences in focus of the various forms of awareness will become clearer in the following sections.

Systemic awareness. Systemic awareness is awareness of facts about memory, in other words, awareness of the memory system and how it works. It has been argued (Cavanaugh & Perlmutter, 1982) that systemic awareness is what was originally meant by the term "metamemory." It involves information that can be put into the form "I know that. . . . " For instance, most people know that recall typically is harder than recognition, that mnemonic devices often are helpful, and that short-term memory capacity is not limitless. This is the kind of awareness that is routinely assessed in memory questionnaires and metamemory interviews. More is known about this category of awareness than any other. (For a more complete discussion of systemic awareness, see Dixon, Chapter 22, this volume.)

Epistemic awareness. The ability to know about the extent and soundness of one's general knowledge base is what is meant by epistemic awareness. In other words, epistemic awareness is knowledge about one's own knowledge base. The notion here is that at times we must make judgments about whether or not we know something, how well we know it, or how sure we are that what we know is correct. Such occasions include eyewitness testimony (e.g., Are we sure it was the defendant we saw?), the feeling of knowing (e.g., Haven't we met before?), awareness of the sources of memory (e.g., Am I remembering it from personal experience or from someone's description?), awareness of the reliability of memory (e.g., If I remember it today, can I count on remembering it next week?), and awareness of changes in knowledge states (e.g., I know things now that I did not know before.). Epistemic awareness occurs during the retrieval process, when the judgment about our knowledge is made (Klatzky, 1984). Two applications of epistemic awareness that have received attention from cognitive-developmental researchers are described in other chapters: expert systems (Charness, Chapter 24, this volume) and the difference between perceived and generated memories (Cohen & Faulkner, Chapter 14, this volume).

On-line awareness. On-line awareness is the type that concerns us most in this chapter. It refers to the awareness of ongoing memory processes and has been described as memory monitoring or, more generally, as executive processes. We can be aware of the *process* of remembering in many different ways. Sometimes it is the awareness of how we are studying, or how we are making a systematic search of memory for some particular fact, or the experience of remembering an episode from our past. At other times, on-line awareness occurs as questions we ask ourselves while doing a memory task; for example, when faced with having to remember an appointment later in the day, we might consciously ask ourselves if the steps we have taken (writing a note) are sufficient.

Categories of awareness compared

There are important distinctions to note about the three types of awareness. They differ not only in terms of their focus but also on another interesting dimension. Note that systemic awareness relates to stored content knowledge about memory. When we experience systemic awareness, we are simply aware of some "fact." It is fundamentally a static phenomenon. Contrast this with the other two types. In them, we are no longer talking about being aware of stored content knowledge. Rather, we are referring to types of awareness in relation to some ongoing cognitive activity, whether it is the outcome of a judgment process (epistemic awareness) or the activity itself (on-line awareness). Although epistemic and on-line awareness may appear static at times (as when the awareness is of the outcome of some series of cognitive events), they really reflect a much more dynamic process that has to do with how these types of awareness come about. Both epistemic awareness and on-line awareness have to do with cognitive operations performed on some kind of stored content, whereas systemic awareness concerns content per se. Finally, epistemic awareness and on-line awareness would seem to require a specific situation involving memory processing in which to operate. It would appear unreasonable to suggest that one is aware that one is memorizing, for example, if in fact there is no memorization taking place. Systemic awareness, on the other hand, can be readily experienced without on-going memory processing, as has been repeatedly demonstrated in survey and interview studies, which present participants with hypothetical situations concerning memory (e.g., Suppose you needed to remember your umbrella. How would you do it?).

The lack of independence of the different types of awareness should also be stressed. Each affects the others. For example, suppose one has a tip-of-the-tongue experience (recognizes a familiar face, cannot recall the name, but knows that it is known), an instance of epistemic awareness, and begins to search the knowledge base. Systemic awareness (e.g., being aware that thinking about related events often aids retrieval) could help focus the search. Meanwhile, on-line awareness could help keep track of how well the search is going. The point is that whereas the divisions suggested earlier provide a heuristic that enables us to consider and account for several important developmental phenomena, we must not lose sight of the fact that in the person's head the types of awareness form an interacting set.

The focus of the remainder of this chapter is on how people experience on-line awareness and on how this experience is related to age across adulthood. In our consideration of this topic, several questions should be kept in mind. What are some of the conditions under which on-line awareness occurs? How often and how reliably do people experience it? How does on-line awareness change with age? Of what practical importance is it? How can we account for the patterns that we observe? How should we investigate it? These and other issues will be treated as we go. Throughout the discussion, emphasis will be on developmental trends and on implications for practical, everyday memory situations.

In summary, awareness of memory can take three forms: systemic awareness (awareness of facts about memory), epistemic awareness (awareness of the validity of knowledge), and on-line awareness (awareness of ongoing memory processing). Although the distinctions among them are somewhat arbitrary, the three categories highlight the point that we are aware of different aspects of memory and that they may have different developmental courses.

On-line awareness: Predicting performance

Recall that on-line awareness refers to one's conscious knowledge of what one is currently doing cognitively (e.g., what one is currently thinking about). If we accept the assumption that our cognitive systems have a way of keeping track or monitoring ongoing thought, then on-line awareness is our conscious experience of that monitoring. There is no implication, of course, that we are always aware of everything that is going on. On the contrary, we are aware of only a fraction of the monitoring process; see Lachman and Lachman (1980) and Langer (1981) for extensive discussions of this point. The present discussion is limited to only those times when we are aware. Additionally, I believe that the monitoring process itself is a dynamic one, with continual flow of information to and from various knowledge bases and other parts of the memory system. As indicated earlier, the point is that the various categories of awareness set important boundary conditions and constraints on each other.

On-line awareness has been examined from a limited number of perspectives in adult developmental research. Almost all of them are variations on one simple theme: predicting how well one will do on a memory task. Generally speaking, there are two major ways that performance predictions are obtained. One technique requires that people predict how well they think they will perform on a task prior to actually doing it. In the other method, predictions are obtained after participants have seen the task (e.g., studied the list). Both approaches are based on the idea that predicting performance demands monitoring of current memory processing and, in the case of having a chance to study, self-testing of how well one believes that an item has been learned. Research based on the two different approaches has resulted in two different views of age-related developmental trends.

Predictions without experience

In general, studies examining the accuracy of predictions made prior to actually performing the task have documented a tendency for older adults to overestimate how well they will do (Bruce, Coyne, & Botwinick, 1982; Coyne, 1983; Mason, 1981; Murphy, Sanders, Gabriesheski, & Schmitt, 1981). That is, older adults typically predict that they will be able to remember more items than they will actually recall.

Nondevelopmental aging research does not support the overestimation finding. Camp, Markley, and Kramer (1983) asked older adults to predict recall from a 15-item list of words that were high in imagery, frequency, concreteness, and meaningfulness. Older adults underestimated their performance when they were asked to think about the strategies that they might use. Similarly, Berry, West, and Scogin (1983) found that older adults underestimated performance for both laboratory and everyday memory tasks, although accuracy was better for everyday tasks. Berry and associates also found that the best memorizers were the people with the best on-line awareness; the correlation between prediction accuracy and performance was .60.

Predictions after experience

A much different picture emerges when the participants study the list first, for example, and then make judgments (e.g., through confidence ratings) about whether or not they will remember the item. Results from several studies using this approach (Lovelace, Marsh, & Oster, 1982; Perlmutter, 1978; Rabinowitz, Ackerman, Craik, & Hinchley, 1982) have demonstrated that older adults are just as accurate in predicting their recall and recognition performance as younger adults. (It should be noted that, on average, people of all ages overestimate performance on recall tests and underestimate performance on recognition tests, a phenomenon that should be examined more closely by those wishing to understand systemic awareness.)

A second method used to investigate performance prediction after having task experience involves a combination of the feeling-of-knowing paradigm and retrieval from tertiary memory. The method involves having participants respond to questions that force them to make inferences about pieces of general information that typically are not already stored (e.g., What horror-movie character would starve in northern Sweden in the summer?). Reports of the processing involved in answering are sometimes obtained. Age differences have not been found in studies examining this issue (Lachman & Lachman, 1980; Lachman, Lachman, & Taylor, 1982; Lachman, Lachman, & Thronesberry, 1979). A more complete discussion of these studies is provided by Camp (Chapter 25, this volume).

Factors influencing predictions

In view of the research findings we have reviewed, there are two conflicting data sets that lead to two opposing conclusions about the pattern of age-related differences in predicting performance. Older adults clearly are hindered if they must predict before having some experience with the task, but may do just as well as younger adults if experience is allowed. Why should this be? Is it really just a matter of experience (e.g., being able to study for a bit) that makes the difference? It appears that this is true, but that raises another sticky issue. Just what is it about experience with the task that makes the difference? The answer to this question is not so obvious.

A few investigators have attempted to uncover some of the determinants of older adults' estimations. Most of these studies have pointed to interactions between task demands and person (knowledge) factors as the critical elements. It must be kept in mind, however, that no one study has considered more than a handful of factors at a time.

Recall that older adults are at a disadvantage when no clear task knowledge or task demands are provided before making predictions. One consistent finding from metamemory research is that older adults seem to be less aware of the nature of task demands and how they influence performance (e.g., differential difficulty of recall versus recognition tests) (Dixon, Chapter 22, this volume). On the basis of these data, one factor that may be responsible for overestimation of performance is a basic lack of metamemorial knowledge about the nature of the task demands. If one does not realize that a task is difficult, one may predict performance on the assumption that it is easy, leading to an overestimation of actual performance.

In contrast, what and how much older adults know about specific aspects concerning their own personal abilities (another category of systemic awareness) do not differ from those for younger adults (Cavanaugh, 1986–87). Interestingly, in situations that involve a large component of knowledge of personal abilities, older adults do not tend to overestimate their performance (Berry et al., 1983; Camp et al., 1983). It appears that to the extent a situation taps personal knowledge, or is familiar (Berry et al., 1983), systemic awareness affects the prediction decision. This finding provides one possible explanation for the lack of age differences in some research. It may be that the tasks presented in these cases tapped extensive systemic awareness related to personal memory ability that was used to make realistic predictions.

In summary, research on developmental differences in performance prediction has documented two distinct patterns. When provided with very little or no information about the task, younger adults are more accurate than older adults at predicting how well they will do. However, when participants are given some experience with the task, older adults and younger adults are equally accurate. These findings highlight the importance of relevant experience as a factor in predicting how well one will do.

Practical memory: On-line awareness revisited

Thus far, on-line awareness has been described as predicting one's performance. But this is not the only way nor perhaps the best way to view it. Let us return to the opening scenario for additional vantage points. It is apparent that on-line awareness refers broadly to the whole experience of knowing that we are doing something cognitively at a given moment. So, realizing that I have three committee meetings that I must not forget and checking the clock from time to time involve on-line awareness. Note that nowhere in this example does the idea of performance prediction appear (in the sense reviewed earlier). The omission is intentional. On-line awareness does not appear as performance prediction in everyday, practical memory, at least not very often. It happens more like it was portrayed in the example: a fleeting awareness of something that needs to be remembered, a feeling that we know what we are thinking about, an awareness of the need to keep track of what is going on in our heads so that we can do what needs to be done, a realization of when things are going right or wrong, and so on.

Tulving (1985) has raised a very provocative notion in this regard. He states categorically that the very act of remembering *requires* awareness. Tulving partitions memory into three systems: procedural, semantic, and episodic. It is the episodic system (responsible for mediating personally experienced events) that relates to remembering, hence directly to inherent awareness. He argues that episodic memory maps onto "autonoetic" consciousness, that is, self-knowing. It is autonoetic awareness that is responsible for the subjective feelings associated with the experience of remembering. In contrast, Tulving believes that our awareness of semantic knowledge (the system responsible for the symbolically representable knowledge about the world) is subjectively different. To denote the difference, he refers to awareness of semantic memory as "noetic"; that is, it is characterized by "knowing," rather than remembering. Subjectively, the experiences are quite different. "Remembering" is felt to be potent, or more compelling; "knowing" feels fuzzier.

The importance of Tulving's ideas for the present discussion lies mainly in two areas. First, most of the kinds of things we need to monitor either prospectively or retrospectively in everyday life involve the episodic system (e.g., dentist appointment, taking an umbrella to work). If Tulving is correct in linking remembering and awareness, this means that we will be aware of what is going on, no matter how briefly. When we are aware of our monitoring of episodic memory, autonoetic consciousness and on-line awareness are synonymous. In other words, on-line awareness occurs every time we retrieve something from episodic memory. This must be the case. Even if only for a moment, we are aware of the fact that we are remembering an appointment; such things simply do not happen unconsciously.

Second, Tulving's notion of noetic consciousness seems to be similar to both systemic and epistemic awareness. All of these ideas refer to "knowing" rather than "remembering," because systemic awareness is knowing about memory, whereas epistemic awareness is knowing about the adequacy of our knowledge base. Whether or not the relationship between these concepts is also based on the fact that systemic awareness and epistemic awareness both involve semantic memory only is unclear; no discussion of the issue has been undertaken in the literature.

Tulving's position forces cognitive-developmentalists to rethink memory research efforts, especially those that involve the episodic system. A reevaluation and refocusing effort means that we must take a much broader perspective in future research. Taking this broader perspective will allow us to tackle the key issues better than ever before: mapping the patterns of age differences in the various types of awareness; exploring developmental changes in the relationship between degree of awareness and memory performance across adulthood; investigating the factors responsible for individual differences in awareness. To achieve this broader perspective, it will be necessary to take several alternative viewpoints of on-line awareness. It is to this topic we now turn.

Alternative views of on-line awareness

Investigators of adults' memory development have not examined on-line awareness in alternative ways to any great extent. Most of what we know from a memory perspective comes mainly from a few diary studies (Cavanaugh, Grady, & Perlmutter, 1983; West, 1984). Although the evidence is indirect, we shall see from these studies that older and younger adults may be aware of similar things concerning memory that lead them to plan to remember in similar ways (e.g., use the same kinds of strategies). However, the on-line awareness experience appears to differ qualitatively with age concerning forgetting.

Memory diaries. In order to examine age differences in everyday memory experiences, Cavanaugh and associates (1983) had non-college-student younger and older adults keep diaries of their memory experiences 1 day per week for 4 consecutive weeks. Participants were asked to describe each use of memory aids and each memory failure as soon as possible after it occurred by making entries in pocket-size notebooks. For each episode of forgetting or of using a memory aid, individuals were instructed to record the time of day, place, what the incident involved, and its importance. For episodes of forgetting, participants were also told to indicate their personal feelings about the memory failure and what they did when they realized they had forgotten something. For episodes of using memory aids, they were also told to note the type of aid used and how far into the future the to-be-remembered incident was to occur.

The results revealed no overall differences in the frequency of use of memory aids as a function of age. In addition, no differences were seen regarding the type of aids used; both age groups used external aids (e.g., lists, calendars, spouses) far more often than internal aids (e.g., rehearsal, imagery). A lack of differences also was found for the time of day that memory aids were used, the importance of the information to be remembered, and the time into the future that the information was to be remembered.

In sharp contrast, several age-related differences were found for the forgetting data. Older adults reported almost twice as many instances of forgetting, and they reported forgetting more names, routines, and objects, in particular. No overall differences emerged when the importance ratings were examined. However, older adults were significantly more upset about forgetting at all levels of self-rated importance. Finally, memory failures tended to occur most frequently when people were out of their normal routine, tired, required to retrieve information that had not been used recently, were not concentrating, or were under stress. Interestingly, older adults most often mentioned problems occurring when they were out of their normal routine or being asked for information not used recently, whereas younger adults most often reported failures when they were under stress.

These data are admittedly preliminary. But they do force us to consider several things. First, the evidence obtained by Cavanaugh and associates corroborates that obtained by others (Harris, 1980), indicating that in everyday life, people tend not to use the memory strategies investigated most intensively (e.g., imagery), but prefer external strategies (e.g., making lists). These data also call into question the conclusion drawn by many reviewers of the memory-strategy literature that older adults do not use memory strategies spontaneously as often as younger adults. It may be true regarding internal mnemonics, but may not be true about external mnemonics, a finding replicated by West (1984) in a subsequent study. Finally, the results also point to the need for more intensive research aimed at understanding the subjective experience of remembering and the role that on-line awareness plays in it.

Prospective memory. Another way to examine on-line awareness is to investigate the processes involved in planning for future retrieval. This topic, termed "prospective memory," has a large component of monitoring and control processes, which means that on-line awareness is implicated. Sinnott (Chapter 20, this volume) provides a thorough review of this literature. The key feature of this research is that on-line awareness is a very important element in prospective memory. For example, lack of awareness of good planning may make it difficult to remember information when it is needed, and absentmindedness is characterized by a lack of awareness of what one is doing. Although it appears that prospective memory research has implications for understanding age differences in on-line awareness, very little of this work has been done with older adults; so its complete contribution cannot be assessed as yet. For our purposes, the most important point from this literature concerns the connection between awareness and forgetting – without awareness, one is rather oblivious to memory failures. Typically, such forgetting without awareness is termed absentmindedness.

Awareness and forgetting

Of all the possible questions one can ask concerning awareness and memory aging, I believe that the most intriguing one relates awareness and forgetting. The question is this: If we fail to retrieve information at the time we should do so, and we are not aware of our failure, is it a true episode of personal forgetting? In other words, does someone (either ourselves or someone else) need to be aware of our memory failure for it to be called forgetting? If the answer to this question is yes, then it would appear that forgetting represents another case of the inextricable link between memory (or, in this case, memory failure) and awareness. It also means that absentmindedness and forgetting are two different things. If these speculations are true, then it also seems that on-line awareness should be the key link involved in both remembering and forgetting.

These issues are not idle philosophical exercises. To the extent that they implicate awareness as a necessary condition for forgetting, then understanding on-line awareness becomes a necessary condition for understanding memory and its development in the fullest sense. Those of us concerned with how on-line awareness is related to age need to consider this idea carefully. Recall that older adults have been shown to report more instances of forgetting and to demonstrate a higher concern about it in everyday life (Cavanaugh et al., 1983; Poon, 1985). Are these findings indicative only of purely quantitative, inevitable changes in memory processing qua processing? Or could they be at least in part a reflection of age-related increases in on-line awareness? Might there be a systematic and normative increase with age in the amount of on-line awareness we experience? Such an increase likely would result in more frequent realization of memory failures. It could be speculated that once this happened, the level of concern about failing memory would rise, which could result in still more monitoring, leading to more awareness, and so on. This scenario provides a plausible account of the widely reported increase in memory complaints with age that is largely unrelated to memory performance (Poon, 1985) and the increase with age in concern about forgetting (Cavanaugh et al., 1983).

Note that it does not follow from these speculations that a rise in awareness is necessarily accompanied by a rise in the actual rate of forgetting. Several things could be happening. For example, there may be little increase in the actual rate of forgetting, but a large increase in awareness of failures that previously went unnoticed. Or there could be a normative moderate increase in both forgetting and awareness of it. Or the increase in monitoring and its results could cause a subsequent increase in actual forgetting. The point is that we need not infer large increases in actual forgetting with age just because that is what people say happens. Rather, we must begin to uncover the extent to which increases in awareness of forgetting influence the subjective reporting of it, independent of its rate. Perhaps by pursuing this idea we can begin to understand the reasons for the apparent lack of relationship between memory complaints and memory performance.

In summary, Tulving (1985) has argued that remembering in everyday life requires awareness. His conceptualization of awareness can be subsumed into the present scheme and should be extended to include forgetting. Research involving memory diaries and prospective memory has shown that there may be a developmental shift in the importance of on-line awareness, especially in terms of awareness of forgetting. It is argued that the increase in memory complaints that often is seen as adults age may be the result of increased awareness of memory failures, not necessarily a reflection of an actual increase in the rate of forgetting.

A proposed research agenda

Given the thrust of this review, it should come as no surprise that we need considerably more work on developmental aspects of on-line awareness. We are especially in need of information about four things: What is the nature of the subjective experience of on-line awareness for adults of different ages? What is the role of on-line awareness in planful, prospective memory as people age? How are forgetting and on-line awareness related, and does this relationship change developmentally? How does the interaction between on-line awareness and other types of awareness change with age?

As indicated earlier, on-line awareness is an important aspect of everyday, practical memory. It is on-line awareness that reminds us to get to a meeting or that one's time is running out during a presentation. But what we do not know is whether or not the *subjective* experiences of these things are similar for younger and older adults. Does everyone think about and feel the same kinds of things? Does on-line awareness for two individuals happen at similar times and under similar circumstances? What makes it happen?

Second, we need to learn much more about the role that on-line awareness plays in prospective memory. We know something about how the prediction function works in a few circumscribed situations, but very little about other equally important issues. For example, does the ability to keep track of ongoing cognitive activity (e.g., monitor the time for an upcoming dinner date) vary as a function of age? Are older adults differentially aware of the times when they use deliberate memory strategies (e.g., making lists), as compared with young adults? These questions can be cast in a number of frameworks, from cognitive psychological ones, such as production systems (Anderson, 1976), to social cognitive ones, such as Langer's distinction (1981) between mindlessness and mindfulness. Regardless of the framework, more work needs to be directed at uncovering how on-line awareness helps us remember.

Likewise, we need a better understanding of forgetting, both empirically and theoretically. As developmentalists interested in adults, we should take a special interest in this topic. After all, forgetting is the focus of most people's understanding of memory development and aging, at least in an everyday context. One does not hear very many people talking about changes in the use of mnemonics with age; people tend to talk about forgetting. But what *is* forgetting? It is not just the flip side of remembering, according to most cognitive theorists. It is a poorly understood process, one with few well-thought-out theories. Consequently, it is time that researchers in adult developmental memory begin to increase their efforts toward understanding forgetting, both objectively and subjectively. As argued earlier, we need to determine whether or not part of the increase in reported forgetting is due to a connection between forgetting and the amount of on-line awareness.

Finally, we need to map out the kinds of interactions that exist among the different types of awareness. We need to see whether or not certain of them operate at different times or under different situations. We need to understand whether or not deficiencies in one area are compensated for by another.

How might we tackle these tasks? The answer lies in pursuing two goals simultaneously: applying better methods and developing theoretical models. The key is to mount a series of intensive, descriptive-exploratory studies aimed at fully understanding on-line awareness and how it varies with age. The approach would combine carefully organized self-report research (e.g., diaries, questionnaires, interviews) with laboratory studies in order to map out the nature of on-line awareness and its boundary conditions. Both of these approaches could include elements of existing methods from nondevelopmental cognitive and social-cognitive research (e.g., talk-aloud methods, confidence ratings), as well as clinical interview and assessment techniques. Such a multifocused attack would provide the basic information needed for future follow-up investigations of the factors responsible for on-line awareness. In these efforts, most attention should be paid to the kinds of memory situations we face in everyday life.

But the real key to understanding where on-line awareness fits in memory development ultimately lies in developing theoretical models to guide our research. Currently, we do not have a single theory from which we can generate testable predictions of how on-line awareness develops across adulthood. All we have are a few descriptive tidbits. That, perhaps, is the glaring weakness in the field, a weakness that must be corrected. There have already been a few beginnings [for some examples, see Poon (1985)], some of which I shall use for my point of departure. Bear in mind, however, that each of the topics I have discussed is fruitful territory for such theoretical endeavors.

In the following sections are discussions of some directions that we could take. They are aimed at stimulating new and innovative approaches to the problem of awareness and memory. First, I shall outline a model that includes the major points raised throughout this chapter that can be used to formulate formal, testable intuitions about the context in which awareness operates in memory. This model is a revision and extension of one presented previously (Cavanaugh, Kramer, Sinnott, Camp, & Markley, 1985). Second, some ideas on the specific types of research needed to examine the role and development of awareness and memory will be offered. This section will focus on how we might use new approaches to old questions; readers interested in more formal critiques of research methods in this area should consult Cavanaugh and Perlmutter (1982), Dixon (Chapter 22, this volume), and Ericssen and Simon (1984).

Some theoretical suggestions

Developing an adequate theoretical framework depends on examining the role of awareness in memory from several perspectives, as argued earlier. The outcome of this examination will be a framework that includes awareness explicitly, specifies where on-line awareness fits into the system, and identifies the main influences on on-line awareness. Of course, specifying these aspects necessitates advancing a more general account of memory processing as well. The next section briefly outlines a theoretical framework that takes all of these points into account.

A model proposal

Elsewhere (Cavanaugh et al., 1985), I have outlined a first approximation to a model for the selection of memory strategies. In that model, several variables influence the decision to use particular kinds of memory strategies. These variables include Experience, Task Demands, Situational Context, Knowledge, Personality, Beliefs, and Motivation. Feedback from the strategy-selection decision and memory performance was included as one way that the system could learn and, more important, develop.

Although this model provides a framework within which one can conceptualize how decisions to use particular memory strategies are made, it has several limitations. Most important, the model focuses on the selection of memory strategies. Despite the importance of this activity, it is clear from the present discussion that many other aspects of memory and forgetting need to be included. Consequently, the model should address these issues, or at least be flexible enough to allow for future modifications.

In order to have a more complete account of memory experience, I believe that additional constructs are necessary. To tie these in with the earlier discussion, they would include such things as how memory situations are perceived by the individual, environmental input (e.g., corroborative feedback concerning the frequency of forgetting), and intellectual factors. Depending on what the focus of the investigation would be, the criterion variable could be performance on a memory task, or the subjective experience of the person. In either case, an appropriate model would be sufficiently flexible so as to be adaptable to remembering or forgetting experiences.

An example of a more complete model is presented in Figure 23.1. In considering it, several things should be noted. The directional flow of memory processing is clearly based mostly on theoretical speculation rather than on hard empirical evidence. The reasons for this, of course, have been argued in the previous sections; the research addressing the issues has yet to be done. Second, I have attempted to present a general framework that applies to several different kinds of memory situations. Third, the connections between the various steps in the process and awareness are made explicit. This is especially important because I believe that an important shift occurs with age in how we focus on the different categories of awareness. Finally, it argues that memory processing is not simply a matter of cold processing of information in a computerlike fashion. Instead, it proposes that memory processing is affected by a host of factors that are related to personality (e.g., personality structure, efficacy judgments, and motivation) and social context.

As presently conceived, the proposed model offers a framework in which future research on memory awareness can be conceived and interpreted. Most important, it offers many testable ideas on how various aspects of the memory system work and are interrelated. This alone represents a major step forward, even if it turns out that the proposed model is inadequate. Moreover, it provides a focus for research examining whether or not particular connections develop at different times, whether or not certain connections are more important at some times than at others, or whether or not some connections disappear with age.

One important developmental aspect to test in the model concerns the relative importance of the links involving awareness. It is my belief that there is a change from systemic-awareness dominance in young adulthood to on-line-awareness

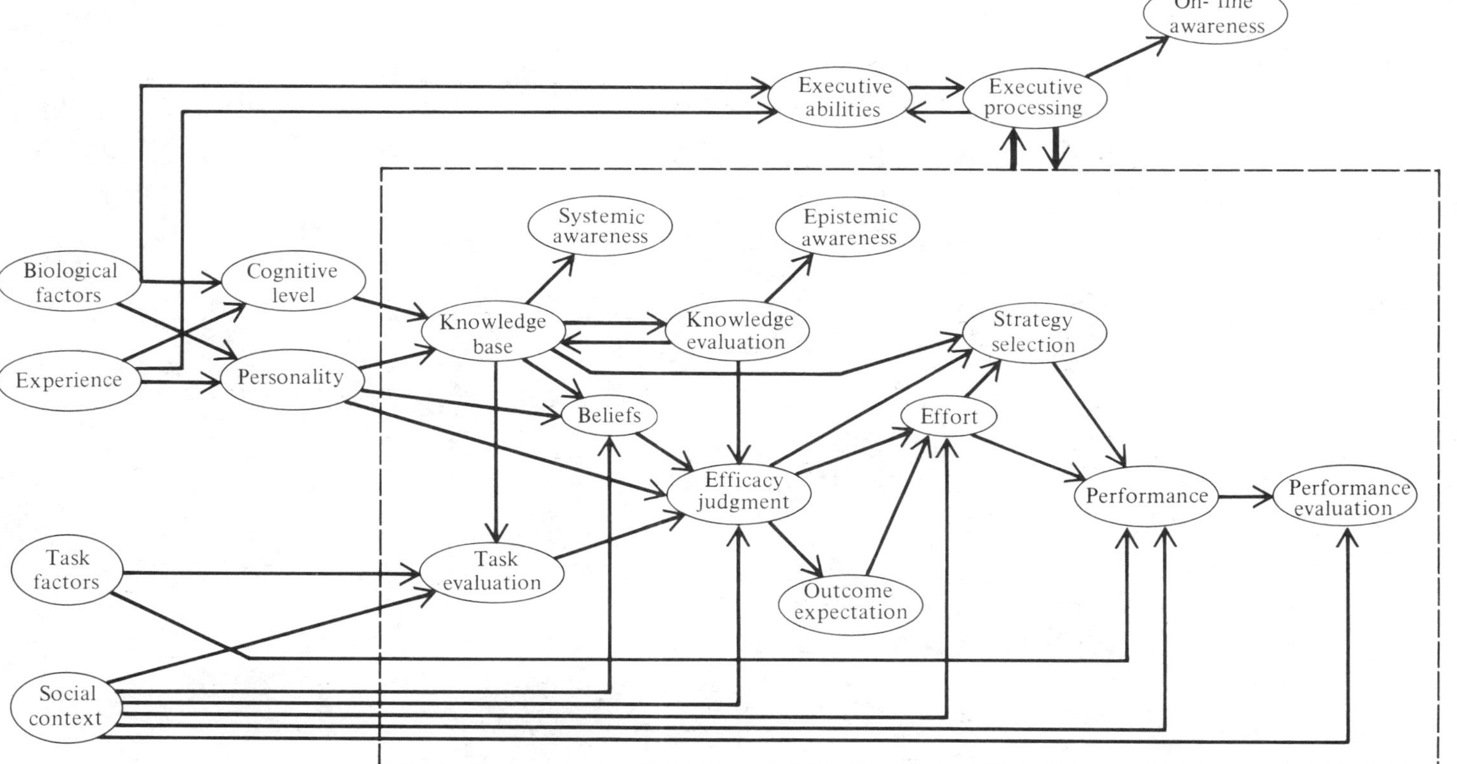

Figure 23.1. Conceptual model of the relationships involving memory and awareness. The model represents the complex state of affairs concerning the central role of self-reflection and evaluation at any one point in time. Note that Executive Processing constitutes those Executive Abilities that are currently being used. Additionally, Executive Processing influences and is influenced by all of the constructs inside the broken-line box. This model is an expansion of one presented earlier (Cavanaugh et al., 1985).

dominance in old age. In causal modeling terms, this change means that the magnitudes of the coefficients for paths involving systemic awareness should decrease with age, whereas those involving on-line awareness should increase with age. In practical terms, what it means is that we go from being concerned about knowing facts about memory (e.g., the most effective way to memorize) to being concerned about whether or not we are in fact remembering.

This hypothesized shift fits with research reviewed by Dixon (Chapter 22, this volume) and West (Chapter 30, this volume) showing that in some respects older adults tend not to demonstrate as much content knowledge as younger adults about some aspects of memory. However, as pointed out earlier in this chapter, when it comes to keeping track of ongoing processing, older adults are at least as good most of the time, and in some cases they may be even more sensitive. Given the nature of the other relationships in the proposed model, one would also predict age differences at any point past the knowledge-base level; indeed, there is considerable evidence for such differences in many task situations, as noted by most of the authors in this volume.

Where would we most likely see the impact of the shift to on-line awareness dominance? The model predicts that Efficacy Judgment is where the action is. Theoretically, young adults' personal competency judgments should be based on prior knowledge, whereas older adults' judgments should be based more on prior actions. Additionally, the influence of Social Context on Beliefs, and subsequently on Efficacy Judgments, should increase with age, but especially in those individuals who accept the stereotype of memory failure. This latter situation would help account for the lack of a consistent relationship between memory complaints and memory performance, because Efficacy Judgment represents only one of many mediated influences on performance.

Overall, the proposed model points out the fact that awareness and memory are vastly more complicated than one would suspect given the extant literature. The fact that personality, among other things, influences memory performance certainly makes things complex. But what this complexity does is force us to consider how memory development fits into the broader scheme of adult development, something that memory-development researchers have been largely reluctant to do; studies by Lachman (Lachman & McArthur, 1986) and by Langer (1981) are notable exceptions.

The broader picture

A long-range goal for researchers dealing with on-line awareness ought to be putting it in the broader perspective of adult development and aging. Many of the ideas discussed here are reminiscent of ideas discussed in other literatures. For example, I speculated that there may be an increase in on-line awareness with age that is reflected in increased monitoring of forgetting. This increase could be seen as an increase in self-reflection in the memory domain. From the personality-development literature, we know that there is an age-related increase in interiority (Neugarten, 1977) that is reflected in several behaviors, from increased introspection, as part of the move toward ego integrity (Erikson, 1980), to the life review or reminiscence process. Consequently, the potential increase in on-line awareness may be the memory component of a more general movement inward.

Going a step further, the normative developmental patterns observed for on-line awareness may add to our understanding of the differences between normal and abnormal aging. Perhaps the behaviors seen in depression concerning complaints about memory difficulties are related to changes in on-line monitoring. The degree to which on-line awareness is operating "correctly" could be one reason for the difference between a depressed person's emphasis on a memory problem and another patient's seeming denial. Maybe some types of psychopathology are characterized by abnormally increased levels of awareness of how many times we think (or actually notice that) memory fails. This potential increase could be due to being abnormally more vigilant, to a change in underlying neurological processes, or to some complex interaction among memory processes and the prevailing social stereotypes linking age, memory loss, and "senility." Similar speculations are offered by Cohen and Faulkner (Chapter 14, this volume), indicating that there is growing concern about the interface between research on normative developmental changes in memory and various forms of psychopathology.

At this point it is too early to draw any firm conclusions about where the development of on-line awareness fits in the grand scheme of things. Nor do the examples raised here exhaust the points of contact. Nevertheless, we need to keep in mind the eventual need to place this area in context and continue to work toward this goal.

Methodological issues

One of the things that should be apparent from our earlier discussion is that there are various ways to study on-line awareness. Such diversity is good, but we must not lose sight of the need to use reliable and valid methods. Unfortunately, we have almost no information about the soundness of the methods currently being used to investigate on-line awareness. Clearly, the first thing that needs to be done is to establish the reliability and validity of our methods (Ericssen & Simon, 1984).

There are several measures of on-line awareness that provide important information, but currently they either are underused or are narrowly identified with a particular way of defining awareness. Chief among these are confidence ratings, talk-aloud methods, and interviews.

Confidence ratings are currently used predominantly by researchers interested in performance prediction and the feeling-of-knowing phenomenon. However, they could be used with any operationalization of on-line awareness. For example, confidence ratings could be used in conjunction with diaries; the degree of confidence that a particular way of planning for future retrieval will work could be obtained for each entry.

Talk-aloud methods have been used most often in the problem-solving literature. However, some of the data obtained in these studies provide a good measure of on-line awareness. For example, Giambra (1984) used this method to study task-unrelated thought intrusions. One should build on Giambra's work by having participants provide accounts of their thinking (both task-related and unrelated) in many situations. These records could, for example, provide insights into the cognitive processes resulting in older adults' overestimations. Ericssen and Simon (1984) provide a thorough critique of this method and how it can be used to describe thinking.

In-depth interviews can be extremely helpful in mapping out interesting issues and clarifying other data. Asking several adults to describe their experiences with on-line awareness in considerable detail would provide a number of interesting issues to pursue that might have escaped us otherwise. Additionally, including an interview at the conclusion of a study will allow the researcher to explore important issues about memory with the participants without affecting their performance and will aid in clarifying the participants' responses, if needed. This step is essential if our goal is to understand what is going on in the participants' heads; see Lincoln and Guba (1985) for more on the need for follow-up interviews.

The ideal study of on-line awareness would include several of these and other methods (e.g., performance prediction, questionnaires, diaries). Only by combining several methods will we improve our understanding of on-line awareness and its place in memory aging. However, simply putting two or three methods together is not all that is necessary. We need to choose the best methods for the job and use those that will yield the best data based on our theoretical perspective. In short, we need to move toward theory-driven selection of methods to complement the currently dominant problem-driven approach.

In summary, a model is proposed that explicitly outlines the place of awareness in memory. Additionally, it is shown that memory is heavily influenced by a host of factors related to social context, personality, and judgments about one's ability. Clearly, the picture is complex, but the model offers testable intuitions about the locus of key developmental change. In particular, it is predicted that there is a shift from systemic-awareness dominance to on-line-awareness dominance with increasing age. It is also argued that there is a need to place memory development in the broader context of adult development in view of the considerable overlap among the forces that shape both. Finally, it is pointed out that a multimethod approach to the study of memory and awareness needs to be taken, an approach that is well grounded in theory.

Conclusions

The main point of this chapter is that awareness is a key component of memory that needs to be included in research. Although the focus is on the importance of on-line awareness, it should be recognized that both systemic and epistemic awareness need to be considered as well.

Perhaps the most important conclusion that can be drawn is that much of memory aging may have more to do with what people are noticing about themselves than with structural changes per se. It may be more fruitful to begin researching what the typical adult thinks is happening to him or her than to focus exclusively on more "objective" assessments. At the very least, researchers trying to map the developmental course of memory need to consider the major roles played by personality and related factors. In the end, it may be that each of us is more responsible for what happens to our memory over time than we ever imagined. It may be that what we think is true is what really matters the most.

References

Anderson, J. R. (1976). *Language, memory, and thought*. Hillsdale, NJ: Lawrence Erlbaum.

Berry, J., West, R., & Scogin, F. (1983). *Predicting everyday and laboratory memory skill*. Paper presented at the annual meeting of the Gerontological Society, San Francisco.

Binet, H. (1903). *L'etude experimentale de l'intelligence*. Paris: Schleicher.

Bobrow, D. G., & Collins, A. (1975). *Representation and understanding: Studies in cognitive science*. New York: Academic Press.

Bruce, P. R., Coyne, A. C., & Botwinick, J. (1982). Adult age differences in metamemory. *Journal of Gerontology, 37*, 354–357.

Camp, C. J., Markley, R. P., & Kramer, J. J. (1983). Spontaneous use of mnemonics by elderly individuals. *Educational Gerontology, 9*, 57–71.

Cavanaugh, J. C. (1986–87). Age differences in adults' self-reports of memory ability: It depends on how and what you ask. *International Journal of Aging and Human Development, 24*, 271–277.

Cavanaugh, J. C., Grady, J. G., & Perlmutter, M. (1983). Forgetting and use of memory aids in 20 to 70 year olds' everyday life. *International Journal of Aging and Human Development, 17*, 113–122.

Cavanaugh, J. C., Kramer, D. A., Sinnott, J. D., Camp, C. J., & Markley, R. P. (1985). On missing links and such: Interfaces between cognitive research and everyday problem solving. *Human Development, 28*, 146–168.

Cavanaugh, J. C., & Perlmutter, M. (1982). Metamemory: A critical examination. *Child Development, 53*, 11–28.

Coyne, A. C. (1983). *Age, task variables, and memory knowledge*. Paper presented at the annual meeting of the Gerontological Society, San Francisco.

Ericsson, K. A., & Simon, H. A. (1984). *Protocol analysis: Verbal reports as data*. Cambridge, MA: M.I.T. Press.

Erikson, E. H. (1980). Elements of a psychoanalytic theory of psychosocial development. In S. I. Greenspan & G. H. Pollack (Eds.), *The course of life. Vol. 1: Infancy and early childhood* (pp. 11–61). Washington, DC: Department of Health and Human Services.

Giambra, L. M. (1984). *Frequency of task-unrelated thought intrusions as a function of age: A laboratory study*. Paper presented at the annual meeting of the Gerontological Society, San Antonio.

Harris, J. E. (1980). Memory aids people use: Two interview studies. *Memory and Cognition, 8*, 31–38.

Hilgard, E. R. (1980). Consciousness in contemporary psychology. *Annual Review of Psychology, 31*, 1–26.

Klatzky, R. L. (1984). *Memory and awareness*. New York: Freeman.

Lachman, J. L., & Lachman, R. (1980). Age and the actualization of world knowledge. In L. W. Poon, J. L. Fozard, L. S. Cermak, D. Arenberg, & L. W. Thompson (Eds.), *New directions in memory and aging* (pp. 285–308). Hillsdale, NJ: Lawrence Erlbaum.

Lachman, J. L., Lachman, R., & Thronesberry, C. (1979). Metamemory throughout the adult life span. *Developmental Psychology, 15,* 543–551.

Lachman, M. E., & McArthur, L. Z. (1986). Adulthood age differences in causal attributions for cognitive, physical, and social performance. *Psychology and Aging, 1,* 127–132.

Lachman, R., Lachman, J. L., & Taylor, D. W. (1982). Reallocation of mental resources over the productive life span: Assumptions and task analyses. In F. I. M. Craik & S. Trehub (Eds.), *Aging and cognitive processes* (pp. 278–308). New York: Plenum.

Langer, E. J. (1981). Old age: An artifact? In J. L. McGaugh & S. B. Kiesler (Eds.), *Aging: Biology and behavior* (pp. 255–282). New York: Academic Press.

Lincoln, Y. S., & Guba, E. G. (1985). *Naturalistic inquiry.* Beverly Hills, CA: Sage.

Lovelace, E. A., Marsh, G. R., & Oster, P. J. (1982). *Prediction and evaluation of memory performance by young and old adults.* Paper presented at the annual meeting of the Gerontological Society, Boston.

Mandler, G. (1975). Consciousness: Respectable, useful, and necessary. In R. L. Solso (Ed.), *Information processing and cognition* (pp. 229–254). Hillsdale, NJ: Lawrence Erlbaum.

Mason, S. E. (1981). *Age group comparisons of memory ratings, predictions, and performance.* Paper presented at the annual meeting of the Gerontological Society, Toronto.

Miller, G. A. (1980). Computation, consciousness, and cognition. *Behavioral and Brain Sciences, 3,* 146.

Murphy, M. D., Sanders, R. E., Gabriesheski, A. S., & Schmitt, F. A. (1981). Metamemory in the aged. *Journal of Gerontology, 36,* 185–193.

Natsoulas, T. (1981). Basic problems of consciousness. *Journal of Personality and Social Psychology, 41,* 132–178.

Neisser, U. (1979). Review of *Divided Consciousness* by E. R. Hilgard. *Contemporary Psychology, 24,* 99–100.

Neugarten, B. L. (1977). Personality and aging. In J. E. Birren & K. W. Schaie (Eds.), *Handbook of the psychology of aging* (1st ed., pp. 626–649). New York: Van Nostrand Reinhold.

Perlmutter, M. (1978). What is memory aging the aging of? *Developmental Psychology, 14,* 330–345.

Poon, L. W. (1985). Differences in human memory with aging: Nature, causes and clinical implications. In J. E. Birren & K. W. Schaie (Eds.), *Handbook of the psychology of aging,* (pp. 427–462). New York: Van Nostand Reinhold.

Rabinowitz, J. C., Ackerman, B. P., Craik, F. I. M., & Hinchley, J. L. (1982). Aging and metamemory: The roles of relatedness and imagery. *Journal of Gerontology, 37,* 688–695.

Tulving, E. (1985). Memory and consciousness. *Canadian Psychology, 26,* 1–12.

Underwood, G. (1982). *Aspects of consciousness. Vol. 3: Aspects of awareness and self-awareness.* London: Academic Press.

West, R. (1984). *Do the elderly know what they know? An analysis of memory monitoring and prediction.* Unpublished manuscript, Washington University.

24 Age and expertise: Responding to Talland's challenge

Neil Charness

This chapter is intended to serve as a tutorial on expertise. As a result, it represents a very selective review of studies in order to sketch what I believe to be the main trends in the study of expertise as they may apply to research on aging. For a fine general overview of this topic, see Hoyer (1985). To start with, it is useful to recall a point raised by George Talland about 20 years ago. Talland noted a feature of aging that many investigators have since commented on, namely, that there are many older people in our society who function well, and some who function in expert fashion. He put it this way:

> I am still puzzled by the contrast of the athlete who, at thirty, is too old for the championship and the maestro, who, at eighty, can treat us to a memorable performance on the concert stage. . . . Are our aged masters freaks of nature, paragons of self-discipline, or do they demonstrate the inadequacy of our present notions about the effects of age on human capacities? (Talland, 1965, p. 558)

I shall try to respond to Talland's challenge by assessing what we have learned in recent years about expertise and how the joint study of age and expertise can shed new light on issues important to both fields.

Age and expertise are both individual-difference variables. Levels of both variables are selected rather than manipulated experimentally. This leads to difficult problems when making inferences about the effects of age, or expertise, on performance. Theorists have worried about this a great deal in gerontology, though hardly at all in the area of skill, perhaps because of a basic difference in thrust. In the skill area, the underlying assumption is that skill differences are due to learning, not genetics; see, for example, Ericssen (1985) on skilled memory. In

This chapter was written while the author was supported by a grant from the Natural Sciences and Engineering Research Council of Canada (NSERC A0790) and by a Leave Fellowship from the Social Sciences and Humanities Research Council of Canada (SSHRCC 451–84–4284). I am grateful to A. T. Welford and J. Cerella for comments on an earlier draft.

the aging area, until the current concern with cohort explanations was aroused, the assumption was that age effects were attributable to the normal unfolding of the genetic program governing species-specific decline in physical and mental functioning. To use a heuristic I have discussed elsewhere (Charness, 1985a), skill effects were assumed to be due to "software" changes, age effects to "hardware" changes.

There is some justification for a skills theorist to assume that learning underlies skill differences. Many theorists have noted that virtually all types of skill acquisition are fit by the same function, a power curve (Newell & Rosenbloom, 1981). This universality in the time course of improvement suggests that anyone can acquire skill if given the motivation to practice. Further, there have been a few recent examples of selecting normally intelligent people to engage in longitudinal laboratory studies of skill acquisition; perhaps not too surprisingly, these people acquired rather extraordinary skill, a result similar to that found earlier by other investigators around the turn of the century (Ericssen, 1985).

On the other hand, it must be admitted that practice is *necessary but not sufficient* for acquiring high levels of skill. Each of us probably can cite at least one case where a friend or acquaintance put in many long hours (though perhaps in inefficient ways) at tennis, bridge, or typing and never achieved world-class standing. There are comparable cases in the laboratory [see the case of a digit-span trainee in Ericssen (1985)]. There are individual differences in learning rates that probably reflect "hardware" (genetic) constraints.

Nonetheless, the consistency of findings for practice being the major predictor of skill level argues that any genetic differences are likely to be small relative to learning-opportunity differences. This position is less likely to be true when looking at the interaction of age and practice for performance.

Age and professional performance

As many sociologists have pointed out, work seems to be the major role-determining force in a person's life. One of the first questions asked on meeting someone new (at least for adults who do not appear to be too old) is, "What do you do?" Hence, it is little wonder that assessing the effects of arbitrary retirement, with the perceived loss of a major role, is a current concern of sociologists, psychologists, and other social scientists. Whether or not people should be forced to retire, is a compelling topic for investigation, as is the question how age affects job performance (Davies & Sparrow, 1985). To make a long story short, there is little evidence to suggest that age per se (as opposed to a confounding factor such as obsolescence of knowledge) accounts for much of the variance in job performance, whether one deals with sales or engineering. Hunter and Hunter (1984) reviewed predictors of entry-level job performance and showed that age had an average validity coefficient of –.01. Nonetheless, the possible confounding of self-selection factors makes it difficult to arrive at any definitive conclusions. We have to rely on artificial laboratory research on novel cognitive and physical tasks for a thorough assessment of possible age declines, as well as on the archival studies that Lehman (1953) made famous.

Most of the literature on aging and physical and mental performance suggests that as tasks become more demanding, age decline is more apparent. This rather robust finding is sometimes termed the age–complexity hypothesis (Cerella, Poon, & Williams, 1980), and it finds support in studies of tasks ranging from reaction time (Salthouse, 1985) to running (Stones & Kozma, 1985). A similar relationship between age and professional performance can be seen in Lehman's data. (It probably was this relationship that prompted Talland's comment about athletes.)

Lehman showed that world-class performance in a diversity of endeavors – ranging from sedentary occupations such as writing or composing music to sports activities such as wrestling and weight lifting – occurred with greater frequency in young adults than in older adults. He demonstrated numerous inverted U-shaped functions relating performance to age, almost always finding that peak performances occurred most frequently for people who were in their thirties. No one disputes the data, though many dispute his interpretation. One of the confounding factors that clouds interpretation is the exponential increase in world population and hence the bias for young people, who form the greatest proportion of the population, to make most of the major discoveries or advances (Cole, 1979).

Again, recent longitudinal and cross-sectional archival investigations bear out the inverted U-shaped function (Cole, 1979), but demonstrate that age per se is not a powerful predictor of performance, accounting for less than 10% of the variance. Thus, there is a weak relationship between age and peak professional performance, and it tends to follow the laboratory results, showing an increase in performance from the teens into the twenties and thirties and a decline thereafter. Where refined measures of skill level have been developed, as is the case with the Elo chess rating scale (Elo, 1965, 1978), the longitudinal decline seems to be about one-half of a standard deviation from peak performance in the thirties to performance levels in the sixties. Because chess players usually give up tournament chess by their sixties or before, it is entirely possible that much more severe declines would be observed. The longest active career in chess for a strong grandmaster is that of 74-year-old Samuel Reshevsky (~1927 to the present). His best 5-year average was only about one standard deviation above his 1984 rating. Further, according to Elo (1978), the generational improvement in grandmaster performance is about one-half standard deviation over the last century. (This half-standard-deviation longitudinal improvement provides a quantitative answer, incidentally, to the question how far we can advance by virtue of "standing on the shoulders of giants.")

In summary, Lehman's data seem to portray accurately a decline in creative performance as a function of age. Nonetheless, longitudinal investigations have shown the decline to be slight, and they argue that age per se is not a very good predictor of individual differences in performance. Left unexplored, however, is

Table 24.1. *Sources of individual differences in performance*

Hardware	Software
1. Asymptotic speed of elementary information processes (e.g., recognition, matching two symbols for identity)	Nonasymptotic speed of an elementary information process (e.g., after moderate practice)
2. Working memory capacity measured in number of chunks	Chunk size (e.g., elements per chunk)
3. Time to create a new chunk in long-term memory (consolidation rate: seconds per chunk)	Number and type of symbol structures in long-term memory (e.g., extent and format of knowledge base of data and programs)

whether or not the degree of decline might not accelerate in old age, though self-selection processes and societal retirement requirements may make it difficult to gather the relevant data. Cerella and Poon (1983), in a provocative theoretical paper, argue that biological factors do undergo exponential decay.

Incidentally, even the very small amount of age-related decline discerned in these studies is meaningful. If there were no changes in a person's cognitive machinery with age, one would expect monotonic-increasing functions in performance with age, if only because people would be expected to increase their knowledge base over a lifetime of working in a professional domain.

Understanding individual differences: Information-processing framework

It is useful to examine potential sources of individual differences from an information-processing perspective; see Charness (in press) for a more detailed discussion. As seen in Table 24.1, we can divide up differences into two classes: (1) hardware, constraints due to invariant aspects of a person's cognitive architecture, and (2) software, differences due to the particular set of (nonphysically traumatic) circumstances that one has experienced over a lifetime. The former are viewed as relatively invariant, except for physical trauma to the brain. The latter are seen as relatively malleable, open to short-term intervention, where "short" can be measured as minutes to hours, that is, the length of a typical experiment in psychology.

A much more detailed set of principles for defining the performance of the human information-processing system is suggested by Card, Moran, and Newell (1983). They sketch out about 10 principles and associated parameters for processing (see their Chapter 2 and Figure 2.2). Their parameters for basic operations (e.g., the ~100-msec "cycle time" for the cognitive processor) span a "Fastman-to-Slowman" range that was derived virtually exclusively from young-adult data. Thus, these ranges probably should be modified to reflect changes with age ("Youngman" to "Oldman"?) in processing speed. Using the heuristic provided by Cerella (1985), the estimates of Card and associates for basic perceptual operations should be multiplied by about 1.2, and cognitive operation times should be multiplied by about 1.7, to approximate the performance of the average 60-year-old person.

Skill review

With so many potential loci for individual differences to be manifested, it becomes difficult to decide the nature-versus-nurture question with regard to skill (or age). Researchers in the skill area have relied on the *interaction effect* to assign responsibility to nurture rather than nature. That is, they have sought two parallel experimental conditions: one where a skill effect was present and another where it was not. The clinical literature calls this the search for dissociation effects.

An example from the domain of chess skill is the following. Chase and Simon (1973), following earlier work by de Groot (1966), showed that when a structured middle-game chess position is reproduced after a 5-sec look, the accuracy of piece placement depends on chess skill level. Without the control condition, it would be impossible to decide whether chess masters have better *general* memory capacity than poorer players or whether they have superior memory only for domain-related material. The control condition consisted of showing the same number of pieces randomly assigned to chessboard locations. Reproduction accuracy for randomly arranged chess pieces was not related to chess skill level. A novice did as well as a master in remembering. The conjunction of these two findings indicates that chess masters do *not* have superior general memory capacity, but they do have better memory for familiar or game-related configurations of pieces. As we shall see, this basic finding of a domain-specific memory advantage has been replicated numerous times. Although it is still possible to argue for a genetic, brain-related advantage for masters, it is not too parsimonious to expect nature to have devised specialized neural circuits for legal chess positions and to have endowed only those destined to become chess masters with more of these circuits.

The demonstration of an *interaction effect* (e.g., skill level × experimental conditions) can be an effective deterrent to the riposte that experts are born, not made. What serves as an effective parallel condition is a problem that must be met by the experimenter's ingenuity coupled with a theory about task performance.

Experts are better than novices on many dimensions of performance. The most significant of these are speed and accuracy. Experts solve problems in their domains more quickly and more accurately. In fact, most experiments demonstrate a speed–error complementarity, rather than the traditional speed–error trade-off.

Faster, more accurate performance can be attributed to advantages in the speed of elementary operations, more domain-relevant information (both declarative and procedural knowledge), and, as a result, more refined programs for operating on the "problem space" (Newell & Simon, 1972) in which a problem is represented internally by the would-be solver.

Speed of elementary processes

As computer advertisements for the latest microprocessors are fond of pointing out, if the central processor operates at a higher clock speed, a given program will run faster. That is, if the fetch–execute cycle is shorter, more operations can be crammed into the same unit of time. A good analogy for human processing is reading speed. Someone who can extract the meaning of a word more quickly will, on average, read at a faster pace than his or her slower-decoding counterpart.

The experimental task chosen by those who study verbal ability is not lexical access, but a subcomponent of this, letter decoding. Hunt and his colleagues (Hunt, 1978) have shown that the reaction time to decide that a capital letter has the same name as its lowercase counterpart (e.g., e = E, despite the shape difference) is a good predictor of verbal ability, after subtracting out the time taken to decide that two uppercase or lowercase identical letters are the same. It takes less time to decide that a "name identity" exists for more (verbally) intelligent people. Theory suggests that this is an instance of the more general process of accessing an abstract code.

The expectation is that when an elementary process such as this occurs thousands of times in a larger task (e.g., reading), the very small time advantage will cascade into large performance differences favoring more skilled encoders. It was natural for investigations of skilled performance to home in on early perceptual encoding processes to explain skill differences.

A good case in point is a study by Bean (1938) on music reading. He built a tachistoscope into a piano and briefly flashed (190 msec) short melodies and chords to pianists varying in skill who had to play them. Reanalysis of his Table 1 (p. 29) shows that if the 10 professionals are tied for top experience rank and the 30 nonprofessionals are ranked according to years of musical training, span correlates with musical experience (Spearman rank correlation) .6 for melodies, .7 for polyphonic melodies, and .4 for chords. This perceptual advantage for more skilled musicians (in this case over nonmusicians) was replicated by Sloboda (1976, 1978) when he required subjects to write pitch symbols on a staff. The advantage for skilled musicians disappeared when the duration of the stimulus was 20 msec, but by 50 msec the musicians already showed an advantage in coding absolute contour of the notes. Clifton (1986) has also shown more specifically that sight-reading skill (average time per note for an unfamiliar music piece) is predicted by success at recalling music notation after a 2-sec look, even within a group of musicians with equivalent musical training who presumably perform similarly on non-sight-read pieces.

Similar rapid encoding advantages for more skilled performers have been demonstrated for chess players, as discussed earlier, electronics technicians (Egan &

Schwartz, 1979), bridge players (Charness, 1979, 1983; Engle & Bukstel, 1978), go players (Reitman, 1976), programmers (McKeithen, Reitman, Rueter & Hirtle, 1981; Shneiderman, 1976), sports players (Allard & Burnett, 1985), and those in many other skill domains. Most interpretations of the encoding advantage for more skilled practitioners center around the notion of a chunking advantage. The evidence suggests that better performers can match larger patterns in their domain of expertise to a "vocabulary" of stored chunks. Assuming that information must be held in a limited-capacity working memory, those who can unitize (chunk) more elements will be able to maintain more information and thereby report more after a brief exposure. More direct measures of chunking and chunk size were developed in Chase and Simon (1973) and by Reitman and colleagues (Reitman, 1976; McKeithen et al., 1981).

Knowledge-base differences

The processing-speed advantage is seen to depend on the size of the vocabulary of domain-dependent patterns that the expert possesses. One estimate of the vocabulary size for an expert arises from some simulation work by Simon and Gilmartin (1973) on the chess recall task. They estimate that the master chess player has a vocabulary of around 50,000 chess chunks that are immediately recognizable. Obviously, chess masters know much more than how to recognize chess subpatterns; so their total domain-dependent knowledge base probably is an order of magnitude larger. Having 50,000 recognizable chunks is not that tall an order (though it evidently takes between 1,000 and 10,000 hours to acquire). Using random selection of words from large dictionaries, Oldfield (1963) demonstrated that typical college undergraduates have word-recognition vocabularies of at least that size.

Thus far, we have been discussing what could be called memory for facts, or declarative knowledge. Experts know both *what* to do and *how* to do it. That is, they also have much of their knowledge represented by procedures that enable them to execute mental activities directly, with minimal search. It is assumed that novices have very general problem-solving procedures that they can use to manipulate their facts. They use means–ends reasoning (Newell & Simon, 1972) to guide their search for a solution.

Recent models of skill acquisition make a strong case for a progressive change in the representation of knowledge from declarative to procedural. See Anderson's theory (1982) of skill acquisition and Pirolli and Anderson's extension (1985) to learning to program recursive functions.

A good example is given for solving physics problems by Simon and Simon (1978). As people acquire skill, they develop very specific procedures for operating on their representation of the problem, often simulated with "production rules" that are tailored to many unique problem states. Thus, in many cases they do little searching in the problem space. Simon and Simon's expert did a forward search, simply substituting values for equation variables until the solution more or less popped out. As Chi, Feltovich, and Glaser (1981) have shown, physics experts represent problems in terms of high-level physics principles, such as the laws of conservation of energy and momentum, which help to guide their search through the problem space. Novices seem to attend to surface features of the problems and have to engage in the more "logical" means–ends search through the equation space. Experts not only have more knowledge but also have that knowledge organized differently, usually hierarchically.

There is an occasional exception to the rule that experts have a more differentiated knowledge base. Murphy and Wright (1984) showed that clinical psychologists and experienced child-care workers had more overlap in diagnostic categories for childhood adjustment problems than did novice undergraduates. The experts did generate more features for each category, but features overlapped more categories, probably reflecting the fuzzy nature of real-world diagnostic categories.

To complicate matters further, the format of the representation being used (e.g., verbal, visual, motoric) may change with level of expertise, as a study on abacus experts doing mental calculation has shown (Hatano, Miyake, & Binks, 1977). In that study, when concurrent tasks were required, different patterns of interference were obtained. Moderately skilled abacus calculators, who used a kinesthetic representation, ran into trouble when their fingers were kept occupied, but this additional task did not affect highly skilled operators who were using a mental abacus that was no longer tied to finger movements. A more recent study by Stigler (1984) has shown how both latency and error patterns can reveal which representation is being used for mental calculation.

Even when the representation being used is restricted to one format, the dimensions may be weighted differently at different levels of skill. A dissertation by Romanow, cited by Marteniuk and Romanow (1983), showed that as skill in reproducing a complex movement was acquired, higher-order components of movement parameters were more heavily weighted. People seemed to attend first to displacement information, then to velocity, then to acceleration. In short, there are many dimensions along which experts may differ from novices.

Attentional resources and expertise

There is widespread acceptance for the view that as people acquire skill, their processing becomes more automatic, and hence they have more capacity to devote to other tasks. A striking example of how two seemingly incompatible tasks can be integrated comes from a study by Hirst, Spelke, Reaves, Caharack, and Neisser (1980), in which after much practice people could take dictation and read other material at the same time. In the sports domain, Allard and Burnett (1985) reviewed experiments showing that skilled softball batters either improved their batting performance with a relevant concurrent visual task or were unaffected by an irrelevant auditory detection task, whereas less skilled batters showed large decrements.

Those of us who have tried a new task certainly recall how there seemed to be too much to attend to at first, but as we improved, we could carry out all kinds of time-sharing successfully, as in the case of driving a car and adjusting the fan, the radio, the mirror, and so forth. Much of the work on automaticity bears out this view; see Logan's review (1985) of automaticity and skill, and Plude and Hoyer's review (1985) of automaticity and aging. As Logan points out, increases in automaticity do not necessarily imply loss of control, in that the initiation and some monitoring of automatic processes are under effortful control.

Despite this view, there is evidence that skilled individuals sometimes are more heavily engaged in a task, in the sense that activation of their knowledge base may make them less able to monitor other environmental events. Britton and Tesser (1982) showed that people who knew more about the domain that they were processing (e.g., chess, content of a paragraph in a comprehension task) were *slower* to respond to an auditory probe than were those with less knowledge. Evidently, it is possible for the expert to become "lost in thought."

Costs of expertise

In addition to Britton and Tesser's demonstration (1982) of the disadvantage of being more expert, several other cases have come to light. Arkes and Freedman (1984) have shown that because experts know more about a given subject, they can be led to infer incorrectly that a sentence has been presented, whereas a novice has no trouble rejecting the same sentence in a recognition task. Experts were more likely to recognize falsely a new sentence as old when it was a synonym for an old one. They were also more likely to accept an inference sentence as old when it was supported by the text they read, though more likely to reject one that did not fit. Experts appear freer to go "beyond the information given," as Arkes and Freedman point out.

Similarly, Adelson (1984) showed that when expert programmers were given an inappropriate set before studying a simple program, they were less accurate than novices were in answering concrete-level questions about the program. The experts were almost always superior when answering abstract-level questions. Evidently, experts prefer to try to comprehend programs at an abstract level, emphasizing what a program does, rather than at the more concrete level of attending to what each line in the program does. Experts can be led to attend to low-level detail, and when they do so, their question answering on concrete details is as good as that of novices.

These results fit with the view that novices tend to focus on surface features of a problem, whereas experts tend to abstract representations that encode higher-level features. The results also fit with the view that as processing becomes automatic, experts lose conscious access to the processes that generate intermediate-level results and cannot report how they got the result. A good example of this is the problem that skilled typists have in naming which finger is used for a given key on the keyboard, without imagining themselves hitting the key. Novices usually can report the finger, but still have trouble getting there quickly. There are some costs associated with becoming expert, as well as the better-known benefits.

In summary, it is worthwhile to sound a note of caution about the range of differences found between experts and novices. Experts exceed novices in many respects, and it is dangerous to assume that a difference we observe is the only one or even the most important one. Consider, for example, the differences in memory for chess positions that most chess researchers have observed. It is likely that chess masters did not set out to develop a vocabulary of 50,000 chess chunks; rather, incidental to their efforts to learn about chess, they acquired such a vocabulary. It is also quite conceivable that one could sit down with a chess book and learn to become skilled at reproducing chess positions from memory, without increasing one's skill at playing chess. Recognizing that we have seen a problem before and knowing how to solve it can be independent processes.

The fact that there has been such consistency in finding a knowledge-base difference across a diverse set of domains strengthens the hypothesis that expertise depends heavily on acquiring a large knowledge base. Nonetheless, the fact that skilled volleyball players seem to be best at rapid ball detection (Allard & Starkes, 1980), whereas skilled basketball players show the usual superior memory for structured game positions (Allard, Graham, & Paarsalu, 1980), reminds us how the task environment constrains the process of becoming an expert. In some cases, sheer speed is important. In others, specific knowledge of what to do next suffices.

Age and expertise

There is a burgeoning literature that addresses the issue of how age and expertise jointly determine performance; see, for example, the recent review by Charness (1985b) on problem-solving tasks. Interestingly, most of the literature on aging and text comprehension deals with this issue indirectly, because most older adults have had a lifetime of experience at comprehending language; see the reviews by Meyer and Rice (Chapter 12, this volume) and Spilich (1985) on discourse-comprehension tasks. The study by Stine, Wingfield, and Poon (Chapter 13, this volume) shows how knowledge of syntax and semantics can permit older listeners to compensate for general slowing and successfully comprehend rapidly presented speech.

The critical issue here is how the older expert compensates for apparent general changes in processing speed and working memory capacity to maintain performance. That is, what are the compensatory mechanisms that older experts employ? Further, are there tasks in which no compensation is possible? Current disputes over mandatory-retirement regulations for airline pilots and other professionals are obviously based around the latter issue. Another critical issue is how best to train the older adult to acquire new skills (also asked under the guise of the problem of job retraining).

It is worth looking at two examples where the question of compensation has been raised: chess (Charness, 1981a, 1981b, 1981c) and typing (Salthouse, 1984). Chess is a game that depends heavily on the ability to think ahead (search), which in turn makes demands on working memory for keeping track of positions searched and their evaluations. It appears that humans are very selective searchers, typically evaluating no more than 5 or 6 base moves (moves for the player who is selecting a move) out of the 30–50 possible legal moves for any board situation. This incredible selectivity is a hallmark of human problem solving. People use heuristics to cut down the potentially enormous search space to manageable size. Selectivity in chess search is believed to be due to pattern-driven move generation. That is, the master *recognizes* that one of a small set of plausible moves is called for in a given situation. Nonetheless, follow-up search is still necessary, and the depth and extent of search are positive functions of the player's skill level.

It is believed that plausible move generation is tied to the size of a chess player's vocabulary of recognizable chess chunks. That is why the chess recall task is theoretically valuable, because it indexes vocabulary size. I have shown that when equivalently skilled chess players who are young and old do a brief-exposure recall task, the young players recall more chess pieces (Charness, 1981c). This result implies either that older players achieved their level of skill differently than did young ones (somewhat implausible given the cohort insensitivity of chess) or that older players have lost the ability to access some of these patterns as rapidly as they once could. I have also shown that older players are inferior to equivalently skilled younger ones when recalling incidentally learned chess positions (Charness, 1981a). Further, they recall such positions using a larger number of smaller chunks, again implicating loss of access to stored patterns as a possible effect of age.

Curiously, older players were no worse than equally skilled younger ones in choosing the best move from four chess positions. That is, they were as good as their chess ratings said they were. They did vary in the way in which they searched. Older players searched less extensively (fewer total moves explored), though they searched equally deeply (looked as far ahead). They also examined fewer initial moves and, most important, conducted their search in less time, on average, than did their younger counterparts. That is, they found equally good moves in less time than equally skilled younger players.

Thus, we have the paradoxical situation that older players have less efficient memory processes, as judged by recall tasks, but more efficient search processes, as judged by move selection. What compensatory mechanisms do older players rely on? The data rule out the idea that they generate better plausible moves (Charness, 1981b). Their less extensive search may be due to a better sense of what a chess position holds for a given side (their level of aspiration may be more realistic). They may also have been more confident of the results of search and thus have forgone the verification that younger players needed to do.

This still leaves us with the paradox of how older players with diminished memory resources were able to search as deeply as younger players. Depth of search is much like a memory-span task. That is, players search ahead until they reach a point where they are no longer confident that they can evaluate the imagined position properly. They then return to the base position (the position physically present on the board in front of them) and start their search again. This style of search was termed "progressive deepening" by de Groot (1978).

I think we have to look to newer conceptualizations of working memory to understand this result, such as that proposed by Chase and Ericssen (1982) and Ericssen (1985). They demonstrated through training studies that college undergraduates could learn to expand their digit span to 80+ digits; yet at the same time, their consonant span remained at 7. That is, working memory capacity can expand beyond the traditional limits of three to five chunks of rehearsable information by virtue of the development of *domain-specific* retrieval structures that can index recently activated semantic-memory structures. It evidently takes about 100 hours to build up these elaborate hierarchical retrieval structures and to speed up the encoding processes that chunk incoming information. Preliminary results from research conducted by workers at the Max Planck Institute (Smith, 1985) suggest that old adults can learn to stretch their working memory capacity using similar mnemonic techniques.

Returning to the chess-search paradox, it is quite possible to view the uninhibited search capabilities of older chess players in the same light. That is, over the thousands of hours that they have spent searching for moves, they, too, may have developed elaborate retrieval structures that enable them to chunk sequences of moves, thereby enabling them to search deeply. Further experimentation will be necessary to evaluate this possibility.

The case of compensatory mechanisms for skilled typists seems much clearer. Salthouse (1984) showed that there was a significant correlation between age and choice reaction time in a group of typists varying in age and skill level (.46 and .62 in two samples). Yet, in these same samples, typing speed was uncorrelated with age (–.06, .07). Further, Salthouse also showed that other speed measures (such as tapping speed, digit–symbol substitution) exhibited age-related declines.

How do other typists maintain typing speed when their reaction time is declining? The answer appears to be that older typists look farther ahead. The eye–hand span was positively related to age (.50, .53). Further analysis of the time span (a time-related variant of eye–hand span) showed that on average, typists of age 60 have about a quarter to a third of a second longer than typists of age 20 to prepare for impending keystrokes. By giving themselves more planning time, older typists can compensate for diminished reaction time. Typing is not a reaction-time task, because, as Salthouse points out, most of the gains in speed come from overlapping processing operations. This ingenious set of experiments demonstrates the first clear-cut example of "wisdom" on the part of older people. It also demonstrates the degree to which compensatory mechanisms are domain-specific, because in theory, the same look-ahead strategy could have improved performance on digit–symbol substitution.

Age and skill acquisition

The preceding section pointed out that older people can function at very high levels of performance despite declines in the hardware that supports cognitive functioning generally. In effect, it answered Talland's query by showing that when people can draw on domain-specific knowledge, and when they have developed appropriate compensatory mechanisms, they can treat us to memorable performances, whether on the keyboard of a typewriter, on a piano, or on the podium of an orchestral stage. When the task environment does not afford the same predictability or opportunity to plan ahead, however, as is the case in fast-moving sports environments, degradation in hardware cannot be compensated for by more efficient software. Thus, it is not surprising that athletes may no longer be in their prime past the thirties in some sports, though I think it is only fair to note that many of them still can give memorable performances (e.g., Jack Nicklaus winning the 1986 Masters golf tournament at age 45).

In this section, we shall look at training studies in an attempt to create a new metric for assessing age decline. It is probably fair to say that the debate whether or not age decline is a myth has ended, with most people acknowledging that performance changes, usually negatively, as people age. The debates over methodology (whether to use cross-sectional, longitudinal, or sequential designs) and statistics (whether to use *F*, *p*, or effect-size variants such as η^2, ω^2, r^2 to gauge the importance of age differences) go on. It is to the latter issue that studies of modifiability, championed early by Baltes, Schaie, and their colleagues (Baltes, Dittmann-Kohli, & Dixon, 1984; Baltes & Willis, 1982), provide a useful perspective.

My claim is that the best index of the importance of an age effect is how much practice, measured in minutes per year of age difference, is necessary to bring an older person to the same (or better) performance level as that exhibited by a younger adult initially. I shall review several studies on the digit–symbol substitution task, because it is one of the psychometric tests that is most sensitive to age.

In one study, Grant, Storandt, and Botwinick (1978) attempted to assess how incentive and practice (five blocks of four trials) affected the performances of young (22 years) and old (70 years) people. The ANOVA revealed a highly significant ($F = 133$) and large ($\omega^2 = .65$) effect of age, a highly significant ($F = 61$) and modest ($\omega^2 = .06$) effect of practice, and no effect of incentive. As Newell and Rosenbloom (1981) have noted, practice data are well fit by simple power functions of this form: performance on trial $T = aT^b$, where a is a constant (typifying initial performance) and b is the exponent indexing improvement. Thus, if we plot the logarithm of trial number against the logarithm of performance (e.g., proportion correct or reaction time), we obtain a straight line whose slope is the exponent and whose intercept (the antilogarithm of the intercept) is the constant. A more complete power function has three parameters: the initial level of performance, the learning rate, and the asymptotic level of performance. It may be that hyperbolic fits are better, as Cerella and Lowe (1984) have argued, but given the low number of trials and the excellent fit with the simple power law, it is not worth worrying here. At any rate, collapsing across incentive conditions yields the following equations:

Old: Digits copied = 15.8 block number$^{.165}$, $r^2 = .99$.
Young: Digits copied = 26.3 block number$^{.136}$, $r^2 = .99$.

Solving for block number, the old group would be expected to equal the initial level of the young group by block 23. That is, 92 trials would be needed by the old group to attain the initial level of performance of the young group. Given that each trial was 50 sec in duration (30 sec per trial and 20 sec intertrial interval), that level would be reached in a little more than an hour of practice (77 min). That is, the 48-year age gap in performance would be alleviated by less than 2 min of practice per year of age difference.

No claim is made that if both groups were to continue practicing, the older group would converge on the same asymptotic level of performance as the young. Murrell's $N = 3$ study (1970) yielded an affirmative answer to this for simple and choice reaction time, though the old subject was in her fifties. Cerella and Lowe (1984) showed in their survey of studies that there would be a predicted gap between young and old of around 22% at asymptotic performance levels. In their review, they found that the learning rate (rate-of-improvement parameter) did not vary consistently with age. They ultimately argued from these data that about two-thirds of the initial age deficit is due to factors other than experience differences.

In another digit–symbol substitution study, where the codes were changed on a daily basis, Beres and Baron (1981) showed strong improvement for both an old (69 years) and a young (23 years) group of women over 5 days involving 100 trials of practice. Estimating mean daily performance from their data yields the following functions:

Old: Number of symbols copied = 22.7 days$^{.08}$, $r^2 = .97$.
Young: Number of symbols copied = 29.9 days$^{.09}$, $r^2 = .99$.

Using the mean day-1 performance of the young (30 symbols copied) as the target, it can be seen that the old group would be expected to reach this level after 33 days of practice, or 660 trials. Here, too, a trial lasted 30 sec, with an intertrial interval of 20 sec. Thus, after about 9.2 hours of practice, the old group should reach the mean day-1 performance level of the young group. If, on the other hand, trial-1 performance (26.5) rather than trial-10 performance is taken as the target, the data show that the old group reached this level by day 5, after 200 trials.

Using the theoretical function and solving for the mean daily trial-1 performance level of 26.5, the result is that 6.9 days of practice are predicted to be necessary, that is, 1.9 hours of on-task practice. This yields the estimate of 2.5 min per year of age difference, a figure remarkably close to that estimated from the Grant and associates (1978) study, where the code did not change from block to block. Even the 9.2-hour figure is not particularly high, when considering it in the context of daily television viewing time, a 40-hour work week, or the estimated 1,000–10,000 hours necessary to achieve a high level of skill in a semantically rich domain such as chess.

Perhaps the most complete recent data base on practice effects was gathered by Salthouse and Somberg (1982), who practiced eight young (23 years) and eight old (69 years) subjects for over 50 sessions. Using one of the three tasks, the Sternberg memory-search task data, and eliminating trials where the procedure was changed, the following simple power-function fits are obtained:

Old: Reaction time $= 908\ \text{session}^{-.17},\ r^2 = .96.$
Young: Reaction time $= 480\ \text{session}^{-.07},\ r^2 = .60.$

A power fit to the young-group data is not very good, because it severely underestimates the session-1 reaction time (predicting 480 msec, where 599 msec was the actual value). Fortunately, in the actual data base, the old group reached the initial level of the young group between sessions 9 and 10 (this is a conservative estimate, because at that point the old group's error rate was below that of the young group on their first session).

Although there is no report of time per trial, conservatively, a trial should take between 5 and 10 sec. There were 100 trials in each session beyond the first. Thus, after about 950 trials and 2 hours of practice, the old group met (exceeded) the initial performance of the young. For a mean age difference of 46 years, the leveling point occurs after less than 2.6 min of practice per year of age difference.

Finally, it is worth looking at some preliminary data from one of my own studies (Charness & Campbell, in press). We taught 16 young (24 years), middle-aged (41 years), and old (67 years) adults an algorithm to square two-digit numbers mentally, over five sessions. Mean performance levels can be seen in Figure 24.1. Here, too, the simple power law provides an excellent fit to the group means:

Young: Response time $= 8.29\ \text{session}^{-.44},\ r^2 = .994.$
Middle: Response time $= 15.32\ \text{session}^{-.54},\ r^2 = .998.$
Old: Response time $= 19.4\ \text{session}^{-.44},\ r^2 = .994.$

Again, although there are large initial differences between groups, the gap is predicted to be closed by about the seventh session for the old adults, after about 7 hours of practice. Because the actual on-task time was about 15 to 20 min per session, on average, the 43-year age difference in performance would be alleviated in a bit more than 3 min of practice per year of age difference.

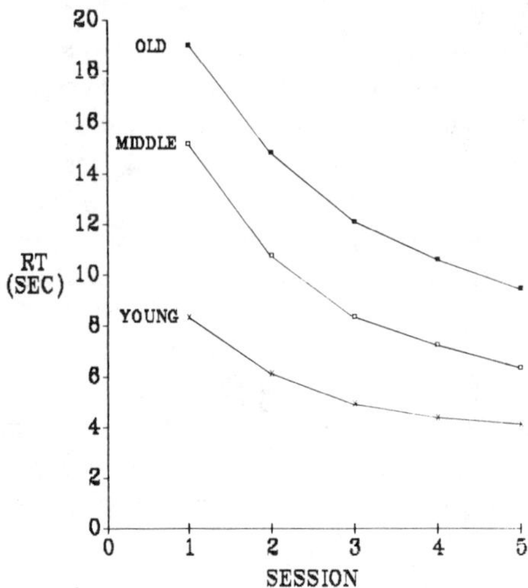

Figure 24.1. Mean correct reaction times across sessions for young (age 24), middle-aged (age 41), and old (age 67) adults squaring numbers (1–99) mentally.

In summary, it appears that there is a magic number for this new metric on the importance of initial age differences in performance. Namely, 3 min of practice per year of age difference is all that it takes to eliminate age effects, using the benchmark of the initial performance level of young adults. Put more crudely, by giving up one night of television watching and practicing a typical laboratory task, an older adult will perform as well as an unpracticed young adult.

Conclusions

The skills-research area has pointed increasingly in the direction of applied work, as seen in the emphasis on education-related issues (e.g., work on physics problem solving) and the issue of human factors in computer technology (Card et al., 1983). Research on aging has not been particularly concerned with applied issues, despite an eloquent plea by Fozard and Popkin (1978), with the exception of the area of industrial gerontology. A strong case has been made from psychology's inception that interesting theoretical issues can be addressed within an applied framework (Bryan & Harter, 1899).

A good start is provided by the search for invariants, such as the processing-time constants that Cerella (1985) uncovered. Unfortunately, such constants are likely to be associated with large standard errors of estimate when predicting the behavior of an older person, simply because older groups are more variable than younger groups for measures such as reaction time. Nonetheless, the enterprise is worthwhile, even necessary, because many design decisions for equipment specifications will depend increasingly on the parameters outlined by applied human-factors groups such as Card and associates (1983). I see little evidence to date that standards are set with an older population in mind, probably because short-range planning does not permit developers to see older adults as a target user group.

Another fruitful avenue that should be adopted from skills research is the generation of detailed models of individual cases, an approach advocated for gerontologists by Giambra and Arenberg (1980). It is probably only with the development of such detailed models and the attempt to extend them to the same individuals doing other tasks, as well as to other individuals, that there is any hope of separating out hardware and software factors in aging.

The street need not be a one-way street. One of the virtues of aging research is that its practitioners are aware of the extent of individual differences and are attuned to the possibility that hardware factors are likely to play an important role. Too often in the skills area, genetic/hardware explanations of differences are ruled out without the proper checks. Further, longitudinal studies of skill acquisition are only now beginning to be seen as important, whereas they have always been the ideal in gerontology. Perhaps because of the difficulty of getting representative samples and the variability in performance of older people, gerontological studies tend to use much larger sample sizes than skills studies. Somewhere between the two extremes of large-N studies using powerful multivariate analysis and $N = 1$ studies using simpler statistics lies the happy medium of in-depth studies that will have modest generalizability.

In short, there is the opportunity for "hybridizing" research on skills and that on aging. Both variables can account individually for large chunks of the individual-difference variance in human performance. Jointly they can do a much better job.

References

Adelson, B. (1984). When novices surpass experts: The difficulty of a task may increase with expertise. *Journal of Experimental Psychology: Learning, Memory and Cognition, 10,* 483–495.

Allard, F., & Burnett, N. (1985). Skill in sport. *Canadian Journal of Psychology, 39,* 294–312.

Allard, F., Graham, S., & Paarsalu, M. E. (1980). Perception in sport: Basketball. *Journal of Sport Psychology, 2,* 14–21.

Allard, F., & Starkes, J. L. (1980). Perception in sport: Volleyball. *Journal of Sport Psychology, 2,* 22–33.

Anderson, J. R. (1982). Acquisition of cognitive skill. *Psychological Review, 89,* 369–406.

Arkes, H. R., & Freedman, M. R. (1984). A demonstration of the costs and benefits of expertise in recognition memory. *Memory and Cognition, 12,* 84–89.

Baltes, P. B., Dittmann-Kohli, F., & Dixon, R. A. (1984). New perspectives on the development of intelligence in adulthood: Toward a dual-process conception and a model of selective optimization with compensation. In P. B. Baltes & O. G. Brim (Eds.), *Life-span development and behavior* (Vol. 6). New York: Academic Press.

Baltes, P. B., & Willis, S. L. (1982). Plasticity and enhancement of intellectual functioning in old age. In F. I. M. Craik & S. Trehub (Eds.), *Aging and cognitive processes.* New York: Plenum Press.

Bean, K. L. (1938). An approach to the reading of music. *Psychological Monograms, 226,* 1–80.

Beres, C. A., & Baron, A. (1981). Improved digit symbol substitution by older women as a result of extended practice. *Journal of Gerontology, 36,* 591–597.

Britton, B. K., & Tesser, A. (1982). Effects of prior knowledge on use of cognitive capacity in three complex cognitive tasks. *Journal of Verbal Learning and Verbal Behavior, 21,* 421–436.

Bryan, W. L., & Harter, N. (1899). Studies of the telegraphic language. The acquisition of a hierarchy of habits. *Psychological Review, 6,* 345–375.

Card, S. K., Moran, T. P., & Newell, A. (1983). *The psychology of human–computer interaction.* Hillsdale, NJ: Lawrence Erlbaum.

Cerella, J. (1985). Information processing rates in the elderly. *Psychological Bulletin, 98,* 67–83.

Cerella, J., & Lowe, D. (1984). *Age deficits and practice: 27 studies reconsidered.* Paper presented at a meeting of the Gerontological Society of America, San Antonio.

Cerella, J., & Poon, L. W. (1983). *Life cycles: How grim the reaper?* Paper presented at a meeting of the Gerontological Society of America, San Francisco.

Cerella, J., Poon, L. W., & Williams, D. M. (1980). Age and the complexity hypothesis. In L. W. Poon (Ed.), *Aging in the 1980s: Psychological issues* (pp. 322–392). Washington, DC: American Psychological Association.

Charness, N. (1979). Components of skill in bridge. *Canadian Journal of Psychology, 33,* 1–16.

Charness, N. (1981a). Aging and skilled problem solving. *Journal of Experimental Psychology: General, 110,* 21–38.

Charness, N. (1981b). Search in chess: Age and skill differences. *Journal of Experimental Psychology: Human Perception and Performance, 7,* 467–476.

Charness, N. (1981c). Visual short-term memory and aging in chess players. *Journal of Gerontology, 36,* 615–619.

Charness, N. (1983). Age, skill, and bridge bidding: A chronometric analysis. *Journal of Verbal Learning and Verbal Behavior, 22,* 406–416.

Charness, N. (1985a). Introduction to aging and human performance. In N. Charness (Ed.), *Aging and human performance.* New York: Wiley.

Charness, N. (1985b). Aging and problem solving performance. In N. Charness (Ed.), *Aging and human performance.* New York: Wiley.

Charness, N. (in press). Talent: A cognitive framework. In L. Obler & D. Fein (Eds.), *The neuropsychology of talent and special abilities.* New York: Guilford Press.

Charness, N., & Campbell, J. I. D. (in press). Acquiring skill at mental calculation in adulthood.

Chase, W. G., & Ericsson, K. A. (1982). Skill and working memory. In G. H. Bower (Ed.), *The psychology of learning and motivation* (Vol. 16). New York: Academic Press.

Chase, W. G., & Simon, H. A. (1973). The mind's eye in chess. In W. G. Chase (Ed.), *Visual information processing* (pp. 215–222). New York: Academic Press.

Chi, M. T. H., Feltovich, P. J., & Glaser, R. (1981). Categorization and representation of physics problems by experts and novices. *Cognitive Science, 5,* 121–152.

Clifton, J. (1986). *Cognitive components of music reading and sight reading performance.* Unpublished doctoral dissertation, University of Waterloo.

Cole, B. (1979). Age and scientific performance. *American Journal of Sociology, 84,* 958–977.

Davies, D. R., & Sparrow, P. R. (1985). Age and work behaviour. In N. Charness (Ed.), *Aging and human performance.* New York: Wiley.

Egan, D. E., & Schwartz, E. J. (1979). Chunking in recall of symbolic drawings. *Memory and Cognition, 7,* 149–158.

Elo, A. E. (1965). Age changes in master chess performances. *Journal of Gerontology, 20,* 289–299.

Elo, A. E. (1978). *The rating of chess players. Past and present.* New York: Arco Publishing.

Engle, R. W., & Bukstel, L. (1978). Memory processes among bridge players of differing expertise. *American Journal of Psychology, 91,* 673–689.

Ericsson, K. A. (1985). Memory skill. *Canadian Journal of Psychology, 39,* 188–231.

Fozard, J. L., & Popkin, S. J. (1978). Optimizing adult development. Ends and means of an applied psychology of aging. *American Psychologist, 33,* 975–989.

Giambra, L. M., & Arenberg, D. (1980). Problem solving, concept learning and aging. In L. W. Poon (Ed.), *Aging in the 1980s: Psychological issues* (pp. 253–259). Washington, DC: American Psychological Association.

Grant, E. A., Storandt, M., & Botwinick, J. (1978). Incentive and practice in the psychomotor performance of the elderly. *Journal of Gerontology, 33,* 413–415.

Groot, A. D. de (1966). Perception and memory versus thought: Some old ideas and recent findings. In B. Kleinmuntz (Ed.), *Problem solving: Research, method and theory* (pp. 19–50). New York: Wiley.

Groot, A. D. de (1978). *Thought and choice in chess* (2nd ed.). The Hague: Mouton Publishers.

Hatano, G., Miyake, Y., & Binks, M. G. (1977). Performance of expert abacus operators. *Cognition, 5,* 47–55.

Hirst, W., Spelke, E. S., Reaves, C. C., Caharack, G., & Neisser, U. (1980). Dividing attention without alternation or automaticity. *Journal of Experimental Psychology: General, 109,* 98–117.

Hoyer, W. J. (1985). Aging and the development of expert cognition. In T. M. Shlechter and M. P. Toglia (Eds.), *New directions in cognitive science.* Norwood, NJ: Ablex.

Hunt, E. (1978). Mechanics of verbal intelligence. *Psychological Review, 85,* 109–130.

Hunter, J. E., & Hunter, R. F. (1984). Validity and utility of alternative predictors of job performance. *Psychological Bulletin, 96,* 72–98.

Lehman, H. C. (1953). *Age and achievement.* Princeton, NJ: Princeton University Press.

Logan, G. D. (1985). Skill and automaticity: Relations, implications, and future directions. *Canadian Journal of Psychology, 39,* 367–386.

McKeithen, K. B., Reitman, J. S., Rueter, H. H., & Hirtle, S. C. (1981). Knowledge organization and skill differences in computer programmers. *Cognitive Psychology, 13,* 307–325.

Marteniuk, R. G., & Romanow, S. K. E. (1983). Human movement organization and learning as revealed by variability of movement, use of kinematic information, and Fourier analysis. In R. A. Magill (Ed.), *Memory and control of action* (pp. 167–198). Amsterdam: North Holland.

Murphy, G. L., & Wright, J. C. (1984). Changes in conceptual structure with expertise: Differences between real-world experts and novices. *Journal of Experimental Psychology: Learning, Memory and Cognition, 10,* 144–155.

Murrell, K. F. H. (1970). The effect of extensive practice on age differences in reaction time. *Journal of Gerontology, 25,* 268–274.

Newell, A., & Rosenbloom, P. S. (1981). Mechanisms of skill acquisition and the law of practice. In J. R. Anderson (Ed.), *Cognitive skills and their acquisition.* Hillsdale, NJ: Lawrence Erlbaum.

Newell, A., & Simon, H. A. (1972). *Human problem solving.* Englewood Cliffs, NJ: Prentice-Hall.

Oldfield, R. C. (1963). Individual vocabulary and semantic currency: A preliminary study. *British Journal of Social and Clinical Psychology, 2,* 122–130.

Pirolli, P. L., & Anderson, J. R. (1985). The role of learning from examples in the acquisition of recursive programming skills. *Canadian Journal of Psychology, 39,* 240–272.

Plude, D. J., & Hoyer, W. J. (1985). Attention and performance: Identifying and localizing age deficits. In N. Charness (Ed.), *Aging and human performance.* New York: Wiley.

Reitman, J. (1976). Skilled perception in go: Deducing memory structures from inter-response times. *Cognitive Psychology, 8,* 336–356.

Salthouse, T. A. (1984). Effects of age and skill in typing. *Journal of Experimental Psychology: General, 13,* 345–371.

Salthouse, T. A. (1985). Speed of behavior and its implications for cognition. In J. E. Birren & K. W. Schaie (Eds.), *Handbook of the psychology of aging* (2nd ed., pp. 400–426). New York: Van Nostrand Reinhold.

Salthouse, T. A., & Somberg, B. L. (1982). Skilled performance: Effects of adult age and experience on elementary processes. *Journal of Experimental Psychology: General, 111,* 176–207.

Shneiderman. B. (1976). Exploratory experiments in programmer behavior. *International Journal of Computer and Information Sciences, 5,* 123–143.

Simon, H. A., & Gilmartin, K. (1973). A simulation of memory for chess positions. *Cognitive Psychology, 5,* 29–46.

Simon, D. P., & Simon, H. A. (1978). Individual differences in solving physics problems. In R. Siegler (Ed.), *Children's thinking: What develops?* Hillsdale, NJ: Lawrence Erlbaum.

Smith, J. (1985). *Skilled digit memory in old age: A test of reserve capacity.* Paper presented at a meeting of the International Society for the Study of Behavioral Development, Tours, France.

Spilich, G. J. (1985). Discourse comprehension across the life span. In N. Charness (Ed.), *Aging and human performance.* New York: Wiley.

Stigler, J. W. (1984). "Mental abacus": The effect of abacus training on Chinese children's mental calculation. *Cognitive Psychology, 16,* 145–176.

Stones, M. J., & Kozma, A. (1985). Physical performance. In N. Charness (Ed.), *Aging and human performance.* New York: Wiley.

Talland, G. A. (1965). Initiation of response, and reaction time in aging, and with brain damage. In A. T. Welford & J. E. Birren (Eds.), *Behavior, aging, and the nervous system* (pp. 526–561). Springfield, IL: Charles C. Thomas.

25 World-knowledge systems

Cameron J. Camp

Definition of world knowledge

I distinctly remember an event that took place when I was a graduate student. I was giving an older gentleman in a retirement home the Information subtest of the Wechsler Adult Intelligence Scale (Wechsler, 1955) and asked the question, "How far is it from Paris to New York?" My respondent waited a moment and then said in a steady and deliberate voice, "Well, Lindbergh flew there in about 36 hours, with an average air speed of about 100 m.p.h., so I'll say that it's about 3600 miles." His response surprised me, for I had asked many younger adults this question, but had never encountered either this level of accuracy or this particular approach to deriving the answer. This older gentleman had retrieved facts from what appeared to be an impressive base of knowledge about his life and world (i.e., "world knowledge") and additionally had created a new piece of information to be retained for future use. Three interrelated questions immediately came to mind: (1) How is this knowledge base created? (2) What processes influence the utilization of this knowledge base? (3) How does human aging influence these mental structures and processes? The search for answers to these questions has led to a series of studies in a relatively new but rapidly growing area of research. This chapter represents an attempt to chart what we think we know, the problems that such studies have encountered, and some things we may want to know in our attempts to better answer these questions.

In the first place, world knowledge has been defined in a variety of different ways. Lachman and Lachman (1980, p. 287) defined world knowledge as a per-

The preparation of this chapter and the research reported in it were partially supported by NIA grant 1 RO1 AG 02427-01A1 and by grants from the graduate research councils of the University of New Orleans and Fort Hays State University. The author gratefully acknowledges the extensive assistance provided by Dianne Meder, Wally Parish, Kay Gobin, Mary Williams, and Bruce Dorval, as well as those individuals attending the Talland conference and the Second Harvard Conference on Adult and Adolescent Thought and Perception for their valuable suggestions. Finally, the author wishes to thank Roy and Janet Lachman for their encouragement and wisdom.

manent base of information that an individual acquires over a lifetime from both educational and day-to-day experiences. Howard defines world knowledge as information dealing with the properties of the world, both physical and social (1983, p. 310). It has sometimes been referred to as tertiary or very long term memory. World knowledge is a combination of personal experiences and generic information that is stored without a record of where and when it was acquired (Kausler, 1982; Tulving, 1972). Tulving (1985), for example, sees episodic memory as a specialized subsystem of semantic memory. Others view personal or episodic memory and generic or semantic memory as relatively distinct, though interconnected, systems. See Chang (1986) for a general review of models of semantic memory.

Schank (1975) restricts his definition of world knowledge to the domain of generic knowledge, but he provides some interesting thoughts on the migration of information from the episodic domain of knowledge to the generic. He argues that world knowledge consists of episodes whose central themes have been encountered so often that it is impossible to trace their origins. For example, consider the question, "What is the largest city in Great Britain?" If you know the answer, ask yourself the following: "When and where did I first encounter this question and its answer? When and where did I last encounter this question and its answer?" Though the correct answer to the question has been stored, episodic information about encountering the question and its answer often is not readily available. Thus, this piece of information is no longer an episodic memory (Schank, 1975, p. 180).

Schank sees repetition as the vehicle that allows stored information to lose its personal contexts. (Bahrick, 1979; Linton, 1982). Over time, repeated encounters with similar information in similar environmental contexts leads to the creation of "scripts," which contain the routinized information distilled from past experiences. Lachman, Lachman, and Taylor (1982, p. 302) use a similar idea to describe an aspect of life-span cognitive development. They point out that early life may be viewed as a time of storing new types of episodes, and later life is spent interpreting episodes encountered in the environment as instances of familiar ones. What may eventually become generic information may still be primarily episodic in early life.

Hoyer (1985, p. 80) describes similar processes in the transition from "novice" to "expert." He sees cognitive expertise as a learning process that requires the steady accumulation of information over time. He notes that knowledge scripts become automatized after much practice, thus freeing up capacity-limited control processes. Finally, he describes the process by which experts deal with exceptional cases – by drawing inferences and using integrative and constructive processes. A discussion of the use of expert knowledge is provided by Charness (Chapter 24, this volume).

But personal memories often are useful sources of information when dealing with the world. Valuable knowledge can be embedded within idiosyncratic, non-boring, or "low-frequency" episodes stored in memory. Older adults often interrupt experiments to explain how our world-knowledge stimuli relate to specific personal episodes or reminiscences. They love to tell about how a past episode enabled an answer to a question to be selected (e.g., "I remember once using a pair of tweezers to unscrew a device located inside of a bicycle tire valve."). Remembering this episode can help solve the same problem at a later date. Therefore, we include both episodic and generic information bases in our definition of world knowledge. World knowledge will therefore be defined as all information acquired by individuals in real-world settings outside of the context of the research laboratory.

In summary, various definitions of world knowledge have been presented. World knowledge has been learned before a research participant enters a research laboratory. Some knowledge involves personal memories, whereas other information is relatively free of personal contexts. Repeated encounters with specific information causes that knowledge to lose its episodic nature. Because living presents a greater likelihood of repeatedly encountering a piece of information over time, the amount of knowledge that is not episodic probably increases as individuals grow older. Both types of information are included in this chapter's definition of world knowledge.

Environmental inputs are first matched against current world knowledge. When an incomplete match is found, constructive/inferential processes are generated in order to comprehend the novel information or answer a question. Decisions about matches between incoming information and stored information are determined by "executive" processes such as "metamemory." The reader is referred to Chapter 22 by Dixon (dealing with a review of the questionnaire method of studying metamemory) and Chapter 23 by Cavanaugh (dealing with the importance of awareness in memory and aging research) for more detailed discussion of this topic. The initial findings of research dealing with world knowledge and aging will be described next.

What we think we know

Overview

In this section, some of the conclusions that have been drawn about world-knowledge systems will be discussed. What little knowledge is presently available exists because of a slowly accelerating attack on the idea that memory research can effectively ignore the types of memories that most individuals use in daily living. The historical influences on research activities involving world knowledge therefore will be reviewed. Utilization of world knowledge involving the use of fact retrieval, inferential reasoning, and metacognition knowledge systems will be discussed. The growth of knowledge will be examined, followed by a discussion of the influence of motivational forces (specifically, curiosity and depression) on utilization of world-knowledge systems. Finally, the relationship between utilization of world-knowledge systems and the beliefs that individuals of different ages have regarding world-knowledge utilization will be discussed.

Historical influences

Ebbinghaus's attempts to study "natural memory" involved active efforts to exclude the influence of world knowledge, and especially generic memory, on memory performance. As a partial result of his efforts, this field has only recently begun to see intensive research by a large number of memory researchers. Memory research carried on in the behavioristic tradition likewise opted for laboratory-based research rather than "world-based" research, with the creation and decay of new associations being a prime focus of study. Previously learned information was not as amenable to precise measurement and often was viewed as a source of "interference." Neisser (1982, chap. 1) argues that many current theories of memory suffer the same paucity of ecological validity.

An interesting exception to this trend has been intelligence testing. Here, at least, there has been interest in how to make water boil, what yeast does in dough, and so forth. It should therefore come as no surprise that one of the first experimental efforts to measure world knowledge in old age was an attempt to measure intelligence in older adults by dealing with problems indigenous to them (Demming & Pressey, 1957). Their test was based on information useful in solving the problems posed by everyday life, such as legal terms or how to use the yellow pages of the telephone book. Interestingly, they found a rise in scores in middle age and later years in the same individuals who showed declining test scores on conventional tests.

Neisser (1982, chap. 1) offered a clear challenge to researchers studying memory. He called for a more "naturalistic" approach to memory research in which the contents and processes of memories used in real-world settings should be the focus of attention. Research that has attempted to respond to this challenge often has retained its laboratory setting but has shifted its content and focus. Much of this research is quite recent, and the conclusions to be drawn are necessarily tentative. Nevertheless, a start has been made.

Utilizing world knowledge

Remembering facts. Studies involving the retrieval of factual information from tertiary memory generally have found either no age effects or higher levels of performance in older adults compared with the young (Fozard, 1980; Lachman et al., 1982). These findings extend to measures of vocabulary and other crystallized-intelligence measures (Horn, 1982).

Inferential reasoning. Most of the initial research of inferential reasoning in old age was conducted within the research context of text comprehension. For example, Cohen (1981) and Cohen and Faulkner (1981) reported that older adults did not draw inferences from text as efficiently as did younger adults, and they showed a similar deficit for retention of inferences made from text. Belmore (1981) and Light, Zelinski, and Moore (1982) also found age-related deficits in retention of inferences and ability to make inferences at delayed recall. However, when facts were available for viewing, age deficits in making inferences from text disappeared. Light and associates (1982) concluded that problems in inferential reasoning associated with old age might be due to poor retention of new factual information and/or reduced working memory capacity, rather than reasoning deficits per se. Because all of this research was based on reasoning from new information, these studies involved not only reasoning but also the learning of new information. Even in this context, however, not all studies have shown differences between younger and older adults in making inferences from text (Cavanaugh, Kramer, Sinnott, Camp, & Markley, 1985; Hess & Arnould, 1986; Walsh & Baldwin, 1977).

Research using stimuli designed to tap world knowledge has generated a somewhat similar pattern of results. When the task demands on working memory were low, no age deficits were found in answering world-knowledge questions designed to elicit inferential reasoning (Camp, 1981; Camp & Pignatiello, 1984). When the task demands on working memory were increased (e.g., by increasing the number of alternatives in a question-answering task), older adults became less accurate in answering questions, as compared with younger adults (Camp, 1981; Camp & Pignatiello, 1984). (These findings will be discussed in more detail in the section dealing with beliefs about world-knowledge systems.) Again, however, not all researchers have found age deficits in answering such questions, even when using multiple alternatives as potential answers (Lachman et al., 1982).

Metacognition and world knowledge. Metacognitive systems for world knowledge also seem either to remain stable or to increase in efficiency as individuals age (Lachman, Lachman, & Thronesberry, 1979). This is true for fact retrieval (Lachman et al., 1979, 1982), as measured by confidence ratings and the feeling-of-knowing phenomenon, in addition to measures of the amount of time spent searching for information that is not immediately recalled. It is also true for inferential reasoning, as measured by estimates of the amount of inferential reasoning necessary to select an answer to a question (Camp, 1981; Camp & Pignatiello, 1984; Lachman et al., 1982).

A caution. This view of world-knowledge systems may be optimistic. Given that much of the research that supports this view involves "no difference" studies, it is extremely important to be wary of ceiling or floor effects when using stimuli designed to measure world knowledge. Still, many of the studies supporting views of little or no decline in memory for world knowledge seem to be free of these confounds.

Growth of world knowledge

Lachman and Lachman (1980) found evidence that the efficiency with which information is extracted from world-knowledge systems remains stable throughout adulthood, whereas the size of the knowledge base increases. Kausler (1982, p. 264) stated that a large amount of generic information is acquired during childhood, but that new information is added to the generic-knowledge store throughout the life span, and such information is extremely resistant to forgetting. Fitzgerald and Lawrence (1984, p. 697), in a study concerning autobiographical memory in groups of individuals ranging from 11 to 75 years of age, concluded that the memory systems of older and younger adults acquire new information at similar rates and retain it for similar periods of time. Thus, the size of the domain of world knowledge seems to increase with age. There is some disagreement over the rate at which the size of this knowledge base increases over time. Factors that influence the rate of knowledge accretion over long time periods in real-world settings also need extensive investigation.

Motivational forces and world-knowledge systems

Curiosity. Motivational forces also influence the rates of knowledge accretion and knowledge utilization. Curiosity in children has been seen as an adaptive characteristic for our species. Knowledge acquisition is intrinsically reinforcing. But at what age does this built-in reinforcer cease to function, if ever? Few researches have studied curiosity across the adult life span. The first data relevant to this question were gathered by Giambra (1974, 1977). He used a 344-item imaginal-proccesses inventory to study daydreaming in adults of different ages. This inventory had two subscales designed to measure different types of curiosity and another subscale designed to measure boredom. Contrary to negative stereotypes, age generally was not related to curiosity measures in Giambra's studies. Boredom, however, was consistently related to age, with level of boredom decreasing with advancing age.

We have begun a series of experiments to examine curiosity in younger and older adults. Our findings indicate that although younger adults may have higher levels of "sensation seeking," age differences are negligible when desire to obtain new information is measured (Camp, 1986; Camp, Dietrich, & Olson, 1985; Camp, Rodrigue, & Olson, 1984). In addition, our observations during experiments, informal observations such as the rise in popularity of games involving memory for world knowledge or "trivia," examinations of the cognitive tasks contained in television quiz shows, and so forth, indicate that knowledge retrieval is enjoyed by most individuals, regardless of age. This is especailly true for information that has not been used for some time. Interesting research could be initiated using games of memory for trivia or by examining the records of performance of contestants on certain television game shows. Until now, we primarily have attempted to simulate such experiences in the laboratory in order to make research more palatable to our participants. There probably are some fascinating archival research projects waiting to be conducted with the behavior of contestants on television quiz shows.

Depression. Another approach to the study of motivational influences on the use of world knowledge has involved the study of depression. Niederehe (in press) presented world-knowledge questions to both younger and older adults. Within each age group, depressives (taken from an outpatient population and screened for organic brain dysfunction) were compared with nondepressives. Participants were matched on education level. In testing situations using free recall, cued recall, and recognition, older adults outperformed younger adults. Depression was not a significant factor.

Recently, we have begun to study depression through the use of mood-induction procedures (Camp, 1985; Pignatiello, 1985; Pignatiello, Camp, & Rasar, 1986). Our college-student subjects read a series of statements or listened to music selections that were intended to induce various moods: depressed, neutral, or elated. They were then presented a series of world-knowledge questions in a multiple-choice format. In two studies using sentences as stimuli and one study using music, mood has not been found to be related to number of correct responses or reaction times for answering world-knowledge questions. In these studies, we used questions that induced either fact retrieval or inferential reasoning, because inferential reasoning might require more cognitive effort than fact retrieval (based on the finding that longer reaction times have been associated with inferential reasoning than with fact retrieval for answering questions in a recognition memory format). This factor had been suggested by Niederehe (in press) as a potential reason for the lack of a depression effect in his study. However, this within-subjects factor did not interact with depression in any of our studies, though it proved to be a potent main effect for reaction times. Thus, the initial research findings do not support the contention that depression is associated with reduced ability to utilize world-knowledge systems. Niederehe suggested that depression might be involved with decisions to *initiate* cognitive processes; this idea will be discussed later. For a general review of the role of depression and elation in biasing memory, see Blaney (1986).

Stereotypes

Confidence ratings for question answering. In spite of an increasing accumulation of evidence that world-knowledge utilization does not significantly decline in late life, negative stereotypes regarding the decline of memory functioning and aging persist and are widespread. In another study, we asked 40 young, 40 middle-aged, and 40 older adults to make both specific and global judgments concerning "remembering" (fact retrieval) and "figuring out" (inferential reasoning) (Camp & Pignatiello, 1984; Pignatiello & Camp, 1984). These individuals answered 120 world-knowledge questions, 60 of which were intended to induce fact retrieval and 60 of which were intended to induce inferential reasoning. An example of a fact-retrieval question: "What is the capital of Lebanon?" (Beirut). An example of an inferential-reasoning question: "What piece of playground equipment would be most useful in weighing a sack of potatoes?" (seesaw). [A list of 60 previously used fact-retrieval and inferential-reasoning items has been published elsewhere (Camp, Lachman, & Lachman, 1980). A list of the 120 stimulus items used by Camp and Pignatiello is available on request.] Questions were presented in a true/false context (one answer shown that had to be judged as a correct or incorrect answer to the question) and multiple-choice context (four alternatives). We assumed that the complexity of the tasks would vary as a function of two factors. Increasing the number of alternatives would increase task complexity. Also, the inferential-reasoning initiators would involve more cognitive processing than fact-retrieval initiators, at least in terms of requiring longer reaction times to obtain correct answers (Camp, 1981; Camp et al., 1980; Camp & Pignatiello, 1984). Thus, three levels of complexity emerged: (1) fact-retrieval questions in a true/false context (least complex); (2) true/false inferential-reasoning questions or fact-retrieval questions with four alternatives; (3) inferential-reasoning initiators with four alternatives (most complex). At complexity level 1, older adults answered more items correctly than younger adults and were also more confident in their responses than younger adults. At complexity level 2, no age differences were found in either the number of correct responses or the confidence ratings. These outcomes may reflect good metamemorial performance at all age levels, a finding that other researchers using these types of stimuli have reported (Lachman et al., 1979, 1982). At complexity level 3, younger adults answered significantly more items correctly than did older adults, but no age effects were found for confidence ratings.

Similarly, Lachman and Jelalian (1984) compared the predictions of older adults and younger adults for performance on a fluid-intelligence task (letter series) and a crystallized-intelligence task (vocabulary). She found that both young and elderly adults were fairly accurate in monitoring their intellectual abilities, but elderly adults more frequently overestimated their performance, particularly on the test for which they performed more poorly (p. 581).

These results seem to indicate that if negative stereotypes about aging and memory are held by older adults, such stereotypes do not produce lower levels of confidence for specific answers to questions. This is similar to a finding of Niederehe and Camp (1985) in a study in which depressed and nondepressed elderly adults were asked to give ratings of their performance in a recognition memory task, as well as global ratings of memory ability. Neither ability to recognize targets nor performance ratings were related to depression, though depressives did rate themselves significantly lower on global measures of memory ability. But why were there no age differences in confidence ratings for inferential questions, even under conditions in which older adults answered *fewer* questions correctly (complexity level 3)? Do *positive* stereotypes about aging (such as ideas about becoming "wiser" with age) influence confidence for item-specific judgments, whereas negative stereotypes do not? Are older adults simply more stable in their self-judgments than younger adults?

In order to address some of these issues, we next attempted to measure global beliefs for fact retrieval and inferential reasoning in the same individuals who had already answered our world-knowledge questions. We wished to know how such global beliefs might be related to confidence ratings for specific items.

Global beliefs. After completing the tasks mentioned earlier, our participants made global judgments about "remembering" and "figuring out." We asked individuals to compare themselves to other cohorts in relative ability to use these two cognitive processes. For example, an older adult would be asked, "When it comes to remembering facts (or figuring out), how do you compare with most people 20 years (or 40 years) younger than yourself? Are you worse, about the same, or better?" We also asked individuals to compare their cohort versus other cohorts. Finally, we asked that individuals compare their current levels of ability against their past (for older adults) or future (for younger adults) levels of performance.

Our results were quite intriguing. Younger adults, in general, believed that cognitive abilities remained stable into middle age and then declined in old age, regardless of the type of comparison being made. Middle-aged adults, in general, shared this pattern of beliefs, with one exception. Our middle-aged participants believed that within themselves, the ability to "figure out" had *improved* since their youth and would not decline in their old age. Our older adults believed that their cohort was worse than other cohorts for both cognitive processes. These older adults also viewed *themselves* to be equal in ability for both cognitive processes compared with younger cohorts. Finally, these older individuals believed that they themselves had become worse at fact retrieval since their own youth, but had improved in their ability to make inferences since their own youth.

We view these outcomes for our older adults as possibly indicating the internalization of both negative and positive global beliefs or stereotypes about aging and cognition. The negative stereotype is that advancing age produces a decline in memory (associated with "remembering"), and the positive stereotype is that advancing age brings about increased wisdom (associated with "figuring things out"). Until we have a longitudinal data base that can be used to determine the accuracy of these beliefs, we shall not know the utility of maintaining them.

We think that these stereotypes may have influenced confidence ratings in the following manner. When an experimental task is not too difficult, and stored information can be easily matched with incoming information, accurate metacognitive functions will monitor the matching process and control confidence ratings. But under conditions of high uncertainty and/or task complexity (such as the presentation of inferential questions with multiple alternatives), metacognitive functions will simply monitor the fact that the task requires a great deal of cognitive effort and that there is no match to be found between past experience and the available alternative answers. In these circumstances, decisions as to the accuracy of selected answers and decisions as to how much cognitive effort to allocate to the task may be made on the basis of global beliefs. In this particular instance, a positive stereotype will lead to overly high confidence and perhaps to an underestimation of the amount of processing necessary to select an accurate answer. The general principle involved therefore seems to be that metacognition functions relatively independent of global stereotypes, except under conditions of high task complexity and/or uncertainty.

In summary, research involving world knowledge does not readily reflect the picture of declining ability with advancing age found in more traditional memory research. World-knowledge systems seem to grow over time, and world-knowledge utilization seems to be both effective and remarkably resistant to factors such as aging and depression. Furthermore, the interest in acquiring new information to add to the world-knowledge store does not seem to diminish over time. Stereotypes about world-knowledge utilization are both positive and negative, but seem to have little influence on confidence measures except under conditions of high task complexity and/or uncertainty.

Issues in the measurement of world knowledge

In this section, a number of issues and related problems arising from attempts to measure world-knowledge systems are discussed. These issues include selection of stimulus materials, attempts to measure the efficiency of usage and the size of world-knowledge systems, and the role of social contexts in utilization of world-knowledge systems. Difficulties inherent in current methods of studying world-knowledge systems are reviewed.

Selection of measures

Different topic areas. The immediate problem facing the researcher wishing to work with world-knowledge systems is the selection of appropriate measures. But the measures deemed appropriate will vary widely according to the goals of the researcher. One approach has been to use questions sampled from a variety of topic areas (Botwinick & Storandt, 1974; Camp, 1981; Camp & Pignatiello, 1984; Lachman & Lachman, 1980; Perlmutter, 1978). This has the advantage of giving an index of breadth of knowledge, but may not give an accurate description of an individual whose knowledge base is extensive but specialized. Individuals with little formal education may fit this description (Neisser, 1982, Chapter 1).

Current events. Current events sometimes are included in pools of world-knowledge questions (Botwinick & Storandt, 1974, 1980; Camp et al., 1980; Lachman & Lachman, 1980; Niederehe, in press; Perlmutter 1978; Poon, Fozard, Paulshock, & Thomas, 1979; Storandt, Grant, & Gordon, 1978; Warrington & Silberstein, 1970). An almost uniform finding in these studies is that older adults show no deficits in answering such questions and often outperform younger adults. One difficulty with such items is that "current" events quickly become "historical" events. Thus, current-events items will become progressively more difficult for younger adults with successive usage. (Try asking an 18-year-old the name of the U.S. spy ship seized by North Korea, or the name of the woman who was killed in Ted Kennedy's car on Chapaquidick Island.) Similarly, events that are "historical" for younger generations today have personal relevance (and may involve episodic information) for older generations. For example, freshmen who entered college in 1987 were born after Neil Armstrong first walked on the moon. Current events, therefore, will always contain inevitable cohort disparities.

Tertiary memory. Larry Squire and his colleagues have investigated tertiary memory using questions about more specific topics, such as TV shows (Squire, Chance, & Slater, 1975) and racehorses (Squire & Slater, 1975). In both studies, older adults exhibited maximum levels of performance. Bartlett and Snellus (1980) found similar results comparing middle-aged and older adults' memories for melodies. In these studies, only older adults had been uniformly exposed to the critical information as adults. Botwinick (1984, pp. 328–9) described this issue as the problem of measuring knowledge versus memory. The use of "dated" information items favors older adults, thus making the study of tertiary "memory" something of a misnomer when younger adults are studied.

Vocabulary. Vocabulary measures can face similar problems. Barrett and Wright (1981) gave a free-recall test to younger and older adults using words that were relevant to older generations (e.g., flapper) or to younger generations (e.g., joint). Though young adults (as usual) had higher overall recall scores, older adults outperformed younger adults in recalling words more familiar to their generation. This result was replicated in a later study (Barrett & Watkins, 1986). Barrett has also published a set of age-specific word-familiarity norms (Barrett, 1983).

Picture naming. Other researchers have used picture naming as a means of measuring world knowledge. Thomas, Fozard, and Waugh (1977) presented pictures to younger and older adults while recording naming speed under three conditions. The conditions involved naming an object after first being shown an appropriate prompt (its printed name), an inappropriate prompt, or no prompt. Naming latency for the appropriate-prompt condition was fastest for all age groups and was assumed to involve the retrieval of the appropriate name from primary memory. Naming latencies for the no-prompt and inappropriate-prompt conditions were identical and were assumed to involve retrieval from tertiary memory. Naming latencies increased as a function of age, but in all three conditions, naming latency increased at a constant amount over age.

Thomas and associates also found that frequency of word usage was the single best predictor of naming speed. This led to a second study by Poon and Fozard

(1978). They presented pictures of objects commonly used 50 to 70 years earlier (e.g., spittoon), objects unique to contemporary times (e.g., dune buggy), and objects commonly used during both time periods (e.g., shoes from a 1910 catalogue and shoes from a 1974 catalogue) to older and younger adults. Younger adults were fastest at naming objects unique to recent time periods, older adults were fastest at naming objects unique to past time periods and older versions of common objects, and no age differences were found for current versions of common objects.

These studies demonstrate that familiarity with information is a critical variable when studying world-knowledge systems. What is normative for one generation may not be familiar or normative for another. Attempts to measure the size or content of world-knowledge systems must take into account the unique domains of information acquired over time within both cohorts and individuals.

Measures of world-knowledge utilization

Efficiency ratio. Attempts to measure world-knowledge utilization have taken several different approaches. Lachman and Lachman (1980) measured the number of world-knowledge questions answered by individuals of different age groups in a free-recall format and a multiple-choice format. For each person, this measure of "total knowledge" was then compared with the number of items that could be recalled to obtain a measure of the efficiency of world-knowledge utilization (i.e., efficiency = recalled information/total knowledge). This measure showed no age effect. The benefit of using such a ratio is that such a measure is based on the amount of information available, regardless of the size of the knowledge base. The difficulty with this measure is that it is not a true ratio, in the sense that the function does not have an absolute zero point.

Equating item familiarity. Another approach is to attempt to equate familiarity of information so that the information tested should be equally familiar to all generations (Poon & Fozard, 1978). Niederehe (in press) devised a set of world-knowledge questions that were extensively pretested to screen out items that were age-biased in either the free-recall format or recognition-memory format. (Interestingly, age effects were found for these questions in the actual study, with older adults outperforming younger adults.)

A problem with this procedure is that the screening device (equating accuracy among different age groups in answering stimulus questions) virtually assures that no age effects will be found in subsequent studies with similar populations where accuracy is the dependent measure. The technique does allow a researcher to determine if some factor (such as depression, stress, etc.) produces lower performance in samples that have different levels of the factor than are found in normative samples. It also allows a researcher to determine if a factor such as depression influences different cohorts to the same degree. Assuring that experimental samples differ from normative samples only on the one factor of interest is the greatest difficulty with this approach.

An alternative to this approach is to equate stimulus items for age familiarity and then use a measure other than accuracy to determine efficiency of knowledge utilization in normative older and younger samples. The picture-naming research described earlier, by Fozard and his colleagues, used this method. Poon and Fozard (1978) attempted to measure retrieval from tertiary memory after eliminating the contribution of the perceptual-motor component of response speeds. They concluded that the age effect in picture-naming latency is almost entirely attributable to slowness in the perceptual-motor component of the naming latency, not the memory-search component. In our previously mentioned studies using induced moods (Camp, 1985; Pignatiello, 1985), we had matched the difficulty of fact-retrieval and inferential-reasoning questions in terms of accuracy; yet these different types of questions still produced significantly different reaction times. We had hoped that this technique would produce interaction effects between mood condition and question type for reaction times. Though our interaction effects were not significant, the group-by-task design has long been a staple of gerontological research. See Kausler (1982) for an extended discussion of age-by-task interaction designs.

Reaction-time measures. Researchers measuring reaction times in question-answering tasks have found older adults to be slower at answering such questions, independent of whether the older adults were answering more items correctly than the young, answering fewer items correctly, or displaying equal accuracy (Camp, 1981; Camp & Pignatiello, 1984; Lachman et al., 1982). Slower reaction times with increasing age in question-answering tasks have also been shown to be independent of measures of psychomotor components, such as time to respond to simple visual patterns (Camp, 1981) or reading speed (Camp & Pignatiello, 1984).

Learning new information. Another approach to the study of efficiency of retrieval from world-knowledge systems has been based on learning within laboratory settings. In an attempt to create an analogue of real-world learning, researchers have presented pictures (Fozard, Waugh, & Thomas, 1975) and line drawings (Mitchell, 1984) to adults of different ages and then tested recognition memory for these visual stimuli at different intervals after initial presentation. Fozard and associates found that most of the decline in recognition memory over time occurred within 4 weeks, at which time age effects were seen favoring younger adults. However, age was not a significant predictor of forgetting after a 2.5-year interval. Mitchell tested for recognition after 1 hour and again after 1 year. He also varied the number of exposures to his line drawings, as well as the number of intervening stimuli between initial presentation and the test for recognition (i.e., a lag effect). After an interval of 1 hour, both repetition and lag effects were found, but no age effects were present. After 1 year, repetition effects were still seen, but the lag effect and age effect were not significant. These studies clearly support the contention that retrieval from tertiary memory seems unimpaired across age levels. Retention of verbal information needs to be tested under similar conditions in order to determine the generalizability of these results.

Age of memories. The preceding two studies attempted to equate date of acquisition of information across age groups. An alternative technique has been to test for the retrieval of information that has resided for differing amounts of time within memory. Warrington and Sanders (1971), in addition to using a questionnaire of past events, presented pictures of famous individuals cut out from a newspaper. They found that performance dropped with increasing age, though recall deficits were more pronounced than recognition deficits. Bahrick, Bahrick, and Wittlinger (1975), working with older and younger adults, tested for memory of both names and faces of classmates from high school yearbooks. Younger adults outperformed older adults in both recalling and recognizing names. Recognition of faces was not affected by age. Bahrick (1979) later tested for recall of street names in places people had attended college. Much decline was found in the first year after leaving college, with less decline in subsequent years. These studies support the unsurprising conclusion that visual information is retained better than verbal information over long time periods and that recognition performance levels are higher than recall for such information. Aging was related to some loss in the retrievability of information, depending on whether or not the information tested was personally relevant, visual versus verbal, and so forth.

Botwinick noted that these studies share a common methodological problem in that the age of the memory is confounded with the age of the research participants (1984, p. 327). Bahrick (1983) attempted to control for this problem by varying both the age of subjects and the age of memories. College teachers of different ages attempted to recall, recognize, and match pictures and names of students who had taken or were currently taking their classes. The names of the students were taken from class lists dating back 8 years, 4 years, 1 year, and 2 weeks. Interestingly, he found name recognition to be better than portrait recognition. He ascribed this outcome to a lower level of original learning of students' names, compared with the learning of names of classmates in his original study. After reviewing his data, Bahrick concluded that aging of the memory trace may adversely influence performance independent of the age of the research participant, at least in his sample (p. 32).

Rehearsal of world-knowledge items. Other problems can influence outcomes in the study of world-knowledge utilization. Older adults often amaze new visitors with tales of their remote past, thus enhancing the belief that the older individual "has a remarkable memory." However, such behaviors often represent the retrieval of well-rehearsed and oft-repeated stories. Multiple rehearsals of "old" information through reminiscing is an issue that has received scant attention in the research literature. Along these same lines, the repetition of "old" information through TV reruns of shows made in the 1950s, the rise in popularity of trivia games, and so forth, may further confound attempts to study retrieval of information from world-knowledge systems.

Size of knowledge-base estimates and inferential reasoning. Another problem involves the assumption that the size of the knowledge base increases with advancing age, whereas accessibility to such information remains relatively intact. If this assumption is correct, older adults may be able to answer questions via inferential reasoning more readily than younger adults, because older cohorts will have more "raw material" (i.e., stored information) to use in constructing inferences. This could cause overestimation of the size of the knowledge base in older cohorts, vis-à-vis the young, as well as perhaps mask any deficits in the ability to retrieve such information that might increase as a function of advancing age. It is even possible that the knowledge base decreases with age, whereas inferential ability increases, though this seems a bit unlikely. Thus, studies that attempt to estimate the size of an individual's knowledge base must also take into account the processes used to generate responses from the knowledge base.

Real-world settings. Perhaps the ultimate problem facing researchers interested in studying world knowledge and everyday cognition is how to study knowledge acquisition and retrieval outside of the laboratory. Some valuable initial attempts have been made in this area. Cavanaugh, Grady, and Perlmutter (1983) had older individuals keep diaries of instances of forgetting. West (1985) embedded tests of over 15 practical memory tasks within a 1-hour interview. Barrett and Estes (1984) created a mental-activity scale that was given to adults of different ages. Mental activity was measured by having adults describe their activities on an hourly basis over a 24-hour period. Activities were then classified into 14 categories, ranging from sleeping (lowest amount of conscious mental activity) to learning and problem solving (highest levels of conscious mental activity). A mental-activity score was then derived from this information, and older adults had lower scores than younger adults. This represents one of the first empirical means of testing the assumption that the way to a meaningful and rewarding old age is to remain mentally active throughout life.

Anschutz, Camp, Markley, and Kramer (1985) trained older adults to use the method of loci to memorize a grocery list. Participants then were taken grocery shopping at a nearby supermarket, and performance was measured by the number of items placed in a grocery cart and purchased with money earned from participating in the study. Across a wide variety of individual differences in formal education, health status, and so forth, performance in this task was nearly perfect and remained so at retest 1 month later. Perhaps the most important thing that we learned from the study was that external factors greatly influenced the behavior of our sample. These individuals resided in an apartment complex for elderly adults. They soon became celebrities within the complex. Lines of well-wishers would see them off on their grocery-shopping excursions. Participants in the study began to train spouses and friends who were not in the study. Participants offered encouragement to each other, as well as assurances that the task would be enjoyable and not too difficult. Our participants performed exceptionally well, with almost all demonstrating perfect performance in the grocery-shopping task. An older man who forgot one grocery item was chided by female participants. He responded by redoubling his efforts at mastering the training, and he was superior to other participants at generalizing the training at a final testing session using word lists. We simply had not anticipated the impact that our intervention would have on the social milieu of our participants, nor the milieu's sometimes crucial role in influencing performance.

The role of social contexts

If we are to understand everyday cognition across adulthood, we must eventually try to understand it within social contexts, where support and assistance are available from others. The need to study world-knowledge utilization within a social context is not a new idea. It has been over 50 years since Vygotsky initially suggested that intelligence should not be measured by tests that force an individual to perform tasks alone and without assistance. Vygotsky (1962, 1978) claimed that such an approach distorted our measures of competence. Instead, he recommended studying an individual's "zone of proximal development" (i.e., things that could be accomplished with assistance).

In this spirit, Hulicka (1982, p. 349) reported that two elderly adults, a brother and sister, let her read letters they had written to one another as young adults. Hulicka then created a 20-item test for each person based on what they had known at one time about trips, family problems, and so forth. Ten questions were asked of each individual. The brother had four correct answers, and the sister had three (they were 80 and 75 years of age, respectively). The brother and sister then met for the first time in several years and began to talk about their childhood. The 10 new questions were then given to each of them. Both then answered correctly 9 of the new questions and 9 of the old. The ability to remember information was critically influenced by the ability to interact with another person. Remembering often (usually?) takes place within a social context. This study demonstrates that such contexts can be integrated into memory research.

In summary, various methodological issues inherent in world-knowledge research have been examined. Central problems are that the knowledge base is different for each individual, and the size and content of this knowledge base change over time. This makes comparisons between individuals quite difficult. Attempts to deal with these issues have enjoyed limited success. Another problem is that laboratory-based research has continued to ignore the influence of social contexts on memory, even though world knowledge is acquired and utilized within such contexts. Until more "naturalistic" research is undertaken, Neisser's original challenge (1982, chap. 1) will not be fully met.

Some things we want to know

In this section, various topics for future research are discussed. These include studying the influences of environmental contexts, attributions, physiological disorders, affective factors, and selectivity in both remembering and learning on world-knowledge utilization. Finally, the topic of wisdom is reviewed.

Environmental contexts

There are many questions left unanswered concerning world-knowledge acquisition and utilization by adults. In which naturally occurring contexts are fact retrieval and especially inferential reasoning utilized by adults? What factors influence their initialization? I remember showing an undergraduate this question: "What letters are associated with the number 6 on the telephone dial?" An answer next appeared, which the participant quickly judged to be true, and the participant next rated his response as a "wild guess." At that point, I said, "What would you do if I offered you $10,000 for the correct answer?" He immediately initiated an appropriate strategy and gave the correct answer. In this situation, the requisite information to answer this question was accessible, knowledge of how to create the answer was present, and yet the correct strategy was not used. The participant recognized that doing so would require cognitive effort, and he was unwilling to expend such effort. Are such behaviors common? Do they occur more frequently in different age groups? Do stereotypes influence initialization of these processes? If we wish to understand everyday cognition, we must seek the answers to these questions. A recent study by Sinnott (1986) gives us some hints about possible answers to some of these questions. She presented adults of different ages a series of questions about everyday memory, operationalized as memory for experiences from a 3-day period in which they served as research subjects. She found that incidental memory was negatively influenced by increasing age, but not prospective/intentional memory. She speculated that perhaps as adults grow older and memory or attentional resources decline, memorial processing is first allocated to input social commitments and other salient information, leaving less memorial processing available for incidental learning.

Attribution

A related issue deals with understanding the interaction of attribution and cognition. Is attribution of success or failure different for fact retrieval and inferential reasoning? If so, are these patterns similar in different age groups? In a previously mentioned study, Lachman and Jelalian (1984) compared older and younger adults' causal attributions for test performance on a fluid-intelligence test and a crystallized-intelligence test. Younger adults scored higher on the fluid test, and older adults scored higher on the crystallized test. Both age groups were more likely to attribute successful performance to ability, and unsuccessful performance to task difficulty. Do negative stereotypes influence our attributions?

Hulicka (1982, p. 342) relates a story about an older woman who made an excellent meal, except for the use of Clorox instead of vinegar in the salad dressing. Her dinner guests immediately attributed this behavior to a cognitive deficit. However, an early house guest assisting with the housework had erroneously put the Clorox in the cupboard where the vinegar was kept. The two containers were very similar in appearance. The woman had reached into the cupboard for the vinegar and had not looked at the label. Because she had made the salad dressing many times, she had not tasted it, nor had she been able to smell Clorox. The impairment that caused her to serve this concoction to her guests was olfactory, not cognitive. Interpersonal and intergenerational attributions regarding cognitive functioning may be critical components of everyday cognition.

Factors adversely affecting world-knowledge utilization

Physiological factors. What factors are associated with the loss of ability to effectively utilize world-knowledge systems? Brain damage due to stroke, closed-head injury, and so forth, are obvious causes. But neurological assessment techniques often lag behind the cutting edge of cognitive psychology. Both areas benefit from collaborative interchange, as Squire's research so readily demonstrates (Squire, 1980). Disease processes often are implicated (e.g., cardiovascular disease). Terry Barrett (Barrett & Estes, 1984; Barrett & Watkins, 1986) measured word recall in a semantic-memory task using healthy adults of different ages, as well as middle-aged and older adults with histories of cardiovascular problems. He found that the presence of cardiovascular disease had a debilitating effect on recall performance, especially in older adults, and he concluded that such effects might also be present in other types of memory tasks.

Memory lapses are sometimes seen after surgery, especially cardiac surgery in older adults. Savageau, Stanton, Jenkins, and Frater (1982a) and Savageau, Stanton, Jenkins, and Klein (1982b) reported finding substantial declines in neuropsychological test scores for many open-heart-surgery patients, though these declines were no longer present after 6 months. Willner and associates (1983) found that the degree of cognitive impairment was related to the type of arterial filtration used during cardiopulmonary bypass surgery. Willner and Rabiner (1982) found that postoperative mortality was related to preoperative condition. Patients demonstrating a *combination* of both psychopathology and cognitive disorders (PCD syndrome) are much more likely to die after surgery than are patients with only one of these conditions. Research looking into the effects of cardiovascular disease on the utilization of world knowledge would seem to be most timely.

Another disease that has pervasive impact on the use of world knowledge is Alzheimer's disease. The past decade has seen truly remarkable increases in public awareness, news coverage, and research concerning Alzheimer's disease. This heightened awareness has led to increased interest in memory functioning. When my father (a salesman) forgets a name, he now looks at me and mutters, "Must be Alzheimer's." His dark humor is an attempt to deal with a perceived threat to both health and self-concept.

Affective factors. Larry Thompson and Delores Gallagher, at a discussion session on depression and memory held at the 1984 annual convention of the Gerontological Society of America, described memory complaint as a symptom that was common for both depression and the first stage of Alzheimer's disease. They mentioned a clinical rule of thumb in distinguishing between the two sources of such complaints. When asked about specific types of memory impairment (e.g., forgetting appointments, forgetting locations), depressed individuals often will not give positive instances of specific impairment. Patients with Alzheimer's disease will. A large-scale study to verify these observations empirically would be quite worthwhile. Research relating impairment in the utilization of world-knowledge systems to the progressive stages of Alzheimer's disease, as well as research into means of differentiating the symptoms of Alzheimer's disease from those of other disorders, will become increasingly salient to gerontology and society as a whole.

Affective factors. A general observation is that high levels of stress often are associated with absentmindedness, and so forth. Our laboratories currently are analyzing pilot data looking at the relationships among a variety of stress measures (e.g., measures of type A versus type B personalities, stress in day-to-day living, etc.) and the utilization of world-knowledge systems across the adult life span.

Depression often is linked to increased complaints about memory failure, as mentioned earlier. Kahn and Miller (1978) noted that depression in older adults also is related to complaints about memory for recent events being more impaired than memory for remote events (another stereotype about memory and aging). They wrote that one of the major reasons for the acceptance of this stereotype is its repeated assertion by the aged themselves, in spite of the fact that research has not supported the stereotype. Kahn and Miller stated that the claimed memory impairment for recent events may have adaptive significance as a means of denying current unpleasant matters. In many institutionalized older adults, this can take on an extreme form, referred to as "unorientation." Kahn and Miller described the phenomenon as a selectivity of responding. An unoriented person may be able to answer general-information questions or nonthreatening personal questions, but will become apathetic or will respond "don't know" when answering questions that have an unpleasant personal significance (e.g., "Where are you now?") (1978, pp. 282–3). World-knowledge utilization would seem to be a useful measure in attempting to distinguish between depression and forms of true dementia.

In a related vein, thought disorders such as schizophrenia would seem to be obvious causes of impaired utilization of world-knowledge systems. However, researchers studying memory from a world-knowledge framework have not yet explored this idea in any depth.

Selective remembering and learning

The preceding description of unorientation demonstrates that the ability to forget selectively (or at least to claim this) can have some adaptive value. I remember attending a paper session on memory and aging at a convention of the Gerontological Society in 1981. An older delegate listened patiently to a number of presentations. Finally, the gentleman could contain himself no longer and rose to address the assembly, asking the following question: ''Does anyone here know anything at all about the ability to forget useless information? Older folks seem to be better at this than younger ones.'' His query was met with silence. [At this time, I know of only one study dealing with directed forgetting and aging. Pavur, Comeaux, and Zeringue (1984) found that older adults were not significantly different from younger adults in the effects that directed forgetting instructions produced in recall for word lists.] However, if we again assume that the size of the world-knowledge base increases over time, it may become increasingly more difficult over time to encounter truly novel information, especially if there are environmental restrictions on the type and amount of information available (e.g., living in a nursing home). We have commented on these speculations elsewhere (Cavanaugh et al., 1985). If that is the case, the expectations of older adults might be different from those of younger adults vis-à-vis the likelihood of encountering novel or ''useful'' information. This, in turn, could influence processes such as willingness to engage in elaborative encoding, and so forth. At some point, the interrelationship between world-knowledge systems and learning in late life must be explored.

Wisdom

Finally, at some point we need to deal with sources of positive stereotypes about aging, such as the growth of wisdom. Perhaps, as Socrates noted, the growth of wisdom is facilitated by an awareness of how little one knows (Meacham, 1982). Perhaps ''wisdom'' refers to the ability to scan domains of information and find gaps, inconsistencies, or points in need of elaboration. I remember once coming into my advisor's office as a graduate student to ask a mundane question about how many subjects to use in a pilot study. After listening to the question, my advisor thought for a moment and said, ''What our discipline needs is a psychological analogue of Planck's constant. That will be the breakthrough.'' At the time, I found his answer unsatisfying, but over the years I keep turning it over in my mind. I now consider him exceptionally wise. Or perhaps, as Arlin (1975, 1985) has suggested, old age involves a new stage of cognitive development, a stage of question asking. Individuals in this stage have the ability to view knowledge from a broad perspective, seeing where the gaps in information have developed and scouting new areas to be explored.

Baltes and his colleagues (Dittmann-Kohli & Baltes, in press; Smith, Dixon, & Baltes, 1985) offer five features that characterize wisdom and/or wisdom-related tasks: (1) expertise in a selected domain of knowledge; (2) contextual richness in problem definition and solution; (3) the fundamental pragmatics of life: (4) uncertainty of problem definition; (5) relativism in judgment and recommendation concerning action. They define wisdom as knowledge and judgment about important but uncertain matters of life, or as expertise in a knowledge domain labeled as the fundamental pragmatics of life, and they have recently begun an attempt to devise laboratory-type tasks designed to study wisdom.

Clayton (1982) has taken a similar stance. She views wisdom as the ability to grasp the contradictory, changing, paradoxical aspects of human nature. She therefore sees the function of intelligence as determining *how* to accomplish life tasks, whereas the function of wisdom involves determinations of the impacts of actions on oneself and others (i.e., *Should* one pursue a particular course of action?).

Boucouvalas (1985; personal communication) has related the recent literature and research on wisdom to the areas of philosophy, theology/religion, and poetry/prose. She presents a case for the importance of wisdom in a future society. Her current research in the area involves a more phenomenological approach than that of the Baltes group and should provide an excellent complementary perspective to their research.

In any event, an exploration of the utility of aging for our species and the possible cognitive benefits that could accrue over time would be most valuable. Mergler and Goldstein (1983) claim that physiological and cognitive changes in late life make older adults uniquely able to carry out certain tasks (e.g., oral transmission of information, such as storytelling). This, in turn, is said to increase the possibility of group survival. Perhaps it is time to initiate the setting of new goals for late life. It may eventually be far better to hope to become wise rather than to either deny the aging process or decry "inevitable" decline. Marcel (1954) stated this case nicely. He noted that wisdom must be the end product of a slowly developed maturity, and maturity presupposes patience and continuity. Therefore, if respect for age has declined in "modern" times, this must be associated with a devaluation of wisdom itself (p. 40).

In summary, we have explored a series of topics for future research. Environmental contexts, motivation, attribution, physiological and affective factors, and self-generated decisions regarding the allocation of attention and effort all seem to be potentially important influences on the utilization of world-knowledge systems. In addition, wisdom has been discussed as a possible end product of a lifetime of using world-knowledge systems. New research into the nature of wisdom may help bring about changes in society's view of the effects of aging on cognitive functioning.

Conclusion

The study of world-knowledge systems is still in its infancy. Its birth came about through the recognition that the study of memory processes is incomplete if the influence of memory content on such processes is excluded. It has grown and been sustained by an increased interest in demonstrating the ecological validity of memory research. The existence of this volume is ample evidence that such an interest is both current and widespread. The measures developed thus far to map out this domain of knowledge are crude, but it is hoped that time will bring increased sophistication to the methodology of this area.

This chapter was written in an attempt to outline the types of research that have been accumulating in this field. Many important questions about world-knowledge systems have yet to be asked, much less answered. By raising a series of unanswered questions in this chapter, one hopes that similar question-finding activities will follow in the minds of other researchers. Once the number of such questions reaches a "critical mass," the relevance and importance of this area will become more evident, inspiring even greater efforts to find answers to questions about world-knowledge systems.

References

Anschutz, L., Camp, C. J., Markley, R. P., & Kramer, J. J. (1985). Maintenance and generalization of mnemonics for grocery shopping by older adults. *Experimental Aging Research, 11*, 157–160.

Arlin, P. K. (1975). Cognitive development in adulthood: A fifth stage? *Developmental Psychology*, 602–606.

Arlin, P. K. (1985). *Strategy and structure in postformal thinking*. Paper presented at the symposium Beyond Formal Operations 2: The Development of Adolescent and Adult Thought and Perception, Cambridge, MA.

Bahrick, H. P. (1979). Maintenance of knowledge: Questions about memory we forgot to ask. *Journal of Experimental Psychology: General, 108*, 296–308.

Bahrick, H. P. (1983). Memory for people. In J. E. Harris & P. E. Morris (Eds.), *Everyday memory*. London: Academic Press.

Bahrick, H. P., Bahrick, P. O., & Wittlinger, R. P. (1975). Fifty years of memory for names and faces: A cross sectional approach. *Journal of Experimental Psychology: General, 104*, 54–75.

Barrett, T. R. (1983). Word familiarity norms for two generations of adults. *Psychological Documents, 13*, 21.

Barrett, T. R., & Estes, B. B. (1984). *When aging does not produce memory deficits*. Paper presented at the 30th annual meeting of the Southeastern Psychological Association, New Orleans, LA.

Barrett, T. R., & Watkins, S. K. (1986). Word familiarity and cardiovascular health as determinants of age-related recall differences. *Journal of Gerontology, 41*, 222–224.

Barrett, T. R., & Wright, M. (1981). Age-related facilitation in recall following semantic processing. *Journal of Gerontology, 36*, 194–199.

Bartlett, J. C., & Snellus, P. (1980). Lifespan memory for popular songs. *American Journal of Psychology, 93,* 551–560.

Belmore, S. M. (1981). Age-related changes in processing explicit and implicit language. *Journal of Gerontology, 36,* 316–322.

Blaney, P. H. (1986). Affect and memory: A review. *Psychological Bulletin, 99,* 229–246.

Botwinick, J. (1984). *Aging and behavior* (3rd ed.). New York: Springer.

Botwinick, J., & Storandt, M. (1974). *Memory, related functions, and age.* Springfield, IL: Charles C. Thomas.

Botwinick, J., & Storandt, M. (1980). Recall and recognition of old information in relation to age and sex. *Journal of Gerontology, 35,* 70–76.

Boucouvalas, M. (1985). *On wisdom.* Paper presented at the annual conference of the Virginia Association of Adult and Continuing Education, Blacksburg, VA.

Camp, C. J. (1981). The use of fact retrieval versus inferential reasoning in young and elderly adults. *Journal of Gerontology, 36,* 715–721.

Camp, C. J. (1985). *Effects of depressed mood on fact retrieval and inferential reasoning.* Unpublished manuscript, University of New Orleans.

Camp, C. J. (1986). I am curious-grey: Information seeking and depression across the adult lifespan. *Educational Gerontology, 12,* 377–386.

Camp, C. J., Dietrich, M. S., & Olson, K. R. (1985). Curiosity and uncertainty in young, middle aged, and older adults. *Educational Gerontology, 11,* 401–412.

Camp, C. J., Lachman, R. L., & Lachman, R. (1980). Evidence for direct-access and inferential retrieval in question answering. *Journal of Verbal Learning and Verbal Behavior, 19,* 583–596.

Camp, C. J., & Pignatiello, M. F. (1984). *Utilization of fact retrieval and inferential reasoning in young, middle-aged, and elderly adults.* Paper presented at the 30th annual meeting of the Southeastern Psychological Association, New Orleans, LA.

Camp, C. J., Rodrigue, J. R., & Olson, K. R. (1984). Curiosity in young, middle aged, and older adults. *Educational Gerontology, 10,* 387–400.

Cavanaugh, J. C., Grady, J. G., & Perlmutter, M. (1983). Forgetting and the use of memory aids in 20 to 70 year olds' everyday life. *International Journal of Aging and Human Development, 17,* 113–122.

Cavanaugh, J. C., Kramer, D. A., Sinnott, J. D., Camp, C. J., & Markley, R. P. (1985). On missing links and such: Interfaces between cognitive research and everyday problem solving. *Human Development, 28,* 146–168.

Chang, T. M. (1986). Semantic memory: Facts and models. *Psychological Bulletin, 99,* 199–220.

Clayton, V. (1982). Wisdom and intelligence: The nature and function of knowledge in the later years. *International Journal of Aging and Human Development, 15,* 315–321.

Cohen, G. (1981). Inferential reasoning in old age. *Cognition, 9,* 59–72.

Cohen, G., & Faulkner, D. (1981). Memory for discourse in old age. *Discourse Processes, 4,* 253–265.

Demming, J. A., & Pressey, S. L. (1957). Tests "indigenous" to the adult and older years. *Journal of Counseling Psychology, 2,* 144–148.

Dittmann-Kohli, F., & Baltes, P. B. (in press). Towards a neofunctionalist conception of adult intellectual development: Wisdom as a prototypical case of intellectual growth. In C. Alexander & E. Langer (Eds.), *Beyond formal operations: Alternative endpoints to human development.* New York: Oxford University Press.

Fitzgerald, J. M., & Lawrence, R. (1984). Autobiographical memory across the lifespan. *Journal of Gerontology, 39,* 692–698.

Fozard, J. L. (1980). The time for remembering. In L. W. Poon (Ed.), *Aging in the 1980's: Psychological issues* (pp. 273–290). Washington, DC: American Psychological Association.

Fozard, J. L., Waugh, N. C., & Thomas, J. C. (1975). Effects of age on long-term retention of pictures. In *Proceedings of the Tenth International Congress of Gerontology* (Vol. 2, p. 137).

Giambra, L. M. (1974). Daydreaming across the lifespan: Late adolescent to senior citizen. *International Journal of Aging and Human Development, 5,* 115–140.

Giambra, L. M. (1977). Adult male daydreaming across the lifespan: A replication, further analysis, and tentative norms based upon retrospective reports. *International Journal of Aging and Human Development, 8,* 197–228.

Hess, T. M., & Arnould, D. (1986). Adult age differences for explicit and implicit sentence information. *Journal of Gerontology, 41,* 191–194.

Horn, J. L. (1982). The theory of fluid and crystallized intelligence in relation to concepts of cognitive psychology and aging in adulthood. In F. I. M. Craik & S. Trehub (Eds.), *Aging and cognitive processes.* New York: Plenum Press.

Howard, D. V. (1983). *Cognitive psychology: Memory, language, and thought.* New York: Macmillan.

Hoyer, W. J. (1985). Aging and the development of adult cognition. In T. M. Schlecter & M. P. Toglia (Eds.), *New directions in cognitive science.* Norwood, NJ: Ablex.

Hulicka, I. M. (1982). Memory functioning in late adulthood. In F. I. M. Craik & S. Trehub (Eds.), *Aging and cognitive processes.* New York: Plenum Press.

Kahn, R. L., & Miller, N. E. (1978). Adaptational factors in memory function in the aged. *Experimental Aging Research, 4,* 273–290.

Kausler, D. H. (1982). *Experimental psychology and human aging.* New York: Wiley.

Lachman, J. L., & Lachman, R. (1980). Age and the actualization of world knowledge. In L. W. Poon, J. L. Fozard, L. S. Cermak, D. Arenberg, & L. W. Thompson (Eds.), *New directions in memory and aging; Proceedings of the George A. Talland memorial conference* (pp. 285–312). Hillsdale, NJ: Lawrence Erlbaum.

Lachman, J. L., Lachman, R., & Thronesberry, C. (1979). Metamemory through the adult lifespan. *Developmental Psychology, 15,* 543–551.

Lachman, M. E., & Jelalian, E. (1984). Self-efficacy and attributions for intellectual performance in young and elderly adults. *Journal of Gerontology, 39,* 577–582.

Lachman, R., Lachman, J. L., & Taylor, D. W. (1982). Reallocation of mental resources over the productive lifespan. In F. I. M. Craik & S. Trehub (Eds.), *Aging and cognitive processes.* New York: Plenum Press.

Light, L. L., Zelinski, E. M., & Moore, M. (1982). Adult age differences in reasoning from new information. *Journal of Experimental Psychology: Learning, Memory and Cognition, 8,* 435–447.

Linton, M. (1982). Transformation of memory in everyday life. In U. Neisser (Ed.), *Memory observed: Remembering in natural contexts.* San Francisco: W. H. Freeman.

Marcel, G. (1954). *The decline of wisdom.* London: Harvill Press.

Meacham, J. A. (1982). Wisdom and the context of knowledge: Knowing that one doesn't know. In D. Kuhn & J. A. Meacham (Eds.), *On the development of developmental psychology* (pp. 111–134). Basel: Krager.

Mergler, N. L. & Goldstein, M. D. (1983). Why are there old people? *Human Development, 26,* 72–90.

Mitchell, D. B. (1984). *Aging and repetition effects in recognition: The same old story.* Paper presented at the 30th annual meeting of the Southeastern Psychological Association, New Orleans, LA.

Neisser, U. (1982). *Memory observed: Remembering in natural contexts.* San Francisco: W. H. Freeman.

Niederehe, G. (in press). Depression and memory impairment in the aged. In L. Poon (Ed.), *Handbook for clinical memory assessment of older adults.* Washington, DC: American Psychological Association.

Niederehe, G., & Camp, C. J. (1985). Signal detection analysis of recognition memory in depressed elderly. *Experimental Aging Research, 11,* 207–213.

Pavur, E. J., Comeaux, J. M., & Zeringue, J. A. (1984). Younger and older adults' attention to relevant and irrelevant stimuli in free recall. *Experimental Aging Research, 10,* 59–60.

Perlmutter, M. (1978). What is memory aging the aging of? *Developmental Psychology, 14,* 330–345.

Pignatiello, M F. (1985). *A comparison of mood induction techniques: Effects on cognitive and physiological functioning.* Unpublished master's thesis, University of New Orleans.

Pignatiello, M. F., & Camp, C. J. (1984). *Internalized cognitive processing stereotypes and aging.* Paper presented at the 37th annual scientific meeting of the Gerontological Society of America, San Antonio, TX.

Pignatiello, M. F., Camp, C. J., & Rasar, L. A. (1986). Musical mood induction: An alternative to the Velten technique. *Journal of Abnormal Psychology, 95,* 295–297.

Poon, L. W., & Fozard, J. L. (1978). Speed of retrieval from long-term memory in relation to age, familiarity, and datedness of information. *Journal of Gerontology, 33,* 711–717.

Poon, L. W., Fozard, J. L., Paulshock, D. R., & Thomas, J. C. (1979). A questionnaire assessment of age differences in retention of recent and remote events. *Experimental Aging Research, 5,* 401–411.

Savageau, J. A., Stanton, B. A., Jenkins, C. D., & Frater, R. W. M. (1982a). Neuropsychological dysfunction following elective cardiac operation. II. A six month reassessment. *Journal of Thoracic and Cardiovascular Surgery, 84,* 595–600.

Savageau, J. A., Stanton, B. A., Jenkins, C. D., & Klein, M. D. (1982b). Neuropsychological dysfunction following elective cardiac operation. I. Early assessment. *Journal of Thoracic and Cardiovascular Surgery, 84,* 585–594.

Schank, R. C. (1975). The role of memory in language processing. In C. Cofer (Ed.), *The structure of human memory.* San Francisco: W. H. Freeman.

Sinnott, J. D. (1986). Prospective/intentional and incidental memory: Effects of age and passage of time. *Psychology and Aging, 1,* 110–116.

Smith, J., Dixon, R. A., & Baltes, P. B. (1985). *Expertise: A research tool for investigating aspects of wisdom.* Paper presented at the symposium Beyond Formal Operations 2: The Development of Adolescent and Adult Thought and Perception, Cambridge, MA.

Squire, L. R. (1980). The neuropsychology of amnesia: An approach to the study of memory and aging. In L. W. Poon, J. L. Fozard, L. S. Cermak, D. Arenberg, & L. W. Thompson (Eds.), *New directions in memory and aging: Proceedings of the George A. Talland memorial conference* (pp. 433–450). Hillsdale, NJ: Lawrence Erlbaum.

Squire, L. R., Chance, P. M., & Slater, P. C. (1975). Assessment of memory for remote events. *Psychological Reports, 37,* 223–234.

Squire, L. R., & Slater, P. C. (1975). Forgetting in very long term memory as assessed by an improved questionnaire technique. *Journal of Experimental Psychology: Human Learning and Memory, 104,* 50–54.

Storandt, M., Grant, E. A., & Gordon, B. C. (1978). Remote memory as a function of age and sex. *Experimental Aging Research, 4,* 365–375.

Thomas, J. C., Fozard, J. L., & Waugh, N. C. (1977). Age-related differences in naming latency. *American Journal of Psychology, 90,* 499–509.

Tulving, E. (1972). Episodic and semantic memory. In E. Tulving & W. Donaldson (Eds.), *Organization of memory* (pp. 382–404). New York: Academic Press.

Tulving, E. (1985). How many memory systems are there? *American Psychologist, 40,* 385–398.

Vygotsky, L. S. (1962). *Thought and language.* Cambridge, MA: M.I.T. Press.

Vygotsky, L. S. (1978). *Mind in society.* Cambridge, MA: Harvard University Press.

Walsh, D. A., & Baldwin, M. (1977). Age differences in integrated semantic memory. *Developmental Psychology, 13,* 509–514.

Warrington, E. K., & Sanders, H. I. (1971). The fate of old memories. *Quarterly Journal of Experimental Psychology, 23,* 432–442.

Warrington, E. K., & Silberstein, M. (1970). A questionnaire technique for investigating very long term memory. *Quarterly Journal of Experimental Psychology, 22,* 508–512.

Wechsler, D. (1955). *Manual for the Wechsler Adult Intelligence Scale.* New York: The Psychological Corporation.

West, R. L. (1985). *Practical memory functioning in the elderly.* Paper presented at the Second National Forum on Research in Aging, Lincoln, NE.

Willner, A. E., Carmante, L. L., Garvey, J. W., Wolpowitz, A., Weisz, D., Rabiner, C. J., & Wisoff, B. G. (1983). The relationship between arterial filtration during open heart surgery and mental abstraction ability. In *Proceedings of the American Academy of Cardiovascular Perfusion* (Vol. 4, pp. 56–65).

Willner, A. E., & Rabiner, C. J. (1982). The psychopathology and cognitive disorder syndrome (PCD) in open-heart surgery patients: Consequences for psychiatric outcome and mortality. In R. N. Malateshu & L. C. Hartlage (Eds.), *Neuropsychology and cognition* (Vol. 2, pp. 661–673). The Hague: Martinus Nijhoff.

26 Comments on aging memory and its everyday operations

Donald H. Kausler

My comments focus on three broad issues that enter prominently into much of the content of the chapters in this section: the conceptualization of aging's effects on memory proficiency, the generalizability of laboratory memory performances to everyday memory performances, and the concept of expertise and its implications for aging's effects on everyday memory performances.

Aging's effects on memory proficiency

General-decrement principle

The nature of research on adult age differences in everyday memory performances is likely to be influenced greatly by one's conceptualization of aging's effects on memory proficiency. The conceptualization that has dominated laboratory research on adult age differences in memory proficiency may best be described in terms of a general-decrement principle. The carryover of this principle to research on everyday memory performances has obvious important implications. It surely will preclude attempts by investigators to discover components of everyday memory that are immune to age-related decrements in proficiency or to explore means of alleviating or reducing age-related decrements for those components that are age-sensitive.

According to this principle, irreversible decrements in memory proficiency are inevitable consequences of the organism's biological degeneration from early to late adulthood, resulting either in a decrease in cognitive resources (Hasher & Zacks, 1979) or in a "slowing down" of cognitive processes (Salthouse, 1980) during old age. Much of the emphasis in contemporary aging-memory research is on testing the validities of these theoretical accounts of why memory proficiency declines with aging. Evidence supporting a given theory consists in fulfilling predictions for laboratory-based phenomena that are derived from that theory.

In effect, old adults function at a process level characteristic of less proficient young adults. Interestingly, this position suggests that insights into the memory functioning of elderly adults can be gained without actually studying elderly adults. An individual-differences approach to the study of memory processes in the young-adult population should yield substantial understanding of the memory operations that distinguish between young and old performers. An "average" old performer presumably corresponds at the process level to a "below-average" young adult. For example, it may be postulated that the processing resources of the average old adult have been reduced to the level of the below-average young performer. Thus, knowing how the poorer young performer differs from the better young performer should also reveal how the average old performer differs from the average young performer.

Many cognitive geropsychologists will surely wince at the mention of this individual-differences approach to adult age differences in memory proficiency. Nevertheless, the approach is not without merit. If nothing else, it may offer converging validity for the results obtained in traditional aging studies that contrast young and old individuals. Consider, for example, a recent study by Wang (1983) that employed only young adults. Wang compared fast and slow paired-associate learners and discovered that fast learners generated more elaborators (or mediators) quickly during pair-study trials than did slow learners. This distinction between fast and slow young-adult learners is also the major distinction between average young and old paired-associate learners (Hulicka & Grossman, 1967). Moreover, Wang also discovered that the elaborators activated on test trials by fast learners were better reinstatements of the elaborators utilized during study trials than were the test-trial elaborators of slow learners. In effect, this means that fast learners are more capable of recovering the encoding context during retrieval than are slow learners. Translate fast learners to young adults and slow learners to elderly adults and this is exactly the difference postulated by Burke and Light (1981) to distinguish young and old memory performers.

The validity of the general-decrement principle has been challenged in recent years by the dichotomizing of memory processes into effortful and automatic components. The decrement principle applies to the effortful component, but not to the automatic component, at least according to contemporary theorists (Hasher & Zacks, 1979). The concept of effort usually is identified with forms of episodic memory in which both encoding and retrieval processes are presumed to draw on one's limited cognitive resources. However, effortful processing is not necessarily restricted to episodic memory. Theorists speculate that generic, or semantic, memory of the kind analyzed by Bowles, Obler, and Poon (Chapter 15, this volume), also has automatic and effortful components (Posner & Snyder, 1975), just as episodic memory has. Consequently, adult age differences (i.e., age deficits) are expected to be found for the effortful processes of generic memory, but not for the automatic processes (Burke & Yee, 1984).

Unfortunately for those of us who would like to believe that at least some components of the total memory system are spared the inevitable aging decrement, recent evidence indicates that even automatic memory processes experience a modest degree of age-related decline in proficiency. Such a decline may even be true for the prototypic task of automaticity within episodic memory, namely, the frequency judgment task (Kausler, Lichty, & Hakami, 1984). Moreover, the evidence presented by Bowles and associates in Chapter 15 suggests that the age-related decline is also true for at least one form of automatic memory within the generic or semantic system. The implication is that the decrement in proficiency from early to late adulthood should be conceptualized as a continuum that ranges from slight to pronounced.

Contextualism

The general-decrement principle has also been challenged by the recent movement of a number of cognitive geropsychologists toward a contextual conceptualization of aging's effects on memory proficiency. From a contextual position, a decrement in memory proficiency clearly is not the inevitable consequence of aging. In other words, elderly adults may not always correspond to below-average young adults in terms of memory performance. For some tasks, older adults are more likely than younger to be affected by variations in certain contextual conditions. Given appropriate levels of these conditions, the net effect could be reductions in age-related memory deficits, and perhaps even their elimination. Presumably, effective contextual conditions are more likely to be present in everyday memory situations than in their laboratory simulations. However, for other tasks, compensatory contextual conditions may be lacking, resulting in seemingly irreversible age-related memory deficits.

Laboratory demonstrations of memory decrements with aging often may be the result of our failure to consider components of the total cognitive system other than memory processes per se. Included here are a number of possible supplementary processes that may provide contextual enhancement of elderly adults' memory performances. The list includes the following contributions in this volume: the motivation and goals of the performer (J. Hartley, Chapter 11; Meyer & Rice, Chapter 12; Perlmuter & Monty, Chapter 21), the salience of the cognitive demand placed on the performer (Sinnott, Chapter 20), training on the cognitive skills needed by the performer (Charness, Chapter 24; A. Hartley, Chapter 18), continuing maintenance practice on a given cognitive skill (Denney, Chapter 19), expertise and/or an extensive knowledge system (Camp, Chapter 25; Charness, Chapter 24), and perceived versus constructive representations (Cohen & Faulkner, Chapter 14). Many of the contributors to this section have attempted to compensate for this failure by introducing conditions into their laboratory studies that seemingly approximate more closely the conditions of everyday memory performances than is ordinarily the case for laboratory studies of age differences in memory.

Judging from the content of the presentations in this section, the contextual principle is likely to exert a stronger influence on everyday-memory research than will the general-decrement principle. A primary thrust in this research is likely to be the attempt to discover effective means of intervention to overcome deficits in memory performances that may unnecessarily accompany aging. An excellent example of effective intervention with elderly adults is found in Perlmuter's work on perception of control (Chapter 21, this volume). Control of task options enhances performance not only on that specific task but also on other tasks for which control is absent. In agreement with Rabbitt, "we require descriptions of the ways in which people actively optimize their performance to cope with changing task demands, to improve with practice, and to circumvent or minimize growing failures in their own efficiency" (1982, p. 96). That is, indeed, what research on aging and memory should be about. Unless we believe that we have the capability of discovering these ways, there really is no justification for our studies of aging and everyday memory functioning. Implicit in this position is the distinction between competence and performance described by Perlmuter. Our objectives as cognitive geropsychologists surely should be dominated by our attempts to discover means of reducing the gap between performance and competence for elderly people, thereby significantly improving the quality of their lives.

Whether or not interventions influence the magnitude of age differences in performance scores should continue to be of theoretical importance to all of us. In many instances, they probably will not (Kausler, 1982; Perlmuter, Chapter 21, this volume). Young adults also often perform on tasks below their true competence levels, and they are also likely to benefit from intervention. As a result, the magnitude of an age deficit in performance on a given task often is unaffected by an intervention administered to all subjects. However, whatever gain in performance can be accomplished by older adults through intervention has a practical importance that greatly transcends the theoretical standstill created by undiminished overall age differences following interventions.

In summary, research on adult age differences in everyday memory performances is likely to be influenced by the researcher's conceptualizaion of aging's effects on memory proficiency overall. Traditional laboratory research has been guided by a general-decrement principle. This principle argues that the average elderly adult's memory proficiency is inevitably reduced to the level of a below-average young adult. In agreement with this principle, there is evidence indicating that the paired-associate learning processes of "average" elderly adults are functionally identical with those of poorer young-adult paired-associate learners. The general-decrement principle has been challenged in recent years by the separation of memory processes into age-sensitive effortful and age-insensitive automatic components. Another serious challenge is the emergence of contextualism in memory theory and research. Contextualism views some memory performances of older adults as being enhanced by certain conditions, conditions more likely to be present in everyday memory situations than in laboratory simulations of those situations. A major objective of everyday-memory research should be the discovery of these conditions and the means of implementing them during memory performances. Much of the research presented in this section has been concerned with contextual conditions that approximate those found in everyday memory performances.

From the laboratory to the everyday world

Generalizability of laboratory research

Do our laboratory studies of adult age differences in memory proficiency really give us insight into the nature of age differences for everyday memory performances? In agreement with Mook (1983, Chapter 3, this volume), what is at stake in laboratory research on memory is the generalizability to the real world of the conclusions arrived at by that research. Laboratory tasks represent simulations of everyday events, not copies. Critics of laboratory research on memory (Neisser, 1982) often fail to realize that there may be considerable commonality between the processes entering into everyday memory activities and the processes entering into laboratory analogues of those activities.

Consider, for example, laboratory research on paired-associate learning. The name itself is likely to arouse associations of ''irrelevant'' and ''ecologically trivial.'' And yet the processes of paired-associate learning are not unknown in everyday memory performances. We do learn such paired associates as face–name connections and city–sports–team–name connections throughout our daily lives. Surely, the paired-associate processes studied in the laboratory should at least approximate the paired-associate processes engaged in during our daily lives. Accordingly, what we know about age differences in performance on laboratory-based paired-associate tasks should generalize to some degree to age differences in the real world.

Unfortunately, however, often there are complicating factors that seriously challenge the external validity of our laboratory research on adult age differences in memory performances. In fact, this is probably true for paired-associate learning. Here we encounter the problem of an excess of processes in laboratory acquisitions of paired associates by young and old adults. Paired associates are presented in the laboratory as components of a lengthy list. All of the components are to be acquired at virtually the same time. This is unlikely to be the format of paired-associate learning in the everyday world. We may encounter one new face–name combination at a party, and then not encounter another new combination until days or even weeks go by. There is a negative process affecting the acquisition of a single pair embedded within a lengthy list that is absent when the same pair is acquired in isolation. The process is that of interpair interference (Battig, 1968). Most important, this laboratory extra process is likely to be age-sensitive. The net effect is an exacerbation of the age deficit found in the everyday counterpart. A learning condition in which subjects practice single pairs in isolation, and eventually have all pairs combined into a total list, would be expected to benefit elderly subjects more than younger. Note that this is an example of introducing to the laboratory situation a contextual condition from everyday memory functioning that is missing in the laboratory counterpart.

There are occasions, however, when real-world paired-associate learning does approximate the list format employed in the laboratory. For example, some forms of the spatial memorization described by Kirasic (Chapter 16, this volume) may be conceptualized in terms of paired-associate learning. Mastery of what objects may be found in what locations in a supermarket may be thought of in terms of a list of connections between A (location) and B (object). Given such a list, an effective intervention procedure for elderly shoppers would consist of having them master initially a small subset of these connections, then master another small subset, and so on, until the full-scale environment becomes familiar. Much of the devastating adverse effect of interpair interference could again be avoided by the older learner.

A problem occurs for all learners when a familiar spatial array is reorganized, much as a paired-associate list is reorganized in an A–B, A–Br transfer sequence (identical stimulus and response elements in the two lists, but the elements are paired in a different way on the second list than on the first). Performance on an A–Br task is especially difficult for elderly adults (Lair, Moon, & Kausler, 1969). The problem for the elderly learner is likely to be aggravated further when the reorganization is only partial. This happened recently in my community when a popular supermarket went through a major remodeling. At the end of the remodeling, some objects were in new locations, and other objects remained in their old locations. The consequence was the creation of a mixed transfer list containing some old A–B pairs and some new A–Br pairs. The need to discriminate between sets (Kausler, 1974) adds greatly to the difficulty created by the interference from repairing, especially for older adults.

In some instances, performance on an everyday activity may involve an age-sensitive process that is missing in the laboratory analogue of that activity. These circumstances seem to occur in memory for the frequency of occurrence of episodic events. In the laboratory, the episodic events usually are discrete items that vary in their frequencies within a study list. Encoding and retrieval processes for this kind of information are expected to differ only moderately in proficiency between young and elderly adults. Consequently, only a modest age deficit is expected to be found for laboratory performances. In the everyday world, however, memory for frequency information often involves an additional process of abstraction, as well as the process of encoding discrete-item information. Discrete items may have to be analyzed in terms of their membership within superordinate taxonomic categories. Consider, for example, your answer to the question, "How many movie comedies did you see in the past year?" Each movie must be evaluated with respect to its membership in the superordinate category of comedy. This abstraction process is likely to be age-sensitive, leading to a more pronounced age deficit for external criterion scores than for scores on the standard laboratory analogue (Kausler, Hakami, & Wright, 1982).

In the case of memory for prose, there are still other reasons why age differences found in the laboratory may misrepresent age differences found on an external criterion. These reasons were stressed by both J. Hartley (Chapter 11, this volume) and Meyer and Rice (Chapter 12, this volume). Under normal laboratory conditions, subjects of all ages are likely to employ a memorization strategy. An age difference favoring young adults in memory for higher-order propositions is the likely result. By contrast, an "idea" or "gist" strategy is likely to be operative for adults of all ages in their everyday exposures to such prose as a magazine article. With this strategy, little, if any, age deficit may be manifested for scores on an external criterion. Most important, the laboratory situation could be altered to stress the activation of an "idea" strategy comparable to that activated away from the laboratory. If the attempt is successful, the outcome is likely to parallel that found on the external criterion.

Implicit faith in the external validity of laboratory research on adult age differences in memory performances is, of course, insufficient. We greatly need empirical demonstrations of that validity. Unfortunately, the accrual of evidence for external validity has been a terribly slow process. Part of the blame rests on the preoccupation of many laboratory researchers with resolving relatively minor theoretical issues. For example, how important is it to demonstrate whether the age difference in memory for performed activities is attributable to an age deficit in the encoding stage or in the retrieval stage (Kausler, Lichty, & Freund, 1985b)? If the deficit rests mainly in the retrieval stage, then its magnitude should be greatly reduced when memory is tested by recognition rather than by recall. The fact remains, however, that in the everyday world, our memory for our own performed activities ordinarily demands recall, not recognition. Because encoding and retrieval processes are inextricably bound together in our everyday-activity memories, does it really matter where the primary locus of age sensitivity is?

The external-criterion problem

The major villain thwarting our endeavors to establish the external validities of our laboratory studies is our failure to tackle fully the problem of identifying reliable and valid external criteria, that is, "true" assessments of everyday memory performances. The most obvious choice of an external criterion consists of self-reports of everyday memory proficiency in the form of questionnaires, inventories, diaries, and so on. Of interest to us are the correlations between scores on these everyday proficiency measures and measures on laboratory tasks. A number of researchers have indeed employed this method of testing the external validity of laboratory performances. Although some have reported moderate correlations between the two measures (Hulicka, 1982; Sunderland, Harris, & Baddeley, 1983; Zelinski, Gilewski, & Thompson, 1980), others have found almost zero correlation (Broadbent, Cooper, Fitzgerald, & Parkes, 1982; Zarit, Cole, & Guider, 1981). The problems inherent in the use of self-reports as measures of external criteria have been discussed thoroughly elsewhere (Dixon, Chapter 22, this volume; Salthouse & Kausler, 1985); only two of those problems will be considered here.

One problem is the difficulty many people have in assessing objectively the proficiencies of their own memory operations. An important step in solving this problem occurred through the innovative procedure introduced by Sunderland and associates (1983). They obtained ratings of memory proficiency from significant other people who were quite familiar with the subjects, as well as from the subjects themselves. Laboratory scores on a paired-associate learning task were found to correlate more highly with ratings provided by significant others than with ratings provided by the subjects themselves. In my opinion, however, the major problem in the past has been the omnibus nature of most self-reports: Questions requiring ratings of proficiency on a wide range of memory skills and memory problems are simply thrown together. Included are likely to be questions referring to metamemory, generic memory, short-term memory, long-term episodic memory, prospective memory, automatic episodic memory, and so on. The implication is that a memory is a memory, and a given proficiency on any one component is equivalent to the same degree of proficiency on any other component. Clearly, that is not true. The approach taken by Dixon (Chapter 22, this volume) is an important departure from the omnibus tradition. From that approach, an effective instrument for measuring separate components of metamemory is emerging. The use of this instrument should prove to be quite effective in testing the external validity of various laboratory measures of metamemory.

Even with these improvements in self-report measures, we should be directing our efforts to the discovery of alternative forms of external criteria that may prove to be more effective than self-reports. One alternative requires the expansion of laboratory studies to include "extralaboratory" activities that closely approximate everyday memory activities directly relevant to those being investigated in the laboratory. Of interest would be the covariation between laboratory measures and extralaboratory measures. Consider, for example, scores obtained on laboratory tasks dealing with speech comprehension and memory, studies of the kind described by Stine, Wingfield, and Poon (Chapter 13, this volume). A plausible external criterion consists of subjects' memory for the informal remarks made by the investigator at the start of the laboratory task. Similarly, a plausible criterion for studies of prose memory consists of subjects' incidental memory of the content of the consent form they were required to read (Taub & Baker, 1983), and a plausible criterion for studies of temporal memory consists of subjects' incidental memory of when in a series of preexperimental tasks (e.g., meeting the investigator's assistant, signing the consent form, and taking a vocabulary test) each task was performed.

Finally, we clearly need more studies of the kind described by Kirasic (Chapter 16, this volume) and Sinnott (Chapter 20, this volume), in which a laboratory-like task is essentially performed in the subject's everyday world. This happy blend of laboratory-like control and observation in a natural setting is perhaps the ideal solution to the external-criterion problem. Stated somewhat differently, we need more researchers who are willing to use their ingenuity to resolve external-validity issues rather than minor theoretical issues.

In summary, a major issue facing laboratory research on aging's effects on memory is the generalizability of the processes studied in the laboratory to the processes involved in everyday memory performances. In some cases, age-sensitive processes may be involved in laboratory simulations that are absent from the everyday-world counterparts, leading to an overestimation of aging deficits in everyday memory. In other cases, the reverse may be true, resulting in an underestimation of aging deficits in the real world. There are instances, however, in which the processes guiding laboratory performances appear to approximate closely the processes of everyday memory performances. Clearly, more attention needs to be given to the external validity of the results obtained in laboratory research in terms of how well laboratory-based scores covary with assessments of everyday memory proficiency. Especially needed are improved means of evaluating everyday memory performances. Recent advances in self-report evaluations of everyday memory proficiencies should help to solve this problem. Another important direction for researchers to take is to add extralaboratory activities to their laboratory memory studies. If the extralaboratory activities approximate everyday memory activities, then the covariation between laboratory and extralaboratory scores should provide an effective assessment of the external validity of the laboratory findings. Also needed are more aging studies in which a laboratory-like task is performed in the subject's everyday world.

Memory expertise and its limitations

The importance of expertise as a compensatory factor for the loss of certain cognitive skills with aging has been nicely documented by Charness (Chapter 24, this volume). However, it seems apparent that most components of the human memory system, both episodic and generic, are largely unaffected by the development of expertise over the course of the adult life span. If extended practice yields expertise, then we should all be "memory experts" long before we reach late adulthood. The fact is, however, that elderly adults have had 60 years or more of practice on such episodic skills as learning face–name connections, and yet little, if any, expertise is the result. This is especially true in the sense of expertise serving to eliminate, or at least to diminish greatly, the decline of those skills during late adulthood.

On-line awareness and procedural expertise

Perhaps a major reason for the failure of expertise to emerge for these skills is the low level of on-line awareness (Cavanaugh, Chapter 23, this volume) that we ordinarily have of them while they are being utilized. Even the rehearsal of face–name connections probably is accompanied for most of us by little on-line awareness of what rehearsal strategy has been applied and why it has been applied. As Cavanaugh observed, we seem to have far greater awareness of memory's failures than we have of its specific operations. On the other hand, there is good reason to believe that expertise does not necessarily require on-line awareness. It seems unlikely that the compensatory skill manifested by older skilled typists (Salthouse, 1984) involves awareness of that skill's application during typing. The suspected lack of awareness occurs even though the compensatory skill itself seems to demand considerable cognitive effort.

The fact that expertise may involve compensatory skills suggests that expertise in memory need not be restricted to the content of memory, as with chess experts (Charness, Chapter 24, this volume). That is, expertise may also involve procedural memory, or memory of the processes that guide the acquisition of specific content (Tulving, 1983).

It is intriguing to view mnemonic training from the perspective of expertise in procedural memory. An important ingredient of mnemonic training at any age level (West, Chapter 30, this volume; Yesavage et al., Chapter 31, this volume) is to have the participants experience on-line awareness of the to-be-encouraged cognitively effortful rehearsal strategy, such as the use of interacting compounded images. Can such training, if intensive and extensive enough, result in the production of true expertise in the everyday application of a memory skill? Perhaps. If so, will young adults who have been so trained resist the decline in that skill as they grow older? Alternatively, will young adults who are without special training, but who are nevertheless highly skilled in some component of memory, grow old "gracefully" with respect to that skill, at least relative to others less skilled for that same component of memory? Consider, for example, the "fast" versus "slow" paired-associate learners identified by Wang (1983). If only Wang could be convinced of the gerontological importance of continuing to monitor the paired-associate performances of these individuals over the next 40 to 50 years! Alas, this is unlikely to happen. However, it would be of great interest to examine the memory-skill fates of "fast" versus "slow" young-adult learners who were participants years ago in the Baltimore Longitudinal Study and who have continued as participants over the years (Arenberg & Robertson-Tchabo, 1977). Do they indeed show differential rates of loss of learning skill, a differential presumably due to different degrees of expertise?

Automaticity and expertise

Any examination of the potential role played by expertise in negating the ravages of aging on everyday memory skills must consider the possibility that many components of everyday memory are mediated by automatic processes. A prevailing argument (Hasher & Zacks, 1979) is that episodic forms of automatic memory are immune to the benefits of extensive training and practice. If that is true, then it seems unlikely that individuals can intentionally acquire expertise for these skills. Our studies of automatic activity memory, that is, memory for one's own performances on a series of tasks (Kausler & Hakami, 1983; Kausler, Lichty, & Davis, 1985a; Kausler et al., 1985b), suggest that encouraging rehearsal of an activity (i.e., intentional memory) may actually be disruptive to elderly adults. Our old subjects who performed under incidental memory conditions consistently were found to have a slight advantage in memory of their participation over those who performed under intentional memory conditions. Activity memory is therefore a component of episodic memory for which intervention may actually work to the disadvantage of elderly adults. That is, it may be better simply to let nature follow its own course of registering automatically the participation in an activity, imperfect though that registration may be. However, intervention need not be restricted to attempts to train compensatory skills. In the case of activity memory, an important kind of intervention may take the form of assuring that elderly adults participate regularly in a wide range of everyday activities. In the absence of such participation, even an automatic memory skill may undergo considerable atrophy, atrophy that results in the decline of that skill below the level it manifested prior to late adulthood.

The issue of atrophy may also be relevant to automatic generic memory skills. This issue arises in the peculiar asymmetry of automatic processes demonstrated by Bowles and associates (Chapter 15, this volume). The retrieval of semantic concepts using words as stimuli seems to be largely insensitive to aging deficits, whereas the retrieval of words using semantic concepts as stimuli seems to be far less robust. Thus, there is an asymmetry in retrieval proficiency for older adults between name–concept associations and concept–name associations. Such asymmetry is reminiscent of the asymmetry between S–R and R–S associations that attracted considerable attention in the verbal learning era (Kausler, 1974). Conceivably, the asymmetry is the product of differential opportunities for atrophy of the underlying skills. Most elderly adults are likely to maintain everyday experiences that demand the use of name-to-concept associations. In fact, they may even increase those experiences, relative to earlier in life. These experiences include reading newspapers and magazines, listening to the radio, and watching television. In each case, attention to the verbal input requires activation of name-to-concept associations. By contrast, concept-to-name associations are most likely to be activated during speech production of the kind that enters into normal everyday conversations. The relatively passive living style of many elderly adults is likely to carry with it a reduction of conversational activity, a reduction that could be sufficient to result in some degree of atrophy of the ability to retrieve concept-to-name associations.

In summary, expertise in memory may apply to procedural skills as well as to content skills. The development of expertise in procedural skills should serve to diminish aging decrements in everyday memory proficiency. Perhaps the reason why we seemingly develop little expertise for procedural skills is the absence of on-line awareness of their utilization during the encoding of to-be-remembered information. On-line awareness is possible, however, through effective mnemonic training. Conceivably, young adults so trained can acquire sufficient procedural expertise to sustain proficient memory performances as they grow older. However, the development of procedural expertise is likely to be restricted by the automatic nature of many memory processes. With automatic processes, intervention in the form of preventing atrophy may be the only effective means of reducing whatever decrements occur with aging.

Conclusion

Research on adult age differences in everyday memory performances need not abandon the traditional laboratory approach. However, the focus of that research should be on the analysis of conditions likely to affect the proficiency of everyday memory processes, rather than on tests of either the validities of theories accounting for general decrements in memory with aging or the generalizability to late adulthood of the minor memory phenomena discovered by basic memory researchers. As demonstrated by the contributors to this section, laboratory simulation of these conditions is indeed possible and is likely to enhance considerably our understanding of older adults' everyday memory capabilities. At the same time, the external validity of our laboratory research should not be accepted as a given. Memory researchers clearly need to develop more effective external criteria for assessing everyday memory performances and to demonstrate adequate covariations between these assessments and their laboratory-based assessments of memory performances.

References

Arenberg, D., & Robertson-Tchabo, E. A. (1977). Learning and aging. In J. E. Birren & K. W. Schaie (Eds.), *Handbook of the psychology of aging* (pp. 421–449). New York: Van Nostrand Reinhold.

Battig, W. F. (1968). Paired-associate learning. In T. R. Dixon & D. L. Horton (Eds.), *Verbal behavior and general behavior theory* (pp. 146–171). Englewood Cliffs, NJ: Prentice-Hall.

Broadbent, D. E., Cooper, P. F., Fitzgerald, P., & Parkes, K. R. (1982). The Cognitive Failures Questionnaire (CFQ) and its correlates. *British Journal of Clinical Psychology, 21,* 1–16.

Burke, D. M., & Light, L. L. (1981). Memory and aging: The role of retrieval processes. *Psychological Bulletin, 90,* 513–546.

Burke, D. M., & Yee, P. L. (1984). Semantic priming during sentence processing by young and older adults. *Developmental Psychology, 20,* 903–910.

Hasher, L., & Zacks, R. T. (1979). Automatic and effortful processes in memory. *Journal of Experimental Psychology: General, 108,* 356–388.

Hulicka, I. M. (1982). Memory functioning in late adulthood. In. F. I. M. Craik & S. Trehub (Eds.), *Aging and cognitive processes* (pp. 331–352). New York: Plenum Press.

Hulicka, I. M., & Grossman, J. L. (1967). Age-group comparisons for the use of mediators in paired-associate learning. *Journal of Gerontology, 22,* 46–51.

Kausler, D. H. (1974). *Psychology of verbal learning and memory.* New York: Academic Press.

Kausler, D. H. (1982). *Experimental psychology and human aging.* New York: Wiley.

Kausler, D. H., & Hakami, M. K. (1983). Memory for activities: Adult age differences and intentionality. *Developmental Psychology, 19,* 889–894.

Kausler, D. H., Hakami, M. K., & Wright, R. E. (1982). Adult age differences in frequency judgments of categorical representations. *Journal of Gerontology, 37,* 365–371.

Kausler, D. H., Lichty, W., & Davis, R. T. (1985a). Temporal memory for performed activities: Intentionality and adult age differences. *Developmental Psychology, 21.*

Kausler, D. H., Lichty, W., & Freund, J. S. (1985b). Adult age differences in recognition memory and frequency judgments for planned versus performed activities. *Developmental Psychology, 21,* 647–654.

Kausler, D. H., Lichty, W., & Hakami, M. K. (1984). Frequency judgments for distractor items in a short-term memory task: Instructional variation and adult age differences. *Journal of Verbal Learning and Verbal Behavior, 23,* 660–668.

Lair, C. V., Moon, W. H., & Kausler, D. H. (1969). Associative interference in the paired-associate learning of middle-aged and old subjects. *Developmental Psychology, 1,* 548–552.

Mook, D. G. (1983). In defense of external validity. *American Psychologist, 38,* 379–387.

Neisser, U. (1982). *Memory observed: Remembering in natural contexts.* San Francisco: W. H. Freeman.

Posner, M. I., & Snyder, C. R. R. (1975). Attention and cognitive control. In R. L. Solso (Ed.), *Information processing and cognition* (pp. 55–85). Hillsdale, NJ: Lawrence Erlbaum.

Rabbitt, P. M. A. (1982). How do old people know what to do next? In F. I. M. Craik & S. Trehub (Eds.), *Aging and cognitive processes* (pp. 79–98). New York: Plenum Press.

Salthouse, T. A. (1980). Age and memory: Strategies for localizing the loss. In L. W. Poon, J. L. Fozard, L. Cermak, D. Arenberg, & L. W. Thompson (Eds.), *New directions in memory and aging* (pp. 47–65). Hillsdale, NJ: Lawrence Erlbaum.

Salthouse, T. A. (1984). Effects of age and skill in typing. *Journal of Experimental Psychology: General, 113,* 345–371.

Salthouse, T. A., & Kausler, D. H. (1985). Memory methodology in maturity. In C. J. Brainerd & M. Pressley (Eds.), *Basic processes in memory development: Progress in cognitive development research* (pp. 279–311). New York: Springer-Verlag.

Sunderland, A., Harris, J. E., & Baddeley, A. D. (1983). Do laboratory tasks predict everyday memory? *Journal of Verbal Learning and Verbal Behavior, 22,* 341–357.

Taub, H. A., & Baker, M. T. (1983). The effect of repeated testing upon comprehension of informed consent materials by elderly volunteers. *Experimental Aging Research, 9,* 135–138.

Tulving, E. (1983). *Elements of episodic memory.* Oxford: Clarendon Press.

Wang, A. Y. (1983). Individual differences in learning speed. *Journal of Experimental Psychology: Learning, Memory, and Cognition, 9,* 300–311.

Zarit, S. H., Cole, K. D., & Guider, R. L. (1981). Memory training strategies and subjective complaints of memory in the aged. *Gerontologist, 21,* 158–164.

Zelinski, E. M., Gilewski, M. J., & Thompson, L. W. (1980). Do laboratory memory tests relate to everyday remembering and forgetting? In L. W. Poon, J. L. Fozard, L. Cermak, D. Arenberg, & L. W. Thompson (Eds.), *New directions in aging* (pp. 519–544). Hillsdale, NJ: Lawrence Erlbaum.

Part III

Cognitive enhancement and aging: Clinical and educational applications

27 Introduction to Part III: Approaches to practical applications

Barbara A. Wilson and Leonard W. Poon

In Part III, we consider ways of compensating for everyday memory failures and discuss methods for improving memory. We begin by looking at some of the issues involved, continue with reports of studies designed to enhance memory in the normal elderly, and conclude by examining memory programs for those with acquired brain damage.

The opening chapter in Part III is by Lars Bäckman, of the University of Umea, Sweden. He discusses types of compensation strategies used by older adults in episodic remembering. Bäckman provides a scholarly text that suggests that although the elderly do less well on many memory tasks than younger people, they are nevertheless able to compensate for some of their memory deficits. They do this in three major ways. First, they may pick up on the support provided by experimenters. For example, scores on paired-associate learning tasks can be improved by responding positively to a tester's prompts and cues. Second, compensation may occur through properties inherent in the task itself. Thus, for example, when elderly subjects are asked to recall a series of actions they have watched, their recall is inferior to that of younger subjects, but if the elderly subjects perform the actions themselves, the age effect is eliminated. Third, the elderly may compensate through cognitive support systems. It can be argued, for instance, that elderly chess players compensate for encoding and retrieval deficits by better global evaluation of positions.

Recoding is an important issue in Bäckman's Chapter 28. He discusses the elderly person's need for attentional guidance in order to achieve compensatory memory behavior, compensation when conscious encoding (or rehearsal) is not required, compensation through modifying the level of arousal, and compensation as adaptive behavior.

A further aspect of compensation regarded as important by Bäckman is that of multimodality, an item mentioned again by Robin West later in Part III. It is argued that information coming in through several modalities is more likely to be remembered than when it arrives through a single modality, such as vision, hearing, or touch.

In Chapter 29, Sherry Willis writes about several aspects of cognitive training in later adulthood. Questions are raised about remediation and new learning. The author also asks what abilities have been targeted in cognitive-training research. The answer suggests those abilities that show large age differences, such as problem solving, inductive reasoning, spatial orientation, and response speed.

Wide differences are noted in the timing of the onset of decline and in the particular abilities or skills that are affected. In one of Willis's studies, she looked at a large group of subjects aged 64 to 95 years who had been assessed on reasoning and spatial orientation tasks 14 years earlier. She found that approximately 55% had declined on one or both of these tasks, whereas the other 45% remained stable. The decliners were trained in the skill for which the decline was observed. Those who had declined in both skills were assigned randomly to one of two types of training, as were those who had remained stable. The findings indicated that cognitive training techniques can reverse reliably documented declines in a number of older adults. Such reversal can occur for both reasoning and spatial abilities. Furthermore, training selectively enhanced the performance of those who had remained stable. The magnitude of the training effect was greater for the decliners than for those who had remained stable, and spatial-orientation training had a greater effect on women than on men.

All the subjects in Willis's study were in fair to excellent health, and none had complained of problems. This leaves us uncertain whether or not older adults who do complain of memory problems and who are not in such good health would show a similar pattern. Nevertheless, the results are encouraging and suggest that it is worth conducting a similar study with the confused or frail elderly. However, as we shall see in a later chapter, new learning is much less likely in people whose memory difficulties stem from cerebral lesions.

In Chapter 30, Robin West considers practical memory mnemonics for the aged. She begins by providing a comprehensive review of studies that have examined everyday memory problems of the elderly. The problems include recall of names, faces, and routes, remembering to do things, remembering conversations, and the contents of television programs. As a prelude to her discussion of practical memory training, West makes a plea for better assessment tools for measuring everyday memory, an issue that is taken up by Wilson in a later chapter. West argues that individual differences must also be taken into account.

Few studies have tried to teach mnemonic strategies to the elderly, and even fewer have been concerned with teaching practical real-life tasks. What is needed, says West, is more information on retrieval processes in the elderly and on external aids. The main advantage of many mnemonic methods is that they have their own built-in retrieval mechanisms; for example, thinking of the first location along a route is a retrieval cue for the first item in the method of loci. Furthermore, retrieval methods such as alphabet searching and mental retracing are the only internal methods that are reported frequently in questionnaires and self-reports completed by the elderly.

Similarly, external aids are commonly used in everyday situations, and it is surprising that more work has not been done to increase or improve the use of these aids in memory-impaired populations.

Automatic behaviors and automatic memory strategies are also underinvestigated. We do not yet know enough about age changes in automaticity. West suggests that we should not be teaching multiple techniques for multiple memory tasks in multiple sessions, as this practice overburdens the learning requirements. Instead, it might be better to teach multiple techniques for the same task or else apply the same strategies to multiple tasks. The thorny problem of generalization is also mentioned by West. This problem receives further attention in the next two chapters by Jerome Yesavage and associates and Barbara Wilson.

Chapter 31, by Jerome Yesavage, Danielle Lapp, and Javaid Sheikh, continues the discussion on mnemonics and the elderly. They begin by considering the magnitude of memory deficits seen in the normal elderly and report a decline on cognitive measures from 10% to 40% between the ages of 20 and 70 years, depending on the test and testing methods used.

Yesavage and associates also remind us that many treatment effects that have previously been reported have used experimental material, such as list learning. The mnemonic strategies involved often have been too complicated for the elderly, and there is no evidence that the techniques help outside the experimental situation or that the effects last longer than 1 week.

Other limitations of previous studies include (1) difficulties experienced by older people in producing and remembering images and imagery associations, (2) high anxiety levels interfering with test performance, (3) superficiality of improvements, and (4) shallowness of treatment effects.

Yesavage and associates avoid some of these limitations in the studies reported in their chapter. Three studies are reported in which subjects received preliminary training to prepare them for using mnemonics. One of those studies dealt with teaching techniques to help subjects learn visual imagery before using visual imagery itself. Subjects who did not have the preliminary training did not do so well. Another study included additional encoding in a face–name association task. Again, subjects who were exposed to the additional encoding did better than those who were denied such exposure. In the third study, half the subjects received relaxation training prior to learning, and these, too, recalled more information than those who did not receive the training.

Yesavage and associates conclude by arguing for more consideration to be given to generalization of treatment effects, for more practical applications, for more individually tailored treatment programs, for greater exploration of the effects of affect, motivation, and self-image, and for greater understanding of the interaction between treatment and medication. Many of these issues are taken up in the last three chapters of Part III.

All the chapters in Part III discussed thus far are concerned with the normal elderly living in the community. The final three chapters look at people with organic memory impairments caused by head injury, stroke, or other kinds of brain damage. Barbara Wilson begins her Chapter 32 by pointing out that restoration of memory functioning is rarely a practical goal for brain-damaged adults. Rather, emphasis is placed on bypassing the problems and on finding the most efficient way for each individual to learn new information. Wilson continues by looking at the three major fields of cognitive psychology, neuropsychology, and behavioral psychology to see how they have contributed to the new area of memory therapy.

Wilson offers ways of identifying problems for treatment and includes a short description of a new test that assesses everyday memory skills rather than performance on experimental material. A discussion follows on some of the strategies available to help the memory-impaired. These include environmental adaptations, external aids, internal strategies, rehearsal and repetitive practice, memory games, and reality orientation. Having identified problems for treatment and considered available strategies, Wilson then discusses the selection of appropriate strategies for individuals.

The last part of Wilson's chapter considers evaluation of memory therapy programs. She argues for greater acceptance of a range of methodologies, including those that evaluate an individual's response to treatment, particularly single-case experimental designs and behavioral-assessment procedures. Some good examples of these are described in the final chapter in Part III.

Nadina Lincoln's Chapter 33 deals with the management of memory problems in a hospital setting. Both long-stay and rehabilitation wards are considered. It is pointed out that the approaches taken will differ for those whose impairments are likely to deteriorate (e.g., patients with Alzheimer's disease) and those whose problems are likely to remain static (e.g., following severe head injury). Lincoln concentrates on general medical wards rather than geriatric wards, given the lack of studies in the former field. She begins by considering reality orientation in long-stay wards. The results typically are small gains, with limited generalization to other aspects of behavior. However, the results can be regarded as stepping-stones to other intervention programs. (Reality orientation is considered further in the final chapter.)

Treating patients in groups is discussed, and one study is described. Memory groups are potentially important for remediation of some memory problems and, if successful, could reduce the cost of providing memory therapy to the organically impaired. They could have other benefits not possible in individual therapy, such as lessening the fear of losing one's sanity when exposed to others with similar or worse problems. Tasks can be included that will ensure success for each member of the group. For people used to failure, such success could have considerable indirect therapeutic benefit. It could, of course, be the case that memory groups are not effective means of helping people with memory problems, and relevant studies are awaited with interest. (Groups for relatives of memory-impaired people are described in Chapter 34 by Nicholas Moffat.)

Lincoln reports an interesting questionnaire study conducted with hospitalized stroke patients. The proportion of patients experiencing memory problems was generally low, but they did experience certain problems significantly more frequently than did orthopedic controls. This chapter concludes with a discussion of some of the practical problems encountered when working in a hospital setting. Descriptions of some of the ways these difficulties may be overcome are offered.

In Chapter 34, Nicholas Moffat begins with a consideration of the strains placed on those caring for the memory-impaired elderly. He describes relatives' support groups aimed at reducing stress. Information on dementia and advice on coping with memory problems were the most frequently reported needs among these support groups.

Involving care-givers in treatment is another major concern in this chapter, and we are given some interesting and ingenious solutions to particular problems such as losing things around the house. Moffat takes us beyond pure memory problems when he discusses two examples of treatment for dysgraphia and nominal dysphasia.

Moffat describes his reality-orientation (RO) study that took place in a day hospital. He found that the ability to benefit from RO could be predicted by the level of performance during a baseline period. The ability to predict which particular patients are likely to respond to particular therapies obviously is of great importance in memory therapy.

Moffat's next concern is with the utilization of community services to provide cognitive rehabilitation. There are several advantages to home-based treatment, not least of which is the expression by elderly patients of a preference for it. One of the interesting observations from this discussion is the author's view that home-care services may not have proved particularly effective because the implementation of these services has followed a traditional model of "doing things to the patient" rather than actively involving the patient and his or her relatives in the treatment. In other words, a medical model rather than a behavioral model has been pursued. Moffat concludes his chapter with suggestions on alternative ways of helping the elderly memory-impaired in their homes. These include provision of computers and carefully constructed therapy manuals. Such innovative thinking should be welcomed in an era in which the emphasis has been on cutbacks.

Several issues emerge from the chapters in Part III. The first is that of generalization. This remains one of the crucial issues in rehabilitation, and we must be able to demonstrate successful outcomes in order to offer real assistance to people with memory impairments. Generalization can refer to transfer of information or learning from one patient to another or from one setting to another or from one problem to another. So far, the emphasis has been on discovering successful strategies. We must now find out which particular individuals benefit from these strategies, develop ways of teaching people to use or apply them, and discover which situations are conducive to particular strategies. We must not assume that generalization will occur automatically. The available evidence (at least for the organically impaired) suggests that generalization is unlikely to occur without special efforts being made on the part of the therapist.

A second issue referred to in many of the chapters in Part III is the question whether we should treat the underlying deficit or the problem itself. Sherry Willis believes we should be dealing with problems at an ability level rather than at a task-specific level, whereas the last three authors claim (either explicitly or implicitly) that success is more likely if we tackle the particular problems faced by the memory-impaired. If treating the underlying deficit is the way forward with a particular patient, then obviously that is what we should do, because several problems will be overcome in the process. However, if that is not the way to proceed, then we would be denying a patient the chance of learning some useful, life-enhancing information or skill if we did not offer treatment aimed at overcoming a particular problem. The reasons for the different viewpoints expressed by these authors may have much to do with the different perspectives from which they regard the issue. Sherry Willis works with non-brain-damaged elderly, whereas the others work with neurologically impaired patients. Differences in perspective, experience, and even ideology are such important issues in themselves that some major studies aimed at comparing approaches and settings would be welcomed.

The third major issue in Part III is the purpose of training in mnemonics. Authors present arguments for using mnemonics for improving memory and for learning new information. Again, viewpoints are influenced by different work perspectives resulting from the kinds of patients seen and treated in the different institutions where the authors are employed. A key factor is whether the patient has or has not suffered neurological damage. For the normal elderly, training in mnemonics may well help them deal more effectively with the memory demands they are likely to face in their daily living, particularly if training in this ability is built into their treatment programs. Those people with organic impairments, however, are very unlikely to use or apply mnemonics. For them, mnemonic strategies will be used to teach certain limited amounts of new information. Here, mnemonics often are more effective than rote rehearsal, but it is unrealistic to expect most of these people to use the techniques for novel situations. The concern regarding people with organic impairments is whether or not they can learn anything at all, rather than whether or not they can learn to use mnemonics. Of course, the answer to the former question is positive, because although new learning is slow and difficult for them, it is nevertheless possible. It is likely that mnemonics can make this process a little less slow and difficult.

Further questions relating to mnemonics are raised in Part III by authors who discuss the concepts of memory training and memory therapy. It is suggested that the former is given in order to improve people's memory functioning, or at least to teach them to use their memory skills more effectively. This, again, might be possible with the normal elderly, but it is unlikely to assist the brain-injured. Memory therapy, certainly as it is considered in Great Britain, refers to any treatment that helps people to cope with, to manage, or to bypass their memory problems; it also refers to the employment of strategies for learning new information. It is likely that some confusion over terminology and controversy over concepts have arisen in this debate surrounding the treatment of amnesic patients. Are we at all sure, for instance, that others share our interpretations of terms like "treatment" and "therapy"?

Most people are likely to agree that we cannot restore lost memory functioning in Alzheimer's patients or those patients with a classic amnesic syndrome, but this does not mean that nothing can be done to help reduce the problems faced by these people and their families. Treatment is not solely concerned with restoration of function; it also involves making changes in the environment to make life easier for a patient. Treatment must be defined more broadly in order to encourage the search for materials and processes that will enable patients and their families to lead their lives more efficiently and effectively.

There are several intermediate questions that remain to be answered in the management of memory problems. We do not know, for example, what importance to give to insight or, as often happens, lack of insight. Relatives in the support groups organized by Nicholas Moffat became more depressed after gaining more insight into the nature of and prognosis for the elderly patients' memory problems. Patients themselves frequently underestimate the extent or severity of their memory difficulties, and although clinicians often feel that insight is an important factor in response to therapy, we remain unclear about its precise role.

We are also unclear about the timing of help for memory problems. When is the best time for introducing treatment? There are wide individual differences in the rate of decline in the normal elderly, but if we can preempt the decline by having the resources to introduce treatment prophylactically, we might postpone confusion and save society from some of the expense of caring for the confused elderly. For those sustaining neurological damage, the picture often is less clear, with some patients requiring physical therapy, occupational therapy, and speech therapy, with little or no time left for memory therapy. Furthermore, if such patients are improving, is there any point in trying to reduce the memory problems? Should we wait for stable baselines? If we do, we may miss the most opportune moment for treatment. Obviously, we can obtain answers to such questions only when proper evaluations are the norm in our institutions.

Even if we solve the question of when to begin treatment, we are still left with a series of choices to be made concerning the problems to tackle and their aggregation. We can be guided by the complaints of patients or their relatives, but this has its limitations. As Nadina Lincoln reminds us, patients and relatives do not always recognize the problems. As an alternative, we might look at performance on certain tests. Probably the most effective way is to use a combination of sources, an approach recommended by Barbara Wilson. Most of our authors agree, however, that we should be concentrating on practical problems.

The final issue to highlight in this introduction to part III is that of time/cost effectiveness. An enormous amount of time has gone into the research reported in these chapters. It is hoped that our theoretical understanding of memory and cognitive functioning has increased as a result. However, it is unlikely that the work reported here will lead directly to dramatic improvements in the treatment of memory difficulties faced by either the normal elderly or those with organic problems. Can we therefore justify our efforts? An answer is not immediately forthcoming, and it will continue to elude us until we have found answers to a series of subsiduary questions. These can be summarized in the following manner:

1 How far can we improve memory functioning in the normal elderly?
2 How successful can we be in postponing or slowing down the rate of decline in both normal and brain-damaged elderly people?
3 How much useful information can we teach the organically impaired?

Although much time and effort, as well as money, will have to be spent in pursuing these questions, we should nevertheless remind ourselves of the possible results of seemingly inexpensive inactivity. Many memory-impaired adults face long-term institutional care, and few processes in the health services are more expensive than that. If we give up the search for ways of alleviating memory problems, we shall have to pay larger bills for longer terms of institutional care for growing populations of elderly people.

Even though dramatic changes may not be achieved in the foreseeable future, we should proceed toward realistic goals, adding to our store of knowledge, finding out what works best for each individual in particular circumstances. We can use volunteers or therapy assistants as well as family members to help us. Indeed, we can direct our efforts more toward teaching relatives, investigating suitable environments, and designing more appropriate external aids. It could well be that these approaches will provide us with more satisfactory answers than mnemonics. Our principles should perhaps be similar to those held by psychologists working with people with mental handicaps. They argue that if a handicapped person is not learning, it is because the therapist has not yet found the right way to teach that person.

Part IIIA

Issues and perspectives

28 Varieties of memory compensation by older adults in episodic remembering

Lars Bäckman

In a recent paper (Bäckman, 1985a), I introduced a conceptual frame of reference for research on adult aging and episodic remembering based on the superordinate concepts of compensation and recoding. This chapter constitutes an extension and elaboration of the framework proposed there. One basic point of departure for the discussion here concerns the fact that older adults possess the ability to compensate for various deficits in episodic remembering through different types of contextual and cognitive support. A classification scheme comprising three basic categories of memory compensation in later adulthood is presented: compensation via experimenter-provided support, compensation via inherent task properties, and compensation via cognitive-support systems. These categories deal with proximal interactions between the capabilities of the learner and the actual task demands. It is also suggested that younger adults, because of superior ability in various *recoding operations,* are less dependent on contextual and cognitive support in order to remember successfully. ''Recoding'' is here defined as ''all the processes and operations an individual possesses that, when applied, bring about a richer and more elaborate representation of the initially registered information to be remembered'' (Tulving, 1983).

It is argued that a multifactorial approach is a necessary prerequisite for gaining the best understanding of what happens with memory as one gets older. Accordingly, some aspects of memory compensation in later adulthood other than those falling under the aforementioned categories are described. This includes discussions of (1) older adults' need for attentional guidance, (2) compensation via modification of level of arousal and laboratory anxiety, and (3) compensation as adaptive behavior by older adults. It is hoped that demonstration of memory

Preparation of this chapter was partly supported by grants from the Bank of Sweden Tercentenary Foundation and the Delegation of Social Research in Sweden. I am grateful to Fergus Craik, Roger Dixon, Lars-Göran Nilsson, and Jerker Rönnberg for discussions of some of the ideas presented in this chapter, to three anonymous reviewers for helpful comments on an earlier draft, and to Karen Hill and Ann Louise Söderlund for technical help in the preparation of the manuscript.

compensation by older adults in a variety of different situations and from various levels of analysis will underscore the need for adopting a multifactorial approach to the study of cognitive aging.

In addition, the experimental paradigms that have been employed when the different forms of memory compensation of the elderly have been demonstrated are evaluated in terms of their representativeness of remembering in everyday life. Finally, possible implications of the proposed view of cognitive development in adulthood for the development of memory-training programs are outlined.

The concept of compensation

Reports of interactions between age and type of task or material are commonplace in the literature on aging and memory. These interactions typically are taken as points of departure for attempts at localizing the adult age deficit in episodic remembering. For example, it has been suggested that the elderly suffer from deficits in organization (Hultsch, 1969; Waddell & Rogoff, 1981), visual imagery (Treat, Poon, & Fozard, 1978; Winograd & Simon, 1980), verbal mediation (Hulicka & Grossman, 1967; Hulicka, Sterns, & Grossman, 1967), semantic encoding (Eysenck, 1974; Simon, 1979), retrieval (Erber, 1974; Perlmutter, 1979), speed of processing (Salthouse, 1980; Waugh & Barr, 1980), effortful processing (Attig & Hasher, 1980; Hasher & Zacks, 1979), utilization and integration of contextual information (Burke & Light, 1981; Craik & Rabinowitz, 1984), and storage (Harwood & Naylor, 1969; Wimer & Wigdor, 1958).

Occasionally these views have been treated as alternative hypotheses in determining the locus of the age decrement in episodic remembering (e.g., encoding deficit vs. retrieval deficit, effortful-processing deficit vs. speed-of-processing deficit). However, this may be the time to stop for a moment, take one step back, and view the area in a somewhat broader sense. The age-by-task interactions obtained have two characteristic features: (1) pronounced age differences in favor of younger adults in "nonguided" memory tasks (e.g., free recall, paired-associate learning) and (2) reduced age differences or no differences in tasks in which various types of contextual or cognitive support are provided. This pattern of data supports the concept of compensation. That is, older adults apparently are capable of compensating for plausible neural/sensory/cognitive deficits through a variety of environmental and cognitive aids.

In the present context, the concept of compensation is closely related to those views of remembering that emphasize the interactions between different cognitive processes and the task demands at hand as being the primary objects of study for memory researchers (Bransford, 1979; Craik, 1983, 1985; Hultsch & Pentz, 1980; Jenkins, 1979; Nilsson, 1979, 1984). One implication of such an approach is that contextual factors must be included in the explanation of a given set of data. As applied to research on aging and memory, this means that whenever the concept of compensation is used, the user must specify the properties of the memory tasks for which aging effects occur or do not occur. In other words, the critical contextual prerequisites for compensatory memory behavior by the elderly must be determined. Such an enterprise requires an extensive task analysis (Moscovitch, 1984; Rönnberg & Bäckman, 1984; Rönnberg & Ohlsson, 1985).

Several other aspects of the concept of compensation are important to keep in mind. First, in the context of aging and episodic remembering, the term "compensation" refers to a selective improvement by older adults as a function of some experimental manipulation; that is, the descriptive statement that elderly adults compensate for a memory deficit presupposes an interaction between age and a task variable (Rohwer, 1976; Smith & Winograd, 1978). Accordingly, an empirical outcome showing equal improvements by younger and older adults in task B compared with task A does not qualify as an illustration of compensation by older adults. Such data, which have been obtained in studies on face recognition (Smith & Winograd, 1978), text recall (Light & Anderson, 1983; Zelinski, Light, & Gilewski, 1984), and the effects of prior retrieval on recall (Rabinowitz & Craik, 1986), reflect that both groups subject to study are sensitive to the experimental manipulation proper; the results demonstrate memory enhancement, but they do not tell us anything about the compensatory capabilities of older adults.

Second, given that an organism (in this case, an aging organism) is capable of compensating for a deficit, it seems likely that some of the abilities necessary for a successful solution of a particular task are relatively intact. In this respect, the concept of compensation is related to the concept of production deficiency (Reese, 1976); that is, the ability to carry out a certain cognitive operation is available, but not always spontaneously accessible. Results from other areas of study in memory disorders, such as Alzheimer's disease (Miller, 1977; Moscovitch, 1982), Huntington's disease (Butters, 1980), depression (Ellis, Thomas, & Rodriguez, 1984), and acute alcohol intoxication (Karlsson & Bäckman, 1985), indicate that compensation via contextual or cognitive support is not always possible to demonstrate in cognitively impaired groups.

Third, although evidence for compensatory capabilities is seen in many groups of individuals with memory disorders, the conditions under which this is manifested may vary considerably between groups. Comparisons between different types of amnesic patients illustrate this point nicely; see Hirst (1982) and Squire (1982) for reviews. Therefore, it is necessary to attain group-specific analyses of the types of contextual and cognitive guidance that are utilized by different groups with memory deficits; see Cermak (1982) and Moscovitch (1984) for similar viewpoints in the context of research on amnesia. The present plea for analysis of compensatory task conditions utilized by older adults should be seen in the light of this line of reasoning.

Finally, it should be emphasized that the present framework focuses on the ability of older adults to utilize compensatory task conditions. In many other areas of research in which the concept of compensation has been extensively used (e.g., sensory handicaps, brain injury), the other side of the coin of compensation has been emphasized: namely, the self-initiated compensatory efforts undertaken by individuals with various types of deficits (Bäckman & Dixon, 1986; Dixon & Bäckman, 1986). In those domains of inquiry, compensation usually is inferred when a loss in one ability or component thereof is balanced by a concomitant growth in another (Salthouse, in press).

Generally, the area of aging and episodic remembering has presented very few direct empirical demonstrations of self-initiated compensatory efforts by older adults. Exceptions to this rule are two studies on the use of memory aids: Cavanaugh, Grady, and Perlmutter (1983) reported increased use of internal (e.g., organization, rehearsal) as well as external (e.g., lists, calendars) memory aids in real life in older adults compared with younger adults, whereas Dixon and Hultsch (1983) found this to be true only for external aids. This pattern of results may reflect an attempt by older adults to compensate for objective or perceived memory difficulties. However, as will be discussed later, I think that the two sides of the compensation coin (utilization of compensatory task conditions vs. self-initiated compensation) can be brought together; this is illustrated by some recent memory studies in which presumably ecologically relevant tasks were employed.

Compensation via experimenter-provided support

There are several subcategories of "compensatory triggers" that can be identified within the area of aging and memory. The first subcategory may be labeled compensation via experimenter-provided support. This type of compensation evidently has been the type most often studied in the aging and memory literature. Relevant to this category are all those studies that have demonstrated pronounced age effects in free recall or paired-associate learning tasks (unaccompanied by pretask encoding instructions, cues, and so forth) and reduced effects or elimination of age effects in tasks where the experimenter provided the subjects with instructions, hints, cues, and the like. Such results have been obtained by contrasting the memory performances of young and old adults in "standard-instruction" tasks and their performances in tasks where organizational strategies (Hultsch, 1969, 1971), instructions to use verbal mediators (Hulicka & Grossman, 1967; Hulicka et al., 1967), or imagery instructions (Canestrari, 1968; Thomas & Ruben, 1973; Treat et al., 1978) were provided by the experimenter. Other demonstrations of compensation via experimenter-provided support come from studies showing smaller age differences or elimination of differences when the experimenter supplied copy cues, as in recognition (Erber, 1974; Howell, 1972; Kausler & Hakami, 1983a; Schonfield & Robertson, 1966), or category cues, as in cued recall (Hultsch, 1975; Laurence, 1967), compared with free-recall tasks.

In addition, studies by Smith (1977), Ceci and Tabor (1981), and Shaps and Nilsson (1980), as well as some studies on levels of processing and aging, provide cases in point. Smith (1977) and Ceci and Tabor (1981) failed to find any age differences in memory when category cues were presented together with the to-be-remembered (TBR) items at encoding and retrieval, respectively. Employing the recognition-failure paradigm (Tulving & Thomson, 1973), Shaps and Nilsson (1980) found equivalent cued-recall performances for younger and older adults when strong semantic associates were provided at study (together with the TBR items) and test (as retrieval cues). In contrast, the young outperformed the old when weak associates were provided at encoding and retrieval (Rabinowitz, 1984). Further, a number of "levels" studies that employed orienting tasks prior to recognition tests (Erber, Herman, & Botwinick, 1980; Mason, 1979; White, cited in Craik, 1977) reported invariance across the adult life span. These studies also showed pronounced age effects in favor of younger adults in a variety of control tasks lacking this experimenter-provided support. In a related vein, Bäckman, Mäntylä, and Erngrund (1984) employed a paradigm introduced by Mäntylä and Nilsson (1983) to study encoding–retrieval compatibility in relation to aging. Bäckman and associates (1984) found extremely high levels of recall (92% and 82% for young and old adults, respectively) when subjects were instructed to generate their own cues to the TBR items at encoding and were presented with these self-generated cues at retrieval.

Taken together, the cited studies suggest that old adults are capable of compensating for cognitive deficits by using different types of experimenter-provided support and that there is an adult age difference with respect to the need for contextual support in order to achieve maximal memory performance: The elderly need more than the younger adults (Craik, 1983; Winocur, 1982).

Representativeness of experimental paradigms

Many authors, such as Giambra and Arenberg (1980) and Salthouse (1982), have noted that research on aging and memory has been largely dependent on advances in its mother discipline of basic memory research. One of many consequences of this direction of influence has been the adoption of experimental paradigms and TBR materials. The memory tasks that have been employed when compensation via experimenter-provided support has been demonstrated have represented a selection of standard laboratory memory tasks from the 1960s and 1970s (mostly variations on the word-recall and paired-associate learning themes). During recent years, several theorists (Baddeley & Wilkins, 1984; Kausler, 1983; Neisser, 1982) have argued that many of the most commonly used paradigms in memory research (e.g., recall or recognition of unrelated words) are not representative of the encoding and retrieval requirements of the natural environment, and pleas have been made both to study remembering in natural settings and to employ more ecologically relevant tasks and materials. Analogously, the tasks for which this type of memory compensation have been observed may be criticized for the same lack of ecological relevance. More specifically, how often does an "experimenter" provide us with instructions, hints, or cues in the natural environment, and how often does the natural environment present the same cues at encoding and retrieval? To quote Kinsbourne and Wood (1982), "much if not most episodic remembering proceeds without any overt cueing at all" (p. 210).

To summarize briefly, the interactions between adult age and type of task that have been discussed in this section tell us a great deal about the ability of older adults to utilize compensatory task conditions. It is, however, less clear that these interactions tell us anything about similarities and differences between younger and older adults' memory behaviors in real life.

Compensation via inherent task properties

The second subcategory of compensation is labeled compensation via inherent task properties. This form of compensation is similar to the one discussed in the preceding section in the sense that both are empirically based on interactions between age and the quality and quantity of the information provided in the memory task. With respect to compensation via inherent task properties, however, no hints, cues, or instructions trigger the activation of elderly people's compensatory memory behavior. Instead, the basis for memory compensation is here to be found in inherent properties of certain contextually rich memory tasks. Hence, an important difference between compensation via experimenter-provided support and compensation via inherent task properties is that added verbal information is a critical prerequisite in the former case, but not in the latter. Two types of interactions that demonstrate compensation via inherent task properties are identified. The first type is based primarily on interactions between age and the "quality of task properties." The second type is based primarily on interactions between age and the "quantity of task properties."

Quality of task properties

Several recent studies illustrate memory compensation in the aged through manipulations of the quality of task properties. In three studies from our own laboratory (Bäckman, 1985b; Bäckman & Nilsson, 1984, 1985) we have demonstrated that the aging effect typically observed in free recall of verbal materials is eliminated when the task is to remember series of subject-performed tasks (SPTs), a memory task introduced by Cohen (1981). In experiments employing SPTs, subjects are instructed to perform and remember series of real-life acts. These acts are performed either with objects (e.g., lift the spoon, bounce the ball) or without any objects (e.g., nod in agreement, clap your hands). SPTs differ from standard verbal memory tasks in two basic ways with respect to the possibility of memory compensation in the aged. First, they are multimodal, in the sense that several or all sensory systems are activated during encoding. The experimenter reads out each SPT aloud, thereby presenting the information auditorily. The subject's visual system is, of course, activated throughout the presentation of SPTs. The subject has to carry out the SPTs motorically, and hence the tactual system is involved. Also, some SPTs (e.g., smell the flower, eat the raisin) bring about activity in the olfactory and gustatory modes.

Second, the SPTs are characterized by a variety of features on which encoding may be based. Besides the verbal features, SPTs can be encoded on the basis of color, shape, texture, sounds, motor features, taste features, and smell features. Note that some of these features are nominally present in two modalities (e.g., motor features, shape), whereas others are modality-specific (e.g., color, sounds). These task properties clearly distinguish SPTs from verbal memory tasks in which the presentation is typically unimodal and only semantic, phonemic, and orthographic features are available for encoding; see Bäckman, Nilsson, and Chalom (in press) for further discussion. Although no age differences in immediate and delayed free recalls of SPTs were observed by Bäckman and Nilsson (1984, 1985) or Bäckman (1985b), exactly the same verbal information presented unimodally (Bäckman & Nilsson, 1984), bimodally (with imagery instructions) (Bäckman & Nilsson, 1985), or without active motor manipulation (Bäckman, 1985b) gave rise to pronounced age differences in favor of younger adults.

In a similar vein, Arenberg (1968) and Bäckman (1986) observed attenuated age differences in memory for bimodally (visually and auditorily) presented items and marked age differences for unimodally (visually or auditorily) presented items. Bäckman (1986) noted that a cross-experimental comparison between the studies using SPTs and those of Arenberg (1968) and Bäckman (1986) suggested that age differences in free recall were pronounced when the presentation was unimodal, reduced when the presentation was bimodal, and eliminated when the presentation was multimodal. In other words, the elderly's success in demonstrating compensatory memory behavior appears to increase as a function of the number of modalities activated during encoding.

Further, some recent studies on television recall (Cavanaugh, 1983, 1984) are relevant in this context. Cavanaugh found that differences between younger and older adults in television recall were small, and in some cases zero. Even if no verbal control tasks were included in these studies, it seems reasonable to argue that the data reflect the unique properties of the actual presentation mode, because the bulk of previous studies have demonstrated age differences in favor of younger adults in recall of verbal materials, as reviewed by Kausler (1982) and Salthouse (1982). Encoding of television programs is similar to encoding of SPTs in one critical respect, namely, that a variety of features on which encoding may be based are present in both cases. During encoding of a television program, it is possible to acquire the information on the basis of verbal encoding, but other features are also present, including color, shape, and motor features. Moreover, the plot of the program provides an organizational structure for the encoding of the event. Conceivably, these types of contextual support constitute critical prerequisites for the elderly's success in this memory task.

An ingenious study on spatial memory (Waddell & Rogoff, 1981) and a number of studies on text recall provide further evidence for the validity of this type of compensation via inherent task properties. In the Waddell and Rogoff (1981) study, middle-aged and older women were requested to reconstruct spatial arrays by replacing miniature objects in either a contextually organized panorama or a bank of cubicles not contextually organized. No age differences in spatial recall were obtained in the former task, whereas a pronounced superiority on the part of the middle-aged women was observed in the latter task. Note that, similar to the studies on SPT memory, the TBR items were the same in both tasks employed.

Although quite dissimilar to experiments on spatial recall, there are studies on text recall telling the same story. Research on text recall in adulthood has yielded a somewhat mixed picture (Harker, Hartley, & Walsh, 1982; Hultsch & Dixon, 1984; Hultsch, Hertzog, & Dixon, 1984; Meyer & Rice, 1981; Zelinski et al., 1984), and the presence or absence of age differences in text recall appears to depend on multiple interactions between various subject variables (e.g., age, verbal ability, interests) and contextual variables (e.g., organizational structure of text, encoding instructions, retrieval support) (Hultsch & Dixon, 1983; Hultsch et al., 1984; Simon, Dixon, Nowak, & Hultsch, 1982; Meyer & Rice, Chapter 12, this volume). However, despite this empirical ambiguity, one converging pattern of results within this domain of inquiry is that age differences in recall and in the organization of the text are smaller when the text is well organized than when the text is less well organized (Dixon, 1983; Hultsch & Dixon, 1984). That is, age-related differences in text recall are most likely to occur when subjects have to rely on their self-imposed organization of the materials (Craik, 1983; Hultsch, 1969, 1971; Reese, 1976).

In sum, compensation via the quality of inherent task properties has been observed for (1) multimodal and contextually rich encoding environments and (2) bimodal input conditions and when (3) spatial or (4) propositional organization is inherent in the task; that is, for memory tasks in which the contextual support is high because of their embedded properties.

Quantity of task properties

The other type of compensation via inherent task properties occurs as a function of quantitative changes in the task situation. The vast number of studies demonstrating that older adults benefit more than younger adults when task pacing decreases, that is, when the presentation rate slows down and/or the recall interval increases (Adamowicz, 1978; Arenberg, 1965, 1967; Canestrari, 1963; Cohen, 1979; Eisdorfer, Axelrod, & Wilkie, 1963; Kinsbourne, 1973; Kinsbourne & Berryhill, 1972; Treat & Reese, 1976; Troyer, Eisdorfer, Bogdanoff, & Wilkie, 1967), serve as examples of this form of compensation. Also, the finding that older adults, relative to younger adults, benefit more from three as compared with one study trial (Crew, 1977) falls into this category. This type of compensation via inherent task properties should be contrasted with that previously discussed, because here the environmental basis for the elderly's memory compensation is quantitative (simply more time or more trials) rather than qualitative (e.g., a multimodal and rich encoding context, organizational structure).

Representativeness of experimental paradigms

It is arguable that the types of tasks for which compensation via inherent task properties has been observed are more representative of the requirements of remembering in real life than are the tasks for which compensation via experimenter-provided support has been observed. The reasons for this are obvious. For one thing, it is clear that tasks like memory for action events, television recall, and text recall are typical for the world outside the laboratory. Second, although it is, of course, impossible to completely mimic remembering in real life in a laboratory setting, it still can be argued that multimodal and contextually rich encoding situations are rules rather than exceptions in the natural environment (E. J. Gibson, 1969; J. J. Gibson, 1966).

Compensation via cognitive support systems

The third subcategory of compensation may be called compensation via cognitive support systems. However, practically no research has addressed this presumptive basis for compensatory memory behavior among older adults. The concept of cognitive support systems was used by Bransford (1979) to pinpoint the need for resources available to the rememberer from the environment and from previously acquired skills in order to acquire, activate, or retrieve information successfully. The concept, as used by Bransford (1979) in the context of child development and mental retardation, is therefore broad and general. As applied to the present categorization, it seems to embrace all subcategories proposed heretofore. In a recent study on sensory handicaps, Rönnberg and Lyxell (1985) used the concept of cognitive support systems in a more limited sense when discussing linguistic comprehension abilities and visual memory capacity as potential support systems for efficient speech reading.

By the same token, compensation via cognitive support systems as applied to aging and memory is used to embrace certain potential sources of memory compensation in the aged. The idea behind this form of compensation stems from the fact that age differences often are not observed in studies using semantic-memory tasks, although some semantic-memory tasks in which a successful solution is highly dependent on effortful types of processing reveal age differences in favor of younger adults (Byrd, 1984; Craik & Rabinowitz, 1984). For example, it has been demonstrated that young and old adults perform at the same level in linguistic abstraction and integration tasks (Walsh & Baldwin, 1977; Walsh, Baldwin, & Finkle, 1980), Stroop tasks (Howard, Lasaga, & McAndrews, 1980), lexical decision tasks (Bowles & Poon, 1981; Howard, McAndrews, & Lasaga, 1981), proactive inhibition (PI) release tasks (Elias & Hirasuna, 1976; Mistler-Lachman, 1977; Puglisi, 1980), naming latency tasks (Poon & Fozard, 1978; Thomas, Fozard, & Waugh, 1977), and some metamemorial tasks (Bäckman & Karlsson, 1985; Lachman & Lachman, 1980; Lachman, Lachman, & Thronesberry, 1979; Murphy, Sanders, Gabriesheski, & Schmitt, 1981; Perlmutter, 1978). A critical factor for the similarities in patterns of data for younger and older adults in these studies may be that acquisition of new episodic information typically is not required (Cattell, 1971; Horn, 1982; Kinsbourne, 1980; Pribram, 1969).

Thus, it appears that at least some of the cognitive abilities that are critical to successful performance in semantic-memory tasks are relatively well preserved across the adult life span. Now, consider the possibility that an experimental situation would be created in which the interplay between preserved semantic-memory abilities and episodic remembering was the focus of study. Given the observed age deficits in episodic memory tasks, as reviewed by Craik (1977), Kausler (1982), and Salthouse (1982), and given that episodic remembering may draw heavily on semantic activation, it seems likely that the elderly would benefit disproportionally from the support provided by the preserved semantic-memory abilities acting as cognitive support systems.

In a recent study from our own laboratory (Bäckman & Karlsson, 1986), we approached this issue by examining younger and older adults in two types of memory tasks under incidental learning conditions. The first type of task was a common word-recall task, whereas the other was a word-fragment completion or an anagram task (Jacoby, 1982; Zacks, Hasher, Sanft, & Rose, 1983) in which subjects were requested to complete words with missing letters or to solve anagrams, whereafter recall and recognition of these words were compared with recall and recognition of the control words. Note that Zacks and associates (1983) employed similar task comparisons, but failed to find any differences in memory performance between the tasks using only young subjects. However, if older adults are capable of utilizing cognitive support in the form of problem-solving activity during encoding, we might expect that they would show higher memory performance for those tasks involving word-fragment completion or anagram solving than for the control tasks. Data from the Bäckman and Karlsson (1986) study replicated the results of Zacks and associates (1983) for the younger adults, whereas two groups of older adults (old and old-old) exhibited higher levels of recall for the tasks involving problem-solving activity than for the control tasks. Thus, older adults appear to benefit selectively from this added cognitive activity during encoding.

Rehearsal-independent memory

In a series of recent papers, Kausler and colleagues (Kausler, 1983; Kausler & Hakami, 1983a, 1983b; Kausler, Lichty, & Davis, 1985a; Kausler, Lichty, & Freund, 1985b; Kausler, Lichty, Hakami, & Freund, 1986) have argued that memory researchers (including those interested in adult age comparisons) should pay more attention to the types of information that are assumed to be acquired without conscious encoding operations, that is, rehearsal-independent memory. Kausler (1983) pointed out that the majority of researchers have been too inclined to carry on the Ebbinghaus tradition by testing memory for intentionally learned materials and that most of our acquisition of information in daily life proceeds in the absence of encoding strategies.

In the cited papers, younger and older adults' incidental memory and intentional memory for self-performed activities, namely, conversations (Kausler & Hakami, 1983a) and series of laboratory activities (Kausler & Hakami, 1983b), were tested. In addition, younger and older adults were compared on temporal memory for performed activities (Kausler et al., 1985a), frequency judgments of planned activities (Kausler et al., 1985b), and effects of activity duration on memory for performed activities (Kausler et al., 1986). On common finding in this research was that intentionally memorized information was remembered no better than incidentally acquired information, hence allowing for the conclusion that performed activities are encoded in the absence of strategies (or, alternatively, that employment of strategies does not aid activity memory) (Hasher & Zacks, 1979). Further, adult age differences favoring younger adults were generally reported in these studies. However, in agreement with the notion that older adults are capable of compensating for deficits in episodic remembering via experimenter-provided support, greatly reduced age differences in recognition of activities compared with recall of activities were reported (Kausler & Hakami, 1983a).

Of particular interest in the context of compensation via cognitive support systems of older adults is a study by Kausler and Hakami (1983b). These investigators examined younger and older adults' recall of performed activities, presumably varying on the data-driven–conceptually driven continuum (perceptual-motor, verbal learning, generic memory, problem solving). Pronounced age differences in favor of younger adults were found for recall of less demanding activities (e.g., perceptual-motor), whereas the age groups performed at the same level when recall of more demanding activities (problem solving) was requested. According to Kausler and Hakami (1983b), this result may have occurred because cognitively demanding activities yielded more distinctive memory traces than did less demanding activities, which could be of special importance for the elderly. Note that the results of Bäckman and Karlsson (1986) resemble those of Kausler and Hakami in the sense that both studies suggest that problem-solving activity during acquisition may serve as a cognitive support system for older adults' remembering.

A paradox and its solution

The fact that older adults under some conditions appear to benefit disproportionally from investment of more effort during encoding would seem to run counter to the popular notion that age differences in memory should be most pronounced for effortful memory tasks (Hasher & Zacks, 1979). Why is it that investment of more effort during acquisition in the Kausler and Hakami (1983b) and Bäckman and Karlsson (1986) studies greatly reduced age differences in recall, whereas the bulk of research on episodic remembering and aging (Kausler, 1982; Salthouse, 1982) suggests that the more effortful the task (e.g., increased list length, requirements of divided attention, increased task pacing), the more likely it is that one will observe age differences? The paradox might be resolved by means of task analysis: When effort is assumed to increase as a function of increased list length or a division of attention in traditional episodic memory tasks, this does not necessarily guarantee that the elderly subject will engage in more effortful operations; when the task consists of only a learning and a test phase, it is difficult, if not impossible, to determine the degree of effort invested by the subject independent of performance data. On the contrary, such increases in task difficulty might lead to the old subject investing less of his capacity in the task, feeling that "this goes beyond my capacity," because of inaccurate perception of his abilities in relation to the task demands proper (Dixon, Hertzog, & Hultsch, in press; Hultsch, Dixon, & Hertzog, 1985; Murphy et al., 1981; Rabbitt, 1986).

In contrast, with respect to the paradigms employed by Kausler and Hakami (1983b) and Bäckman and Karlsson (1986), the experimenter controls whether or not the subjects engage in the effortful operations proper (e.g., word-fragment completion, anagram solving) due to the actual task demands. That is, subjects are forced to complete the words or to solve the anagrams; if they do not, they fail to fulfill the task requirements. This lack of control versus control over whether or not the subjects really engage in effortful types of processing might be the answer to the question why an increase in effort produces different outcomes in these cases. In other words, the demand for effort is something else than the effort actually expended.

Skilled performance in chess and typing

Although research focusing on older adults' compensation via cognitive support systems is sparse within the area of episodic remembering, there are studies from other fields of cognitive aging that support the validity of this form of compensation. These studies were concerned with the effects of age and skill in chess and typing performance, respectively. In a series of studies, Charness (1981a, 1981b) demonstrated that skilled, aged chess players were capable of performing at the same level as their younger counterparts in a choose-a-move task and in a speeded end-game evaluation task, despite inferior performance on molecular task components (incidental recall and "chunking" of chess positions). In addition, it was found that older players searched more systematically and less redundantly than did younger players in the choose-a-move and speeded end-game evaluation tasks. On the basis of these data, Charness (1981a, 1981b) suggested that elderly chess players may be capable of compensating for encoding and retrieval deficits via more efficient search of the problem space, a more refined move-generation process, and a better global evaluation of chess positions.

In a similar vein, Salthouse (1984) reported that aged typists performed worse than younger typists in a variety of task-relevant molecular components (perceptual-motor efficiency, choice reaction time, rate of tapping, and digit–symbol substitution rate). In contrast, Salthouse (1984) found no age differences in overall typing rates. Salthouse suggested that this discrepancy might be due to older typists compensating for deficits in basic capacities through more extensive overlapping and anticipation of impending characters, that is, via more effective conceptually driven strategies.

The point to be made is that both these sets of data on skilled performance and aging suggest that compensatory behavior by the aged can be achieved through activation of preserved cognitive abilities (or utilization of new cognitive strategies) acting as support systems (in these cases, overlearned skills and heuristics).

Representativeness of experimental paradigms

It seems reasonable to argue that episodic memory tasks (real or hypothetical) for which older adults evince compensation via cognitive support systems are more ecologically valid than are traditional verbal memory tasks. Problem-solving activity (Zacks et al., 1983; Bäckman and Karlsson, 1986) is strongly associated with and embedded in the process of remembering in many real-life situations, as in the case of a person who handles a switchboard or a computer terminal, as well as when an individual orients spatially in the environment, just to mention a few examples. Actually, it is arguable that there are continuous interactions between problem-solving activities and memory operations in the majority of situations of remembering in everyday life. These interactions could either be such that problem-solving activity draws heavily on operations of remembering or be such that problem solving aids the formation of new representations. Clearly, more research focusing on this interplay seems warranted within the area of aging and memory.

To sum up, in the present treatment the concept of compensation is a superordinate concept that embraces many, but not all, empirical findings within the area of aging and memory. The major purpose of entertaining the concept is to provide a conceptual frame of reference for a vast number of empirical studies and to sort single findings into patterns of data by means of the present classification scheme. The superordinate nature of compensation is indicated by the fact that empirical results regarded as supportive of opposed theoretical explanations of age differences in memory (e.g., organization deficit, semantic-encoding deficit, retrieval deficit, effortful-processing deficit, mental-tempo deficit) are incorporated under the category of compensation and sometimes even under the same subcategory. Note that the present framework is largely based on the very same interactions that have been taken as points of departure in determining the locus of the age deficit in episodic remembering (Smith, 1980); here, however, the focus is on older adults' selective utilization of compensatory task conditions (Bäckman, 1985a, 1986).

The tendency among researchers to view the encoding-versus-retrieval-deficit hypothesis or the effortful-processing-versus-mental-tempo-deficit hypothesis as alternative hypotheses for the localization of the age decline in memory has been criticized by other authors (Craik & Rabinowitz, 1984; Eysenck, 1977). The introduction of the present framework may be seen as an alternative to previous attempts along the lines of localization. For one thing, it seems less likely that age differences in memory can be attributed to a single structure or solely to one stage of remembering (Bäckman, 1985a; Craik & Rabinowitz, 1984; Salthouse, 1982). In addition, there is a high degree of dependence within the field of aging and memory between the theoretical conclusion arrived at and the actual experimental manipulation. That is, when organization is manipulated, an organizational deficit in the aged is inferred; when rate of presentation is manipulated, it is concluded that the elderly suffer from a deficit in rate of processing; and so forth. One way of avoiding such paradigm-specific theorizing may be to analyze the area of aging and memory in terms of more general concepts and to pay some attention to the properties of the memory tasks that do or do not reveal age-related differences.

The concept of recoding

The other theoretical concept proposed in this framework is that of recoding: It is suggested that younger adults, relative to older adults, possess superior ability for different recodings of the information to be remembered. The relation between compensation via contextual or cognitive support and recoding is straightforward: The need for contextual or cognitive support in order to remember successfully decreases as a function of an increased ability of recoding (Burke & Light, 1981).

Tulving (1983) proposed the concept of recoding as being an important element in his broad framework of a General Abstracting Processing System (GAPS). In GAPS, "recoding" refers to every process and operation that occurs after the encoding of the original event and that brings about changes in the originally formed engram. Tulving's view (1983) of recoding holds that an interpolated event between the encoding of the original event and retrieval is a critical prerequisite for the occurrence of recoding. Here (Bäckman, 1985b, 1986; Bäckman & Nilsson, 1984, 1985), it is suggested that the concept of recoding might be enlarged to also encompass changes in the initially registered information that take place when various cognitive operations are carried out in order to maximize memory performance: cognitive operations that are not strongly guided by instructions, cues, or embedded task properties. Hence, it is assumed that self-initiated uses of organizational strategies, visual imagery, rehearsal, and verbal mediators, as well as cross-modal transformations of originally encoded events, constitute subordinates under the category of recoding. Utilization of these mental operations is assumed to bring about a richer and more elaborate memory code, as compared with when they are not applied. Accordingly, skilled use of recoding operations is assumed to maximize memory performance (Ericssen, 1985; Miller, 1956).

Younger adults' relative lack of amelioration in tasks wherein contextual or cognitive support is provided (compared with nonguided tasks) may be attributed to their superior ability for recoding. It has been demonstrated that younger adults benefit less than older adults when instructions to use organizational strategies (Hultsch, 1969; 1971), verbal mediators (Hulicka & Grossman, 1967; Hulicka et al., 1967), or imagery instructions (Canestrari, 1968; Thomas & Ruben, 1973; Treat et al., 1978) are provided. Given that the originally stored information in the nonguided control task is recoded, for example, via organization or visual imagery, it follows that the benefit from the experimenter-provided support will be negligible. Similarly, the described interactions between context-bound/context-free tasks and age in spatial recall (Waddell & Rogoff, 1981) and text recall (Hultsch & Dixon, 1984) may be interpreted as indications of younger adults' superior ability for self-initiated recoding operations: When the ability to recode is high, the need for embedded organizational structure in the task is likely to be smaller.

A number of studies on presentation modality and aging have provided further support for this contention. First, it has been demonstrated that younger adults improve less than older adults when provided with a bimodal presentation (visual and auditory), compared with a unimodal presentation (visual or auditory), of the TBR items (Arenberg, 1968; Bäckman, 1986). Second, it has been shown that younger adults benefit less than older adults from an auditory input, compared with a visual input (Bromley, 1958; McGhie, Chapman, & Lawson, 1965). Both these findings suggest that younger adults have superior ability for cross-modal transformations of the originally encoded information: If one has a high level of ability to recode a unimodal (visual) input to an auditory memory code through rehearsal, or to recode a unimodal (auditory) input to a visual memory code through imagery, then a bimodal presentation may not enhance the level of recall; see Bäckman (1986) for further discussion.

The observed interactions between age and visual/auditory presentation (Bromley, 1958; McGhie et al., 1965) point in the same direction: It has been suggested by several researchers on memory and modality (Craik, 1969; Rönnberg & Ohlsson, 1980; Sperling, 1967) that visual information, as opposed to auditory information, requires an extra translation step (i.e., recoding) in order to achieve an optimal level of recall. Hence, when this type of recoding is required, the recall supremacy of younger adults is most pronounced.

The same reasoning can be applied to younger adults' relative lack of improvement in a multimodal and contextually rich memory task, compared with a less rich and unimodal task (Bäckman & Nilsson, 1984), or a less rich and bimodal task (Bäckman, 1985b; Bäckman & Nilsson, 1985). That is, provided that a poorer encoding format (unimodal or bimodal) is recoded to contain multimodal and rich features, then it is not surprising that a multimodal and rich presentation does not elevate recall (Bäckman, 1985b; Bäckman & Nilsson, 1984, 1985).

Notwithstanding the relative lack of empirical studies on aging and cognitive support systems, the same line of reasoning might be applicable to this area as well. Zacks and associates (1983) reported that younger adults did not differ in recall of sentences preceded by a completion task (i.e., a missing word should be filled in) and recall of sentences not preceded by this cognitive activity.

Data from a recent study by Bäckman and Karlsson (1986) confirm this result for younger adults, whereas groups of old and old-old adults in this study recalled more items preceded by completions, as compared with control items. Hence, it might be suggested that younger adults, because of efficient recoding operations (e.g., rehearsal, imagery, organization), benefit less from added problem-solving activity during acquisition (Kausler & Hakami, 1983b).

Also, those data demonstrating that younger adults benefit less than the elderly from retrieval support in the form of copy cues (Craik, 1971; Erber, 1974; Howell, 1972; Schonfield & Robertson, 1966), category cues (Hultsch, 1975; Laurence, 1967), or cues at both encoding and retrieval (Ceci & Tabor, 1981; Smith, 1977) might be partly explained by assuming that younger adults have superior ability for recoding. The train of thought behind this suggestion is that superior ability to recode might make the TBR information more accessible at retrieval (Tulving, 1974; Tulving & Pearlstone, 1966). Provided that the TBR items become more accessible if recoding operations are performed, it seems likely that the need for extraneous cues will be smaller, compared with items not subjected to recoding operations. Such a suggestion is in agreement with numerous studies demonstrating a continuous interaction between the conditions at encoding and retrieval (Fisher & Craik, 1977; Flexer & Tulving, 1978; Mäntylä & Nilsson, 1983; Stein, 1978; Tulving, 1983; Tulving & Thomson, 1973).

Finally, the well-documented finding that younger adults improve less than older adults when task pacing decreases (Arenberg, 1965; Cohen, 1979; Eisdorfer et al., 1963; Kinsbourne, 1973) may be incorporated under the category of recoding. Given that the TBR items are efficiently recoded, it seems reasonable to assume that "more time" would increase the level of recall to a lesser extent than for non-recoded items.

Older adults' need for attentional guidance

Although the literature strongly suggests that the elderly suffer from a recoding deficit, they are nevertheless capable of performing adequate operations of remembering when guided by environmental or cognitive aids, that is, in situations where recoding operations are less necessary or when the actual task demands provoke recoding through contextual guidance. One interesting question is why the elderly do not entertain these operations spontaneously to the same extent as do their younger counterparts.

Categories of compensation: Similarities among tasks

The tasks for which the aforementioned forms of compensation have been demonstrated share basic properties in that they provoke a focusing of attention. In the case of compensation via experimenter-provided support, the experimenter causes the subjects to pay attention to different features of the TBR information (e.g., superordinate categories, verbal mediators) by informing the subjects that these features exist and may be used as mnemonic aids in order to enhance memory performance. In the case of subject-performed tasks or SPTs (an experimental paradigm for which compensation via inherent task properties has been demonstrated), the experimenter presents sentences in imperative form (e.g., lift the spoon, bounce the ball, stand up), and subjects are instructed to perform these acts accordingly (Bäckman & Nilsson, 1984). Thus, the SPT task is goal-directed: Subjects are forced to focus their attention on performing the acts, with the purpose of remembering them as well as possible (Bäckman & Nilsson, 1985). In a similar vein, those memory tasks for which older adults have evinced compensation via cognitive support systems (e.g., memory for solved anagrams, memory for completed word fragments) force the subjects to take an active part in the task at hand; that is, it is impossible not to focus the attention on the performance of the problem-solving activities (Bäckman & Karlsson, 1986).

Thus, in all these tasks for which compensatory memory behavior by older adults has been observed, the task demands strongly focus the subject's attention on critical features of the learning situation. This attentional guidance is essentially lacking in the tasks for which age differences favoring the young are most likely to be observed (standard free-recall or paired-associate learning tasks). In such nonguided memory tasks, subjects are free to perceive, attend to, and memorize the information in any way they prefer.

The primacy of attention

If a certain group of individuals shows a deficit in the ability to focus attention optimally under nonguided conditions, one should, in all likelihood, expect this group to be especially penalized in nonguided memory tasks (Craik & Simon, 1980). Data on aging and attentional functioning do indeed suggest that older adults suffer from attentional deficits. Of particular interest in this context are those studies demonstrating an age-related decline in the ability to focus selectively on those stimulus features promoting high performance, while simultaneously closing out irrelevant information (Layton, 1975; Rabbitt, 1965; Schonfield, 1974). Further, in addition to behavioral data, neuropsychological data and theorizing (Albert & Kaplan, 1980; Kinsbourne, 1980), as well as recent biochemical findings (Mason & Iverson, 1979; Sara, 1985), suggest that the neural mechanisms and transmitters that are critical to attentional functioning decline rapidly in later adulthood.

Provided that the elderly have impairments in the selective aspect of attention, it is not surprising that age differences in memory are most pronounced for tasks lacking attentional support and are attenuated or eliminated for tasks allowing low degrees of attentional freedom (i.e., tasks revealing memory compensation). Thus, the question why the elderly fail to engage in effective recoding operations spontaneously may be answered partly in terms of older adults having an impairment in the selective aspect of attention. Analogously, it may be suggested that attentional guidance (e.g., instructions, hints, a requirement for motor action, or a requirement for problem-solving activity) constitutes a fundamental prerequisite for older adults' utilization of compensatory task conditions.

Alternative sources of adult age differences in recoding

I would like to emphasize that this should not be taken to mean that we should reject alternative suggestions for sources of the elderly's recoding deficit. There are, indeed, such alternative proposals in the literature. Burke and Light (1981) and Craik and Rabinowitz (1984) suggested that the source of the elderly's difficulty is a failure to elaborate the information to be remembered and to integrate it with contextually specific information. Salthouse (1980, 1982) claimed that a deficit in rate of processing hinders the aged from utilizing effective strategies of remembering, whereas Macht and Buschke (1984) identified the elderly's reduced amount of central processing capacity as the origin of their lack of willingness to spontaneously carry out the operations that promote high memory performance. These suggestions may be as adequate as the one proposed here; choosing one over the other may be a matter of preference of level of explanation. Also, as pointed out by several investigators (Bäckman, 1985a; Craik & Rabinowitz, 1984; Hultsch & Pentz, 1980; Labouvie-Vief & Schell, 1982; Poon, 1985), age differences (and similarities) in memory are best understood in terms of complex interactions between various subject variables (e.g., age, cognitive abilities, motivation) and environmental variables (e.g., task structure, materials, contextual support) (Bransford, 1979; Jenkins, 1979).

Compensation via modification of level of arousal and laboratory anxiety

Hitherto, various contextual and cognitive bases for compensatory memory behavior by the aged have been presented. However, there is also evidence to suggest that the elderly are handicapped with respect to a pool of "noncognitive" factors such as laboratory anxiety, self-confidence, and level of arousal, and there are results suggesting that memory performance by older adults may be enhanced as a function of changes in the level of arousal and increased "familiarity with the laboratory situation."

Age differences in decision criteria

Studies on tone detection (Craik, 1966; Potash & Jones, 1977; Rees & Botwinick, 1971) have investigated whether presumptive age differences in the ability to detect pure tones in the presence of noise reflect impaired sensory functions of the aged or age-related differences in decision-making processes. This problem has been approached by analyzing data in terms of the theory of signal detection (Tanner & Swets, 1954). The results from studies by Craik (1966), Potash and Jones (1977), and Rees and Botwinick (1971) suggest that age differences in sensitivity to stimulus characteristics are small or absent, whereas younger and older adults differ markedly with respect to decision criteria, such that the elderly use much more conservative criteria. That is, older adults have to be very certain that a particular judgment is correct before making a response. According to the aforementioned authors, this age difference may be understood in the light of older adults being more cautious and less self-confident in the laboratory situation than younger adults.

Level of arousal and situational anxiety

Eisdorfer and his research group have conducted a series of interesting verbal learning experiments examining the relationship between level of arousal and retention by younger and older adults. Eisdorfer (1968) reported that errors of omission exceeded errors of commission among the aged to a greater extent than for younger adults. He hypothesized that omission errors represent response inhibition caused by heightened situational anxiety. This hypothesis was supported by the finding that slower presentation rates and increased recall intervals markedly reduced the numbers of omissions among the elderly, whereas the numbers of omissions remained at the same level as for fast presentation rates and short recall intervals. The rationale behind this theorizing is that presentation and response rates have been found to be positively correlated with level of arousal (Arenberg, 1965; Troyer et al., 1967); that is, when task pacing increases, so does level of arousal. Powell, Eisdorfer, and Bogdanoff (1964) examined younger and older adults in a serial verbal learning task in which FFA (free fatty acid) levels, GSR (galvanic skin response), and heart rate were used as indicators of arousal. The older adults exhibited higher levels of arousal than the younger adults, and they also performed more poorly. These data suggest that the elderly are more stressed by the laboratory situation than are younger adults, but they do not provide evidence for a cause-and-effect relationship between a high level of arousal and poor performance.

In order to study this relationship, Eisdorfer, Nowlin, and Wilkie (1970) selected a drug (propranolol) that blocks autonomic nervous system (ANS) activity, but has minimal effect on the central nervous system. One group of elderly subjects received this drug, whereas another group of elderly were given placebo injections before a rote verbal learning task was administered. The experimental group showed a lower level of arousal (as indicated by measures of FFA, GSR, and heart rate) than did the placebo group. More interesting with respect to the cause-and-effect relationship mentioned earlier was the finding that those older adults who received propranolol outperformed the control group on the verbal learning task. These data provide support for the contention that task demands associated with ANS activation may contribute to performance decrements in older adults and that memory enhancement among the aged may be accomplished via modification of level of arousal.

Relaxation in memory training

Moreover, there are studies on memory training of older adults that are relevant in this context. First, relaxation training has been found to improve learning in the elderly, both when it is the only ability trained and when it is included as part of a memory-training program; see Yesavage, Lapp, and Sheikh (Chapter 31, this volume) for a review. Clearly, such data suggest that reduction in ANS activity could serve as an effective compensatory trigger for older adults. Second, results showing quite dramatic memory improvement among older adults with traditional training techniques (Langer, Rodin, Beck, Weinman, & Spitzer, 1979; Schmitt, Murphy, & Sanders, 1981) need not necessarily be interpreted as exclusively due to improvement in the trained cognitive abilities: Repeated confrontation with the learning and test demands may increase familiarity with the test situation and the self-confidence of the elderly, while simultaneously reducing anxiety and level of arousal.

The studies described in this section suggest that it might be fruitful to include various noncognitive factors as potential causes of age differences in episodic remembering. In addition, memory compensation in the aged seems to be possible via manipulation of certain factors not traditionally regarded as cognitive in their nature.

Compensation as adaptive behavior by older adults

Impacts of environmental factors on age differences in memory

Some investigators have argued that assumptions about age differences in cognitive processes do not suffice in order to fully come to grips with age-related differences in memory. Looft and Charles (1971) pointed out that a decline in social interactions in later adulthood may be partly responsible for observed age deficits in cognitive functioning. Gardner and Monge (1977) suggested that older adults are unfamiliar with "school-learned skills," and they also argued that such skills often are critical prerequisites for high memory performance in laboratories. Wiersma and Klausmeier (1965) maintained that the infrequency of new learning episodes might be reflected in "forgetting how to learn" in older individuals. Along the same lines, Perlmutter (1980) commented on the dissociation between episodic and semantic memory tasks in the aging and memory literature by stating that "it is tempting to conclude that the grim picture of age deterioration of memory so often portrayed is really an experimental artifact. That is, perhaps older adults are simply unfamiliar with and intimidated by [episodic] laboratory tasks" (p. 346). In a related vein, Hultsch and Pentz (1980) argued that traditional learning and memory tasks, in which verbatim recall of nonrelated verbal materials is requested, are not perceived as meaningful by many older adults. They pointed out that the incidence of older adults' questions about the relevance of such tasks and their refusals to continue participation are striking as compared with those for younger adults. According to Hultsch and Pentz (1980), this age difference may reflect something more basic than uncooperativeness and obstinacy among the elderly: the lack of meaning from the point of view of the aged (Erickson, Poon, & Walsh-Sweeney, 1980).

Bäckman and Nilsson (1984) suggested that rote learning and verbatim recall of verbal materials correspond with the demands of formal education, which might favor memory performance by young subjects who have recently finished school (Cornelius, 1984; Dixon, Kramer, & Baltes, 1985; Popkin, Schaie, & Krauss, 1983; Schaie, 1978). Analogously, the elderly, who left school decades earlier, may be disadvantaged when such memory tasks are employed. In the Bäckman and Nilsson (1984) paper, data were presented suggesting that age differences in memory are minimized when the memory task is more "age-fair" (in this case, memory for real-life action events).

Dixon (1983) briefly reviewed recent studies on text recall in adulthood and arrived at conclusions similar to those of Bäckman and Nilsson (1984). Although the bulk of studies on text recall and aging show age differences favoring the young (Hultsch & Dixon, 1984; Meyer & Rice, 1983), the magnitudes of the differences appear to be smaller than for traditional word-recall or digit-recall tasks. In addition, some investigators have failed to find any age-related differences in text recall (Harker et al., 1982; Meyer & Rice, 1981), whereas others (Byrd, 1981; Zelinski, Gilewski, & Thompson, 1980) have found this lack of age difference to be true for recall of the main ideas of the text.

According to Dixon (1983), this discrepancy between text-recall tasks and traditional episodic memory tasks may partly depend on text recall being a more representative and age-fair task than word or digit recall, because older adults in all likelihood spend much more time reading texts (e.g., books, letters, periodicals) than memorizing words, digits, or nonsense syllables. By the same token, it might be argued that the observed lack of age differences in television recall (Cavanaugh, 1983, 1984), in contrast to the substantial age decline in recall of most verbal materials, could be attributed to television recall being a more representative and age-fair task.

Utilization of compensatory task conditions and self-initiated compensation

Obviously, these types of data underline the need to take into consideration other factors than the cognitive factors when evaluating age differences in episodic remembering. Hitherto, the discussion of memory compensation has emphasized older adults' utilization of compensatory task conditions or "bottom-up compensation," rather than compensation as a function of some selective compensatory process undertaken by the older adult, or "top-down compensation." As noted at the beginning of this chapter, this bias reflects the fact that, with the exception of some studies on chess (Charness, 1981a, 1981b), typing (Salthouse, 1984), and use of memory aids (Cavanaugh et al., 1983; Dixon &

Hultsch, 1983), no empirical research has been devoted to self-initiated compensation by older adults.

In a series of recent papers, Baltes and colleagues (Baltes, in press; Baltes, Dittmann-Kohli, & Dixon, 1984; Baltes & Willis, 1982) have discussed the issue of self-initiated compensatory efforts by older adults under the label "selective optimization with compensation," described as a main principle of adaptation to old age (Baltes, in press). In short, this principle states that aged individuals more and more selectively engage in intellectual activities wherein high performance still is possible through compensatory efforts (e.g., by investing more time and effort and by giving up other activities). According to this view, the term "compensation" refers to a goal-directed adaptive activity of the older person. However, I strongly believe that Baltes's conceptualization and the various categories of compensation proposed in the present chapter are not mutually exclusive. As stated by Baltes and associates (1984), "it [growthlike change] can occur in some (or most) individuals if conditions are supportive, and further that, if it occurs, it is likely to apply to select cognitive skills and expert knowledge systems" (p. 49).

It may be relevant to view compensation as a goal-directed adaptive activity of the older adult, in the light of age differences in memory being reduced or eliminated in more ecologically relevant memory tasks, but pronounced for tasks more linked to the laboratory or tasks drawing heavily on school-learned skills. That is, it might be that the observed recoding deficit of the elderly is partly a function of recoding operations being relatively redundant in the natural environment (Kausler, 1983) because of its multimodal and rich properties (E. J. Gibson, 1969; J. J. Gibson, 1966). Provided that a multimodal and rich encoding context decreases the need for recoding operations in order for successful remembering to occur (Bäckman, 1985b, 1986; Bäckman & Nilsson, 1984, 1985), then the ability to utilize these contextual aids optimally (as opposed to the ability to recode poor and unimodal events) may be a good example of adaptive behavior (or selective optimization with compensation) by older adults.

However, this issue becomes somewhat complicated when we consider the apparent paradox between research findings on everyday use of recoding operations, such as organization and rehearsal (Cavanaugh et al., 1983), and the bulk of laboratory research on spontaneous use of recoding (Kausler, 1982; Poon, 1985; Salthouse, 1982). Whereas Cavanaugh and associates reported greater use of recoding operations among older adults compared with younger adults, the laboratory results clearly indicate just the opposite.

Conceivably, the task demands of everyday remembering differ from those of laboratory remembering, such that the incentive (which may be viewed as a form of contextual support) for recoding the TBR items before driving to the shopping center to carry out a list of chores is somewhat greater than that for recoding a list of words in the laboratory setting: In those everyday memory situations where recoding operations are likely to be applied, the task is typically self-defined, the TBR items are self-generated, the operations are self-initiated, and the overall goal of remembering is self-selected. In contrast, for most laboratory research on recoding, the prefix "self" should be substituted with the prefix "experimenter." That is, the task is experimenter-defined, the TBR items are experimenter-provided, and so forth.

These discrepancies between what triggers recoding in the real world and in the laboratory (i.e., the goals of remembering) may explain the seemingly paradoxical results in the studies mentioned earlier. As noted in the section on recoding, the bulk of research suggests that older adults can perform adequate recoding operations when informed about the utility of such operations. When recoding operations are applied in real life, their utility may be self-evident, and an experimenter who informs about beneficial effects of recoding may be redundant. However, in this context, it should be pointed out that the mere demonstration of greater use of recoding operations by older adults than by younger adults in real life does not imply that the old are superior to (or even equal to) the young with respect to the effectiveness of recoding.

A recent study by Sinnott (1986) lends further support to the notion that environmental factors play important roles in the presence or absence of age differences in memory. Sinnott found that younger and older adults remembered contextually meaningful information that was needed for future action (i.e., prospective items) equally well (Poon & Schaffer, 1982), whereas the young outperformed the old for less meaningful and incidental information (i.e., information that required proficiently applied recoding operations to be remembered well). According to Sinnott (1986), the high performance of older adults for prospective memory items may reflect an adaptive compensatory mechanism; that is, as basic memory capacities decline, the older individual may invest more time and effort in remembering information that has obvious social links (e.g., visits, telephone calls). Thereby, the individual's commitment as a social being may be maintained, but possibly at the expense of further declines in some basic cognitive capacities (Baltes et al., 1984).

The various suggestions for sources of age deficits in memory and this proposed classification scheme for compensatory behaviors by older adults could be supplemented with the foregoing reasoning about interactions among recoding skills, amount/quality of contextual support, and the goal of remembering (Bransford, 1979; Bäckman, 1985a; Jenkins, 1979), which suggests a potential impact of environmental factors on age-related differences in memory (Poon, 1985).

Possible implications for the development of memory-training programs

It is hoped that the present discussion has shown (1) that age-related differences in episodic remembering may have a variety of sources, ranging from changes in the nervous system, causing a "neural speed loss" (Salthouse, 1980), to distal factors such as the impact of schooling, and (2) that it is possible to demonstrate memory compensation by the aged via manipulation of several factors associated with these different sources. That is, age differences in memory are multifactorial, and so is the compensatory memory behavior of older adults.

Multifactorial training

One obvious implication of this approach is that a memory-training program designed for elderly populations should be multifactorial in order to optimize the effects of training. Accordingly, it seems warranted to train several of those abilities in which age impairment has been observed. This may include, for example, training of the selective aspect of attention and relaxation training, as well as training of recoding operations. As noted, even if there is some evidence to suggest that older adults use recoding operations to a greater extent than younger adults in everyday life (Cavanaugh et al., 1983), this does not necessarily imply that they use them as effectively as the young. As is evident from Yesavage's review (Chapter 31, this volume), the multifactorial approach to training has been recognized and applied by some of those working within the field of practical memory enhancement for older adults. As pointed out by Yesavage, however, such multifactorial approaches make it difficult to gain knowledge about the relative effects of the trained factors when evaluating the outcome. One possible solution to this problem, although probably time-consuming, would be to arrange the training conditions such that group 1 receive training in abilities A, B, and C, groups 2, 3, and 4 receive training in abilities A and B, A and C, and B and C, respectively, groups 5, 6, and 7 receive training in A, B, and C, respectively, and group 8 receive no training, but an equivalent amount of general activity. Such a design would permit conclusions about those abilities most likely to benefit from training, as well as provide information about potential additive (or multiplicative) effects of training.

The purpose of training: General or specific?

The foregoing strategy has one clear limitation. The strategy may be feasible if the purpose is to evaluate different components in a training program or to investigate the "disuse" hypothesis of age differences in memory, that is, whether or not older adults perform more poorly than younger adults in memory experiments because of lack of practice. By including a younger control group, it would be possible to examine potential age differences in sensitivity to training of various cognitive abilities. Both these purposes are general in nature and are not primarily concerned with how to improve 69-year-old Mrs. Miller's deteriorating memory abilities.

Variability between different cohorts of older adults

If the main purpose of training is clinical or practical, rather than experimental, I believe there are some additional aspects that should be taken into consideration. First, there are data showing that differences exist between various cohorts of older adults with respect to the ability to utilize recoding operations. Employing a free-recall task, Bäckman and Karlsson (in press) showed that a group of 73-year-olds improved markedly when receiving organizational instructions, compared with standard instructions, whereas a group of 82-year-olds did not benefit from pre-task organizational instructions. Thus, it appears that there are differences between "younger" and "older" elderly adults in the ability to utilize contextual support in the form of organizational instructions. This might have implications for the implementation of memory-training programs, in the sense that a cognitive ability likely to improve as a function of training in one cohort of older adults may not be amenable to training in another cohort.

This state of affairs becomes even more clear when we consider attempts to enhance memory performance in patients with senile dementia. It is well known from the literature that senile patients typically are insensitive to the types of experimental manipulations that their healthy aged counterparts benefit from, such as deep processing (Corkin, 1982; Wilson, Kaszniak, Bacon, Fox, & Kelly, 1982), organizational instructions (Diesfeldt, 1984; Weingartner et al., 1982), word frequency (Wilson, Bacon, Kramer, Fox, & Kaszniak, 1983), and copy cues (Miller, 1975). Given this failure among senile patients to utilize guidance at encoding and retrieval, traditional memory training emphasizing recoding operations may not be time well invested. A more fruitful avenue for severely impaired elderly individuals could be to concentrate the efforts to enhance memory on external contextual support, such as clear signs in the hospital environment, concrete reminders, colored clocks on the wall, and big and legible name tags on the clothes of the nursing staff (Lincoln, Chapter 33, this volume).

Not only the ability to utilize contextual support varies between cohorts of older adults; Faucheux, Lillie, Baulon, Dupuis, and Bourliere (1985) observed quite dissimilar patterns of arousal in 55-year-old and 70-year-old adults, as indicated by autonomic and cortical measures of stress reactions to mental tasks. Such data have clear implications for relaxation training, in that the so-called optimal levels of arousal in relation to cognitive performance may be different for different groups of older adults.

Variability within different cohorts of older adults

Further, there is evidence to suggest that the sources of memory deficits, as well as the ability to utilize various kinds of recoding operations (and, accordingly, the target abilities to be trained), vary even within groups of elderly adults. Great variability within groups of adults has been observed in imagery (Bäckman & Nilsson, 1985; Ernest, 1977; Galton, 1880) and organization (Bäckman & Nilsson, 1984, 1985). Further, in a recent series of field and laboratory experiments, Bäckman and Molander (1986, in press) observed large differences between older individuals within the same age group with respect to optimal level of arousal in a precision sport (miniature golf). Whereas some players performed optimally when they were very aroused, others showed the best performance under intermediate stress conditions, and still others tended to perform at the highest level when they were underaroused.

Hence, the literature suggests not only differences between different cohorts of older adults but also within-group differences regarding cardinal components in most memory-training programs (e.g., imagery, organization, arousal). In other words, what is most effective for enhancing memory in a training context may vary widely from one old adult to another. Consequently, the "group approach" to memory training, although well suited for detecting age-related laws in sensitivity to training, may be inappropriate when the purpose of training is to improve memory in a certain aged individual (Poon, Walsh-Sweeney, & Fozard, 1980; Robertson-Tchabo, 1980; Winograd & Simon, 1980).

Design of memory-training programs

Tentatively, an individualized training program for the older individual could proceed as follows: First, the individual would be screened on a test battery including critical items such as (1) the ability to apply various types of recoding operations effectively (e.g., organization, visual imagery, cross-modal transformations, semantic associations, rehearsal), (2) the ability to utilize external encoding and retrieval cues, (3) measures of arousal, and (4) self-reports of memory problems in everyday life. The purpose of this screening would be to detect the major memory problems of the individual and to determine which abilities are most likely to respond positively to training. Then, on the basis of the individual's test profile, an optimal compound of target abilities to be trained could be obtained in order to achieve maximal enhancement of memory performance. It should be noted that such an approach would be similar to the multimodal therapy advanced by Lazarus (1981) in the context of treatment of depression and other mental disorders (Poon et al., 1980).

Although it has been argued that "group specificity" and "individualization" are key words in the practical training setting, I believe there is still room for some invariance. One cognitive ability that, in all likelihood, ought to be included in a memory-training program for older adults is the ability to focus attention on the critical stimulus features, that is, those features that promote high memory performance. There are two simple reasons for this need. First, the deficit among older adults in this ability is perhaps the most well-documented finding in the literature of cognitive aging; see Kausler (1982) and Salthouse (1982) for reviews. Second, there are few, if any, situations of remembering where successful performance does not rest on appropriate control of attentional allocation.

Preserved abilities

As a final comment, many, if not all, attempts to improve memory performance among older adults by means of training have departed from the idea that the training should be concerned with those abilities for which an age-related decline has been observed. This may be inevitable. However, a complementary approach might be to focus on those abilities reported to be relatively intact in older adults and to use these well-preserved abilities as triggers for new learning, thereby possibly enhancing the effects of training on deteriorated abilities. Two types of preserved abilities that are relevant in this context may be (1) the ability to utilize an active motor manipulation during encoding as an aid for episodic remembering (Bäckman, 1985b; Bäckman & Nilsson, 1984, 1985) and (2) the ability to utilize problem-solving activity during acquisition to improve recall (Bäckman & Karlsson, 1986; Kausler & Hakami, 1983b).

Conclusion

It is emphasized that adult age differences in episodic remembering are multifactorial in character. The cardinal concepts proposed in this chapter in order to come to grips with adult age differences and similarities in memory are compensation and recoding. It is suggested that younger adults perform better than older adults in the majority of standard laboratory memory tasks because of superior ability in various types of recoding operations. Older adults, however, have the ability to compensate for deficits in episodic remembering through utilization of different forms of environmental and cognitive support; that is, the compensatory memory behavior of the aged is multifactorial as well. The concept of recoding is a processing concept in the sense that it embraces all the cognitive operations an individual possesses that, when applied, bring about a richer and more elaborate representation of the original event. In the present context, the concept of compensation, on the other hand, reflects the fact that older adults benefit disproportionally when the task, the materials, or the experimenter guides the learner.

Despite these differences, the two concepts are similar in many ways. Both are superordinate concepts that encompass a vast number of empirical findings previously regarded as "belonging to" opposed theoretical accounts, and neither of the concepts is concerned with the localization of the age deficit in memory. Because of its emphasis on similar implications of, rather than theoretical conflicts between, these accounts, the classification scheme proposed here and the various applications of recoding may help to bring taxonomic order and structure into the field of aging and memory (Tulving, 1985).

Lockhart (1982) discussed general frameworks of the kind proposed here, as compared with precisely quantified and sharply focused theories. He concluded that broad frameworks may serve two important functions: first, to provide a frame of reference within which certain questions can be shown to be meaningful, while others are shown to be less meaningful; second, to guide the future formation of the data base in a certain area of research. It is hoped that this chapter will at least partly serve these two functions. With respect to the former function, the issue whether or not "true" age differences exist in recognition memory, like the debate as to the exact localization of the age deficit in episodic remembering, may prove to be less fruitful; a careful analysis of the actual task demands might resolve such issues.

A more meaningful research question, according to the present framework, would be to ask which are the contextual and cognitive prerequisites for age differences and similarities in cognitive functioning. One offspring of such a question might be an intensified search for compensatory task conditions as well as self-initiated compensatory efforts utilized by older adults in order to optimize cognitive performance.

Regarding the second function, it is hoped that the formulation of two categories – compensation via inherent task properties and compensation via cognitive support systems – may serve as a point of departure for future research: Provided that the types of tasks that illustrate these forms of compensation are more representative of memory situations in everyday life than are traditional episodic memory tasks, and given the increasing interest among memory researchers for ecologically relevant tasks, the introduction of these two categories could perhaps be of some value as a conceptual basis for future investigation.

References

Adamowicz, J. K. (1978). Visual short-term memory, age, and imaging ability. *Perceptual and Motor Skills, 46,* 571–576.

Albert, M. S., & Kaplan, E. (1980). Organic implications of neuropsychological deficits in the elderly. In L. W. Poon, J. L. Fozard, L. S. Cermak, D. Arenberg, & L. W. Thompson (Eds.), *New directions in memory and aging* (pp. 403–432). Hillsdale, NJ: Lawrence Erlbaum.

Arenberg, D. (1965). Anticipation interval and age differences in verbal learning. *Journal of Abnormal Psychology, 70,* 419–425.

Arenberg, D. (1967). Age differences in retroaction. *Journal of Gerontology, 22,* 88–91.

Arenberg, D. (1968). Input modality in short-term retention of old and young adults. *Journal of Gerontology, 23,* 462–465.

Attig, M., & Hasher, L. (1980). The processing of frequency of occurrence information by adults. *Journal of Gerontology, 35,* 66–69.

Bäckman, L. (1985a). Compensation and recoding: A framework for aging and memory research. *Scandinavian Journal of Psychology, 26,* 193–207.

Bäckman, L. (1985b). Further evidence for the lack of adult age differences on free recall of subject-performed tasks: The importance of motor action. *Human Learning, 4,* 79–87.

Bäckman, L. (1986). Adult age differences in cross-modal recoding and mental tempo, and older adults' utilization of compensatory task conditions. *Experimental Aging Research, 12,* 135–140.

Bäckman, L., & Dixon, R. A. (1986). *Compensation and adaptive cognitive functioning in adulthood.* Paper presented at the 2nd European Conference on Developmental Psychology, Rome, Italy.

Bäckman, L., & Karlsson, T. (1985). The relation between level of general knowledge and feeling-of-knowing: An adult age study. *Scandinavian Journal of Psychology, 26,* 249–258.

Bäckman, L., & Karlsson, T. (1986). *Effects of word fragment completion on free recall: A selective improvement of older adults.* Unpublished manuscript.

Bäckman, L., & Karlsson, T. (in press). On the need and utilization of contextual support in episodic remembering in young adults, 73-year-olds, and 82-year-olds. *Scandinavian Journal of Psychology.*

Bäckman, L., Mäntylä, T., & Erngrund, K. (1984). Optimal recall in early and late adulthood. *Scandinavian Journal of Psychology, 25,* 306–314.

Bäckman, L., & Molander, B. (1986). Adult age differences in the ability to cope with situations of high arousal in a precision sport. *Psychology and Aging, 1,* 133–139.

Bäckman, L., & Molander, B. (in press). Effects of adult age and level of skill on the ability to cope with high-stress conditions in a precision sport. *Psychology and Aging,*

Bäckman, L., & Nilsson, L.-G. (1984). Aging effects in free recall: An exception to the rule. *Human Learning, 3,* 53–69.

Bäckman, L., & Nilsson, L.-G. (1985). Prerequisites for lack of age differences in memory performance. *Experimental Aging Research, 11,* 67–73.

Bäckman, L., Nilsson, L.-G., & Chalom, D. (in press). New evidence on the nature of the encoding of action events. *Memory & Cognition,*

Baddeley, A. D., & Wilkins, A. (1984). Taking memory out of the laboratory. In J. E. Harris & P. E. Morris (Eds.), *Everyday memory, actions and absentmindedness* (pp. 1–18). London: Academic Press.

Baltes, P. B. (in press). The aging of intelligence: On the dynamics between growth and decline. *Scientific American.*

Baltes, P. B., Dittmann-Kohli, F., & Dixon, R. A. (1984). New perspectives on the development of intelligence in adulthood: Toward a dual-process conception and a model of selective optimization with compensation. In P. B. Baltes & O. G. Brim, Jr. (Eds.), *Life-span development and behavior* (Vol. 6). New York: Academic Press.

Baltes, P. B., & Willis, S. L. (1982). Plasticity and enhancement of intellectual functioning in old age: Penn State's Adult Development and Enrichment Project (ADEPT). In F. I. M. Craik & S. E. Trehub (Eds.), *Aging and cognitive processes.* New York: Plenum Press.

Bowles, N. L., & Poon, L. W. (1981). The effect of age on speed of lexical access. *Experimental Aging Research, 7,* 417–425.

Bransford, J. D. (1979). *Human cognition. Learning, understanding, and remembering.* Belmont, CA: Wadsworth.

Bromley, D. B. (1958). Some effects of age on short-term learning and memory. *Journal of Gerontology, 13,* 398–406.

Burke, D. M., & Light, L. L. (1981). Memory and aging: The role of retrieval processes. *Psychological Bulletin, 90,* 513–546.

Butters, N. (1980). Potential contributions of neuropsychology to our understanding of the memory capacities of the elderly. In L. W. Poon, J. L. Fozard, L. S. Cermak, D. Arenberg, & L. W. Thompson, (Eds.), *New directions in memory and aging.* Hillsdale, NJ: Lawrence Erlbaum.

Byrd, M. (1981). *Age differences in memory for prose passages.* Unpublished Ph.D. thesis, University of Toronto.

Byrd, M. (1984). Age differences in the retrieval of information from semantic memory. *Experimental Aging Research, 10,* 29–33.

Canestrari, R. E. (1963). Paced and self-paced learning in young and elderly adults. *Journal of Gerontology, 18,* 165–168.

Canestrari, R. E. (1968). Age changes in acquisition. In G. Talland (Ed.), *Human aging and behavior* (pp. 169–188). New York: Academic Press.

Cattell, R. B. (1971). *Abilities: Their structure, growth, and action.* Boston: Houghton Mifflin.

Cavanaugh, J. C. (1983). Comprehension and retention of television programs by 20- and 60-year-olds. *Journal of Gerontology, 38,* 190–196.

Cavanaugh, J. C. (1984). Effects of presentation format on adults' retention of television programs. *Experimental Aging Research, 10,* 51–53.

Cavanaugh, J. C., Grady, J. G., & Perlmutter, M. P. (1983). Forgetting and use of memory aids in 20- and 70-year-olds' everyday life. *International Journal of Aging and Human Development, 17,* 113–122.

Ceci, S. J., & Tabor, L. (1981). Flexibility and memory: Are the elderly really less flexible? *Experimental Aging Research, 7,* 147–158.

Cermak, L. S. (1982). Future challenges. In L. S. Cermak (Ed.), *Human memory and amnesia.* Hillsdale, NJ: Lawrence Erlbaum.

Charness, N. (1981a). Aging and skilled problem solving. *Journal of Experimental Psychology: General, 110,* 21–38.

Charness, N. (1981b). Search in chess: Age and skill differences. *Journal of Experimental Psychology: Human Perception and Performance, 7,* 467–476.

Cohen, G. (1979). Language comprehension in old age. *Cognitive Psychology, 11,* 412–429.

Cohen, R. L. (1981). On the generality of some memory laws. *Scandinavian Journal of Psychology, 22,* 267–282.

Corkin, S. (1982). Some relationships between global amnesias and the impairments in Alzheimer's disease. In S. Corkin, K. L. Davis, J. H. Growdon, E. Usdin, & R. J. Wurtman (Eds.), *Alzheimer's disease: A report of progress in research.* New York: Raven Press.

Cornelius, S. W. (1984). Classic pattern of intellectual aging: Test familiarity, difficulty, and performance. *Journal of Gerontology, 39,* 201–206.

Craik, F. I. M. (1966). The effects of aging on the detection of faint auditory signals. In *Proceedings of the 7th International Congress of Gerontology* (Vol. 6). Vienna.

Craik, F. I. M. (1969). Modality effects in short-term storage. *Journal of Verbal Learning and Verbal Behavior, 8,* 658–664.

Craik, F. I. M. (1971). Age differences in recognition memory. *Quarterly Journal of Experimental Psychology, 23,* 316–319.

Craik, F. I. M. (1977). Age differences in human memory. In J. E. Birren & K. W. Schaie (Eds.), *Handbook of the psychology of aging* (pp. 384–420). New York: Van Nostrand.

Craik, F. I. M. (1983). On the transfer of information from temporary to permanent memory. *Philosophical Transactions of the Royal Society of London, 302,* 341–359.

Craik, F. I. M. (1985). Paradigms in human memory research. In L.-G. Nilsson & T. Archer (Eds.), *Perspectives on learning and memory.* Hillsdale, NJ: Lawrence Erlbaum.

Craik, F. I. M., & Rabinowitz, J. C. (1984). Age differences in the acquisition and use of verbal information. In H. Bouma & D. G. Bouwhuis (Eds.), *Attention and performance* (Vol. 10). Hillsdale, NJ: Lawrence Erlbaum.

Craik, F. I. M., & Simon, E. (1980). Age differences in memory: The roles of attention and depth of processing. In L. W. Poon, J. L. Fozard, L. S. Cermak, D. Arenberg, & L. W. Thompson (Eds.), *New directions in memory and aging* (pp. 95–112). Hillsdale, NJ: Lawrence Erlbaum.

Crew, F. F. (1977). *Age differences in retention after varying study and test trials.* Unpublished master's thesis, Georgia Institute of Technology.

Diesfeldt, H. F. A. (1984). The importance of encoding instructions and retrieval cues in the assessment of memory in senile dementia. *Archives of Gerontology and Geriatrics, 3,* 51–57.

Dixon, R. A. (1983). How to avoid aging effects in free recall. *Scandinavian Journal of Psychology, 24,* 335–337.

Dixon, R. A., & Bäckman, L. (1986). *The functional role of compensation in memory development in adulthood.* Paper presented at the 94th annual meeting of the American Psychological Association, Washington, DC.

Dixon, R. A., Hertzog, C., & Hultsch, D. F. (in press). The multiple relationships among Metamemory in Adulthood (MIA) scales and cognitive abilities in adulthood. *Human Learning.*

Dixon, R. A., & Hultsch, C. (1983). Structure and development of metamemory in adulthood. *Journal of Gerontology, 38,* 682–688.

Dixon, R. A., Kramer, D. A., & Baltes, P. B. (1985). Intelligence: A life-span development perspective. In B. B. Wolman (Ed.), *Handbook of intelligence: Theories, measurements, and applications.* New York: Wiley.

Eisdorfer, C. (1968). Arousal and performance: Experiments in verbal learning and a tentative theory. In G. Talland (Ed.), *Human aging and behavior* (pp. 189–216). New York: Academic Press.

Eisdorfer, C., Axelrod, S., & Wilkie, F. L. (1963). Stimulus exposure time as a factor in serial learning in an aged sample. *Journal of Abnormal and Social Psychology, 67,* 594–600.

Eisdorfer, C., Nowlin, J., & Wilkie, F. (1970). Improvement of learning in the aged by modification of autonomic nervous system activity. *Science, 170,* 1327–1329.

Elias, C. S., & Hirasuna, N. (1976). Age and semantic and phonological encoding. *Developmental Psychology, 12,* 497–503.

Ellis, H. C., Thomas, R. L., & Rodriguez, I. A. (1984). Emotional mood states and memory: Elaborative encoding, semantic processing, and cognitive effort. *Journal of Experimental Psychology: Learning, Memory, and Cognition, 10,* 470–482.

Erber, J. T. (1974). Age differences in recognition memory. *Journal of Gerontology, 29,* 177–181.

Erber, J. T., Herman, T. G., & Botwinick, J. (1980). Age differences in memory as a function of depth of processing. *Experimental Aging Research, 6,* 341–348.

Erickson, R. C., Poon, L. W., & Walsh-Sweeney, L. W. (1980). Clinical memory testing of the elderly. In L. W. Poon, J. L. Fozard, L. S. Cermak, D. Arenberg, & L. W. Thompson (Eds.), *New directions in memory and aging* (pp. 379–402). Hillsdale, NJ: Lawrence Erlbaum.

Ericsson, K. A. (1985). Memory skill. *Canadian Journal of Psychology, 39,* 188–231.

Ernest, C. (1977). Mental imagery and cognition: A critical review. *Journal of Mental Imagery, 1,* 181–216.

Eysenck, M. W. (1974). Age differences in incidental learning. *Developmental Psychology, 10,* 936–941.

Eysenck, M. W. (1977). *Human memory: Theory, research and individual differences.* Oxford: Pergamon Press.

Faucheux, B. A., Lillie, F., Baulon, A., Dupuis, C., & Bourliere, F. (1985). Adjustment to the stress induced by mental tasks, in middle-aged and elderly men. In *Proceedings of the 13th International Congress of Gerontology* (p. 132, abstract).

Fisher, R. P., & Craik, F. I. M. (1977). The interaction between encoding and retrieval operations in cued recall. *Journal of Experimental Psychology: Human Learning and Memory, 3,* 701–711.

Flexer, A. J., & Tulving, E. (1978). Retrieval independence in recognition and recall. *Psychological Review, 85,* 153–172.

Galton, F. (1880). Statistics of mental imagery. *Mind, 5,* 301–318.

Gardner, E. G., & Monge, R. H. (1977). Adult age differences in cognitive abilities and educational background. *Experimental Aging Research, 3,* 337–383.

Giambra, L. M., & Arenberg, D. (1980). Problem solving, concept learning, and aging. In L. W. Poon (Ed.), *Aging in the 1980's* (pp. 253–259). Washington, DC: American Psychological Association.

Gibson, E. J. (1969). *Principles of perceptual learning and development.* New York: Appleton-Century-Crofts.

Gibson, J. J. (1966). *The senses considered as perceptual systems.* Boston: Houghton Mifflin.

Harker, J. O., Hartley, J. T., & Walsh, D. A. (1982). Understanding discourse – a life span approach. In B. A. Huston (Ed.), *Advances in reading/language research* (Vol. 1). Greenwich, CT: JAI Press.

Harwood, E., & Naylor, G. F. K. (1969). Recall and recognition in elderly and young subjects. *Australian Journal of Psychology, 21,* 251–257.

Hasher, L., & Zacks, R. T. (1979). Automatic and effortful processes in memory. *Journal of Experimental Psychology: General, 108,* 356–388.

Hirst, W. (1982). The amnesic syndrome: Descriptions and explanations. *Psychological Bulletin, 91,* 435–460.

Horn, J. L. (1982). The aging of human abilities. In B. B. Wolman (Ed.), *Handbook of developmental psychology.* Englewood Cliffs, NJ: Prentice-Hall.

Howard, D. V., Lasaga, M. I., & McAndrews, M. P. (1980). Semantic activation during memory encoding across the adult life span. *Journal of Gerontology, 35,* 884–890.

Howard, D. V., McAndrews, M. P., & Lasaga, M. I. (1981). Semantic priming of lexical decisions in young and old adults. *Journal of Gerontology, 36,* 707–714.

Howell, S. C. (1972). Familiarity and complexity in perceptual recognition. *Journal of Gerontology, 27,* 364–371.

Hulicka, I. M., & Grossman, J. L. (1967). Age group comparisons for the use of mediators in paired-associate learning. *Journal of Gerontology, 22,* 46–51.

Hulicka, I. M., Sterns, H., & Grossman, J. L. (1967). Age group comparisons of paired-associate learning as a function of paced and selfpaced association and response times. *Journal of Gerontology, 22,* 274–280.

Hultsch, D. F. (1969). Adult age differences in the organization of free recall. *Developmental Psychology, 1,* 673–678.

Hultsch, D. F. (1971). Adult age differences in free classification and free recall. *Developmental Psychology, 4,* 338–342.

Hultsch, D. F. (1975). Adult age differences in retrieval: Trace-dependent and cue-dependent forgetting. *Developmental Psychology, 11,* 197–201.

Hultsch, D. F., & Dixon, R. A. (1983). The role of pre-experimental knowledge in text processing in adulthood. *Experimental Aging Research, 9,* 17–22.

Hultsch, D. F., & Dixon, R. A. (1984). Text processing in adulthood. In P. B. Baltes & O. G. Brim, Jr. (Eds.), *Life-span development and behavior* (Vol. 6). New York: Academic Press.

Hultsch, D. F., Dixon, R. A., & Hertzog, C. (1985). Memory perceptions and memory performance in adulthood and aging. *Canadian Journal on Aging, 4,* 179–187.

Hultsch, D. F., Hertzog, C., & Dixon, R. A. (1984). Text recall in adulthood: The role of intellectual abilities. *Developmental Psychology, 20,* 1193–1209.

Hultsch, D. F., & Pentz, C. E. (1980). Encoding, storage, and retrieval in adult memory: The role of model assumptions. In L. W. Poon, J. L. Fozard, L. S. Cermak, D. Arenberg, & L. W. Thompson (Eds.), *New directions in memory and aging* (pp. 73–94). Hillsdale, NJ: Lawrence Erlbaum.

Jacoby, L. L. (1982). Knowing and remembering: Some parallels in the behavior of Korsakoff patients and normals. In L. S. Cermak (Ed.), *Human memory and amnesia.* Hillsdale, NJ: Lawrence Erlbaum.

Jenkins, J. J. (1979). Four points to remember: A tetrahedral model of memory experiments. In L. S. Cermak & F. I. M. Craik (Eds.), *Levels of processing in human memory.* Hillsdale, NJ: Lawrence Erlbaum.

Karlsson, T., & Bäckman, L. (1985). Evidence for disruptive effects of alcohol on the transfer of information from temporary to permanent memory. In *Proceedings and Abstracts of the Annual Meeting of the Eastern Psychological Association* (Vol. 56, p. 35, abstract).

Kausler, D. H. (1982). *Experimental psychology and human aging.* New York: Wiley.

Kausler, D. H. (1983). *Episodic memory and human aging.* Paper presented at the 91st annual meeting of the American Psychological Association, Anaheim, CA.

Kausler, D. H., & Hakami, M. K. (1983a). Memory for topics of conversation: Adult age differences and intentionality. *Experimental Aging Research, 9,* 153–158.

Kausler, D. H., & Hakami, M. K. (1983b). Memory for activities: Adult age differences and intentionality. *Developmental Psychology, 19,* 889–894.

Kausler, D. H., Lichty, W., & Davis, R. T. (1985a). Temporal memory for performed activities: Intentionality and adult age differences. *Developmental Psychology, 21,* 1132–1138.

Kausler, D. H., Lichty, W., & Freund, J. S. (1985b). Adult age differences in recognition memory and frequency judgments for planned activities. *Developmental Psychology, 21,* 647–654.

Kausler, D. H., Lichty, W., Hakami, M. K., & Freund, J. S. (1986). Activity duration and adult age differences in memory for activity performance. *Psychology and Aging, 1,* 80–81.

Kinsbourne, M. (1973). Age effects on letter span related to rate and sequential dependency. *Journal of Gerontology, 28,* 317–319.

Kinsbourne, M. (1980). Attentional dysfunctions and the elderly: Theoretical models and research perspectives. In L. W. Poon, J. L. Fozard, L. S. Cermak, D. Arenberg, & L. W. Thompson (Eds.), *New directions in memory and aging* (pp. 113–130). Hillsdale, NJ: Lawrence Erlbaum.

Kinsbourne, M., & Berryhill, J. L. (1972). The nature of the interaction between pacing and the age decrement in learning. *Journal of Gerontology, 27,* 471–477.

Kinsbourne, M., & Wood, F. (1982). Theoretical considerations regarding the episodic–semantic memory distinction. In L. S. Cermak (Ed.), *Human memory and amnesia.* Hillsdale, NJ: Lawrence Erlbaum.

Labouvie-Vief, G., & Schell, D. A. (1982). Learning and memory in late life. In B. Wellman (Ed.), *Handbook of developmental psychology.* Englewood Cliffs, NJ: Prentice-Hall.

Lachman, J. L., & Lachman, R. (1980). Age and the actualization of world knowledge. In L. W. Poon, J. L. Fozard, L. S. Cermak, D. Arenberg, & L. W. Thompson (Eds.), *New directions in memory and aging* (pp. 313–344). Hillsdale, NJ: Lawrence Erlbaum.

Lachman, J. L., Lachman, R., & Thronesberry, C. (1979). Metamemory through the adult life span. *Developmental Psychology, 15,* 543–551.

Langer, E. J., Rodin, J., Beck, P., Weinman, C., & Spitzer, L. (1979). Environmental determinants of memory improvement in late adulthood. *Journal of Personality and Social Psychology, 37,* 2002–2013.

Laurence, M. W. (1967). Memory loss with age: A test of two strategies for its retardation. *Psychonomic Science, 9,* 209–210.

Layton, B. (1975). Perceptual noise and aging. *Psychological Bulletin, 82,* 875–883.

Lazarus, A. A. (1981). *The practice of multi-modal therapy.* New York: McGraw-Hill.

Light, L. L., & Anderson, P. A. (1983). Memory for scripts in young and older adults. *Memory & Cognition, 11,* 435–444.

Lockhart, R. S. (1982). Introduction. *Canadian Journal of Psychology, 36,* 125–129.

Looft, W. R., & Charles, D. C. (1971). Egocentrism and social interaction in young and old adults. *International Journal of Aging and Human Development, 2,* 21–28.

McGhie, A., Chapman, J., & Lawson, J. S. (1965). Changes in immediate memory with age. *British Journal of Psychology, 56,* 69–75.

Macht, M. L., & Buschke, H. (1984). Speed of recall in aging. *Journal of Gerontology, 39,* 439–443.

Mäntylä, T., & Nilsson, L.-G. (1983). Are my cues better than yours? Uniqueness and reconstruction as prerequisites for optimal recall of verbal materials. *Scandinavian Journal of Psychology, 24,* 303–312.

Mason, S. E. (1979). Effects of orienting tasks on the recall and recognition performance of subjects differing in age. *Developmental Psychology, 15,* 467–469.

Mason, S. T., & Iverson, S. D. (1979). Theories of the dorsal bundle extinction effect. *Brain Research Reviews, 1,* 107–137.

Meyer, B. J. F., & Rice, G. E. (1981). Information recalled from prose by young, middle, and old adult readers. *Experimental Aging Research, 7,* 253–268.

Meyer, B. J. F., & Rice, G. E. (1983). Learning and memory for text across the adult life span. In J. Fine & R. O. Freedle (Eds.), *Developmental studies in discourse.* Norwood, NJ: Ablex.

Miller, E. (1975). Impaired recall and the memory disturbance in presenile dementia. *British Journal of Social and Clinical Psychology, 14,* 73–79.

Miller, E. (1977). *Abnormal aging.* New York: Wiley.

Miller, G. A. (1956). The magical number seven plus or minus two. *Psychological Review, 63,* 81–97.

Mistler-Lachman, J. L. (1977). Spontaneous shift in encoding dimensions among elderly subjects. *Journal of Gerontology, 32,* 68–72.

Moscovitch, M. (1982). A neuropsychological approach to perception and memory in normal and pathological aging. In F. I. M. Craik & S. E. Trehub (Eds.), *Aging and cognitive processes.* New York: Plenum Press.

Moscovitch, M. (1984). The sufficient conditions for demonstrating preserved memory in amnesia: A task analysis. In N. Butters & L. R. Squire (Eds.), *The neuropsychology of memory.* New York: Guilford Press.

Murphy, M. D., Sanders, R. E., Gabriesheski, A. S., & Schmitt, F. A. (1981). Metamemory in the aged. *Journal of Gerontology, 36,* 185–193.

Neisser, U. (1982). Memory: What are the important questions? In U. Neisser (Ed.), *Memory observed. Remembering in natural contexts* (pp. 3–20). San Francisco: W. H. Freeman.

Nilsson, L.-G. (1979). Functions of memory. In L.-G. Nilsson (Ed.), *Perspectives on memory research.* Hillsdale, NJ: Lawrence Erlbaum.

Nilsson, L.-G. (1984). New functionalism in memory research. In K. Lagerspetz & P. Niemi (Eds.), *Psychology in the 1990's.* Amsterdam: North Holland.

Perlmutter, M. (1978). What is memory aging the aging of? *Developmental Psychology, 14,* 330–345.

Perlmutter, M. (1979). Age differences in adults' free recall, cued recall, and recognition. *Journal of Gerontology, 34,* 533–539.

Perlmutter, M. (1980). An apparent paradox about memory aging. In L. W. Poon, J. L. Fozard, L. S. Cermak, D. Arenberg, & L. W. Thompson (Eds.), *New directions in memory and aging* (pp. 345–354). Hillsdale, NJ: Lawrence Erlbaum.

Poon, L. W. (1985). Differences in human memory with aging: Nature, causes, and clinical implications. In J. E. Birren & K. W. Schaie (Eds.), *Handbook of the psychology of aging* (2nd ed., pp. 427–462). New York: Van Nostrand Reinhold.

Poon, L. W., & Fozard, J. L. (1978). Speed of retrieval from long-term memory in relation to age, familiarity, and datedness of information. *Journal of Gerontology, 33,* 711–717.

Poon, L. W., & Schaffer, G. (1982). *Prospective memory in young and elderly adults.* Paper presented at the 90th annual meeting of the American Psychological Association, Washington, DC.

Poon, L. W., Walsh-Sweeney, L., & Fozard, J. L. (1980). Memory skill training for the elderly: Salient issues on the use of imagery mnemonics. In L. W. Poon, J. L. Fozard, L. S. Cermak, D. Arenberg, & L. W. Thompson (Eds.), *New directions in memory and aging* (pp. 461–484). Hillsdale, NJ: Lawrence Erlbaum.

Popkin, S. J., Schaie, K. W., & Krauss, I. K. (1983). Age-fair assessment of psychometric intelligence. *Educational Gerontology, 9,* 47–55.

Potash, M., & Jones, B. (1977). Aging and decision criteria for the detection of tones in noise. *Journal of Gerontology, 32,* 436–440.

Powell, A. H., Eisdorfer, C., & Bogdanoff, M. D. (1964). Physiologic response patterns observed in a learning task. *Archives of General Psychiatry, 10,* 192–195.

Pribram, K. H. (1969). The amnestic syndromes: Disturbances in coding. In G. A. Talland & N. C. Waush (Eds.), *The pathology of memory* (pp. 127–160). New York: Academic Press.

Puglisi, J. T. (1980). Semantic encoding in older adults as evidence by release from proactive inhibition. *Journal of Gerontology, 35,* 743–745.

Rabbitt, P. (1965). An age-decrement in the ability to ignore irrelevant information. *Journal of Gerontology, 20,* 233–238.

Rabbitt, P. (1986). *Actual performance vs. self-assessment of competence in aging individuals: A need for corrective actions.* Paper presented at the 2nd European Conference on Developmental Psychology, Rome.

Rabinowitz, J. C. (1984). Aging and recognition failure. *Journal of Gerontology, 39,* 65–71.

Rabinowitz, J. C., & Craik, F. I. M. (1986). Prior retrieval effects in young and old adults. *Journal of Gerontology, 41,* 368–375.

Rees, J. N., & Botwinick, J. (1971). Detection and decision factors in auditory behavior of the elderly. *Journal of Gerontology, 26,* 133–136.

Reese, H. W. (1976). Models of memory development. *Human Development, 19,* 219–303.

Robertson-Tchabo, E. A. (1980). Cognitive-skill training for the elderly: Why should "old dogs" acquire new tricks? In L. W. Poon, J. L. Fozard, L. S. Cermak, D. Arenberg, & L. W. Thompson (Eds.), *New directions in memory and aging* (pp. 511–518). Hillsdale, NJ: Lawrence Erlbaum.

Rohwer, W. D., Jr. (1976). An introduction to research on individual and developmental differences in learning. In W. K. Estes (Ed.), *Handbook of learning and cognitive processes* (Vol. 3). Hillsdale, NJ: Lawrence Erlbaum.

Rönnberg, J., & Bäckman, L. (1984). Attributes of memory tasks. *Umea Psychological Reports* (No. 179).

Rönnberg, J., & Lyxell, B. (1985). On the identification of support systems for speechreading. *Umea Psychological Reports* (No. 183).

Rönnberg, J., & Ohlsson, K. (1980). Channel capacity and processing of modality specific information. *Acta Psychologica, 44,* 235–267.

Rönnberg, J., & Ohlsson, K. (1985). The challenge of integrating animal learning and human memory research. In L.-G. Nilsson & T. Archer (Eds.), *Perspectives on learning and memory.* Hillsdale, NJ: Lawrence Erlbaum.

Salthouse, T. A. (1980). Age and memory: Strategies for localizing the loss. In L. W. Poon, J. L. Fozard, L. S. Cermak, D. Arenberg, & L. W. Thompson (Eds.), *New directions in memory and aging* (pp. 47–66). Hillsdale, NJ: Lawrence Erlbaum.

Salthouse, T. A. (1982). *Adult cognition.* New York: Springer.

Salthouse, T. A. (1984). Effects of age and skill in typing. *Journal of Experimental Psychology: General, 113,* 345–371.

Salthouse, T. A. (in press). Age, experience and compensation. In C. Schooler & K. W. Schaie (Eds.), *Intellectual functioning, social structure, and aging.* Norwood, NJ: Ablex.

Sara, S. J. (1985). Noradrenergic modulation of selective attention: Its role in memory retrieval. *Annals of the New York Academy of Sciences, 444,* 178–193.

Schaie, K. W. (1978). External validity in the assessment of intellectual development in adulthood. *Journal of Gerontology, 33,* 695–701.

Schmitt, F. A., Murphy, M. D., & Sanders, R. E. (1981). Training of older adults' free recall rehearsal strategies. *Journal of Gerontology, 36,* 329–337.

Schonfield, D. (1974). Translations in gerontology – from lab to life: Utilizing information. *American Psychologist, 29,* 796–801.

Schonfield, D., & Robertson, E. A. (1966). Memory storage and aging. *Canadian Journal of Psychology, 20,* 228–236.

Shaps, L. P., & Nilsson, L.-G. (1980). Encoding and retrieval operations in relation to age. *Developmental Psychology, 16,* 636–643.

Simon, E. (1979). Depth and elaboration of processing in relation to age. *Journal of Experimental Psychology: Human Learning and Memory, 5,* 115–124.

Simon, E. W., Dixon, R. A., Nowak, C. A., & Hultsch, D. F. (1982). Orienting task effects on text recall in adulthood. *Journal of Gerontology, 37,* 575–580.

Sinnott, J. D. (1986). Prospective/intentional and incidental everyday memory: Effects of age and passage of time. *Psychology and Aging, 1,* 110–116.

Smith, A. D. (1977). Adult age differences in cued recall. *Developmental Psychology, 13,* 326–331.

Smith, A. D. (1980). Age differences in encoding, storage, and retrieval. In L. W. Poon, J. L. Fozard, L. S. Cermak, D. Arenberg, & L. W. Thompson (Eds.), *New directions in memory and aging* (pp. 23–46). Hillsdale, NJ: Lawrence Erlbaum.

Smith, A. D., & Winograd, E. (1978). Adult age differences in remembering faces. *Developmental Psychology, 14,* 443–444.

Sperling, G. (1967). Successive approximations to a model for short-term memory. *Acta Psychologica, 27,* 285–292.

Squire, L. (1982). The neuropsychology of human memory. *Annual Review of Neuroscience, 5,* 241–273.

Stein, B. S. (1978). Depth of processing re-examined. The effects of precision of encoding and test appropriateness. *Journal of Verbal Learning and Verbal Behavior, 17,* 165–174.

Tanner, W. P., & Swets, J. A. (1954). A decision-making theory of visual detection. *Psychological Review, 61,* 401–409.

Thomas, J. C., Fozard, J. L., & Waugh, N. C. (1977). Age-related differences in naming latency. *American Journal of Psychology, 90,* 499–509.

Thomas, J. C., & Ruben, H. (1973). *Age and mnemonic techniques in paired associate learning.* Paper presented at a meeting of the Gerontological Society, Miami.

Treat, N. J., Poon, L. W., & Fozard, J. L. (1978). From clinical and research findings on memory to intervention programs. *Experimental Aging Research, 4,* 235–253.

Treat, N. J., & Reese, H. W. (1976). Age, pacing and imagery in paired associate learning. *Developmental Psychology, 12,* 119–124.

Troyer, W. G., Eisdorfer, C., Bogdanoff, M. D., & Wilkie, F. L. (1967). Experimental stress and learning in the aged. *Journal of Abnormal Psychology, 72,* 65–70.

Tulving, E. (1974). Cue-dependent forgetting. *American Scientist, 62,* 74–82.

Tulving, E. (1983). *Elements of episodic memory.* Oxford University Press.

Tulving, E. (1985). On the classification problem in learning and memory. In L.-G. Nilsson & T. Archer (Eds.), *Perspectives on learning and memory.* Hillsdale, NJ: Lawrence Erlbaum.

Tulving, E., & Pearlstone, Z. (1966). Availability versus accessibility of information in memory for words. *Journal of Verbal Learning and Verbal Behavior, 5,* 381–391.

Tulving E., & Thomson, D. M. (1973). Encoding specificity and retrieval processes in episodic memory. *Psychological Review, 80,* 352–373.

Waddell, K. J., & Rogoff, B. (1981). Effect of contextual organization on spatial memory of middle-aged and older women. *Developmental Psychology, 17,* 878–885.

Walsh, D. A., & Baldwin, M. (1977). Age differences in integrated semantic memory. *Developmental Psychology, 13,* 509–514.

Walsh, D. A., Baldwin, M., & Finkle, T. J. (1980). Age differences in integrated semantic memory for abstract sentences. *Experimental Aging Research, 6,* 431–444.

Waugh, N. C., & Barr, R. A. (1980). Memory and mental tempo. In L. W. Poon, J. L. Fozard, L. S. Cermak, D. Arenberg, & L. W. Thompson (Eds.), *New directions in memory and aging* (pp. 251–260). Hillsdale, NJ: Lawrence Erlbaum.

Weingartner, H., Kaye, W., Smallberg, S., Cohen, R., Ebert, M. H., Gillin, J. C., & Gold, P. (1982). Determinants of memory failures in dementia. In S. Corkin, K. L. Davis, J. H. Growdon, E. Usdin, & R. J. Wurtman (Eds.), *Alzheimer's disease: A report of progress in research.* New York: Raven Press.

Wiersma, W., & Klausmeier, H. J. (1965). The effect of age upon speed of concept attainment. *Journal of Gerontology, 20,* 398–400.

Wilson, R. S., Bacon, L. D., Kramer, R. L., Fox, J. H., & Kaszniak, A. W. (1983). Word frequency effect and recognition memory in dementia of the Alzheimer type. *Journal of Clinical Neuropsychology, 5,* 97–104.

Wilson, R. S., Kaszniak, A. W., Bacon, L. D., Fox, J. H., & Kelly, H. P. (1982). Facial recognition in dementia. *Cortex, 18,* 329–336.

Wimer, R. E., & Wigdor, B. T. (1958). Age differences in retention of learning. *Journal of Gerontology, 13,* 291–295.

Winocur, G. (1982). The amnesic syndrome: A deficit in cue utilization. In L. S. Cermak (Ed.), *Human memory and amnesia.* Hillsdale, NJ: Lawrence Erlbaum.

Winograd, E., & Simon, E. W. (1980). Visual memory and imagery in the aged. In L. W. Poon, J. L. Fozard, L. S. Cermak, D. Arenberg, & L. W. Thompson (Eds.), *New directions in memory and aging* (pp. 485–506). Hillsdale, NJ: Lawrence Erlbaum.

Zacks, R. T., Hasher, L., Sanft, H., & Rose, K. C. (1983). Encoding effort and recall: A cautionary note. *Journal of Experimental Psychology: Learning, Memory, and Cognition, 4,* 747–756.

Zelinski, E. M., Gilewski, M. J., & Thompson, L. W. (1980). Do laboratory tests relate to self-assessment of memory ability in young and old? In L. W. Poon, J. L. Fozard, L. S. Cermak, D. Arenberg, & L. W. Thompson (Eds.), *New directions in memory and aging* (pp. 519–550). Hillsdale, NJ: Lawrence Erlbaum.

Zelinski, E. M., Light, L. L., & Gilewski, M. J. (1984). Adult age differences in memory for prose: The question of sensitivity to passage structure. *Developmental Psychology, 20,* 1181–1192.

29 Improvement with cognitive training: Which old dogs learn what tricks?

Sherry L. Willis

The term "cognitive training" conjures up the image of young students in a classroom, receiving instruction from a teacher. There is the implicit assumption that the young students did not possess cognitive abilities prior to cognitive training, so that the focus of training is on de novo learning. The critical question is whether or not, as a result of cognitive training, there is *acquisition* of specific knowledge and skills. However, cognitive training is being increasingly employed as a research paradigm across the life span. Questions regarding the purpose and effectiveness of cognitive training at later life stages often are quite different from those relating to the young students. Cognitive training in old age has recently been of particular interest, given the normative pattern of intellectual decline in this developmental period.

This chapter provides a selective review of recent research on cognitive training in later adulthood. The research literature will be reviewed with regard to five major questions: What cognitive abilities have been the targets of cognitive-training research? What is modified as a function of training? How large is the magnitude of the training effect? Who benefits from cognitive training? Are training effects maintained over time? The literature review will focus on the psychometric mental abilities and the cognitive problem-solving skills that have been studied via a training paradigm. The chapters in this volume by Bäckman (Chapter 28), West (Chapter 30), and Yesavage, Lapp, and Sheikh (Chapter 31) review the memory-training literature.

A perspective on cognitive-training research

For the past decade, my colleagues and I have been involved in several programs of cognitive-training research that have examined the modifiability of intellectual performance in later adulthood (Baltes & Willis, 1982; Willis, 1985; Willis & Schaie, 1986). It is our position that the descriptive study of normative

Preparation of this chapter was supported by grants AG03544 and AG05304 from the National Institute on Aging.

trends in intellectual aging should be complemented with research on plasticity or variability in intellectual performance under various types of experimental conditions (Willis & Baltes, 1980). Comprehensive theories of intellectual aging must consider not only mean-level changes in performance but also the range of individual differences in performance and the conditions under which this variability is exhibited. There are three types of variability that are of interest in cognitive-training studies (Baltes & Willis, 1982).

Intraindividual variability

Intraindividual variability is of foremost concern: What is the range of variability in an individual's intellectual performance that can be exhibited as a function of training? Intraindividual change typically has been assessed in terms of pretest–posttest training gain and expressed in terms of standard-deviation units; see Nesselroade, Stigler, and Baltes (1980) and Nunnally (1982) for a discussion of the use of change scores in developmental research. For example, if the mean training-gain score (in t-score units) is 8, then the training gain is on the order of .8 of a standard deviation.

Ideally, pre–post training variability is examined in the context of other data on intraindividual variability available for the population studied. Experimentally induced intraindividual variability is compared with the range of intraindividual variability that has occurred ontogenetically. For example, the investigator can compare the range of intraindividual variability attributable to training with the range of intraindividual variability occurring normatively from middle age to old age; or training variability can be compared with variability from the peak level of performance at some earlier point in development. These types of analyses permit comparison of the range of variability attributable to ontogenetic change versus experimentally induced plasticity. These types of comparisons are useful in developing more complete models of intellectual aging, not only specifying the normative range of development but also providing some indication of the potential range of development. These comparisons are, of course, limited, because plasticity experimentally induced over a very brief time period (e.g., five 1-hour training sessions) is being compared with long-term ontogenetic change occurring over several decades.

If the investigator's goal is to utilize cognitive training as a paradigm for the study of developmental change, then intraindividual variability will be a central concern, and core comparisons will focus on comparing intraindividual variability due to training with longitudinal data on intraindividual variability. An alternative paradigm involves the use of extensive training procedures that make possible comparisons of intraindividual changes across the span of the intervention (Kliegl & Baltes, in press).

Interindividual differences in intraindividual change

The major source of variability examined in most cognitive-training studies has been interindividual differences in intraindividual change, because few training studies have had samples with prior longitudinal data. Comparisons of training and control groups have been the most common types of interindividual differences examined. The range of pretest–posttest variability achieved by the training group is compared with the pretest–posttest changes exhibited by a control/comparison group. Within an experimental design, comparisons of treatment effects are based on the assumption that group differences on all variables expected to be related to the training have been eliminated through either random assignment or statistical control procedures (Campbell & Stanley, 1963). Unfortunately, with the limited sample sizes employed in many studies, adequate control through random assignment may be questionable, and many studies have not reported findings regarding the comparability of various groups.

Examination of other types of interindividual differences in intraindividual change has been seriously neglected (Krauss, 1980). There has been very limited investigation of the sources of individual differences that characterize older adults exhibiting differential training gains. Whereas the majority of training studies in the literature have reported statistically significant mean training improvement, there have been large individual differences in the magnitudes of training improvements. What are the sources of these individual differences? In addition, the majority of training studies have included only one type of training condition (e.g., trainer-directed instruction) and only a pretest–posttest control group. Individual differences in intraindividual variability across multiple training (e.g., practice, computer-assisted instruction, etc.) or control conditions merit further study.

Interability variability

A third type of variability of concern in training research deals with interability variability. Do abilities differ in their susceptibility to training modifiability? Are various training procedures differentially effective for different abilities? Does the nature of performance improvement following training vary by ability? For example, training improvement for some abilities may reflect largely an increase in response speed, whereas improved accuracy may characterize training gains for other abilities. Rarely has training research been conducted in a systematic manner that would permit examination of these types of issues. Although a number of cognitive abilities and processes have been studied via the training paradigm, a given investigator typically has studied only one or two abilities intensively. Comparisons of training effects across abilities have been limited by sampling differences and by lack of comparability of assessment batteries and training procedures.

Abilities and cognitive tasks as targets of training

What abilities and cognitive processes have been studied in training research? The selection of abilities as targets for training has been guided primarily by findings from descriptive, cross-sectional, and longitudinal research on intellectual aging. Abilities for which large and early age differences have been shown have most frequently been chosen as targets for training. Within the classic pattern of intellectual aging, these abilities have been characterized as involving abstract reasoning and speeded responding (Botwinick, 1977). The focus, then, has been on cognitive abilities and skills on which the average performance of the elderly has been shown to be deficient (Denney, 1982).

There have been several reviews of the training-research literature (Baltes & Barton, 1977; Baltes & Willis, 1982; Denney, 1979; Sterns & Sanders, 1980; Willis, 1985; Willis & Schaie, 1981). The training-research literature dealing with problem-solving skills and psychometric abilities is briefly summarized next.

Piagetian and problem-solving tasks

Piagetian tasks. The Piagetian tasks of conservation, classification, spatial egocentrism, and formal operations have been topics of training research. Denney (1974, 1979) has conducted several studies examining the effect of training on the classification criteria employed by the elderly. After observing another person (model) classify stimuli consistently according to dimensions such as shape, color, or size, the elderly were also able to classify consistently according to these criteria. In a spatial-egocentrism training study, Schultz and Hoyer (1976) allowed subjects to view stimuli from different spatial perspectives and gave verbal feedback regarding correctness of responses; training resulted in a significant increase in correct responses. Hornblum and Overton (1976) successfully trained subjects on several surface-area conservation tasks; at posttest, subjects showed improvement on other conservation tasks, suggesting a transfer-of-training phenomenon. These effects were maintained for a 6-week period for a subset of subjects given a delayed posttest. In a study by Tomlinson-Keasey (1972), middle-aged women showed significant improvement on several formal-operations tasks.

Problem-solving tasks. Concept formation has been the primary problem-solving skill studied. Crovitz (1966) found significant improvement on a card-sorting task after subjects observed a model sort the cards several times according to different dimensions. In a concept-formation training study conducted by Sanders, Sterns, Smith, and Sanders (1975), subjects were assigned to one of four conditions: reinforced (monetary) cognitive training, nonreinforced cognitive training, practice with feedback, and a no-treatment control group. At posttest, both the reinforced and nonreinforced training conditions demonstrated greater improvement than did the practice and control conditions. In one of the few studies of long-term maintenance, Sanders and Sanders (1978) found significant training effects 1 year following their study. Meichenbaum (1974) also was able to facilitate performance on a concept-formation task, employing modeling and verbal self-regulatory procedures.

In a series of studies, Denney and associates (Denney & Denney, 1974; Denney, Jones, & Krigel, 1979) studied the manipulation of concept-formation behaviors, using the 20-questions game. Modeling procedures were effective in improving the question-asking efficiency of older subjects. However, Denney (1980) found that other noncognitive treatments were not effective in improving performance on the 20-questions game; these noncognitive conditions included monetary reinforcement, manipulation of self-confidence, and additional time to plan a game strategy.

The modifiability of set induction and behavioral rigidity, which often are related to problem-solving proficiency, has been examined. Studies by Heglin (1956) and Lycette (1973) demonstrated that middle-aged and older adults' tendency to continue to use the same response strategies, even when inappropriate, can be modified with instruction. Levin and Overton (1979) reported that brief instruction on flexibility in thinking (i.e., breaking set) led to improved performance on a spatial-perspective-taking task.

Psychometric abilities

The four psychometric abilities of figural relations, inductive reasoning, spatial orientation, and perceptual speed have received the greatest attention in the training literature.

Figural relations. The fluid ability of figural relations was examined in a series of studies within the Adult Development and Enrichment Project (ADEPT) (Baltes & Willis, 1982; Plemons, Willis, & Baltes, 1978; Willis, Blieszner, & Baltes, 1981). The training involved five 1-hour sessions. Significant training effects were demonstrated for three measures of figural relations (Willis et al., 1981). These training effects were maintained at 1-week, 1-month, and 6-month posttests. Approximately 10 months after the initial training period, subjects were reassessed, and maintenance of the training effects was found. Subjects then participated in five additional training sessions. Additional training resulted in a higher mean level of performance on the figural-relations measures; however, the magnitude of the training gain resulting from additional training was less than that occurring in the first stage of training. At both stages of training, the effects were ability-specific.

Inductive reasoning. Labouvie-Vief and Gonda (1976) examined the manipulation of inductive-reasoning performance, in a study involving four conditions: cognitive-strategy training, a combined strategy training and anxiety-reduction condition, a no-feedback practice condition, and a no-treatment control condition. On the immediate posttest, both cognitive-strategy training conditions demonstrated superior performance to the no-treatment control condition, but did not differ significantly from the no-feedback practice condition. Training effects for the combined training condition were maintained at a 2-week posttest.

Inductive reasoning has also been examined in a series of studies conducted by ADEPT (Baltes & Willis, 1982; Blieszner, Willis, & Baltes, 1981). In an early

ADEPT training study, older adults participated in five 1-hour training sessions on inductive-reasoning problems involving letter-set, number-series, and letter-series tasks. Significant training effects were found on the nearest transfer measure of inductive reasoning at 1-week and 1-month following training. At a 6-month posttest, the no-treatment control group demonstrated significant retest effects such that the training–control-group difference was no longer significant. Because the mean performance of the training group at the 6-month posttest did not differ from their 1-week posttest level, the lack of a significant difference at 6 months appears to reflect a retest effect for the control group, rather than lack of maintenance of the initial training effect.

The effect of a no-feedback practice condition on inductive-reasoning performance was examined in two additional ADEPT studies. In the first study (Hofland, Willis, & Baltes, 1981), subjects participated in eight retest practice sessions. That is, subjects took inductive-reasoning tests under standard timed conditions during each of eight sessions; they received no information regarding their performance. A significant retest effect across trials was found. Examination of the performance pattern across retest sessions indicated that subjects exhibited small, steady gains across consecutive trials. In addition, there was considerable stability in the rank ordering of individuals across trials, suggesting that although there was significant intraindividual improvement, on average, across trials, interindividual differences in levels of performance were maintained across sessions.

An error analysis of trials scores was conducted to examine the nature of retest gains. There was a significant decrease in unattempted test items across trials, indicating that more items were attempted at each succeeding retest session. However, the mean number of commission errors was relatively stable across trials. Therefore, the improvement across trials appears to have been due primarily to an increase in total items attempted, rather than a reduction in commission errors.

Because no apparent performance asymptote appeared to have been reached across the eight trials in the Hofland and associates (1981) practice study, a replication and extension study (Hofland, 1981) was conducted involving 10 no-feedback retest trials. A number of findings from the first study were replicated: (1) A significant retest effect across trials was found. (2) Subjects showed small, steady gains across consecutive trials, with the greatest intertrial gain occurring early, between the pretest and the first retest trial. (3) Rank ordering of individuals' performances across trials was relatively stable. (4) Error analyses indicated a significant decrease in unattempted items across trials. There was a decrease in commission errors also; however, it did not reach statistical significance.

This study also provided additional findings regarding the modifiability of inductive-reasoning performance via practice. First, practice was found to result in significant transfer-of-training effects to a conceptually related measure of inductive reasoning. Second, at posttest, practice effects were examined under a relaxed time condition, as well as under a standard time condition; in the relaxed time condition, practice and no-treatment control groups were given additional time to solve test problems. Mean performances of both practice and control groups improved significantly under the relaxed time condition. However, the practice group maintained a higher performance level. That is, when the groups were given sufficient time to attempt virtually every test item, the practice group answered a significantly greater mean number of items correctly and made significantly fewer commission errors, as compared with the control group.

Baltes and associates (Baltes, Dittmann-Kohli, & Kliegl, 1986) have recently reported a replication and extension of the ADEPT training research with a German sample of elderly. Subjects received five training sessions on inductive reasoning and five training sessions on figural relations in a counterbalanced design. Significant training effects were found for both abilities, and the effects were maintained across 1-month and 6-month posttests. Significant retest effects for the control group were also demonstrated across posttests. Transfer of training was demonstrated to conceptually related measures of inductive reasoning and figural relations. Task analyses also indicated that trained subjects correctly solved more items of various difficulty levels than did control subjects, indicating that the training effect was not restricted to items of low difficulty. Finally, error analyses indicated that although both training and control groups showed significant increases in numbers of items attempted and numbers of correct items, an increase in accuracy of performance (i.e., decrease in commission errors) occurred only for the training group.

Spatial orientation and inductive reasoning. In a recent project, we examined training effects within a longitudinal study design (Schaie & Willis, 1986; Willis & Schaie, 1986). A major purpose of the study was to examine the relative effectiveness of cognitive training in remediating the performances of subjects exhibiting cognitive decline on selected abilities versus improving the performances of subjects with stable levels of prior performance. Elderly participants in the Seattle Longitudinal Study (SLS) were classified as having remained stable or having declined over the previous 14-year period (1970–84) on two mental abilities: spatial orientation and inductive reasoning. Approximately 47% of the sample were classified as having remained stable on both abilities; approximately 31% had declined on only one of the two abilities; 22% had declined on both abilities. Subjects who had declined on only one of the abilities were assigned to a five-session training program focusing on that ability. Subjects who had remained stable on both abilities or who had declined on both abilities were randomly assigned to training on one of the abilities.

We believe that this was the first study to assess training effects at the level of ability factors, rather than at the level of individual test scores (Willis & Schaie, 1986). Significant training effects were found at the factor-score level for both inductive reasoning and spatial orientation. Training effects were ability-specific in that improvement was shown for the two ability factors that were the targets of training, but there were no training effects for any of the other ability factors included in the pretest–posttest battery. In terms of intraindividual change, approximately two-thirds of the sample showed significant pretest–posttest training improvement.

Were there differential training effects for subjects classified as having declined versus those having remained stable over the previous 14-year period? Analyses at the level of factor scores showed no significant differences in the magnitudes of training gains exhibited by stable versus decline subjects. When effects were examined at the level of individual measures, there was a trend for decliners to have gained somewhat more from training than had the stable subjects; this trend was most evident for subjects trained on spatial orientation. Whereas the magnitudes of training gains were roughly comparable for stables and decliners, the two groups did differ in their *levels* of performance at posttest. For the decliners, training improvement represented at least partial remediation to a prior level of performance, whereas for the stables, training improvement reflected a performance level above that previously demonstrated by the subjects over the prior 14-year period.

Of particular interest to us was the effectiveness of training in remediating the performances of decliners (Schaie & Willis, 1986). That is, for what proportion of the decliners was training effective in remediating performance to the level exhibited 14 years previously? The data indicate that at posttest, approximately 40% of the decliners were performing at a level equivalent to or above the level at which they had performed 14 years previously. The proportions of decliners exhibiting remediation were roughly equivalent for inductive reasoning and spatial orientation.

Response speed. Findings from several studies indicate that older adults' speed of responding on a variety of perceptual-discrimination tasks can be significantly increased. Hoyer, Labouvie, and Baltes (1973) examined the modifiability of perceptual speed performance under three conditions: reinforced practice with feedback regarding performance, nonreinforced practice with no feedback, and a no-treatment control. Significant improvement in performance on perceptual speed tasks occurred for both practice conditions; the reinforcement procedure itself appeared to have little effect. No transfer effects were obtained on a battery of psychometric measures administered after training. The lack of transfer from perceptual speed training to intellectual performance was replicated in a study by Hoyer, Hoyer, Treat, and Baltes (1978).

Coyne (1981) examined the effects of practice on forward visual masking for young and older adults. Practice resulted in a reduced susceptibility to forward masking for both age groups. Whereas there was an age effect for the length of the interstimulus interval, the interaction between age and practice was not significant, suggesting that the magnitudes of improvement associated with practice were comparable for the young and older adults.

Several studies (Beres & Baron, 1981; Erber, 1976; Grant, Storandt, & Botwinick, 1978) have examined the effects of practice on performance on the Digit Symbol Substitution subtest of the Wechsler Adult Intelligence Scale (WAIS).

Significant improvement with practice has been exhibited for both young and older age groups. In the most extensive practice condition, Beres and Baron (1981) found that the scores of older women increased from the 25th to the 90th percentile relative to norms for young adults, and these scores were maintained during a follow-up test 10 days later.

Willis, Cornelius, and Baltes (1983) examined the effects of practice on several measures of attention/perceptual discrimination. In addition, transfer of training was examined with an assessment battery involving fluid/crystallized intelligence, perceptual speed, and memory span. Significant training effects occurred for three measures: the Stroop Color Interference task (Stroop, 1935), the Underwood Number Counting task (Underwood, 1975), and the Continuous Paired Associates Recall task (Atkinson & Shiffrin, 1968). These effects were maintained across 1-month and 6-month posttests. In addition to a no-treatment control, a social-contact control group was included to assess the effects of participation in an equivalent number of hours of social contact, but involving no training. No significant training effects occurred for the social-contact control condition. In addition, no transfer of training was found to measures of fluid/crystallized intelligence, perceptual speed, or memory span.

In summary, the training-research literature indicates that cognitive training is effective in significantly improving the performances of older adults on a variety of Piagetian tasks, problem-solving tasks, and psychometric abilities. Although the specific training procedures employed have varied across studies, common elements in training have included behavioral modeling by a trainer, instruction in the use of relevant cognitive strategies, practice with prototypical tasks, and feedback regarding correctness of responses. Training has been found to be effective in both remediating cognitive decline and improving performances of subjects exhibiting no prior decline.

Nature of training effects

Although a review of the training literature strongly supports the notion of plasticity in older adults' intellectual performances, there has been considerable debate and discussion regarding the nature of the training improvement. How are training gains to be interpreted? Reviewers of the literature have tended to focus on three issues: the breadth of training effects, the directionality of these effects, and what specific behaviors are modified as a function of training.

Breadth of training effects

Alternative views have been taken regarding both the expected breadth and the actual breadth of training gains demonstrated. Some have interpreted training effects to be narrow and to reflect little more than "teaching the test." In contrast, others have suggested that training may result in significant alterations in the structural relationships among abilities. For example, Donaldson (1981) has suggested that as a result of training, fluid-ability measures (e.g., figural-relations tasks) may become more characteristic of crystallized intelligence. Findings from several recent studies indicate that neither of these extreme positions is supported by the data.

Latent variables and training

Discussion of the breadth of training effects must begin with recognition that it is a cognitive construct or latent variable (e.g., classification, inductive reasoning) that is the target of intervention research. The primary concern in training research is not a change in performance on a letter-series test or the 20-questions task per se, but rather change in the latent construct that task is said to represent. Latent constructs can be assessed only indirectly via observable tests that have been shown empirically to represent those constructs. Training gains, as measured by these observable tests, however, represent confounding of the variance common to the latent construct and the variance that is unique to that specific measurement instrument. It is change in the common variance that is of primary interest in training. If training improvement reflected primarily change in unique variance, then the critique of "teaching the test" would be valid. When training studies rely on only one test to assess training gains, it is impossible to disentangle changes attributable to common versus unique variance. Subjects' performances on multiple measures representing the latent construct are required to assess change in common variance.

How can training gains attributable to change in the common variance be assessed? One method is to assess training effects at the factorial level, rather than at the level of individual test scores. Ability-factor scores representing variance common to a given latent construct are the dependent variables in these analyses of training effects. Whereas factor-analytic procedures have most commonly been employed in research within psychometric models of intelligence, this method could be usefully employed in research on memory processes or problem-solving abilities and would permit the researchers to examine their findings more precisely at the latent-construct level.

In our recent training studies (Willis & Schaie, 1986) we have found significant training effects at the factorial level for the abilities of inductive reasoning and spatial orientation. These findings are evidence of training gains at the latent-construct level.

Ability-specific training effects

We have found across a number of studies that training effects were specific to the ability that was the focus of training. Demonstration of ability-specific effects requires two conditions: (1) Training effects must be shown for multiple measures of the ability that is the focus of training. Ideally, data will be analyzed at the factorial level, so that training effects at the latent-construct level can be examined. (2) No training effects should occur for measures of other abilities that are not the focus of training. Both conditions must be met for an ability-specific interpretation of training effects. If effects occur for measures of abilities other than that trained, then specification of the nature of training effects at the construct level and in terms of variance common to a particular construct will be more difficult.

Should ability-specific effects, when demonstrated at the construct level, be interpreted narrowly or broadly? We believe that such effects occur at the level that would be expected, given that training procedures typically have been designed to focus on cognitive strategies and behaviors associated with a specific ability or cognitive process. Indeed, the current state of the field of cognitive psychology is such that it would be difficult to develop training procedures aimed for broader effects. In mainstream cognitive psychology, it has proved exceedingly difficult to specify and operationalize executive processes or metacognitive components that are truly generalizable across multiple abilities. Componential analyses typically have been limited to a particular ability construct (Detterman, 1980; Sternberg, 1982). Discussion of metacomponents remains at a theoretical level.

Targeting training effects at an ability-specific level makes sense from the perspective of findings from longitudinal research on intraindividual change in cognitive functioning (Schaie, 1983). There are wide individual differences not only in the timing of the onset of cognitive decline but also in terms of which particular abilities or skills exhibit early change. In young-old age, changes in cognitive functioning tend to be highly specific and individualized. For example, our classification of the change status of elderly participants from the SLS indicated large individual differences, even when two abilities (inductive reasoning, spatial orientation) were considered that should exhibit early decline within the classic pattern of intellectual aging. Almost one-half (46%) of the subjects showed no statistically reliable decline on either ability over the previous 14-year period. Almost a third (31%) of the subjects showed decline on one of the abilities, but not on the other. Because for many older individuals, early ontogenetic changes in cognitive functioning appear to be ability-specific, such an approach to intervention in many cases seems reasonable. A prescriptive, individualized approach to training that will result in ability-specific effects is also compatible with the notion of selective optimization in later adulthood (Baltes, Dittmann-Kohli, & Dixon, 1984). Given older individuals' need and desire to set priorities and selectively utilize their cognitive resources, an ability-specific approach will be useful.

Structural invariance and training effects

Thus far, our discussion of the breadth of training effects has focused on pretest–posttest quantitative change, whether examined at the test-score level or at the latent-construct level. Analyses of training effects have been almost solely concerned with issues of quantitative change. However, our interpretations of findings regarding quantitative change are based on assumptions regarding the structural stability of the measurement framework from pretest to posttest (Donaldson, 1981; Schaie, Willis, Hertzog, & Schulenberg, 1985; Willis & Schaie, 1986). Structural invariance addresses questions such as the following: Are the same latent constructs represented in the assessment battery at pretest and posttest? Are the observable measures still representative of the same latent constructs following intervention? Have the relationships among these constructs remained constant across intervention?

If assumptions regarding structural stability are not met, then interpretation of exactly what was modified as a function of training becomes ambiguous. For example, if Donaldson's suggestion (1981) is correct that educational training procedures resulted in fluid-ability measures becoming more crystallized in character, then our interpretation of the nature of training effects needs to be seriously altered. The existing literature offers strong support for assumptions of structural invariance (Baltes, Cornelius, Spiro, Nesselroade, & Willis, 1980). However, the issue merits empirical investigation.

In recent training research, we examined the pretest–posttest structural stability of a measurement battery representing the five primary mental abilities of verbal meaning, inductive reasoning, spatial orientation, number, and perceptual speed (Schaie et al., 1985). Would training on either inductive reasoning or spatial orientation significantly alter the relationships among these abilities, or the representativeness of tests as "markers" of specific ability factors? We found virtually complete structural stability for the abilities (verbal, number, speed) that were not the targets of training. There were some slight pretest–posttest shifts in the regression weights for measures representing the trained abilities. However, all measures were still representative of the constructs they were selected to mark at pretest, and the shifts in regression weights did not alter interpretation of the ability-specific nature of training effects. These findings are supportive of earlier correlational research on the stability of interability relationships across retest trials (Hofland et al., 1981).

To our knowledge, the study of Schaie and associates (1985) was the first stringent test of structural stability within the context of training intervention. These findings of structural stability were to be expected, given that the psychometric measures employed are highly reliable and have evidenced strong saturations on the particular ability constructs. However, there is need for further examination of structural stability in a training context, particularly with regard to less reliable (i.e., more state-like) constructs. For example, there is some suggestive evidence of changes in the relationship between memory span and other abilities at various stages in the learning curve (Hofland et al., 1981; Labouvie, Frohring, Baltes, & Goulet, 1973).

Directionality of training improvement

Because gerontological training research has focused almost exclusively on those abilities exhibiting early age differences or age-related decline, there has been the implicit assumption that training effects reflect the modifiability/reversibility of cognitive decline. However, longitudinal research findings regarding individual differences in the timing of decline and what abilities show decline suggest that training effects may be multidirectional. That is, training effects may reflect remediation, incrementation, or compensation, depending on a given individual's prior performance history on a specific ability. In our research with SLS participants, approximately 55% of the subjects had exhibited declines over the prior 14 years on one or both of the abilities studied, and thus training effects focused on remediation (Schaie & Willis, 1986). However, approximately 45% of the sample showed no significant decline on either of the abilities studied, and thus training effects represented new performance levels.

Remediating cognitive decline

Are training procedures effective in remediating cognitive decline and in improving the performances of subjects showing no previous decline? To answer this question, training studies must be conducted with subjects with prior longitudinal data, and thus far, very little such research has been conducted. Our training research with SLS subjects examined this question for the abilities of inductive reasoning and spatial orientation (Willis & Schaie, 1986). Findings from this research indicate that there were significant training gains for both stable and decline subjects. When results were examined at the factorial level, there was no significant difference in the mean training gains for stables and decliners.

We have been particularly interested in the effectiveness of training for subjects experiencing significant cognitive decline. To what extent is training effective in remediating decliners' performances to prior performance levels? For 40% of the decliners, training resulted in remediation to the subject's performance level 14 years previously (Schaie & Willis, 1986). These reversal effects were demonstrated for both of the primary abilities (inductive reasoning and spatial orientation) that were the targets of training. We interpret these findings as lending support to the notion of the plasticity of behavior into late adulthood and suggesting that for at least a substantial proportion of the community-dwelling elderly, observed cognitive decline is not irreversible. Part of what has been termed "decline" is likely attributable to disuse and can be subjected to environmental manipulations involving relatively simple educational training techniques.

Although the magnitudes of pretest–posttest training gains were equivalent for stable and decline subjects, training effects have qualitatively different implications for the two groups. Stables and decliners obviously differed on baseline performance at pretest. Consequently, the effects of training resulted in moving the decliners closer to their previous performance levels, whereas training resulted in raising the performances of the stables beyond previously exhibited performance levels. Thus, the mean levels of performance at posttest differed significantly for the two groups.

Without prior longitudinal data, it is not possible to address issues regarding the directionality (i.e., remediation, incrementation) of training effects. Given current cohort differences in ability performance levels, many older adults may be disadvantaged when compared with younger age cohorts, even though showing no significant ability decline. Because most studies have not had subject samples with prior longitudinal data, the more appropriate focus for training research is on the magnitude or range of training gains, rather than on the directionality of the training effects.

Specific behaviors and skills modified via training procedures

The most commonly used dependent variables in gerontological training research have been the number of correct responses and/or the speed of responding. However, these indices provide only limited insight into what specifically is modified as a function of training. An increase in correct responses may occur in several ways. For example, as a result of training, the subject may respond more quickly, therefore attempting more problems and answering a greater number of items correctly. However, the number of commission errors may also increase, such that there will be no change in level of accuracy. On the other hand, training may result in little increase in the number of items attempted, but there may be a significant decrease in commission errors, so that accuracy as well as the number of correct responses will increase.

Error analyses

More microlevel assessments, particularly componential and error analyses, have proved useful in examining the qualitative nature of training improvement. For example, in their study on spatial egocentrism, Schultz and Hoyer (1976) found that training improvement occurred as a result of a significant reduction in perceptual judgment errors (wrong responses), but not in egocentric responses per se. In fact, this sample of elderly people made relatively few egocentric judgments, even prior to training.

Error analyses conducted in conjunction with a series of training studies focusing on the fluid abilities of inductive reasoning and figural relations suggest that various treatment procedures may be differentially effective in increasing performance accuracy. Baltes and associates (1986) found a significant increase in number of correct responses for both a cognitive-training group and a pretest–posttest control group; thus, both cognitive training and simple retest exposures are effective in increasing correct responding. However, ability-specific cognitive training was also effective in decreasing the proportion of commission errors, thus increasing the level of accuracy. In contrast, the pretest–posttest control group exhibited an increase in commission errors. These findings are supported by results from two studies examining extensive retest experience (Hofland, 1981; Hofland et al., 1981). Older subjects experiencing multiple retest sessions with no feedback regarding performance exhibited significant increases in total number of items attempted and in the number of correct responses. However, the proportion of commission errors did not significantly decrease. When the pretest–posttest control group was given additional time to solve test items, there was a significant increase in number of correct responses, but also an increase in commission errors, a finding similar to that for the control group in the study of Baltes and associates (1986). Thus, whereas an increase in correct responses can be elicited by simple retest procedures, improvement in accuracy of performance appears to be related to specific cognitive-training procedures.

Our recent research suggests that the qualitative nature of training improvement may vary with the particular ability that is the target of training. Performance on fluid abilities, such as figural relations and inductive reasoning, typically is characterized by a sizable number of commission errors. Therefore, an important aspect of fluid-ability training is a reduction in the proportion of commission errors. In contrast, descriptive research on spatial orientation indicates that the rate of commission errors is relatively low. The major source of individual differences (including age differences) is in the speed of mental rotation (Cerella, Poon, & Fozard, 1981; Cooper & Shepard, 1973). Thus, one would predict that effective training on spatial orientation would result in a significant increase in the number of items attempted, reflecting increased speed of mental rotation, but that there would be relatively little change in error rate. Error analyses of our study of spatial-orientation training support this prediction. Significant performance improvement is associated primarily with an increase in the number of items attempted (Willis, 1985).

In summary, this section on the nature of training effects has addressed three issues: breadth of training effects, directionality of training effects, and specific behaviors modified via training. Recent training research indicates that training effects are broad, in that they can be demonstrated at the level of the latent construct (e.g., ability factor); however, effects are specific (limited) to the ability trained. Training effects at the construct level have been demonstrated in the context of structural invariance in the measurement framework. With regard to the second issue, training has been found effective both for subjects exhibiting prior decline on the ability trained and for subjects showing no prior decline. Finally, the specific behaviors modified as a function of training appear to vary with the particular ability being trained. That is, for abilities characterized by high rates of commission errors, training may reflect largely a decrease in errors, whereas for other abilities (e.g., spatial orientation) in which speed of mental rotation is the critical component, training improvement may reflect change in this component.

Magnitude of training effects

How large are the training effects reported in the literature? Assessment of the magnitudes of training effects requires the specification of a criterion against which effects can be compared. Training effectiveness may be assessed in terms of the criterion of intraindividual change or in terms of the magnitude of interindividual differences in intraindividual change.

Intraindividual change

If intraindividual change is the primary concern, as we argue it should be, then training improvement needs to be compared with the individual's performance at some earlier time, prior to training. Ideally, if longitudinal data are available, then the individual's posttest performance can be compared with his or her performance at some earlier point in development. In our recent training research with SLS participants, we conducted a number of analyses to determine the training effects on the abilities of inductive reasoning and spatial orientation, using subjects' performances on these abilities 14 years prior to training. The effects of training on average performance levels were examined separately for three age cohorts (Schaie & Willis, 1985). The average ages for these cohorts at the time of training (in 1984) were 67, 74, and 81 years. For all of these age cohorts, statistically significant average declines had been noted by age 67 for the two abilities studied. A cohort's average level of performance 14 years prior to training was first compared with the average performance level for subjects receiving only pretest–posttest assessment (i.e., retest effects) and second compared with that for subjects receiving cognitive training, in addition to pretest–posttest assessment. For *spatial orientation,* retest experience alone was sufficient to remediate the 14-year average decline for the younger (67 years) and middle (74 years) age cohorts. For the oldest cohort (81 years), cognitive training resulted in remediation of average decline. For the younger cohort (67 years), cognitive training raised the average performance level significantly above that observed 14 years previously.

Similar findings occurred for *inductive reasoning*. Retest effects alone were sufficient to remediate the youngest cohort (67 years) to the average performance level 14 years previously. Cognitive training remediated the 14-year average decline for the oldest cohort (81 years) and raised the average performance levels of the youngest and middle cohorts significantly above their average performance levels 14 years previously. Thus, for the young-old, simple retest experience appears to be an effective remediation procedure. For the old-old, more length and structured cognitive-training procedures appear to be required for remediation.

The power of a longitudinal approach to training research, however, lies in the potential for assessing training effectiveness at the individual level, as well as at the group (average) level. When intraindividual change is examined for particular individuals, what proportion of subjects exhibit significant training effects? In our research, we found that approximately 40% of subjects exhibiting prior decline could be remediated to or above their performance levels 14 years previously (Schaie & Willis, 1986). The proportions of subjects showing remediation were comparable for the inductive-reasoning and spatial-orientation abilities.

When the criterion was shifted to pretest–posttest training gain, we found that over half of decliners exhibited significant training improvement. Prior level of performance was a less useful criterion for assessing training improvement for subjects showing no cognitive decline on the ability trained. However, when pretest–posttest training gain was used as the criterion, we found that over half of the stable subjects trained on inductive reasoning showed significant improvement, whereas 40% of stable subjects trained on spatial orientation showed significant pretest–posttest gain.

Interindividual differences in intraindividual change

In the majority of training studies lacking prior longitudinal data, the magnitudes of training effects have been assessed in terms of interindividual differences in intraindividual change: The pretest–posttest training gain of the training group has been compared with that of a control group. When the magnitude of training improvement was examined in terms of standard-deviation units, several studies reported effect magnitudes on the order of .50 to 1.00 standard deviations (Baltes et al., 1986; Hornblum & Overton, 1976; Willis et al., 1981; Willis & Schaie, 1986).

How do these estimates of training gains compare with the magnitudes of age-related declines, as estimated from longitudinal data sets? Recent estimates of the magnitude of age-related declines derived from Schaie's longitudinal study (Schaie & Willis, 1985) indicate that from the age where decline can first be reliably demonstrated to age 74, the magnitude of decline is on the order of one-half of a standard deviation for fluid abilities, such as spatial orientation and inductive reasoning. The cumulative decrement to age 81 amounts to approximately .75 of a population standard deviation. Thus, the magnitude of training improvement reported in several studies compares favorably with the effect size for age-related decline.

If analyses of training effects are to focus primarily on interindividual differences in intraindividual change, the selection of appropriate comparison/control groups becomes critical. The researcher must consider questions such as these: What types of comparisons are of interest? What variables are (are not) controlled for by selection of a particular control group? When training and control groups are randomly selected from the same population, there is the assumption that the effects of all variables expected to be related to the treatment effects have been eliminated (Campbell & Stanley, 1963; Krauss, 1980). Thus, group differences may be attributed to treatment effects.

Age-comparative studies

We find interpretation of training effects involving younger-age comparison groups particularly troublesome. Age-comparative research, whether descriptive or interventive in focus, typically has violated critical assumptions of quasi-experimental design, in that age, of course, cannot be randomly assigned. Rarely have age-comparative studies given careful consideration to comparability of age groups on variables such as education, testing experience, health, and sensory impairment, all of which have been shown to be related to intellectual performance.

In many age-comparative studies, younger and older groups have been compared in terms of their *levels* of performance at posttest. When a significant age difference in performance levels has been found, the authors have concluded that such age differences have not been due primarily to environmental variables, because training intervention (often involving less than an hour) has not eliminated average performance differences. However, for many of the cognitive variables that have been the focus of training research, cohort differences have been reported that have been as large as or larger than the magnitude of age-related change (Schaie, 1983). Even if training is effective in remediating age-related decline for a significant proportion of subjects, it is to be expected that age differences attributable to cohort differences will remain. Age comparisons of levels of performance are, then, particularly vulnerable to multiple confounds. Age comparisons of pretest–posttest change scores probably are the most defensible units of comparison; see Nunnally (1982) for a discussion of change scores. The absence of a significant interaction between age and treatment (assuming a treatment main effect), as reported in several studies, suggests considerable plasticity of intellectual functioning in later adulthood, in that the training gain for the older group was as great as the training gain for the younger group.

In summary, the magnitude of training effects must be assessed with regard to a criterion. We have argued that the individual's performance at some earlier time, prior to training, is the most appropriate criterion, because intraindividual change is the primary concern in the study of behavior plasticity. However, most training research has employed a control group as the criterion, and thus the focus is on interindividual differences in intraindividual change. Several studies have reported effect magnitudes on the order of .50 to 1.00 standard deviation (SD).

Individual differences in training effectiveness

We come now to the issue that is of greatest concern to the older adult, and often to the clinician. Who benefits from training procedures? That is, what are the individual-difference variables associated with training improvement? Ironically, this is an issue that has received little attention in the training literature; see Yesavage, Lapp, and Sheikh (Chapter 31, this volume).

Given the current propensity toward age-comparative designs in research on intellectual aging, chronological age has been one of the common individual-difference variables examined. Researchers have hypothesized that if age differences reflect primarily experiential/environmental differences, then the elderly should exhibit greater training effects than younger age groups. There appears to be the implicit assumption that younger age groups are nearer their maximal potential levels of performance than are older adults and therefore should show smaller training gains. However, longitudinal research indicates that peak levels of performance on many abilities are not attained until the thirties (Schaie, 1983); thus, the typical college-age comparison group may be a full decade from their peak performance levels. Moreover, the limited trials involved in most training studies have not provided an adequate test of maximal performance levels for either age group (Kliegl & Baltes, in press).

The findings are limited and mixed regarding chronological age as a predictor of training improvement within the period of later adulthood. In their training research on the fluid abilities of figural relations and inductive reasoning, Baltes and associates (1986) reported that subjects under 70 years of age exhibited a larger training gain (.1 SD) than did subjects over the age of 70. However, those authors considered these age effects to be rather small, compared with the magnitude of the main effect of training. In our training research on inductive reasoning and spatial orientation, we found that covarying on age, education, and income did not significantly alter the training outcomes (Schaie & Willis, 1986). However, as reported earlier, we found that more intensive and more lengthy training procedures were needed to remediate age-related declines for older cohorts (average age 81) than for younger cohorts (average age 67).

There is some evidence that training may be particularly effective for subjects who have experienced decline on the target ability. Although there was no significant difference between stables and decliners in the magnitude of training gain at the factorial level for either inductive reasoning or spatial orientation, we did find greater training improvement for decliners when training effects were examined at the level of individual tests (Schaie & Willis, 1986; Willis & Schaie, 1986). In particular, subjects who had declined on spatial orientation showed greater training gains. Likewise, training improvement on spatial orientation was greater for females, specifically females who had declined (Schaie & Willis, 1986; Willis, 1985). However, greater training improvement by decliners was not a function of regression toward the mean effects (Schaie & Willis, 1986). Nor did subjects suffering decline function at a lower baseline performance level than stable subjects; stable and decline subjects did not differ in performance level 14 years prior to training (Schaie & Willis, 1986). Baltes and associates (1986) reported that there was a trend for subjects with lower initial levels of performance to exhibit greater training improvement. Lower initial performance levels may reflect decline at some point prior to training.

It should be noted that the training studies cited in this literature review involved community-dwelling elderly who were in fair to excellent health. We do not wish to imply that the cognitive-training procedures utilized in these studies would necessarily be effective with elderly suffering from neuropathologies or severe chronic illnesses. Findings were not as positive from the limited research examining the effectiveness with clinical populations of the brief training procedures employed in the literature cited earlier. However, more intensive intervention procedures have been used effectively to modify more limited areas of behavioral functioning in clinical populations (Wilson & Moffat, 1984; Wilson, Chapter 32, this volume).

In summary, examination of the individual-difference variables associated with training outcomes is one of the most neglected areas in training research and merits further study. Key variables examined have included age, prior decline status, gender, and health. The relative importances of these variables as predictors of responsiveness to training are not well documented at present.

Maintenance of training effects

The temporal durability of training effects is an important issue for both theoretical and practical reasons. The utility of training efforts is greatly diminished unless behavioral proficiency is maintained over time. However, the designs of most training studies have not included delayed posttests. Several studies have reported maintenance of training effects several weeks after training (Beres & Baron, 1981; Blieszner et al., 1981; Hornblum & Overton, 1976; Labouvie-Vief & Gonda, 1976). Maintenance of effects 6 months after training on several fluid abilities has been reported by Baltes and associates (1986) and Willis and associates (1981, 1983). Finally, sustained effects have been reported at 10 months and 1 year following training by Baltes and Willis (1982) and Sanders and Sanders (1978), respectively.

A number of methodological issues are involved in assessing the durability of effects. Delayed posttests provide additional practice on the target measures and thus often serve as a minor form of intervention. In our ADEPT training research involving 1-week, 1-month, and 6-month posttests, we observed increases in levels of performance for both the training and control groups from the 1-week to the 1-month posttest. These retest effects may be particularly sizable for the control group. In the study of Blieszner and associates (1981), the mean performance level of the training group was stable from 1 week to 6 months after training; however, the control group exhibited a significant retest effect across delayed posttests, such that the training–control-group difference was no longer significant at 6 months. Simple retest practice can be a powerful procedure for boosting performance of no-treatment controls at delayed posttests.

When treatment–control-group differences diminish across time, it is important to examine the extent to which the effect reflects decay of training or potent retest gains. One procedure for disentangling treatment maintenance and retest effects is to include multiple control groups, staggering the timing of the initial posttest across groups.

Maintenance of training effects typically has been assessed in terms of mean number of correct responses. However, error analyses have suggest that although both cognitive training and retest experiences result in increases in total number of items attempted and number of correct responses, cognitive training also has the effect of increasing the accuracy level (i.e., decreasing commission errors), whereas the commission-error rate may actually increase under simple retest procedures (Baltes et al., 1986; Hofland et al., 1981). Therefore, analyses of maintenance effects need to include procedures such as error analyses to examine more closely what behaviors are maintained across time.

Although we consider maintenance an extremely important concern, it is important to recognize that the question of the range of behavioral plasticity is a separate issue from that of maintenance. Demonstration of the reversibility of performance decline does not require that these effects be maintained over time. The question of reversibility is addressed most pointedly at the initial posttest. Should we expect training effects to be infinitely durable? No. Research on life-style antecedents of cognitive change indicates that in the natural environment, different types of life styles are associated with maintenance and decline of cognitive functioning (Gribbin, Schaie, & Parham, 1980; Stone, 1980). Maintenance of intellectual performance in healthy older adults is associated with an active life style involving high levels of environmental stimulation. In contrast, decline in intellectual functioning is associated with a restrictive life style, often involving the loss of family supports. If, following training, the individual returns to a life style associated with deleterious cognitive effects, should maintenance of training gain be expected?

Maintenance of cognitive gain following training would seem to require the incorporation of certain critical experiential variables into the life space of the older adult. We, as scientists, know relatively little about the person and environmental variables associated with maintenance of intervention effects. Examination of the more applications-oriented intervention literature on topics such as weight reduction, drug addiction, and cigarette smoking indicates relatively meager success with regard to maintenance of effects. The procedures required to maintain effects may be in many ways qualitatively different from the intervention strategies employed to induce the initial change in behavior. For example, we would not suggest that older adults continue to take periodic cognitive-training booster sessions for the remainder of their lives.

Research on which activities of daily living are related to maintenance of high levels of performance on specific abilities or cognitive processes may prove useful. Just as has been argued with regard to the life-event literature (Hultsch & Plemons, 1979), it probably will be the salient dimensions characterizing these activities, rather than the specific activities per se, that are important. Intervention research in the natural environment can then explore whether or not inclusion of these experiential dimensions in daily living results in maintenance of performance on those abilities associated with these dimensions.

In summary, the few studies that have examined the temporal durability of training effects indicate maintenance at 6-month and 1-year intervals following training. Maintenance of intervention effects for lengthy periods following training would seem to require modifications in the subject's life space that would foster and facilitate utilization of the effective cognitive behaviors acquired during training.

Future perspectives and conclusions

A well-documented finding in descriptive research on intellectual aging is the increasing range of individual differences with age. We believe that one of the most critical next steps in cognitive-training research is movement from a normative to a differential approach to training. The need for a differential approach to the study of aging (in general) was described some years ago (Thomae, 1976), and though often discussed and lauded, it is still the exception when it is adequately reflected in empirical research. Cognitive-training research offers a microcosm for examining some of the more salient individual-difference variables as they interact with training outcomes.

Examination of the interactions between individual differences and training improvements is important in at least two respects. First, it extends our understanding of the nature of training improvement. In our own research, we have been examining the differentiation of training improvement due to remediation of cognitive decline versus training gain reflecting new performance levels in subjects experiencing no prior decline.

Second, examination of individual-difference variables may prove useful in targeting those populations most likely to benefit from training. The fact that a sizable proportion of subjects who had shown prior decline exhibited significant training gains provides empirical support for educational programs for the elderly. Further research is needed on those individual-difference characteristics that distinguish those decliners who showed significant training improvement and those who did not.

Thus, findings from a differential approach to training not only have potential for contributing to basic knowledge on cognitive aging but also should have utility for more applied concerns with regard to clinical and public-policy issues. In order to facilitate optimal functioning and care for the growing proportion of the elderly, we must proceed to ask, Which old dogs can learn what tricks?

References

Atkinson, R. C., & Shiffrin, R. M. (1968). Human memory: A proposed system and its component processes. In K. W. Spence & J. T. Spence (Eds.), *Advances in the psychology of learning and motivation: Research and theory* (Vol. 2). New York: Academic Press.

Baltes, M. M., & Barton, E. M. (1977). New approaches toward aging: A case for the operant model. *Educational Gerontology, 2,* 383–405.

Baltes, P. B., Cornelius, S. W., Spiro, A., Nesselroade, J. R., & Willis, S. L. (1980). Integration versus differentiation of fluid/crystallized intelligence in old age. *Developmental Psychology, 16,* 625–635.

Baltes, P. B., Dittmann-Kohli, F., & Dixon, R. A. (1984). New perspectives on the development of intelligence in adulthood: Toward a dual-process conception and a model of selective optimization with compensation. In P. B. Baltes & O. G. Brim, Jr. (Eds.), *Life-span development and behavior* (Vol. 6, pp. 33–76). New York: Academic Press.

Baltes, P. B., Dittmann-Kohli, F., & Kliegl, R. (1986). Reserve capacity of the elderly in aging-sensitive tests of fluid intelligence: Replication and extension. *Psychology and Aging, 1,* 172–177.

Baltes, P. B., & Willis, S. L. (1982). Enhancement (plasticity) of intellectual functioning in old age: Penn State's Adult Development and Enrichment Project (ADEPT). In F. I. M. Craik & S. E. Trehub (Eds.), *Aging and cognitive processes* (pp. 353–389). New York: Plenum Press.

Beres, C., & Baron, A. (1981). Improved digit substitution by older women as a result of extended practice. *Journal of Gerontology, 36,* 591–597.

Blieszner, R., Willis, S. L., & Baltes, P. B. (1981). Training research in aging on the fluid ability of inductive reasoning. *Journal of Applied Developmental Psychology, 2,* 247–265.

Botwinick, J. (1977). Intellectual abilities. In J. E. Birren & K. W. Schaie (Eds.), *Handbook of the psychology of aging* (pp. 580–605). New York: Van Nostrand Reinhold.

Campbell, D. T., & Stanley, J. C. (1963). *Experimental and quasi-experimental designs for research.* Chicago: Rand McNally.

Cattell, R. B. (1971). *Abilities: Structure, growth and action.* Boston: Houghton Mifflin.

Cerella, J., Poon, L., & Fozard, J. (1981). Mental rotation and age reconsidered. *Journal of Gerontology, 35,* 620–624.

Cooper, L. A., & Shepard, R. N. (1973). Chronometric studies of the rotation of mental images. In W. Chase (Ed.), *Visual information processing.* New York: Academic Press.

Coyne, A. C. (1981). Age differences and practice in forward visual masking. *Journal of Gerontology, 36,* 730–732.

Crovitz, E. (1966). Reversing a learning deficit in the aged. *Journal of Gerontology, 21,* 236–238.

Denney, N. W. (1974). Evidence for developmental change in categorization criteria for children and adults. *Human Development, 17,* 41–53.

Denney, N. W. (1979). Problem solving in later adulthood: Intervention research. In P. B. Baltes & O. G. Brim, Jr. (Eds.), *Life-span development and behavior* (Vol. 2). New York: Academic Press.

Denney, N. W. (1980). The effect of manipulation of peripheral, noncognitive variables on the problem-solving performance of the elderly. *Human Development, 23,* 268–277.

Denney, N. W. (1982). Aging and cognitive changes. In B. B. Wolman (Ed.), *Handbook of developmental psychology.* Englewood Cliffs, NJ: Prentice-Hall.

Denney, N. W., & Denney, D. (1974). Modeling effects on the questioning strategies of the elderly. *Developmental Psychology, 10,* 400–404.

Denney, N. W., Jones, F., & Krigel, S. (1979). Modifying the questioning strategies of young children and elderly adults. *Human Development, 22,* 23–36.

Detterman, D. K. (1980). Understand cognitive components before postulating metacomponents. *Behavioral and Brain Sciences, 3,* 589.

Donaldson, G. (1981). Letter to the editor. *Journal of Gerontology, 36,* 634–636.

Erber, T. J. (1976). Age differences in learning and memory on a digit-symbol substitution task. *Experimental Aging Research, 2,* 45–53.

Grant, E., Storandt, M., & Botwinick, J. (1978). Incentive and practice in the psychomotor performance of the elderly. *Journal of Gerontology, 33,* 413–415.

Gribbin, K., Schaie, K. W., & Parham, I. (1980). Complexity of life style and maintenance of intellectual abilities. *Journal of Social Issues, 21,* 47–61.

Heglin, H. J. (1956). Problem solving set in different age groups. *Journal of Gerontology, 11,* 310–317.

Hofland, B. F. (1981). *Practice effects in the intellectual performance of the elderly: Retesting as an intervention strategy.* Unpublished doctoral dissertation, Pennsylvania State University, University Park.

Hofland, B. F., Willis, S. L., & Baltes, P. B. (1981). Fluid intelligence performance in the elderly: Intraindividual variability and conditions of assessment. *Journal of Educational Psychology, 73,* 573–586.

Hornblum, J. N., & Overton, W. F. (1976). Area and volume conservation among the elderly: Assessment and training. *Developmental Psychology, 12,* 68–74.

Hoyer, W. J. (1974). Aging as intraindividual change. *Developmental Psychology, 10,* 821–826.

Hoyer, W. F., Hoyer, W. J., Treat, N. J., & Baltes, P. B. (1978). Training response speed in young and elderly women. *International Journal of Aging and Human Development.*

Hoyer, W., Labouvie, G., & Baltes, P. B. (1973). Modification of response speed and intellectual performance in the elderly. *Human Development, 16,* 233–242.

Hultsch, D., & Plemons, J. (1979). Life events and life-span development. In P. B. Baltes & O. G. Brim, Jr. (Eds.), *Life-span development and behavior* (Vol. 2). New York: Academic Press.

Kliegl, R., & Baltes, P. B. (in press). Theory-guided analysis of mechanisms of development and aging through testing-the-limits and research on expertise. In C. Schooler & K. W. Schaie (Eds.), *Cognitive functioning and social structure over the life course*. Norwood, NJ: Ablex.

Krauss, I. (1980). Between and within-group comparisons in aging research. In L. W. Poon (Ed.), *Aging in the 1980s* (pp. 542–551). Washington, DC: American Psychological Association.

Labouvie, G., Frohring, W., Baltes, P., & Goulet, L. (1973). Changing relationship between recall performance and abilities as a function of stage of learning and timing of recall. *Journal of Educational Psychology, 64*, 191–198.

Labouvie-Vief, G., & Gonda, J. N. (1976). Cognitive strategy training and intellectual performance in the elderly. *Journal of Gerontology, 31*, 327–332.

Levin, B., & Overton, W. (1979). *Perspective-taking and mental set among the aged: Assessment and training*. Paper presented at a meeting of Society for Research in Child Development.

Lycette, W. H. (1973). Effects of training in overcoming set responses in mature adults. *Dissertation Abstracts, 33B*, 6064.

Meichenbaum, D. (1974). Self-instruction strategy training: A cognitive prosthesis for the aged. *Human Development, 17*, 273–280.

Nesselroade, J. R., Stigler, S. M., & Baltes, P. B. (1980). Regression toward the mean and the study of change. *Psychological Bulletin, 88*, 622–637.

Nunnally, J. (1982). The study of human change: Measurement, research strategies, and methods of analysis. In B. B. Wolman (Ed.), *Handbook of developmental psychology*. Englewood Cliffs, NJ: Prentice-Hall.

Overton, W. F., & Newman, J. (1982). Cognitive development: A competence-activation/utilization approach. In T. Field, A. Houston, H. Quay, L. Troll, & G. Finley (Eds.), *Review of human development*. New York: Wiley.

Plemons, J., Willis, S., & Baltes, P. B. (1978). Modifiability of fluid intelligence in aging: A short-term longitudinal training approach. *Journal of Gerontology, 33*, 224–231.

Sanders, J. C., Sterns, H. L., Smith, M., & Sanders, R. E. (1975). Modification of concept identification performance in older adults. *Developmental Psychology, 11*, 824–829.

Sanders, R. E., & Sanders, J. C. (1978). Long-term durability and transfer of enhanced conceptual performance in the elderly. *Journal of Gerontology, 33*, 408–412.

Schaie, K. W. (1983). The Seattle Longitudinal Study: A twenty-one year investigation of psychometric intelligence. In K. W. Schaie (Ed.), *Longitudinal studies of adult psychological development*. New York: Guilford Press.

Schaie, K. W., & Willis, S. L. (1982). Life span development. In H. E. Mitzel (Ed.), *Encyclopedia of educational research* (5th ed.). New York: Macmillan.

Schaie, K. W., & Willis, S. L. (1985). *Differential ability decline and its remediation in late adulthood*. Paper presented at the annual meeting of the American Psychological Association, Los Angeles.

Schaie, K. W., & Willis, S. L. (1986). Can decline in adult intellectual functioning be reversed? *Developmental Psychology, 22*, 223–232.

Schaie, K. W., Willis, S. L., Hertzog, C., & Schulenberg, J. (1985). *Effects of cognitive training upon primary mental ability structure*. Paper presented at the annual meeting of the American Psychological Association, Los Angeles.

Schultz, N. R., & Hoyer, W. J. (1976). Feedback effects on spatial egocentrism in old age. *Journal of Gerontology, 31*, 72–75.

Sternberg, R. (Ed.). (1982). *Advances in the psychology of human intelligence* (Vol. 1). Hillsdale, NJ: Lawrence Erlbaum.

Sterns, H. L., & Sanders, R. E. (1980). Training and education in the elderly. In R. E. Turner & H. W. Reese (Eds.), *Life-span developmental psychology: Intervention*. New York: Academic Press.

Stone, V. (1980). *Structural modeling of the relations among environmental variables, health status and intelligence in adulthood*. Unpublished doctoral dissertation, University of Southern California, Los Angeles.

Stroop, J. R. (1935). Studies of interference in serial verbal reactions. *Journal of Experimental Psychology, 18,* 643–662.

Thomae, H. (1976). *Patterns of aging.* Basel: Karger.

Thurstone, L. L. (1938). *Primary mental abilities.* University of Chicago Press.

Tomlinson-Keasey, C. (1972). Formal operations in females from eleven to fifty-six years of age. *Developmental Psychology, 6,* 364.

Underwood, G. (1975). *Attention and memory.* New York: Pergamon Press.

Willis, S. L. (1985). Towards an educational psychology of the adult learner. In J. E. Birren & K. W. Schaie (Eds.), *Handbook of the psychology of aging* (2nd ed., pp. 818–847). New York: Van Nostrand Reinhold.

Willis, S. L., & Baltes, P. B. (1980). Intelligence in adulthood and aging: Contemporary issues. In L. W. Poon (Ed.), *Aging in the 1980s* (pp. 260–272). Washington, DC: American Psychological Association.

Willis, S. L., Blieszner, R., & Baltes, P. B. (1981). Intellectual training research in aging: Modification of performance on the fluid ability of figural relations. *Journal of Educational Psychology, 73,* 41–50.

Willis, S. L., Cornelius, S. W., & Baltes, P. B. (1983). Training research in aging: Attentional processes. *Journal of Educational Psychology, 75,* 257–270.

Willis, S. L., & Schaie, K. W. (1981). Maintenance and decline of adult mental abilities: II. Susceptibility to experimental manipulation. In F. Grote & R. Feringer (Eds.), *Adult learning and development.* Bellingham, WA: Western Washington University.

Willis, S. L., & Schaie, K. W. (1986). Training the elderly on the ability factors of spatial orientation and inductive reasoning. *Psychology and Aging, 1,* 239–247.

Wilson, B., & Moffat, N. (Eds.). (1984). *Clinical management of memory problems.* Rockville, MD: Aspen.

Part IIIB

Enhancement approaches

30 Planning practical memory training for the aged

Robin L. West

It is a challenge to address the practical memory needs of older individuals, because psychologists know little about the daily memory demands faced by older adults or the strategies they use to cope with these demands. Recent efforts to investigate "ecological" memory performance have been driven by the desire to maintain experimental control and the desire to examine tasks similar to those studied in the laboratory. This research has rarely been guided by any theoretical or practical evaluation of the memory needs of older adults. Rather, each investigator has identified a task that has appeared to resemble some practical memory situation; that is, it has face validity as an ecological task. In light of this dearth of theorizing or data, I am faced with the dilemma of recommending a program of practical memory training without knowing precisely what the practical memory needs of older persons might be. This review begins, therefore, with an effort to characterize the everyday memory concerns of older adults and to define strategies and tasks that appear to be good candidates for intervention. The chapter concludes with some general recommendations to guide the development of memory-training programs. These recommendations derive from the first part of the chapter, which considers *what* should be trained, as well as from the memory-training literature that considers *how* interventions should be designed.

Strategies and tasks

Tasks

Memory complaints. Subjective memory assessments can help researchers to determine the types of tasks with which older adults have difficulty and to identify their self-perceived strengths and weaknesses as strategic memorizers. The value of self-reports as accurate indicators of the frequency or severity of problems has been questioned (Dixon, Chapter 22, this volume; Herrmann, 1982; Morris, 1984), but the goal here is not to evaluate older adults' prediction accuracy. The predictive failure of such measures may be due to the use of laboratory memory tasks as criterion tests, rather than practical memory measures (Bennett-Levy & Powell, 1980; Berry, West, & Scogin, 1983; Pettinati, Brown, & Mathisen, 1985; Riege, 1982; Sunderland, Watts, Baddeley, & Harris, 1986). Even if a subjective report is not an accurate predictor of task performance, those domains of memory associated with frequent complaints may be the best domains for intervention.

Self-report studies using interviews and questionnaires have attempted to determine the most common, worrisome memory problems of older adults. Unfortunately, responses to specific items have not been reported for the questionnaires with the best psychometric properties (Dixon & Hultsch, 1983; Zelinski, Gilewski, & Thompson, 1980). Often, investigators choose their own items, and items are rarely selected with the older-adult life style in mind. Usually, each investigator analyzes the data into factors or attempts a logical division of the data into factors or attempts a logical division of the items into scales, and these divisions are not always comparable from study to study (Bennett-Levy & Powell, 1980). However, to the extent that agreement occurs across questionnaires, it may be possible to characterize the typical everyday memory concerns of older adults.

On global questions about memory difficulties, the problems experienced most frequently by normal elderly people were forgetting words, names, and object locations, losing the thread of a conversation, and forgetting what they were about to do (Pettinati et al., 1985). With similarly global questions, Zarit (1979) found that a majority of his older adults reported at least some trouble with words, names, immediate memory, memory for recent events, and remembering daily tasks.

Specific memory failures were identified in other studies. Older adults reported more difficulty with short-term memory and remembering recent events that had happened within the last few days (Riege, 1982). Older adults in Sunderland's study reported more problems with words, recalling conversations and object locations, forgetting to take objects, forgetting when something happened, and failing to recall whether or not a task had been completed (Sunderland et al., 1986). Lovelace's subjects (1984) reported more problems in conversation and in completing their actions. No age differences were found in the reported incidences of absentmindedness related to shopping (Reason & Lucas, 1984). On memory diaries, older people described more trouble than the young with recalling names, routine behaviors that needed to be carried out, and objects (remembering to take something with them), but there were no age differences in regard to forgetting locations, facts, appointments, or numbers (Cavanaugh, Grady, & Perlmutter, 1983).

The results of various factor-analytic studies have not been consistent, even when the same questionnaire has been used. On the SIME, which consists of eight forgetting factors, rote-memory ability (recalling information that has been repeated previously) and recent-memory ability declined with age in one study (Chaffin & Herrmann, 1983, exp. I). In a second study, the old reported less difficulty than the young with absentmindedness (including immediate-memory items) and forgetting errands (Chaffin & Herrmann, 1983, exp. II). In a third study, the ability to remember names and recent events declined with age (Chaffin & Herrmann, 1983, exp. III). Also using the SIME, White and Cunningham (1984) found more memory problems for the old than for the young on six factors: names, rote memory, absentmindedness, people, retrieval problems, and conversations.

Conclusions regarding the self-report research are limited by the fact that the various studies covered different domains of tasks. In some cases, data for specific items were reported, and in other cases, scale scores were reported. In some cases the relevant evidence was based solely on age comparisons, whereas in other cases the general frequency of memory failures was reported. Although the common threads are hard to find, one obvious difficulty for older adults is forgetting names (Cavanaugh et al., 1983; Chaffin & Herrmann, 1983, exp. III; Pettinati et al., 1985; White & Cunningham, 1984; Zarit, 1979). It is not surprising that this particular task has received considerable attention in the memory-training literature (Yesavage, Lapp, & Sheikh, Chapter 31, this volume).

In addition to remembering names, older individuals have problems with immediate memory (this includes forgetting what one was about to do) and conversations and have difficulty recalling recent events (secondary memory). Age differences in absentmindedness have been reported, but not in all studies (Chaffin & Herrmann, 1983; Reason & Lucas, 1984). The data on prospective memory (i.e., remembering to complete a task in the future) are inconsistent for remembering appointments (Cavanaugh et al., 1983; Riege, 1982), errands, daily tasks, or routines (Cavanaugh et al., 1983; Chaffin & Herrmann, 1983; Lovelace, 1984; Sunderland et al., 1986; Zarit, 1979). Remembering whether or not a task has already been done is related to prospective memory success and may cause problems for some older adults (Lovelace, 1984; Sunderland et al., 1986).

Age differences. In addition to the self-report data, empirical evidence about everyday memory can help to identify tasks and strategies that should be the focus of training efforts. Ideally, a practical memory task will have (1) content that is practical (e.g., real people are introduced, not slides), (2) encoding conditions that are practical (e.g., a grocery list is written down before making a trip to the store, rather than a list of test items read by an experimenter), (3) retrieval conditions that are practical (e.g., the person walks back through the building to find the exit, and does not draw the path on a piece of paper), and (4) motivations that are practical (e.g., the individual needs to know what he has done, rather than simply trying to remember in order to pass a memory test). These requirements can rarely be met while maintaining essential experimental control. In fact, it is hard to imagine a practical motivation for any memory activity examined in a research setting, because once the investigator intervenes to define what should be remembered, the motivation for memorizing has been altered. As Reed writes:

> For *what* is selected and processed as well as *how* it is remembered are specific to the individual rememberer. The selection of input is determined by the individual's interests

and needs. . . . Whether it is accessible to retrieval and, if so, the form in which it is retrieved are also obviously individualized. (Reed, 1979, p. 17)

The tasks that have been examined in the practical memory literature have attempted to approach the ideal; they often have met one or two of these conditions, but rarely have met all four.

Although the age gap in performance is less consistent on the everyday-memory measures than on traditional laboratory tests, there are areas in which age differences are pervasive. Age-related declines are evident in prose memory, especially memory for details (Hultsch & Dixon, 1984), and spatial memory, including object locations and orientation in large-scale unfamiliar spaces (Kirasic, Chapter 16, this volume). Secondary memory for faces appears to decline with age on recognition tests (Ferris, Crook, Clark, McCarthy, & Rae, 1980; Mason, 1983; Smith & Winograd, 1978), on which older adults consistently have higher false-alarm rates. Tertiary recognition of faces and names, however, does not show significant change with age (Bahrick, 1984; Bahrick, Bahrick, & Wittlinger, 1975). Cued name recall (with a photograph as the cue), on the other hand, shows age-related deficits in secondary (Mason, 1981) as well as tertiary memory (Bahrick, 1984; Bahrick et al., 1975). The data on tertiary free recall of names are mixed (Hanley-Dunn & McIntosh, 1984; Schonfield & Stones, 1979; Warrington & Sanders, 1971).

Age differences have rarely been found for remote memory (Erber, 1981) or prospective memory tasks (Sinnott, Chapter 20, this volume). The data on memory for performed activities are mixed (Bäckman, Chapter 28, this volume; Cohen & Faulkner, Chapter 14, this volume; Kausler, 1985). In other domains of practical memory, such as shopping-list recall or autobiographical memory, there have been only a few studies investigating age differences (Berry et al., 1983; Cavanaugh, 1983; Crook, Ferris, & McCarthy, 1979; Franklin & Holding, 1977; Kausler & Hakami, 1983a; McCarthy, Ferris, Clark, & Crook, 1981; McCormack, 1979; Rubin, Wetzler, & Nebes, 1986). Overall, the results suggest that new learning or episodic memory is problematic for older adults, even when the test conditions are similar to everyday tasks. Except for cued name recall, no tertiary memory task has consistently demonstrated age differences.

Strategies

For practical memory tasks, ''strategy'' should be broadly defined to encompass any method or technique that enhances memory performance, including internal strategies, such as organization and verbal elaboration, and external strategies, such as writing notes and using calendars. To avoid excessive repetition in this chapter, ''strategy'' will be used interchangeably with ''method,'' ''technique,'' ''memory aid,'' and ''mnemonic.''

Strategy knowledge can guide the development of training programs. It would be foolhardy to train an efficient mental visualizer to do imagery, unless of course he had never tried this method in a particular domain and needed guidance.

Memory interventions can be designed (1) to teach effective strategies that are unfamiliar or (2) to build on the older adult's strengths, that is, to improve the effectiveness of a known technique. Whichever approach is used, the trainer should know which mnemonics are already applied in daily life.

Current usage. A number of investigators have asked older adults to report on their strategy usage for laboratory tasks (Camp, Markley, & Kramer, 1983; Canestrari, 1968; Hulicka & Grossman, 1967; Rankin, Karol, & Tuten, 1984; Weinstein, Duffy, Underwood, MacDonald, & Gott, 1981), but few have examined practical memory tasks. External strategies are the most common type of memory aid in everyday situations. In a diary study, 72% of the memory aids mentioned were external (Cavanaugh et al., 1983). Older adults used memory aids more often than young people for prospective tasks – remembering appointments and routines and taking objects with them. The strategic aids reported most often by both age groups were lists and calendars, followed by preparation (using visual external cues) and notes (Cavanaugh et al., 1983). In another diary study completed recently in our laboratory, by West and Bloodworth, young, middle-aged, and older adults were asked to make three entries each day for a week, reporting the memory strategies they used. No age differences in types of strategy usage occurred; about half of the methods described by all age groups were external aids.

Harris (1980) reported that the external aids employed most often by housewives were appointment books, calendars, and shopping lists and that they utilized these methods significantly more often than did students. Internal strategies were rarely employed, but both groups reported occasional usage of mental retracing and alphabetic searching. Lovelace (1984) interviewed older adults to evaluate strategy usage. Mental retracing was the only internal aid used with any frequency. Among 11 methods mentioned, external aids ranked in the top 5 in terms of regular usage. Older adults in another study were asked to describe the internal strategies they would employ for particular everyday memory tasks. Verbal elaboration and rote memorization were reported more often than organization, imagery, or physical/perceptual analysis (Weinstein et al., 1981).

In summary, the strategies utilized most often in daily life were external aids such as lists and calendars. The only internal method cited regularly by the subjects was mental retracing, although rote repetition and elaboration were evident on structured tasks (Weinstein et al., 1981). It is possible that our training efforts should focus on these commonly used methods, because these methods work well. Alternatively, it may be that these techniques are employed out of ignorance or laziness, because more powerful strategies are unfamiliar and/or difficult to put into practice. Empirical investigations of strategic processing should also guide strategy-selection decisions.

Implications from empirical research. To examine the data on strategies that might facilitate performance for the elderly, three areas will be covered: spatial memory, activity memory, and memory for names and faces. In some cases, the research evidence points directly to a strategic intervention that might help the older "learner." In other cases, the strategies recommended here are derived indirectly from the empirical data and will need to be examined in future research.

Spatial memory. Everyday research in this area includes memory for object locations in an array, on a map, or in a room (Light & Zelinski, 1983; Ohta & Kirasic, 1983; Perlmutter, Metzger, Nezworski, & Miller, 1981; Puglisi, Park, Smith, & Hill, 1982; Waddell & Rogoff, 1981; West & Walton, 1985) and recall of configurations, routes, and landmarks in large-scale space (Kirasic, Chapter 16, this volume). There have been a few studies pointing to mnemonic methods that might enhance recall of object locations. In recent in-home interviews, participants were asked to identify the exact current locations of common personal articles such as one's keys. Significant age differences were observed only for recalling the location of one's scissors – older adults were more accurate than young adults and adolescents (West & Walton, 1985). Subjects who were confidently accurate had regular places for their personal articles. Obviously, items that are regularly returned to specific locations are unlikely to be lost.

There is evidence that organized arrays of objects may be easier for older adults to recall than unorganized arrays (Waddell & Rogoff, 1981) and that older adults' attempts to use organized retrieval of object locations are not as effective as those of the young (Charness, 1981b; Waddell & Rogoff, 1981). Perhaps older adults should be encouraged to organize household items systematically. Until the new locations are learned, written descriptions of locations can be reviewed regularly, perhaps with an expanded rehearsal technique (Moffat, Chapter 34, this volume). It also appears that a well-learned pattern or arrangement will not easily be forgotten. Kirasic found, for instance, that older adults were able to locate store items as well as the young in unfamiliar supermarkets, even though some other aspects of spatial knowledge showed deficits (Kirasic & Allen, 1985). This is probably because supermarket layouts do not vary that much from store to store (e.g., dairy, meat, and produce sections usually are around the outside edges), and the layout of a new store can be deciphered by fitting it into a known pattern of store organization. Older adults ought to be encouraged to use comparable household arrangements whenever they move, in order to reduce some of the memory demands involved in resettling.

To enhance retrieval of current locations of items, individuals need to learn ways to link items to locations. Well-known mnemonics will suffice for this memory activity. Older adults can take an extra few seconds when something is put down (e.g., glasses are placed on the television set) to use interactive imagery (e.g., "see" the glasses wrapped around the TV) or verbal elaboration (e.g., "I watch the TV's glass picture through my glasses") to encode the link.

It is not clear how often older adults need to learn their way around new environments. Clearly, older adults have difficulty in unfamiliar areas (Kirasic, Chapter 16, this volume). Because it is not a daily task for most people – maneuvering in familiar environments is far more common – older adults do not report that they are having difficulty with large-scale spatial memory. For those who are concerned about it, the strategic recommendations are not easy to pin down:

1. Should older adults rely on spatial inferences or spatial memory? Ohta and his colleagues (Ohta, Walsh, & Krauss, 1981) asked subjects to view three model buildings (placed on a turntable) from seven specific perspectives, or to study each building separately. The young recognized the correct slides more often than the old in both conditions, although the older subjects made 50% fewer errors in the second condition than in the first (Ohta et al., 1981). Because the first task emphasized memory for specific perspective views, these authors concluded that older adults perform better by making spatial inferences than by memorizing specific views. In another study, however, perspective taking was better after all perspective positions were previewed (Herman & Coyne, 1980).

2. Do older adults need to learn how to integrate spatial information presented sequentially? When an area is viewed via videotape, the subject has to create an internal configuration of the entire area by integrating the sequenced information on the videotape. Integration is not required when the entire area is explored. Older adults' performances were worse after a simulated videotaped tour than after inspection of an entire model city in one case (Walsh, Krauss, & Regnier, 1981), but not in another (Ohta & Kirasic, 1983).

3. What kind of mental-rotation strategy should older adults use? Imagined self-movement increased memory scores in one study (Kirasic, 1980), whereas imagined movement of the array worked better in another (Herman & Coyne, 1980). Such inconsistencies do not provide guidance for strategic recommendations.

One technique that may facilitate memory for large-scale spaces is organization. In comparison with younger adults, older adults were less organized in making neighborhood maps (Walsh et al., 1981) and in recalling landmarks (Evans, Brennan, Skorpanich, & Held, 1984) and demonstrated less organized configurational knowledge (Ohta et al., 1981). Older adults can be encouraged to plot a small area on a grid system to get an organized picture of where things are located. Because familiar areas are more easily remembered (Kirasic, 1980), individuals should be encouraged to compare new areas with known areas in terms of spatial organization (e.g., many cities share a particular street design).

Familiarity is clearly influential in spatial memory. Older adults performed better in locating landmarks that they had encountered more often (Herman & Bruce, 1981), and regular movement in specific environments enhanced recall of those environments (Bahrick, 1979; Walsh et al., 1981) and eliminated age differences in recall (Sinnott, 1984). Scene recognition, route planning, and behavioral efficiency (taking the shortest route) inside a familiar grocery store did not vary with age, whereas age differences in scene recognition and scanning methods did occur in an unfamiliar supermarket (Kirasic & Allen, 1985). Older adults' distance and directional estimates between target sites within a laboratory array were significantly less accurate than estimates made by the young. For target sites within their hometown, on the other hand, their performances were comparable to those of the young (Kirasic & Allen, 1985).

Why is spatial memory better in familiar environments? Self-paced acquisition, distributed practice, and overlearning are likely to occur in those environments. Older adults can be taught to use these methods in learning new environments. Frequent movement in new areas should aid spatial memory. Older adults can practice walking through or drawing maps of a new area. They can identify landmarks and then visualize these structures repeatedly in perspective with known landmarks, and they can add landmark identifiers to maps to facilitate configurational learning.

Activity memory. A variety of tasks can be included within the domain of activity memory: episodic recall of activities already performed (Bäckman, Chapter 28, this volume; Cohen & Faulkner, Chapter 14, this volume; Kausler, 1985; Ratner & Bushey, 1984; Sinnott, 1986), recall of instructions that describe activities to be carried out (Botwinick & Storandt, 1974; West & Walton, 1985), recall of activities performed in vivo (Sinnott, 1986; West & Walton, 1985), and prospective memory (Sinnott, Chapter 5, this volume). The strategy recommendations often vary as a function of task type.

The research on memory for performed activities has raised some interesting questions about rehearsal, organization, and task familiarity. Kausler (1985) emphasizes that the lack of difference between incidental and intentional recall conditions in his studies indicates that encoding of activities is effortless and rehearsal-independent. It is apparent that serial rehearsal contributes very little to the recall of performed activities (Bäckman, Chapter 28, this volume; Kausler, Lichty, & Davis, in press). At the same time, retrieval of such activities is effortful (Kausler, 1985), and organization may facilitate recall (Bäckman, Chapter 28, this volume). Older adults might be encouraged, then, to use organization to enhance recall of activities by planning similar activities for the same time (prospective memory). This will make it easier to remember to do the tasks and to recall that the tasks have been completed.

Kausler has suggested that distinctiveness may enhance activity memory (Kausler & Hakami, 1983b). If that is the case, older adults can be taught to use verbal elaborative or imaginal strategies to make specific activities more memorable. This technique will be especially useful for recalling whether or not a routine activity has been completed. If distinctive encoding can make each day's locking of the door memorable, the older adult will not need to compulsively check to ensure that the task has been accomplished (West, 1985).

Prospective tasks can be remembered with interactive imagery or verbal elaborations that link errands or appointments. Hierarchical organization of activities according to goals may also be appropriate for prospective memory and retrospective retrieval (Meacham, 1982), because higher-level goals are more easily recalled than details (Ratner & Bushey, 1984) and may be used as cues for the details. Time monitoring can also be beneficial (Ceci & Bronfenbrenner, 1985;

Harris & Wilkins, 1982). External aids are key elements in accurate prospective memory (Moscovitch, 1982; Poon & Schaffer, 1982). West (1984) used prospective memory tasks with adolescents, young adults, and older adults. The research participants were asked to phone an answering machine one night and leave a message indicating how they remembered to call, as well as to mail a postcard (2 days later) containing a message about how they remembered. Older adults performed better than young adults in remembering to do the task (likely to be rehearsed externally) and performed worse than the young in remembering to include the required message (likely to be rehearsed internally). External aids obviously can be used to remember that a task has been completed (that item is crossed off a list, the timer is not running, the pill bottle is not on the counter), as well as to remember to do the task in the first place.

Task familiarity appears to affect activity recall. Recall of simple everyday tasks does not show age differences (Bäckman & Nilsson, 1984), whereas recall of previously performed cognitive tasks does vary with age (Kausler, Lichty, & Freund, 1985). Cognitive tests that include arithmetic problems are remembered better than tests consisting of unfamiliar tasks such as paired-associate learning (Kausler & Hakami, 1983b). What makes familiar activities easier to remember? Perhaps mental or kinesthetic imagery of such activities is easier. Older adults might be able to improve their ability to recall all kinds of activities by practicing imagery mnemonics.

Memory for names and faces. The research on memory for names and faces includes studies of episodic memory for names and/or faces presented in the laboratory and studies of remote memory for faces and names acquired in vivo. Facial-recognition data show little age change in terms of misses and significant age increases in false alarms on laboratory stimuli (Ferris et al., 1980; Smith & Winograd, 1978). In the real world, the false alarm is the safest kind of error to make. (Strangers rarely mind if one walks up and says, "Have I met you somewhere before?" Acquaintances may resent it if one fails to recognize them.) The self-report data indicated that facial recognition is not much of a problem for adults (Bennett-Levy & Powell, 1980). Consequently, older adults may not need to learn new methods for face recognition. The best methods to use are to identify distinctive features and to evaluate the face in terms of personality or friendliness (Smith & Winograd, 1978; Warrington & Ackroyd, 1975; Winograd, 1978).

Name–face matching and cued name recall appear to be problems for older adults, even when the information is acquired in vivo (Bahrick et al., 1975). Studies of in vivo learning provide some clues to appropriate training. In an investigation of memory for high school classmates, the names of close friends and romantic interests were recalled more often than were other classmates. Also, forgetting in cued name recall appeared to be due to forgetting the association or relationship one had had with a classmate. If the association was recalled, the name was recalled, suggesting that social context can serve as a mnemonic cue for a name (Bahrick et al., 1975).

Tertiary memory research also showed that older adults' "savings" on a name-recall task were comparable to those of the young during relearning (Bahrick, 1984), that distributed practice and overlearning can help adults retain associated names and faces (Bahrick et al., 1975), that highly familiar names can be recalled after many years (Schonfield & Stones, 1979; Warrington & Sanders, 1971), and that lists of names of familiar individuals are easier for older adults to recall than are lists of unfamiliar individuals (Hanley-Dunn & McIntosh, 1984). These data suggest that distributed practice and overlearning can be beneficial (Morris, 1979). Older adults can be encouraged to use lists for names and review and/or relearn the names at regular intervals. Each time the list is practiced, there should be some savings (i.e., relearning should occur faster than original learning). Where possible, individuals can make appearance notes on the list so that they can match facial features with names during review sessions (West, 1985).

Visual-imagery mnemonics are definitely valuable for learning names (Yesavage et al., Chapter 31, this volume). Verbal elaboration may also improve memory, because semantic orienting facilitates facial recognition for older adults as much as for younger adults (Smith & Winograd, 1978). Also, identification of distinctive facial features is a useful strategy (Winograd, 1978). Combining these two beneficial methods, older adults might be trained to do name-appropriate semantic orienting. If Mr. Winter's smile is his most distinctive feature, the individual can ask himself, as he examines the face, "Does Mr. Winter have a winning smile?" Verbal elaboration can be employed to match the name with the person's distinctive feature. If Wade Callum is always smiling, one might remember that "he is happy as a clam (Callum) wading (Wade)." Efficient use of these techniques will require repeated practice sessions, similar to those needed for verbal elaboration and imagery. Such semantic and verbal strategies should be included in training as well as imagery techniques (Cermak, 1980; Winograd & Simon, 1980).

In summary, it is obvious that there is much to be done in the area of practical memory training. Researchers are just beginning to understand the factors that influence age differences in performance and are far away from defining specific strategic interventions with any confidence. Age-related deficits are evident on a wide range of practical memory tasks, but if older adults are asked about their memory problems, they complain more about names and faces, conversations, and primary and secondary memory difficulties. A training program aimed at common complaints should focus on those particular problems.

The selection of strategies depends on one's goals. Training can be designed to maximize successful application of known strategies, in which case elaborative associations, mental retracing, and external aids should be included. Alternatively, training can be designed to teach strategies that can be widely applied and are known to lead to success, such as organization and imagery. Strategies can be trained as memory tools that can be applied generally or as techniques that apply in specific circumstances. Organization enhances memory, but it may need to be taught as a domain-specific memory aid, because organizing spatial knowledge can be very different from organizing prospective memory tasks. Familiarity facilitates memory, but its impact may also be domain-specific. Unfortunately, it is not yet clear how to translate knowledge about the influence of familiarity into strategic interventions.

General recommendations

Assessment and individual differences

Many issues related to assessment and individual differences have been discussed elsewhere, including the importance of subject characteristics and motivation (Erickson, Poon, & Walsh-Sweeney, 1980; Poon, 1980; Poon, Fozard, & Treat, 1978; Poon, Walsh-Sweeney, & Fozard, 1980; Robertson-Tchabo, 1980; Treat, Poon, Fozard, & Popkin, 1978). Two additional assessment issues will be considered here.

One limitation of training efforts at this time is the lack of assessments of everyday memory. Measures are available for examining age differences in memory for activities (Kausler & Hakami, 1983b), environments (Kirasic & Allen, 1985), prose (Meyer & Rice, 1981), grocery lists (McCarthy et al., 1981), and television programs (Cavanaugh, 1983), but there are no comprehensive batteries comparable to the widely used Wechsler Memory Scale (Wechsler, 1945). However, test development in this area has begun (Poon, 1980; West & Walton, 1985; Wilson & Moffat, 1984b). As this research progresses, the everyday memory demands of the older adult need to be evaluated. It is quite possible, for example, that older adults never memorize 10 new names in one setting, and a test for that skill may be inappropriate.

The usual approach to assessment has been to examine test scores, but it is just as important to measure strategies. Poor performance may be due to any number of factors: (1) failure to use a known technique, (2) inefficient use of an appropriate strategy, (3) use of an inappropriate or weak method, and (4) lack of any strategy knowledge. We need to be more sophisticated about measuring encoding and retrieval processes, because interventions tailored for individuals may be more successful. Inconsistent strategy producers may be aided by practice alone, whereas nonusers require a more powerful intervention (Asarnow & Meichenbaum, 1979). After training, a nonuser can apply a newly learned technique without changing his level of performance if he applies the strategy ineffectively or periodically. Postassessments that focus on performance levels alone will not identify this very important change in behavior that may ultimately lead (with more practice) to higher test scores.

Measures of encoding and retrieval processes can be direct or indirect. Clustering, for instance, is a direct measure of categorical organization (Schmitt, Murphy, & Sanders, 1981). Rehearsal can be measured by observations of lip movements, overt processing, and primacy effects (Sanders, Murphy, Schmitt, & Walsh, 1980). Think-aloud procedures may be used to identify attempts to organize, imagine, associate, or elaborate. In an examination of object-location memory, older adults can be given the opportunity to place items in rooms on a diagram. Strategic placement will be indicated by the extent to which items are placed in associated rooms (e.g., the towel is placed in the bathroom). Clock-watching (Ceci & Bronfenbrenner, 1985) and note-writing can be assessed as prospective memory strategies. The speed with which images or associations are generated may be one indicator of processing efficiency, as well as the quality of the images or associations (Hartley, 1982). Comparable postassessments of strategy effectiveness can quantify processing advances that are not reflected by significant performance changes.

Generalization and maintenance

The overriding goal of any memory intervention program should be to demonstrate that trained strategies can be maintained and can be applied to tasks other than the particular one used in training. Few studies with older adults have accomplished either of these goals (Poon, 1985; Poon et al., 1980; Scogin, Storandt, & Lott, 1985). Generalization and maintenance can be distinguished, although often they are affected by the same factors (Borkowski & Cavanaugh, 1979). For instance, motivation and social reinforcement can affect both (Poon, 1980; Treat et al., 1978). Other influential factors are ease of strategy usage, focus of training, and training effectiveness.

Ease of usage. If it is the case that older adults have reduced processing resources (Craik & Byrd, 1982), strategies with heavy processing demands may be avoided. Instead, the older adult may employ strategies that are less burdensome (Cohen & Faulkner, 1983; Robertson-Tchabo, 1980). The trainer can choose, then, to teach strategies that require less resources (e.g., teach older adults to create one interactive image to recall a few errands, rather than teaching them the more demanding peg system). Alternatively, the trainer can make the strategy automatic so that it will be easier to use and less demanding.

Hasher and Zacks (1979) suggested that automatic behaviors do not change with age. Tasks may become automatic (Shiffrin & Schneider, 1977) or may be automatic by their very nature (Hasher & Zacks, 1979; 1984). Age differences have been evident on tasks defined as automatic by Hasher and Zacks (Kausler, 1985). In contrast, it has not yet been demonstrated that tasks on which adults have *acquired* automaticity will remain stable across the adult life span, although there are indications that this may be the case (Charness, 1981a, 1981b; Murrell & Humphries, 1978; Poon & Fozard, 1978).

If the original characterization of automaticity is correct, acquired automatic behaviors should not be affected by age-related capacity limitations, because they require minimal processing resources (Hasher & Zacks, 1979). Then, the goal of training should be to generate automatic usage of good memory strategies through extensive and repeated practice. Both generalization and maintenance will be more likely if this can be done.

Focus of training. Generally speaking, memory training is much like what the mathematics teacher does in the classroom. She says, "Here is an algebra problem; go solve it with algebra. Here is a trigonometry problem; go simplify the sines and cosines. Here is a geometry problem; calculate the angle." What she does not do, and what is not done typically during memory training, is to say, "Here are some problems. I've taught you some formulas, decide which formula you should apply and then get the answer." Strategies typically are taught and practiced on one task (Rose & Yesavage, 1983) without any discussion of the decision rules that allow the individual to select an appropriate processing method. It needs to be made explicit that strategies are the means to the goal of memorizing and that *every* decision to memorize ought to be accompanied by a strategy-selection process (West, 1985).

Generalization should be an explicit goal of training. Practice sessions can focus only on one method, but once a technique is mastered, the subjects ought to be invited to apply it to other tasks during training sessions or at home. Subjects should be told the critical features of tasks on which the trained processes can be used. For instance, interactive imagery will be useful on any memory task that requires a link between two or more items: paired associates, shopping lists, errand lists, objects and their locations, persons that need to be seen (appointments) and the times to see them (using clock images). If a strategy facilitates performance on more than one type of task, it probably will be practiced more often in daily life and may be maintained longer for that reason.

Alternatively, generalization can be built into the training itself. Planning for broader types of training should be done cautiously – it is just as likely that it is not effective to teach older adults multiple techniques for multiple memory tasks in multiple sessions. That could overburden slow-learning older adults, although some success has been achieved under those conditions (Zarit, Cole, & Guider, 1981a; Zarit, Gallagher, & Kramer, 1981b). An alternative approach, providing an opportunity to establish convergent validity, might be to teach the same memory strategy in multiple task situations. Organizational techniques are appropriate for remembering grocery lists, routes, errands, pills, number series, or facts from prose. One group trained to use this strategy for two different tasks can be compared with a group trained to use verbal elaboration for two tasks, or a group trained to use interactive imagery. The impact of training can be measured by examining performance on those two tasks, as well as generalization to other practical memory tasks. Homework assignments should encourage participants to identify memory tasks in their own environments to which the strategy can be applied.

Training effectiveness. Strategies that are very well learned are more likely to lead to improved scores on immediate testing and to better maintenance and generalization. The experimenter must see that all features of a technique are mastered and that the subjects are well aware of their increased memory success after training.

Component analysis of a strategy, before training, is recommended. For maximum benefit, each component can then be trained. For example, the image–name matching method employed for training cued name recall (Yesavage, et al., Chapter 31, this volume) has several aspects to it: (1) Identify an individual's prominent feature (a perceptual process should be). (2) Identify an imageable key word in the name (a concrete word embedded in the name is discovered through verbal mediation). (3) Convert the key word to an image (mental imagery). (4) Imagine the person's face, with the key-word image by the prominent feature (interactive mental imagery). If execution of any one of these steps is weak, the subject is unlikely to use the method very well a month or two after training. Also, one key to generalization is to recognize that strategy components can be applied elsewhere. Interactive mental imagery (step number 4) is clearly advantageous for other memory tasks, as is verbal mediation (step number 2). If these steps are not mastered independently, the subject cannot generalize and use one step for a different type of task (Borkowski & Buchel, 1983).

Fading techniques can be applied to ensure that the strategy can be employed without the trainer looking over the subject's shoulder: Each individual step is trained. The experimenter explains how to apply all of the steps together, with examples. The experimenter cues each step, in order, for the next few practice exercises. The experimenter cues the subject to utilize the technique on the next few examples. Then he provides no cue for some trials, but asks for strategy descriptions after recall. Finally, no cue is given, and no strategy query is made. This procedure can reinforce spontaneous self-directed application of the strategy, as in self-instructional procedures (Meichenbaum, 1977).

Interventions must have built-in mechanisms to provide feedback. This feedback ought to be given by the experimenter after or during postassessments, emphasizing that test scores on trained tasks are increasing. Feedback on strategy effectiveness has been necessary to achieve maintenance in studies with retarded children (Asarnow & Meichenbaum, 1979; Borkowski & Buchel, 1983). Subjects should also be encouraged to use behavior checklists at home before and after training to monitor memory successes and failures. Such in vivo demonstrations of success may be more powerful motivators to continue strategic behaviors and to attempt to apply newly learned techniques to a range of memory tasks.

Strategies

Gerontologists have only scratched the surface of practical memory training. Of the basic methods taught by mnemonists that are known to improve performance (Cermak, 1975; Higbee, 1977; Lorayne & Lucas, 1974), only two have been used in more than a couple of studies: the method of loci (Anschutz, Camp, Markley, & Kramer, 1985; Robertson-Tchabo, Hausman, & Arenberg,

1976; Rose & Yesavage, 1983; Yesavage & Rose, 1984) and the image–name matching method (Yesavage et al., Chapter 31, this volume). Others, such as the peg system (Mason & Smith, 1977) and the PQRST (Wilson & Moffat, 1984a), have been largely ignored. Little attention has been paid to techniques that are clearly beneficial in the laboratory, such as elaboration (Hulicka & Grossman, 1967), organization (Hultsch, 1969), and rehearsal (Schmitt et al., 1981).

Very few studies have worked with practical memory tasks. Training has focused too much on trying to improve the ability of older adults to recall lists of words or paired associates with visual imagery (Poon et al., 1980). The only practical memory task that has been trained extensively is cued name recall (Yesavage, Rose, & Bower, 1983). That research has yielded valuable data, but future training efforts should focus on more everyday tasks and on a broader range of encoding and retrieval processes.

Task-specific strategies were examined earlier. Here, the emphasis shifts to types of strategies that can be applied generally. Two methods that have received little attention, in spite of their potential value, are verbal elaboration and self-instruction. Two other training areas that have been totally neglected are retrieval techniques and external aids.

Verbal coding. In spite of early indications that verbal elaboration might be a strategy that older adults would employ (Canestrari, 1968; Hulicka & Grossman, 1967), efforts to train elaborative techniques have been very limited. This is surprising given the evidence that older adults maintain their ability to recall high associates (Rabinowitz, Craik, & Ackerman, 1982) and to perform intelligence-test tasks that rely on using verbal information from semantic memory (Botwinick, 1977). Also, the evidence suggests that their semantic-memory networks are comparable to those of young adults (Howard, McAndrews, & Lasaga, 1981). Verbal-elaboration strategies will train older adults to access the considerable semantic knowledge they have to serve their memory.

Self-monitoring. The dearth of self-instructional training is puzzling, because these methods were recommended 10 years ago (Treat et al., 1978), and efforts to utilize this paradigm have met with some success (Adams, Rebok, & King, 1981; Labouvie-Vief & Gonda, 1976). Diverse pieces of evidence suggest that self-instructional techniques can provide a powerful means to teach older adults how to monitor and control on-task strategic processing:

1. Many of the complaints of older adults may reflect a failure to maintain attention to the task at hand – immediate memory problems, forgetting what they are about to do, forgetting where objects have been placed, failing to recall what has been said in conversation by themselves or by others. Older adults can profit from paying greater attention to their own memorizing behavior, especially if they have been using overlearned memory routines (Langer, 1978). One way to improve the performance of older adults might be to increase their self-awareness of on-task memory processing.

2. Studies of metamemorial monitoring show age-related deficits (Cavanaugh, Chapter 23, this volume). Older adults do not initiate newly learned strategic methods (Poon et al., 1980); they overestimate their abilities (Bruce, Coyne, & Botwinick, 1982); they stop studying before they are ready to recall (Murphy, Sanders, Gabriesheski, & Schmitt, 1981). If on-task monitoring is taught directly, older adults are more likely to apply the metamemorial knowledge they have.

3. A focus on self-regulation may be a prerequisite to systematic practical application of memory aids. The experimenter cannot stand behind the individual to cue strategic processing. To initiate and execute the strategy oneself, an encoding and retrieval plan needs to be internalized. Self-instructions offer a useful mechanism for doing that. Furthermore, the most successful demonstration of generalization and maintenance of training among retarded children, according to Kramer, Nagle, and Engle (1980), was one that taught self-regulation to the children (Brown, Campione, & Barclay, 1979). Also, self-instructional techniques that emphasize discovery learning improve children's generalization more than does didactic training (Cohen & Meyers, 1984). It remains to be seen whether or not self-instructional methods will have the same positive impact on older adults.

Retrieval. The scarcity of retrieval-training studies is particularly troublesome for two reasons: (1) Much of everyday memory involves incidental memory (Kausler, 1985). (2) Retrieval deficits are evident in aging (Burke & Light, 1981; Craik & Rabinowitz, 1985). When encoding has been incidental, there are no special encoded cues to access during retrieval. Thus, with incidental learning, recall relies solely on appropriate retrieval techniques.

Even when encoding is intentional and strategies are used to support encoding, some kind of retrieval plan is still necessary (Bower, 1970a). Will older adults be able to reconstruct the categories, distinctive features, semantic associations, or environmental cues that were identified during strategic encoding? Although there are indications that some search processes may not decline substantially with age or may be automatic (Eriksen, Hamlin, & Daye, 1973; Lachman & Lachman, 1980), when the search fails, effortful age-dependent processes may be needed to bring the information back to mind (Kausler & Hakami, 1983b). Older adults certainly report problems of this nature when automatic semantic-memory searches do not produce a word or name (Bowles & Poon, 1985). Also, research suggests that supportive memory guidance needs to be provided at both encoding and retrieval for older adults to benefit from the support (Craik & Simon, 1980; West & Cohen, 1985; Perlmutter & Mitchell, 1982; Craik & Rabinowitz, 1985). It is no accident that the most effective training methods are those in which the strategy itself has inherent retrieval mechanisms (e.g., for the method of loci, one thinks about the first well-known location along a path to remember the image of some object mentally placed in that location) (Bower, 1970b).

There are indications that older adults would be receptive to retrieval training. The only internal strategies reportedly used frequently by middle-aged and older adults are not encoding strategies, but retrieval strategies such as alphabetic search and mental retracing (Harris, 1980). Although older adults may already utilize mental retracing, their mental retracing may not be as organized or systematic as it could be to promote consistent memory success. Thus, the elderly can be taught to remember information using methods based on the principle of encoding specificity (Reddy & Bellezza, 1983; Tulving & Thomson, 1973). They can learn how to work back through association networks to recall the encoded information. Older adults can be trained to reinstate encoding conditions by thinking back to the initial context: recalling their mood (Bower, 1981), distinctive features of the information or setting that may remain clear (Jacoby & Craik, 1979), related information (Peeck, 1982), or the gist of the event, and then working back in a hierarchical fashion to the details (Ratner & Bushey, 1984; Wood, 1972). Hierarchical retrieval may be particularly effective with prospective memory tasks (Brewer & Dupree, 1983; Meacham, 1982).

Methods that enhance retrieval may also be taught in order to facilitate memory for the trained strategy per se. For instance, older adults should be encouraged to use distributed practice or expanded-interval rehearsal (Moffat, Chapter 34, this volume) to maintain the mnemonics they have learned.

External aids. If the goal is to increase memory success for older adults, external memory aids provide a powerful complement to internal strategies, and they are clearly advantageous in everyday situations (Cavanaugh et al., 1983; Harris, 1980; Moscovitch, 1982; West, 1984). External strategies that may be broadly applied and are compatible with existing memory practices can be used for training. It would not be desirable, however, to emphasize these techniques to the exclusion of all internal methods, because some practical memory tasks require internal memory.

Older adults may not be using external mnemonics in the best possible way. Cavanaugh and his colleagues discovered, for example, that older adults reported using external aids more often than young adults to remember objects, but at the same time they reported more incidents that involved forgetting objects than did younger adults (Cavanaugh et al., 1983). West and Walton (1985) found that external aids were used only for a few everyday memory tasks, when they could have been used productively for many more. Just as organization is sometimes carried out haphazardly by older adults (Smith, 1980), their application of external strategies may be inefficient. External aids essentially provide support for internal memory (Wilson & Moffat, 1984b). To use note-writing successfully, for example, the individual has to remember to write the note, to write sufficient specific details, to place the note where it can be easily found or seen as a cue, and to consult the note when it is needed. Failure on any one of these steps will result in ineffective utilization of notes.

Other external aids also have practical value: calendars, address and telephone books, pill boxes, a pill "clock" reminder system, selected memory places for objects, specific object cues in the environment (e.g., leaving out a coat to take to the cleaners), and general reminders such as timers or strings (West, 1985).

Harris (1978) points out that the most appropriate external cues are specific to the task, portable and easy to use, applicable to a wide range of tasks, active rather than passive reminders, and time-tied to the task rather than temporally distant, as forgetting can occur very rapidly (Harris & Wilkins, 1982).

In summary, assessments for memory training need to place more emphasis on measurement of strategic processing during everyday memory tasks. In this way, researchers can examine the impact of training on strategies as well as performance. Techniques that are very well learned will be more likely to be maintained and generalized, especially if the value of the method is made very apparent to the participants. Strategies that are easy to use, more automatic, or less demanding of processing resources are more likely to be used extensively to meet practical needs. Intervention programs can focus more on generalization, in part by building generalization into the training (e.g., by practicing on a variety of different tasks). In addition to specific mnemonics appropriate for single tasks, teaching of retrieval methods, external aids, and self-monitoring behaviors can be beneficial to the older adult.

Conclusions

In planning training programs for everyday memory, the investigator should consider a number of factors: (1) the memory demands of older adults, particularly tasks that present problems for individuals (recalling names, maintaining attention to information in immediate memory, remembering object locations, landmarks, and routes in unfamiliar surroundings); (2) strategies that older adults might benefit from using, including organization, distributed practice and overlearning, retrieval processing, external aids, verbal elaboration, and self-monitoring of on-task behavior; (3) approaches that will enhance maintenance and generalization.

Future intervention efforts should assess and train more everyday skills, teach a wider variety of strategies that build on the older adult's existing memory strengths, and help older adults to develop decision rules for when and why to apply effective memory strategies in their everyday environments. Before older adults will use trained strategies consistently for everyday tasks, they will need to see that the strategy is attainable, that it improves their ability in their daily environment, that the technique is not easily forgotten, and that, once learned, it is not too difficult to put in practice. When techniques can be easily applied to one's daily life, and clearly lead to success, the success serves as its own motivator for maintenance and generalization of strategic processing.

References

Adams, C. C., Rebok, G. W., & King, M. H. (1981, November). *Facilitating intellectual functioning in older adults: A metacognitive approach.* Paper presented at a meeting of the Gerontological Society of America, Toronto.

Anschutz, L., Camp, C. J., Markley, R. P., & Kramer, J. J. (1985). Maintenance and generalization of mnemonics for grocery shopping by older adults. *Experimental Aging Research, 11*, 157–160.

Asarnow, J. R., & Meichenbaum, D. (1979). Verbal rehearsal and serial recall: The mediational training of kindergarten children. *Child Development, 50*, 1173–1177.

Bäckman, L., & Nilsson, L. G. (1984). Aging effects in free recall: An exception to the rule. *Human Learning, 3*, 53–70.

Baddeley, A., Lewis, V., & Nimmo-Smith, I. (1978). When did you last . . . ? In M. M. Gruneberg, P. E. Morris, & R. N. Sykes (Eds.), *Practical aspects of memory* (pp. 77–83). London: Academic Press.

Bahrick, H. P. (1979). Maintenance of knowledge: Questions about memory we forgot to ask. *Journal of Experimental Psychology: General, 108*, 296–308.

Bahrick, H. P. (1984). Memory for people. In J. E. Harris & P. E. Morris (Eds.), *Everyday memory, actions and absentmindedness* (pp. 19–34). London: Academic Press.

Bahrick, H. P., Bahrick, P. O., & Wittlinger, R. P. (1975). Fifty years of memory for names and faces: A cross-sectional approach. *Journal of Experimental Psychology: General, 104*, 54–75.

Bellezza, F. S. (1982). Updating memory using mnemonic devices. *Cognitive Psychology, 14*, 301–327.

Bennett-Levy, J., & Powell, G. E. (1980). The Subjective Memory Questionnaire (SMQ). An investigation into the self-reporting of "real-life" memory skills. *British Journal of Social and Clinical Psychology, 19*, 177–188.

Berry, J., West, R., & Scogin, F. (1983, November). *Predicting everyday and laboratory memory skill.* Paper presented at a meeting of the Gerontological Society of America, San Francisco.

Borkowski, J. G., & Buchel, F. P. (1983). Learning and memory strategies in the mentally retarded. In M. Pressley & J. P. Levin (Eds.), *Cognitive strategy research: Psychological foundations* (pp. 103–128). New York: Springer-Verlag.

Borkowski, J. G., & Cavanaugh, J. C. (1979). Maintenance and generalization of skills and strategies by the retarded. In N. R. Ellis (Ed.), *Handbook of mental deficiency: Psychological theory and research* (2nd ed., pp. 569–617). Hillsdale, NJ: Lawrence Erlbaum.

Botwinick, J. (1977). Intellectual abilities. In J. E. Birren & K. W. Schaie (Eds.), *Handbook of the psychology of aging* (pp. 580–605). New York: Van Nostrand Reinhold.

Botwinick, J., & Storandt, M. (1974). *Memory related functions and age.* Springfield: Charles C. Thomas.

Bower, G. H. (1970a). Organizational factors in memory. *Cognitive Psychology, 1*, 18–46.

Bower, G. H. (1970b). Analysis of a mnemonic device. *American Scientist, 58*, 496–510.

Bower, G. H. (1981). Mood and memory. *American Psychologist, 36*, 129–148.

Bowles, N. L., & Poon, L. W. (1985). Aging and retrieval of words in semantic memory. *Journal of Gerontology, 40*, 71–77.

Brewer, W. F., & Dupree, D. A. (1983). Use of plan schemata in the recall and recognition of goal-directed actions. *Journal of Experimental Psychology: Learning, Memory, and Cognition, 9*, 117–129.

Brown, A. L., Campione, J. C., & Barclay, C. R. (1979). Training self-checking routines for estimating test readiness: Generalization from list learning to prose recall. *Child Development, 50*, 501–512.

Bruce, P. R., Coyne, A. C., & Botwinick, J. (1982). Adult age differences in metamemory. *Journal of Gerontology, 37*, 354–357.

Burke, D. M., & Light, L. L. (1981). Memory and aging: The role of retrieval processes. *Psychological Bulletin, 90*, 513–546.

Camp, C. J., Markley, R. P., & Kramer, J. J. (1983). Spontaneous use of mnemonics by elderly individuals. *Educational Gerontology, 9*, 57–71.

Canestrari, R. E., Jr. (1968). Age changes in acquisition. In G. A. Talland (Ed.), *Human aging and behavior* (pp. 169–188). New York: Academic Press.

Cavanaugh, J. C. (1983). Comprehension and retention of television programs by 20- and 60-year olds. *Journal of Gerontology, 38,* 190–196.

Cavanaugh, J. C., Grady, J. G., & Perlmutter, M. (1983). Forgetting and use of memory aids in 20- to 70-year-olds' everyday life. *International Journal of Aging and Human Development, 17,* 113–122.

Ceci, S. J., & Bronfenbrenner, U. (1985). "Don't forget to take the cupcakes out of the oven": Prospective memory, strategic time-monitoring, and context. *Child Development, 56,* 152–164.

Cermak, L. S. (1975). *Improving your memory.* New York: McGraw-Hill.

Cermak, L. S. (1980). Comments on imagery as a therapeutic mnemonic. In L. W. Poon, J. L. Fozard, L. S. Cermak, D. Arenberg, & L. W. Thompson (Eds.), *New directions in memory and aging: Proceedings of the George A. Talland memorial conference* (pp. 507–510). Hillsdale, NJ: Lawrence Erlbaum.

Chaffin, R., & Herrmann, D. J. (1983). Self-reports of memory abilities by old and young adults. *Human Learning, 2,* 17–28.

Charness, N. (1981a). Aging and skilled problem solving. *Journal of Experimental Psychology: General, 110,* 21–38.

Charness, N. (1981b). Visual short-term memory and aging in chess players. *Journal of Gerontology, 36,* 615–619.

Cohen, G., & Faulkner, D. (1983). Age differences in performance on two information-processing tasks: Strategy selection and processing efficiency. *Journal of Gerontology, 38,* 447–454.

Cohen, R., & Meyers, A. W. (1984). The generalization of self-instructions. In B. Gholson & T. L. Rosenthal (Eds.), *Applications of cognitive-developmental theory* (pp. 95–112). New York: Academic Press.

Craik, F. I. M., & Byrd, M. (1982). Aging and cognitive deficits: The role of attentional resources. In F. I. M. Craik & S. Trehub (Eds.), *Aging and cognitive processes* (pp. 191–212). New York: Plenum Press.

Craik, F. I. M., & Rabinowitz, J. C. (1985). The effects of presentation rate and encoding task on age-related memory deficits. *Journal of Gerontology, 40,* 309–315.

Craik, F. I. M., & Simon, E. (1980). Age differences in memory: The roles of attention and depth of processing. In L. W. Poon, J. L. Fozard, L. S. Cermak, D. Arenberg, & L. W. Thompson (Eds.), *New directions in memory and aging: Proceedings of the George A. Talland memorial conference* (pp. 95–112). Hillsdale, NJ: Lawrence Erlbaum.

Crook, T., Ferris, S. H., & McCarthy, M. (1979). The misplaced objects task: A brief test for memory dysfunction in the aged. *Journal of the American Geriatrics Society, 27,* 284–287.

Dixon, R. A., & Hultsch, D. F. (1983). Structure and development of metamemory in adulthood. *Journal of Gerontology, 38,* 682–688.

Erber, J. T. (1981). Remote memory and age: A review. *Experimental Aging Research, 7,* 189–199.

Erickson, R. C., Poon, L. W., & Walsh-Sweeney, L. (1980). Clinical memory testing of the elderly. In L. W. Poon, J. L. Fozard, L. S. Cermak, D. Arenberg, & L. W. Thompson (Eds.), *New directions in memory and aging: Proceedings of the George A. Talland memorial conference* (pp. 379–402). Hillsdale, NJ: Lawrence Erlbaum.

Eriksen, C. W., Hamlin, R. M., & Daye, C. (1973). Aging adults and rate of memory scan. *Bulletin of the Psychonomic Society, 1,* 259–260.

Evans, G. W., Brennan, P. L., Skorpanich, M. A., & Held, D. (1984). Cognitive mapping and elderly adults: Verbal and location memory for urban landmarks. *Journal of Gerontology, 39,* 452–457.

Ferris, S. H., Crook, T., Clark, E., McCarthy, M., & Rae, D. (1980). Facial recognition memory deficits in normal aging and senile dementia. *Journal of Gerontology, 35,* 707–714.

Franklin, H. C., & Holding, D. H. (1977). Personal memories at different ages. *Quarterly Journal of Experimental Psychology, 29,* 527–532.

Hanley-Dunn, P., & McIntosh, J. L. (1984). Meaningfulness and recall of names by young and old adults. *Journal of Gerontology, 39,* 583–585.

Harris, J. E. (1978). External memory aids. In M. M. Gruneberg, P. E. Morris, & R. N. Sykes (Eds.), *Practical aspects of memory* (pp. 172–179). London: Academic Press.

Harris, J. E. (1980). Memory aids people use: Two interview studies. *Memory & Cognition, 8,* 31–38.

Harris, J. E., & Wilkins, A. J. (1982). Remembering to do things: A theoretical framework and an illustrative experiment. *Human Learning, 1,* 123–136.

Hartley, J. T. (1982, November). *Semantic characteristics of older and younger persons' visual images.* Paper presented at a meeting of the Gerontological Society of America, Boston.

Hasher, L., & Zacks, R. T. (1979). Automatic and effortful processes in memory. *Journal of Experimental Psychology: General, 108,* 356–388.

Hasher, L., & Zacks, R. T. (1984). Automatic processing of fundamental information. *American Psychologist, 39,* 1372–1388.

Herman, J. F., & Bruce, P. R. (1981). Spatial knowledge of ambulatory and wheelchair-confined nursing home residents. *Experimental Aging Research, 7,* 491–496.

Herman, J. F., & Coyne, A. C. (1980). Mental manipulation of spatial information in young and elderly adults. *Developmental Psychology, 16,* 537–538.

Herrmann, D. J. (1982). Know thy memory: The use of questionnaires to assess and study memory. *Psychological Bulletin, 92,* 434–452.

Herrmann, D. J., & Neisser, U. (1978). An inventory of everyday memory experiences. In M. M. Gruneberg, P. E. Morris, & R. N. Sykes (Eds.), *Practical aspects of memory* (pp. 35–51). London: Academic Press.

Higbee, K. L. (1977). *Your memory: How it works and how to improve it.* Englewood Cliffs, NJ: Prentice-Hall.

Howard, D. V., McAndrews, M. P., & Lasaga, M. I. (1981). Semantic priming of lexical decisions in young and old adults. *Journal of Gerontology, 36,* 707–714.

Hulicka, I. M. (1982). Memory functioning in late adulthood. In F. I. M. Craik & S. Trehub (Eds.), *Aging and cognitive processes* (pp. 331–351). New York: Plenum Press.

Hulicka, I. M., & Grossman, J. L. (1967). Age-group comparisons for the use of mediators in paired-associate learning. *Journal of Gerontology, 22,* 46–51.

Hultsch, D. F. (1969). Adult age differences in the organization of free recall. *Developmental Psychology, 1,* 673–678.

Hultsch, D. F., & Dixon, R. A. (1984). Memory for text materials in adulthood. In P. B. Baltes & O. G. Brim, Jr. (Eds.), *Life-span development and behavior* (Vol. 6, pp. 77–108). New York: Academic Press.

Jacoby, L. L., & Craik, F. I. M. (1979). Effects of elaboration of processing at encoding and retrieval: Trace distinctiveness and recovery of initial context. In L. S. Cermak & F. I. M. Craik (Eds.), *Levels of processing in human memory* (pp. 1–22). Hillsdale, NJ: Lawrence Erlbaum.

Kausler, D. H. (1982). *Experimental psychology and human aging.* New York: Wiley.

Kausler, D. H. (1985). Episodic memory: Memorizing performance. In N. Charness (Ed.), *Aging and human performance.* Chichester, UK: Wiley.

Kausler, D. H., & Hakami, M. K. (1983a). Memory for topics of conversation: Adult age differences and intentionality. *Developmental Psychology, 19,* 889–894.

Kausler, D. H., & Hakami, M. K. (1983b). Memory for activities: Adult age differences and intentionality. *Developmental Psychology, 19,* 889–894.

Kausler, D. H., Lichty, W., & Davis, R. T. (in press). Temporal memory for performed activities: Intentionality and adult age differences. *Developmental Psychology.*

Kausler, D. H., Lichty, W., & Freund, J. S. (1985). Adult age differences in recognition memory and frequency judgments for planned versus performed activities. *Developmental Psychology, 21,* 647–654.

Kirasic, K. C. (1980, November). *Spatial problem solving in elderly adults: A hometown advantage.* Paper presented at a meeting of the Gerontological Society of America, San Diego.

Kirasic, K. C., & Allen, G. L. (1985). Aging, spatial performance, and spatial competence. In N. Charness (Ed.), *Aging and human performance*. Chichester, UK: Wiley.

Kramer, J. J., Nagle, R. J., & Engle, R. W. (1980). Recent advances in mnemonic strategy training with mentally retarded persons: Implications for educational practice. *American Journal of Mental Deficiency, 85,* 306–314.

Labouvie-Vief, G., & Gonda, J. N. (1976). Cognitive strategy training and intellectual performance in the elderly. *Journal of Gerontology, 31,* 327–332.

Lachman, J. L., & Lachman, R. (1980). Age and the actualization of world knowledge. In L. W. Poon, J. L. Fozard, L. S. Cermak, D. Arenberg, & L. W. Thompson (Eds.), *New directions in memory and aging: Proceedings of the George A. Talland memorial conference* (pp. 285–311). Hillsdale, NJ: Lawrence Erlbaum.

Langer, E. J. (1978). Rethinking the role of thought in social interaction. In J. H. Harvey, W. Ickes, & R. F. Kidd (Eds.), *New directions in attribution research* (Vol. 2, pp. 35–58). Hillsdale, NJ: Lawrence Erlbaum.

Light, L. L., & Zelinski, E. M. (1983). Memory for spatial information in young and old adults. *Developmental Psychology, 19,* 901–906.

Lorayne, H., & Lucas, J. (1974). *The memory book.* New York: Ballantine Books.

Lovelace, E. A. (1984, August). *Reported mnemonics and perceived memory changes with aging.* Paper presented at a meeting of the American Psychological Association, Toronto.

McCarthy, M., Ferris, S. H., Clark, E., & Crook, T. (1981). Acquisition and retention of categorized material in normal aging and senile dementia. *Experimental Aging Research, 7,* 127–135.

McCormack, P. D. (1979). Autobiographical memory in the aged. *Canadian Journal of Psychology, 33,* 118–124.

Mason, S. E. (1981, November). *Age group comparisons of memory ratings, predictions, and performance.* Paper presented at a meeting of the Gerontological Society of America, Toronto.

Mason, S. E. (1983, November). *Age and sex as factors in facial recognition and identification.* Paper presented at a meeting of the Gerontological Society of America, San Francisco.

Mason, S. E., & Smith, A. D. (1977). Imagery in the aged. *Experimental Aging Research, 3,* 17–32.

Meacham, J. A. (1982). A note on remembering to execute planned actions. *Journal of Applied Developmental Psychology, 3,* 121–133.

Meichenbaum, D. (1977). *Cognitive-behavior modification: An integrative approach.* New York: Plenum Press.

Meyer, B. J. F., & Rice, G. E. (1981). Information recalled from prose by young, middle, and old adult readers. *Experimental Aging Research, 7,* 253–268.

Morris, P. E. (1979). Strategies for learning and recall. In M. M. Gruneberg & P. E. Morris (Eds.), *Applied problems in memory* (pp. 25–57). London: Academic Press.

Morris, P. E. (1984). The validity of subjective reports on memory. In J. E. Harris & P. E. Morris (Eds.), *Everyday memory, actions and absentmindedness* (pp. 153–172). London: Academic Press.

Moscovitch, M. C. (1982). A neuropsychological approach to perception and memory in normal and pathological aging. In F. I. M. Craik & S. Trehub (Eds.), *Aging and cognitive processes* (pp. 55–78). New York: Plenum Press.

Murphy, M. D., Sanders, R. E., Gabriesheski, O. O., & Schmitt, F. A. (1981). Metamemory in the aged. *Journal of Gerontology, 36,* 185–193.

Murrell, H., & Humphries, S. (1978). Age, experience and short term memory. In M. M. Gruneberg, P. E. Morris, & R. N. Sykes (Eds.), *Practical aspects of memory* (pp. 363–368). London: Academic Press.

Ohta, R. J., & Kirasic, K. C. (1983). The investigation of environmental learning in the elderly. In G. Rowles & R. J. Ohta (Eds.), *Aging and milieu* (pp. 83–95). New York: Academic Press.

Ohta, R. J., Walsh, D. A., & Krauss, I. K. (1981). Spatial perspective-taking ability in young and elderly adults. *Experimental Aging Research, 7,* 45–63.

Peeck, J. (1982). Effects of mobilization of prior knowledge on free recall. *Journal of Experimental Psychology: Learning, Memory, and Cognition, 8,* 608–612.

Perlmutter, M., Metzger, R., Nezworski, T., & Miller, K. (1981). Spatial and temporal memory in 20 and 60 year olds. *Journal of Gerontology, 36,* 59–65.

Perlmutter, M., & Mitchell, D. B. (1982). The appearance and disappearance of age differences in adult memory. In F. I. M. Craik & S. Trehub (Eds.), *Aging and cognitive processes* (pp. 127–144). New York: Plenum Press.

Pettinati, H. M., Brown, M. M., & Mathisen, K. S. (1985, August). *Memory complaints by depressed and normal older adults.* Paper presented at a meeting of the International Congress of Gerontology, New York.

Poon, L. W. (1980). A systems approach for the assessment and treatment of memory problems. In J. M. Ferguson & C. B. Taylor (Eds.), *The comprehensive handbook of behavioral medicine* (Vol. 1, pp. 191–212). New York: Spectrum.

Poon, L. W. (1985). Differences in human memory with aging: Nature, causes, and clinical implications. In J. E. Birren & K. W. Schaie (Eds.), *Handbook of the psychology of aging* (2nd ed., pp. 427–462). New York: Van Nostrand Reinhold.

Poon, L. W., & Fozard, J. L. (1978). Speed of retrieval from long-term memory in relation to age, familiarity and datedness of information. *Journal of Gerontology, 33,* 711–717.

Poon, L. W., Fozard, J. L., & Treat, N. J. (1978). From clinical and research findings on memory to intervention programs. *Experimental Aging Research, 4,* 235–253.

Poon, L. W., & Schaffer, G. (1982, August). *Prospective memory in young and elderly adults.* Paper presented at a meeting of the American Psychological Association, Washington, DC.

Poon, L. W., Walsh-Sweeney, L., & Fozard, J. L. (1980). Memory skill training for the elderly: Salient issues on the use of imagery mnemonics. In L. W. Poon, J. J. Fozard, L. S. Cermak, D. Arenberg, & L. W. Thompson (Eds.), *New directions in memory and aging: Proceedings of the George A. Talland memorial conference* (pp. 461–484). Hillsdale, NJ: Lawrence Erlbaum.

Puglisi, J. T., Park, D. C., Smith, A. D., & Hill, G. W. (1982, November). *Memory for complex spatial information in young and old adults: Automatic or effortful?* Paper presented at a meeting of the Gerontological Society of America, Boston.

Rabinowitz, J. C., Craik, F. I. M., & Ackerman, B. P. (1982). A processing resource account of age differences in recall. *Canadian Journal of Psychology, 36,* 325–344.

Rankin, J. L., Karol, R., & Tuten, C. (1984). Strategy use, recall, and recall organization in young, middle-aged, and elderly adults. *Experimental Aging Research, 10,* 193–196.

Ratner, H. H., & Bushey, N. (1984, August). *Adults' event recall: Putting memory in context.* Paper presented at a meeting of the American Psychological Association, Toronto.

Reason, J., & Lucas, D. (1984). Absent-mindedness in shops: Its incidence, correlates and consequences. *British Journal of Clinical Psychology, 23,* 121–131.

Reddy, B. G., & Bellezza, F. S. (1983). Encoding specificity in free recall. *Journal of Experimental Psychology: Learning, Memory, and Cognition, 9,* 167–174.

Reed, G. (1979). Everyday anomalies of recall and recognition. In J. F. Kihlstrom & F. J. Evans (Eds.), *Functional disorders of memory* (pp. 1–28). Hillsdale, NJ: Lawrence Erlbaum.

Riege, W. H. (1982). Self-report and tests of memory aging. *Clinical Gerontologist, 1,* 23–36.

Robertson-Tchabo, E. A. (1980). Cognitive-skill training for the elderly: Why should "old dogs" acquire new tricks? In L. W. Poon, J. L. Fozard, L. S. Cermak, D. Arenberg, & L. W. Thompson (Eds.), *New directions in memory and aging: Proceedings of the George A. Talland memorial conference* (pp. 511–518). Hillsdale, NJ: Lawrence Erlbaum.

Robertson-Tchabo, E. A., Hausman, C. P., & Arenberg, D. (1976). A classical mnemonic for older learners: A trip that works. *Educational Gerontology, 1,* 215–226.

Rose, T. L., & Yesavage, J. A. (1983). Differential effects of a list-learning mnemonic in three age groups. *Gerontology, 29,* 293–298.

Rubin, D. C., Wetzler, S. E., & Nebes, R. D. (1986). Autobiographical memory across the life span. In D. C. Rubin (Ed.), *Autobiographical memory.* Cambridge University Press.

Sanders, R. E., Murphy, M. D., Schmitt, F. A., & Walsh, K. K. (1980). Age differences in free recall rehearsal strategies. *Journal of Gerontology, 35,* 550–558.

Schmitt, F. A., Murphy, M. D., & Sanders, R. E. (1981). Training older adult free recall rehearsal strategies. *Journal of Gerontology, 36*, 329–337.

Schonfield, D., & Stones, M. J. (1979). Remembering and aging. In J. F. Kihlstrom & F. J. Evans (Eds.), *Functional disorders of memory* (pp. 103–139). Hillsdale, NJ: Lawrence Erlbaum.

Scogin, F., Storandt, M., & Lott, L. (1985). Memory-skills training, memory complaints, and depression in older adults. *Journal of Gerontology, 40*, 562–568.

Shiffrin, R. M., & Schneider, W. (1977). Controlled and automatic human information processing. II. Perceptual learning, automatic attending, and a general theory. *Psychological Review, 84*, 127–190.

Sinnott, J. D. (1984, August). *Everyday memory and solution of everyday problems.* Paper presented at a meeting of the American Psychological Association, Toronto.

Sinnott, J. D. (1986). Prospective/intentional and incidental everyday memory: Effects of age and passage of time. *Psychology and Aging, 1*, 110–116.

Smith, A. D. (1977). Adult age differences in cued recall. *Developmental Psychology, 13*, 326–331.

Smith, A. D. (1980). Age differences in encoding, storage, and retrieval. In L. W. Poon, J. L. Fozard, L. S. Cermak, D. Arenberg, & L. W. Thompson (Eds.), *New directions in memory and aging: Proceedings of the George A. Talland memorial conference* (pp. 23–46). Hillsdale, NJ: Lawrence Erlbaum.

Smith, A. D., & Winograd, E. (1978). Adult age differences in remembering faces. *Developmental Psychology, 14*, 443–444.

Sunderland, A., Watts, K., Baddeley, A. D., & Harris, J. E. (1986). Subjective memory assessment and test performance in elderly adults. *Journal of Gerontology, 41*, 376–384.

Treat, N. J., Poon, L. W., Fozard, J. L., & Popkin, S. J. (1978). Toward applying cognitive skill training to memory problems. *Experimental Aging Research, 4*, 305–319.

Tulving, E., & Thomson, D. M. (1973). Encoding specificity and retrieval processes in episodic memory. *Psychological Review, 80*, 352–373.

Waddell, K. J., & Rogoff, B. (1981). Effect of contextual organization on spatial memory of middle-aged and older women. *Developmental Psychology, 17*, 878–885.

Walsh, D. A., Krauss, I. K., & Regnier, V. A. (1981). Spatial ability, environmental knowledge, and environmental use: The elderly. In L. S. Liben, A. H. Patterson, & N. Newcombe (Eds.), *Spatial representation and behavior across the life span* (pp. 321–357). New York: Academic Press.

Warrington, E. K., & Ackroyd, C. (1975). The effect of orienting tasks on recognition memory. *Memory & Cognition, 3*, 140–142.

Warrington, E. K., & Sanders, H. I. (1971). The fate of old memories. *Quarterly Journal of Experimental Psychology, 23*, 432–442.

Wechsler, D. (1945). A standardized memory scale for clinical use. *Journal of Psychology, 19*, 87–95.

Weinstein, C. E., Duffy, M., Underwood, V. L., MacDonald, J., & Gott, S. P. (1981). Memory strategies reported by older adults for experimental and everyday learning tasks. *Educational Gerontology, 7*, 205–213.

West, R. L. (1984, August). *An analysis of prospective everyday memory.* Paper presented at a meeting of the American Psychological Association, Toronto.

West, R. L. (1985). *Memory fitness over 40.* Gainesville, FL: Triad.

West, R. L., & Cohen, S. (1985). The systematic use of semantic and acoustic processing by younger and older adults. *Experimental Aging Research, 11*, 81–87.

West, R. L., & Walton, M. (1985, March). *Practical memory functioning in the elderly.* Paper presented at the National Forum on Research in Aging, Lincoln, NE.

White, N., & Cunningham, W. R. (1984, November). *The relationships among memory complaint, memory performance, and depression in young and elderly adults.* Paper presented at a meeting of the Gerontological Society of America, San Antonio.

Wilson, B., & Moffat, N. (1984a). Rehabilitation of memory for everyday life. In J. E. Harris & P. E. Morris (Eds.), *Everyday memory, actions and absentmindedness* (pp. 207–233). London: Academic Press.

Wilson, B. A., & Moffat, N. (1984b). *Clinical management of memory problems.* Rockville, MD: Aspen.

Winograd, E. (1978). Encoding operations which facilitate memory for faces across the life span. In M. M. Gruneberg, P. E. Morris, & R. N. Sykes (Eds.), *Practical aspects of memory* (pp. 255–262). London: Academic Press.

Winograd, E., & Simon, E. W. (1980). Visual memory and imagery in the aged. In L. W. Poon, J. L. Fozard, L. S. Cermak, D. Arenberg, & L. W. Thompson (Eds.), *New directions in memory and aging: Proceedings of the George A. Talland memorial conference* (pp. 485–506). Hillsdale, NJ: Lawrence Erlbaum.

Wood, G. (1972). Organizational processes and free recall. In E. Tulving & W. Donaldson (Eds.), *Organization and memory* (pp. 49–91). New York: Academic Press.

Yesavage, J. A., & Rose, T. L. (1984). Semantic elaboration and the method of loci: A new trip for older learners. *Experimental Aging Research, 10,* 155–159.

Yesavage, J. A., Rose, T. L., & Bower, G. H. (1983). Interactive imagery and affective judgments improve face–name learning in the elderly. *Journal of Gerontology, 38,* 197–203.

Yesavage, J. A., Rose, T. L., & Spiegel, D. (1982). Relaxation training and memory improvement in elderly normals: Correlation of anxiety ratings and recall improvement. *Experimental Aging Research, 8,* 195–198.

Zarit, S. H. (1979, November). *Affective correlates of self-reports about memory of older people.* Paper presented at a meeting of the Gerontolgical Society of America, Washington, DC.

Zarit, S. H., Cole, K. D., & Guider, R. L. (1981a). Memory training strategies and subjective complaints of memory in the aged. *Gerontologist, 21,* 158–164.

Zarit, S. H., Gallagher, D., & Kramer, N. (1981b). Memory training in the community aged: Effects on depression, memory complaint, and memory performance. *Educational Gerontology, 6,* 11–27.

Zelinski, E. M., Gilewski, M. J., & Thompson, L. W. (1980). Do laboratory tests relate to self-assessment of memory ability in the young and old? In L. W. Poon, J. L. Fozard, L. S. Cermak, D. Arenberg, & L. W. Thompson (Eds.), *New directions in memory and aging: Proceedings of the George A. Talland memorial conference* (pp. 519–544). Hillsdale, NJ: Lawrence Erlbaum.

31 Mnemonics as modified for use by the elderly

Jerome A. Yesavage, Danielle Lapp, and Javaid I. Sheikh

In recent years, considerable attention has been paid to pharmacologic treatments for senile dementias (Reisberg, Ferris, & Gershon, 1979). Many researchers have also studied memory complaints as a sign of depression in the elderly and have attempted to differentiate them from dementia (Kahn et al., 1975; Kiloh, 1961; Wells, 1979). Little work, however, has been done toward developing practical strategies to help nondepressed elderly people experiencing age-related cognitive decline.

Researchers have documented that nondepressed elderly people may score in the "normal" range on screening tests for senile dementia, though still experiencing age-related cognitive declines, a phenomenon recently described in a series of meetings of the National Institute of Mental Health (NIMH) as "minimal memory impairment" (MMI) (Annapolis and Key West, November 1985). Craik's classic review of memory and aging (1977) and Poon's extensive recent review (1985) list a wide variety of significant and substantial declines in memory function in old versus young "normals." Elders who want to continue to work as long as possible may be appropriately concerned if these "normal" losses lead to reduced ability to function professionally or lead to social embarrassment. The purpose of this chapter is to review the cognitive changes that occur with normal aging, critically discuss prior attempts to reduce these losses, present some recent modifications to these attempts, and then finally focus on the limitations of current studies with implications for future research.

Brief review of prior studies of mnemonics and the elderly

Magnitudes of deficits seen in normal elderly people

Elderly subjects who score in the "normal" range of neuropsychiatric batteries for dementia such as the Mini-Mental State exam of Folstein, the

This research was supported by the Medical Research Service of the Veterans Administration, the Lawrence Welk Foundation, and the Center for the Study of Aging, National Institute of Mental Health (grant MH35182).

Halstead-Reitan exam, or the Luria exam (Eisdorfer, 1978; Folstein, Folstein, & McHugh, 1975; Wood et al., 1979) may still have declined considerably in function from their performances when younger. To obtain an estimate of the magnitude of this MMI with age, one may examine in detail differences in young and old performances on some batteries. For example, norms on the verbal measures of the commonly used Weschler Adult Intelligence Scale (WAIS) decline 13% to 30% from age 20–34 and age 70–74 (Sattler, 1982). Declines for the same age groups on WAIS performance measures range from 25% to 64%. Some argue that these deficits substantially reflect slowed motor performance on timed tests; however, a study in which five timed WAIS subtests were administered with unlimited time to elders showed that performance decrements were reduced in only one of the five tests (Storandt, 1979). Such cognitive decrements are consistent with the declines seen in cross-sectional studies of a variety of experimental memory tasks, including all the subscales on the Guild Memory Test (paired associates, paragraphs, designs, digits, etc.), and memory for prose passages (Craik, 1977; Poon, 1985).

Some investigators (Schaie & Stone, 1982) have cautioned against drawing conclusions from cross-sectional data that may reflect cross-generational differences rather than age-related differences. However, there was a longitudinal study documenting declines of 10% to 38% on a battery of intelligence measures in a 21-year period (Schaie, 1983). Another study of nonverbal memory demonstrated, in both longitudinal and cross-sectional samples, that performance on the Benton Visual Retention Test declined substantially with age (Arenberg, 1978). The magnitudes of differences between age groups were substantial, with subjects at least doubling in their numbers of errors between the thirties and the seventies. Further data from the same study indicate similar declines in some attentional functions (Quilter, Giambra, & Benson, 1983). Although it may be misleading to compare percentage differences on raw test scores when one has not demonstrated a linear relationship between scores and abilities, one should at least be able to say that these changes are not small. In fact, there seems to be evidence that the order of magnitude of "normal" cognitive decline by the time one reaches the seventies is substantial, on the order of 15% to 40% of raw scores, depending on the process tested and the testing method. We now turn to a discussion of studies that have attempted to reverse these "normal" changes.

Sizes of treatment effects in prior studies

Several studies have suggested declines in organizational ability with age (Denney, 1974; Hultsch, 1971; Smith, 1980). This has prompted efforts to study the effects of organizational techniques on age-related cognitive decline. Zarit and his collaborators, using the organizational technique of mnemonic training, found improvement in regard to affect, memory complaints, and ability to do certain memory tasks in elderly subjects (Zarit, Cole, & Guider, 1981a; Zarit, Gallagher, & Kramer, 1981b). However, their subjects did not improve on all tasks in which they were trained, and cognitive improvement did not correlate with affective improvement. In one study, subjects improved only on two list-learning tasks using categorization and visual mediators, but did not improve on name-face recall using visual mediators or on paragraph retention using image associations (Zarit et al., 1981a). Most improvement was seen on immediate posttest scores, and less on delayed posttests. Replication of this study was successful (Zarit et al., 1981a), and improvement was also found on the face-name task after testing was changed to avoid ceiling effects. Improvements of scores from pretests to delayed-recall tests were 20% better for recall of lists of related items, 30% better for recall of lists of unrelated items, and 30% better for name-face recall in treatment versus control groups.

A frequently studied organizational technique is the method of loci (Bower, 1972). This method requires the individual to first name several loci or locations in a familiar building or setting, such as his or her home. Once these locations have been learned to criterion, the individual forms a visual-image association between the first item of a list to be remembered and the first location in the house. Each subsequent item to be remembered is then associated with the next location in the house. To recall the list, the individual takes a mental "walk" around the house, "stopping" at each location to retrieve the visual image associated with it that serves as a retrieval cue for the item to be remembered. This mnemonic has well-documented effects on the recall of lists in both young (Bower, 1972) and old (Robertson-Tchabo, Hausman, & Arenberg, 1976). Although it has been suggested that older subjects may have difficulty using this procedure on their own, Robertson-Tchabo and associates found that older subjects using the technique could improve baseline list-learning scores 79% in comparison with controls (Robertson-Tchabo et al., 1976). In a study conducted by our group, after training in the method of loci, older subjects reached the level of proficiency in list learning demonstrated by younger subjects (Rose & Yesavage, 1983). Specifically, older subjects initially recalled 55% of their 18-item lists, whereas younger subjects recalled some 70%. After 3 days of training, older subjects had increased almost to the initial level of the younger subjects. The younger subjects also increased their scores to almost 90% correct with training. The improvement seen in the older subjects was 27%, which is less than that seen in the groups trained by Robertson-Tchabo and associates (1976). This difference may be due to the more extensive training given the subjects in the study by Robertson-Tchabo and associates.

Limitations of prior studies

The following are some of the potential criticisms of prior studies of mnemonics:

1. The mnemonic techniques employed are so complicated that they are not practical for the elderly. In such schemes, the elderly not only must learn a complicated mnemonic but also must learn how to elaborate on the processing of key

elements of the mnemonic. This is a difficult task that may be of benefit only to subjects who have the educational experience and the motivation to attend several training sessions.

2. A potential limitation of mnemonics based on organization and association of visual images is that older people find it difficult to produce and remember visual images and visual-imagery associations (Hulicka & Grossman, 1967; Mason & Smith, 1977; Pavio 1971; Poon, Walsh-Sweeney, & Fozard, 1980; Winograd & Simon, 1980). This has led to suggestions that memory training based on visual-image associations may be less effective than verbal techniques in the aged (Cermak, 1980).

3. It is well known that high anxiety levels can impair test performances (Spielberger, Gonzales, & Fletcher, 1979). It is also a common observation that the elderly often are very anxious when using new techniques in a testing situation. It is quite conceivable, therefore, that the memory training may not prove as useful to them as it potentially could be.

4. Some recent findings suggest that encoding processing may be more superficial in the elderly than in young people (Craik & Simon, 1980). This may mean that the improvement on the mnemonics may be short-term only, unless some additional methods to enhance the "depth" of processing are taught.

5. Treatment effects sometimes are not large enough to be considered useful.

In summary, a survey of prior studies of mnemonics for the elderly with cognitive deficits suggests that declines of 20% to 40% can occur in cognitive functions for 70-year-old normal elderly people. Although training programs for elderly normals have been shown to improve selected cognitive processes, including memory, to about the same degree that some of these processes have declined, the everyday usefulness and long-term effects of such programs remain poorly documented. In addition, such programs can at times be difficult and anxiety-provoking for the elderly, thereby diminishing their potential effectiveness.

Attempts at modification through the use of preliminary training

Rationale

As explained earlier, the mnemonic systems commonly used often are confusing, complicated, and anxiety-producing for the elderly. It is assumed that preliminary training may prepare them for the task of learning these mnemonics.

Results of three studies using preliminary training

Pretraining in the use of visual imagery. One attempt to improve the performances of elderly subjects on a visual-image-based mnemonic improved the treatment effect by pretraining in visual imagery before teaching the mnemonic (Yesavage, 1983). Two groups of elderly subjects were taught a standard mnemonic to improve a common memory complaint among elders: face-name recall (McCarty, 1980). Before learning the mnemonic, one group (imagery group) was first taught techniques to improve visual-imagery ability, and the other group (control group) was first taught a nonspecific method to improve attitudes. Overall performance on face-name recall was significantly better in the imagery group than in the control group.

These results support the hypothesis that techniques that improve visual-imagery ability may improve overall performance using a visual-image-based mnemonic. Although improvement in recall was seen with imagery training alone, this improvement did not become significantly better than the performance of the control group until after mnemonic training. This is consistent with observations that visual imagery improves memory only when it facilitates organization (Pavio, 1971).

Pretraining in improving elaboration of encoding. Studies have demonstrated that certain instructions facilitate retention of visual materials in young and old subjects (Arenberg, 1977; Bower & Karlin, 1974; Smith & Winograd, 1978; Warrington & Ackroyd, 1975). These studies have shown, for example, that recognition memory for faces is improved by requiring subjects to make semantic judgments about faces as they are viewed. Such findings are readily explained in terms of the amount of elaboration given to a stimulus at encoding; that is, by processing a stimulus in additional, nonredundant ways, one is more likely to remember it later (Craik & Tulving, 1975; Klein & Saltz, 1976). Thus, by instructing elderly subjects not only to form visual images but also to elaborate further verbally on the images that are formed, they are more likely to later recognize the visual images so recorded.

Taking this line of reasoning a step further, one study examined the effectiveness of certain instructions designed to increase the elaboration of processing of visual-image associations used in a mnemonic device (Yesavage, Rose & Bower, 1983). Groups of elderly subjects were taught to learn name-to-face associations using one of three different techniques. In a control group (no image), subjects were taught for each face-name pair to select a prominent facial feature and to transform the surname into a concrete word. Subjects in a second group (image) additionally were taught to employ interactive imagery to form an association between the prominent feature and the transformed name. The third group (image plus judgment) was treated the same as the second except that these subjects were also taught to judge the pleasantness of the image association that was formed. As predicted, improvement following instruction was minimal when no image association was formed, but strong when interactive imagery was used. Moreover, subjects in the image-plus-judgment group remembered more names than those in the image group and showed less forgetting on a measure of delayed recall. This study demonstrates that semantic orienting tasks can be used to enhance the retention of visual-image associations as well as the simpler stimuli used in prior research.

Concentration/relaxation pretraining. Changes in attention have been less well studied in the elderly than changes in memory per se, but they may have substantial importance in explaining memory and other cognitive changes with age (Kinsbourne, 1980). Although attention may be conceptualized in several ways (Cohen & Eisdorfer, 1979; Pribram & McGuiness, 1975; Schneider & Shiffrin, 1977), of particular interest are situations in which the subjects must divide their attention between two tasks. It has been well documented that older subjects have substantial difficulty with divide-attention tasks. Such findings imply a reduced processing capacity with age (Kinsbourne, 1980); that is, the elderly have enough capacity to do one task, but not two tasks. Others have seen a linkage between the limited attentional-processing capacity and findings of limited elaboration during encoding (Craik & Simon, 1980; Hasher & Zacks, 1979).

Data suggest that high anxiety levels impair test performance (Spielberger et al., 1979) and that higher anxiety levels are associated with less reliable recall of eyewitness testimony (Siegel & Loftus, 1978). Though these studies were done in younger subjects, it has been argued that this is a general phenomenon: High levels of anxiety, arousal, and depression all produce distraction and reduce cognitive capacity and performance (Hasher & Zacks, 1979). Some investigators have thus suggested that relaxation techniques might reduce anxiety, thereby improving attention (Rimm & Masters, 1974; Spiegel & Spiegel, 1978). A number of studies have found that techniques such as deep muscle relaxation have some positive effects in the elderly (Labouvie-Vief, 1976; Labouvie-Vief & Gonda, 1976; Poon, Fozard & Treat, 1978; Poon et al., 1980; Treat et al., 1978; Zarit et al., 1981a). For example, Labouvie-Vief has shown that training in anxiety reduction may be as effective as specific mnemonics or a problem-solving approach in improving cognitive function in the normal elderly (Labouvie-Vief, 1976; Labouvie-Vief & Gonda, 1976). Zarit also included relaxation and other methods to improve motivation and attention in a study of memory complaints in the elderly and found similar improvement as compared with training based on organizational techniques (Zarit et al., 1981b).

Our research group recently used a package of techniques attempting to improve attention in groups of elderly as a preliminary to learning certain mnemonics (Yesavage & Rose, 1983). These subjects received a combination of two types of training. Concentration training (CT) included several techniques to enhance attention. For example, in selective attention exercises, subjects attempted to perform list-learning tasks against tape-recorded verbal interference. Subjects were also taught classic progressive muscle relaxation in CT. Mnemonic training (MT) involved the method of loci. Order effects were examined using two groups of subjects. One group received CT followed by MT, whereas the other group received MT prior to CT. It was hypothesized that the CT-MT sequence would improve recall more than the reverse sequence, and the results supported this hypothesis, with the subjects in the CT-MT sequence performing significantly better on list learning at the end of training than those who received the MT-CT sequence. An obvious shortcoming of such studies using a package of therapies to improve concentration, however, is that they do not determine whether or not all training components are necessary to improve performance per se.

Some researchers have argued that lack of reliable and valid attentional measures has constrained studies of the effects of individual differences in attention on memory (Fredericksen, 1980). There is, however, evidence that individual differences in anxiety levels may be important. A recent study has suggested that relaxation training improves memory performance in the elderly suffering from performance anxiety, but only in those with high initial anxiety scores (Yesavage, Rose, & Spiegel, 1982). It has long been argued that the relationship between arousal and performance is curvilinear (i.e., increases in arousal have a beneficial effect on performance when motivation is initially low, but tend to disrupt performance when arousal is initially strong) (Yerkes & Dodson, 1980). Many studies have found evidence for this inverted-U relationship. It has been applied routinely, for example, in studies of test anxiety and achievement motivation (Atkinson & Raynor, 1974). Thus, it may be that attempts to modulate anxiety, motivation, and arousal in the elderly will be most fruitful if they consider the individual's initial levels of such factors, as well as what levels would be appropriate for the given patient.

A recent study replicated and expanded the finding that only subjects with high initial anxiety levels benefit from relaxation (Yesavage, 1983). In this study, two groups of elderly subjects were taught a standard mnemonic to improve face-name recall. On the rationale of trying to reduce performance/test anxiety, half of the subjects (experimental group) received relaxation training before learning the mnemonic, and the remainder (control group) were taught a nonspecific method to improve attitudes. Final performance on face-name recall improved significantly more in the experimental group, and this improvement was significantly correlated with decreased anxiety scores. As in studies of college students with test anxiety, these results indicate that relaxation pretraining may reduce performance/test anxiety in elderly people receiving cognitive training.

In summary, mnemonic systems for the elderly can be modified through the use of preliminary training. Such preliminary training can consist of visual-imagery training, training in improving elaboration of encoding, training in concentration/relaxation, or a combination of these. Studies have documented that addition of such preliminary training techniques can enhance the effect of mnemonics.

Limitations of existing studies and future directions

Despite the positive effects reported in several studies of subjects with cognitive losses of normal aging, a critical review of these studies suggests some limitations and areas for future research.

Effect size and long-term retention of training

The question was raised initially whether or not the effects seen are of sufficient magnitude to warrant the training effort. Data cited suggest that if the memory declines in this normal population are on the order of 30% when compared with young normals, increases of this magnitude are not uncommon immediately after training. Decrements of similar magnitude have also been found on certain measures of fluid intelligence, and the magnitude of the deficit appears to be within the range of training successes reported in these areas (Schaie, 1980). Another issue requiring attention in the field of cognitive training is the general lack of documentation of long-term retention of mnemonics. Some of the most recent work, however, suggests retention of training for several months (Baltes & Willis, 1982). In addition, a recently completed 6-month follow-up study by our research group (Sheikh, Hill, & Yesavage, 1986) documented that elderly subjects can maintain their improvement in cognitive functioning over that period when a combination of pretraining and mnemonic techniques is used. Further research in this area is clearly warranted.

Practicality of task versus ease of quantification

Despite a proliferation of research papers on the theoretical aspects of memory, relatively insignificant effort has been put into developing practical techniques for memory problems. The little work done on practical techniques has focused mostly on ways to enhance learning and memory within the laboratory and has not always been relevant to everyday problems. Although reexamination of a large study of memory complaints by Zelinsky and associates indicates that memory for names and faces is a major problem for the elderly (Zelinsky, Gilewski, & Thompson, 1980), there is little to suggest that recall of lists is a concern. Yet many studies have examined list learning. This is probably because list learning is relatively easy to measure, and there are powerful techniques, such as the method of loci, that can improve this ability. Questions regarding generalizability of improvement from specific task to everyday aspects of memory function have not received enough attention. However, a shift in focus toward developing mnemonics for practical memory problems may be occurring. For example, West (Chapter 30; this volume) addresses this issue quite comprehensively by translating laboratory findings on cognition and aging to recommendations for practical mnemonic strategies. Wilson and Moffat (1984) took a step further in this direction by transforming theoretical constructs from the field of memory and aging into therapeutic techniques for the memory-impaired. It is hoped that such works will pave the way for future research in this direction.

Matching appropriate training to the individual

Most studies have shown wide variability of training results between individuals; yet little is known about the predictors of response to training. Furthermore, most studies have been done in white-middle-class populations. We have no idea of the effectiveness of these techniques in other socioeconomic groups, nor do we know if the memory complaints are the same across socioeconomic strata. It is likely that differences between individuals and across groups are profound and that such variability may be large enough to obscure training effects in many studies (Schaffer & Poon, 1982). Several studies have used treatment packages combining several modalities to compensate for individual variability. Such combined approaches, however, make it difficult to interpret results. For example, although virtually all the studies cited earlier attempted to improve motivation and attention, little attempt was made to distinguish the effects of training on separate aspects of motivation and attention.

In an effort to answer some of these questions, we recently asked the participants in our training courses to fill out the Myers-Briggs Personality Type Indicator (MBTI) (Consulting Psychologists Press, Inc., 577 College Ave., Palo Alto, CA 94306) and the ANSIE Form G, Locus of Control Scale (Duke, Shaheen, & Nowicki, 1974). Preliminary data suggest that the elderly scoring higher on the ''intuitive'' scale of the MBTI showed significantly more improvement as a group than those scoring higher on the ''sensing'' scale. Also, the participants in our groups as a whole tended to score considerably higher on the ANSIE Form G, as opposed to the mean for the geriatric group (the higher the score, the more external the orientation). Additional confirmatory data from our study will be needed before we can discuss the implications of these findings.

Developing tests of appropriate difficulty is a recurrent problem. In the group setting, there are wide differences in abilities even in normal, well-educated middle-class older adults: On an 18-item list-learning task, some may initially learn all items perfectly, whereas others will recall virtually none. Zarit has argued that treatment effects may at times be difficult to document because of ceiling effects on tests (Zarit et al., 1981a). Our own experience has been the same; however, one simply cannot design tests so difficult that all will initially score low, because this discourages elders–another bit of evidence that ''remembering is hopeless.'' Such difficulties argue for intensive-study designs with individually designed tests.

Unknown roles of affect and motivation in learning

The roles of affect and motivation in retraining efforts are particularly poorly understood. It has been well documented that memory complaints are better correlated with depression than with the actual degree of cognitive impairment (Kahn et al., 1975; Duke et al., 1974; Zarit et al., 1981b). Furthermore, a mood-dependent memory effect has been documented (Bower, 1981): simply stated, material learned when one is happy is better recalled when happy, and material learned when one is sad is better recalled when one is sad. In addition, poor self-image and stereotypes of the aged as having poor memory may contribute to impaired performance (Kinsbourne, 1980). The effects on cognitive performance of interventions aimed at improving affect, motivation, and self-image remain unexplored.

Interactions with medications

There has been little study of the effects of medications on cognitive training (Fozard & Popkin, 1978). Medications that have psychostimulant effects might be expected to enhance learning (Weiss & Latiess, 1962) and might make it easier for the elderly to assimilate new techniques. It is worth remembering that psychotropics quite commonly used by the elderly have state-dependent effects on memory (Reus, Weingartner, & Post, 1979) that might lead to impairment of recall with changes in medication type and dosage. Other compounds with anticholinergic effects that are commonly used in the elderly can also be expected to impair learning (Davis & Yesavage, 1979). Future research needs to address these issues.

In summary, the existing studies of cognitive training have had some important limitations, including lack of generalizability of training, lack of practicality of commonly used menmonics, lack of attention to individual differences among subjects, and so forth. Despite these limitations, however, it is encouraging that there are therapies that have been shown to reduce cognitive losses at least in the short term. For specific tasks, the magnitude of improvement from training appears to be similar to the magnitude of decline with age. Future research needs to address the many limitations of existing studies to make cognitive-training methods more effective.

Conclusion

We have critically reviewed studies of cognitive training in the aged, pointed out their positive effects, along with some of their limitations, discussed attempts at modification of mnemonic systems through the use of preliminary training, and suggested future directions for research.

One area in which there are obvious gaps in our knowledge concerns the selection of appropriate treatment for individual memory problems. Such a task will first entail developing appropriate assessment techniques for different problems. To begin with, memory-training programs can benefit from use of assessment devices to differentiate MMI from dementia. Various measures, including measures of verbal intelligence, anxiety, personality, and cognitive style can then be used to separate people who would respond to the different kinds of modified training methods described earlier in this chapter. In the same vein, differentiating the depressed from the demented or the elderly with MMI is important while making initial assessments, as the depressed people will respond better to psychotherapy or medications. Furthermore, using the broad tenets of memory theory, we need to develop specialized training programs for people with severe memory impairments of various origins (senile dementia, head injury, cerebral tumor, dementia, brain surgery, nutritional disorder, cerebral vascular accident, etc.). Controlled studies with the severely memory-impaired have been rare and have failed to take into account modern cognitive theory. Future research needs to modify promising programs form the normal elderly for use with these populations. In short, having well-defined treatment goals based on sound assessment techniques can help break down the seemingly difficult task of designing programs for individual memory problems into achievable, down-to-earth goals.

References

Arenberg, D. (1977). The effect of auditory augmentation on visual retention for young and old adults. *Journal of Gerontology, 32,* 192–195.

Arenberg, D. (1978). Differences and changes with age in the Benton Visual Retention Test. *Journal of Gerontology, 33,* 534–540.

Atkinson, J. W., & Raynor, J. O. (1974). *Motivation and achievement.* Washington DC: V. H. Winston.

Baltes, P. B., & Willis, S. L. (1982). Plasticity and enhancement of intellectual functioning in old age: Penn State's Adult Development and Enrichment Project (ADEPT). In F. I. M. Craik & S. Trehub (Eds.), *Aging and cognitive processes.* New York: Plenum Press.

Bower, G. (1972). Mental imagery and associative learning. In L. Gregg (Ed.), *Cognition in learning and memory.* New York: Wiley.

Bower, G. H. (1981). Mood and memory. *American Psychologist, 36,* 129–148.

Bower, G. H., & Karlin, M. B. (1974). Depth of processing pictures of faces and recognition memory. *Journal of Experimental Psychology, 103,* 751–757.

Cermak, L. S. (1980). Comments on imagery as a therapeutic mnemonic. In L. W. Poon, J. L. Fozard, L. S. Cermak, D. Arenberg, & L. W. Thompson (Eds.), *New directions in memory and aging: Proceedings of the George A. Talland memorial conference* (pp. 507–510). Hillsdale, NJ: Lawrence Erlbaum.

Cohen, D., & Eisdorfer, C. (1979). Cognitive theory and the assessment of change in the elderly. In A. Raskin & L. F. Jarvik (Eds.), *Psychiatric symptoms and cognitive loss in the elderly.* Washington DC: Hemisphere Publications.

Craik, F. I. M. (1977). Age differences in human memory. In J. E. Birren & K. W. Schaie (Eds.), *Handbook of the psychology of aging* (pp. 384–420). New York: Van Nostrand Reinhold.

Craik, F. I. M., & Simon, E. (1980). Age differences in memory: The roles of attention and depth of processing. In L. W. Poon, J. L. Fozard, L. S. Cermak, D. Arenberg, & L. W. Thompson (Eds.), *New directions in memory and aging: Proceedings of the George A. Talland memorial conference* (pp. 95–112). Hillsdale, NJ: Lawrence Erlbaum.

Craik, F. I. M., & Tulving, E. (1975). Depth of processing and the retention of words in episodic memory. *Journal of Experimental Psychology: General, 104,* 268–294.

Davis, K. L., & Yesavage, J. A. (1979). Brain acetylcholine and disorders of memory. In K. L. Davis (Ed.), *Brain acetylcholine and neuropsychiatric disease.* New York: Plenum Press.

Denney, N. W. (1974). Clustering in middle and old age. *Developmental Psychology, 10,* 471–475.

Department of Health, Education, & Welfare (1979). *Mental health and the elderly, report of the president's commission on mental health.* Washington, DC: US Government Printing Office.

Duke, M. P., Shaheen, J., Nowicki, S., Jr. (1974). The determination of locus of control in a geriatric population and a subsequent test of the social learning model for interpersonal distances. *Journal of Psychology and Aging, 86,* 277–285.

Eisdorfer, C. (1978). Psychophysiological and cognitive studies in the aged. In G. Usdin & C. K. Hofling (Eds.), *Aging, the process and the people* (pp. 96–128). New York: Brunner Mazel.

Folstein, M. F., Folstein, S. E., & McHugh, P. H. (1975). Mini-mental state: A practical method for grading the cognitive state of patients for the clinician. *Journal of Psychiatric Research, 12,* 189–198.

Fozard, J. L., & Popkin, S. J. (1978). Optimizing adult development. *American Psychologist, 33,* 975–989.

Frederiksen, J. R. (1980). Some cautions we might exercise in attributing age deficits in memory to attentional dysfunctions. In L. W. Poon, J. L. Fozard, L. S. Cermak, D. Arenberg, & L. W. Thompson (Eds.), *New directions in memory and aging: Proceedings of the George A. Talland memorial conference* (pp. 131–139). Hillsdale, NJ: Lawrence Erlbaum.

Hasher, L., & Zacks, R. T. (1979). Automatic and effortful processes in memory. *Journal of Experimental Psychology: General, 108,* 356–388.

Hulicka, I. M., & Grossman, J. L. (1967). Age-group comparisons for the use of mediators in paired-associates learning. *Journal of Gerontology, 22,* 46–51.

Hultsch, D. F. (1971). Adult age differences in free classification and free recall. *Developmental Psychology, 4,* 338–342.

Kahn, R. L., Zarit, S. H., Hilbert, N. M., et al. (1975). Memory complaint and impairment in the aged. *Archives of General Psychiatry, 32,* 1569–1573.

Kiloh, L. (1961). Pseudo-dementia. *Acta Psychiatrica Scandinavia, 37,* 336–351.

Kinsbourne, M. (1980). Attentional dysfunctions and the elderly: Theoretical models and research perspectives. In L. W. Poon, J. L. Fozard, L. S. Cermak, D. Arenberg, & L. W. Thompson (Eds.), *New directions in memory and aging: Proceedings of the George A. Talland memorial conference* (pp. 113–130). Hillsdale, NJ: Lawrence Erlbaum.

Klein, K., & Saltz, E. (1976). Specifying the mechanisms in a levels-of-processing approach to memory. *Journal of Experimental Psychology: Human Learning and Memory, 20,* 671–679.

Labouvie-Vief, G. (1976). Toward optimizing cognitive competence in later life. *Educational Gerontology, 1,* 75–92.

Labouvie-Vief, G., & Gonda, J. N. (1976). Cognitive strategy training and intellectual performance in the elderly. *Journal of Gerontology, 31,* 327–332.

McCarty, D. L. (1980). Investigation of a visual imagery mnemonic device for acquiring face–name associations. *Journal of Experimental Psychology: Human Learning and memory, 6,* 145–155.

Mason, S. E., & Smith, A. D. (1977). Imagery in the aged. *Experimental Aging Research, 3,* 17–32.

Pavio, A. (1971). *Imagery and verbal processes.* New York: Holt, Rinehart & Winston.

Poon, L. W. (1985). Differences in human memory with aging: Nature, causes, and clinical implications. In J. E. Birren & K. W. Schaie (Eds.), *Handbook of the psychology of aging* (2nd ed., pp. 427–462). New York: Von Nostrand Reinhold.

Poon, L. W., Fozard, J. L., & Treat, N. J. (1978). From clinical and research findings on memory to intervention programs. *Experimental Aging Research, 4,* 235–254.

Poon, L. W., Walsh-Sweeney, L., & Fozard, J. L. (1980). Memory skill training in the elderly: Salient issues on the use of imagery mnemonics. In L. W. Poon, J. L. Fozard, L. S. Cermak, D. Arenberg, & L. W. Thompson (Eds.), *New directions in memory and aging: Proceedings of the George A. Talland memorial conference* (pp. 461–484). Hillsdale, NJ: Lawrence Erlbaum.

Primbram, K. H., & McGuiness, D. (1975). Arousal, activation and effort in the control of attention. *Psychology Review, 82,* 116–149.

Quilter, R. E., Giambra, L. M., & Benson, P. E. (1983). Longitudinal age changes in vigilance over an eighteen year interval. *Journal of Gerontology, 38,* 51–54.

Reisberg, B., Ferris, S., & Gershon, S. (1979). Psychopharmacologic aspects of cognitive research in the elderly. *Interdisciplinary Topics in Gerontology, 15,* 132–152.

Reus, V. I., Weingartner, H., & Post, R. M. (1979). Clinical implications of state-dependent learning. *American Journal of Psychiatry, 136,* 927–931.

Rimm, D. C., & Masters, J. C. (1974). *Behavior therapy: Techniques and empirical findings.* New York: Academic Press.

Robertson-Tchabo, E. A. Hausman, C. P., & Arenberg, D. (1976). A classic mnemonic for older learners: A trip that works! *Educational Gerontology, 1,* 215–226.

Rose, T. L., & Yesavage, J. A. (1983). Differential effects of a list-learning mnemonic in three age groups. *Gerontology (Basel), 29,* 293–298.

Sattler, J. M. (1982). Age effects on Wechsler Adult Intelligence Scale–Revised tests. *Journal of Consulting and Clinical Psychology, 30,* 785–786.

Schaffer, G., & Poon, L. W. (1982). Individual variability in memory training with the elderly. *Educational Gerontology, 8,* 217–229.

Schaie, K. W. (1980). *Cognitive training research in perspective.* Paper presented to the Gerontological Society of America.

Schaie, K. W. (1983). The Seattle Longitudinal Study: A 21 year exploration of psychometric intelligence in adulthood. In K. W. Schaie (Ed.), *Longitudinal studies of adult psychological development.* New York: Guilford Press.

Schaie, K. W., & Stone, V. (1982). Psychological assessment. *Annual Review of Gerontology and Geriatrics, 3,* 329–360.

Schneider, W., & Shiffrin, R. M. (1977). Controlled and automatic human information processing. I. Detection, search and attention. *Psychology Review, 84,* 1–66.

Sheikh, J. I., Hill, R. D., & Yesavage, J. A. (1986). Long-term efficacy of cognitive training for minimal memory impairment: A six-month follow-up study. *Journal of Developmental Neuropsychology.*

Siegel, J. M., & Loftus, E. F. (1978). Impact of anxiety and life-stress upon eyewitness testimony. *Bulletin of the Psychonomic Society, 12,* 479–480.

Smith, A. D. (1980). Age differences in encoding, storage and retrieval. In L. W. Poon, J. L. Fozard, L. S. Cermak, D. Arenberg, & L. W. Thompson (Eds.), *New directions in memory and aging: Proceedings of the George A. Talland memorial conference* (pp. 23–46). Hillsdale, NJ: Lawrence Erlbaum.

Smith, A. D., & Winograd, E. (1978). Adult age differences in remembering faces. *Developmental Psychology, 14,* 443–444.

Spiegel, H., & Spiegel, D. (1978). *Trance and treatment: Clinical uses of hypnosis.* New York: Basic Books.

Spielberger, C,. D., Gonzales, H. P., & Fletcher, T. (1979). Test anxiety reduction, learning strategies, and academic performance. In H. F. O'Neill & C. D. Spielberger (Eds.), *Cognitive and affective learning strategies.* New York: Academic Press.

Storandt, M. (1979). Age, ability level, and method of administering and scoring of the WAIS. *Journal of Gerontology, 34,* 175–178.

Treat, N. J., Poon, L. W., Fozard, J. L., et al. (1978). Toward applying cognitive skill training to memory problems. *Experimental Aging Research, 4,* 305–319.

Warrington, E. K., & Ackroyd, C. (1975). The effect of orienting tasks on recognition memory. *Memory & Cognition, 3,* 140–142.

Weiss, B., & Latiess, V. G. (1962). Enhancement of human performance by caffeine and amphetamines. *Pharmacology Review, 14,* 1–37.

Wells, C. E. (1979). Pseudodementia. *American Journal of Psychiatry, 136,* 895–900.

Wilson, B. A., & Moffat, N. (Eds.), (1984). *Clinical management of memory problems.* Rockville, MD: Aspen Systems Corporation.

Winograd, E., & Simon, E. W. (1980). Visual memory and imagery in the aged. In L. W. Poon, J. L. Fozard, L. S. Cermak, D. Arenberg, & L. W. Thompson (Eds.), *New directions in memory and aging: Proceedings of the George A. Talland memorial conference* (pp. 485–506). Hillsdale, NJ: Lawrence Erlbaum.

Wood, W. G., Elias, M. F., Pentz, C. A., et al. (1979, November). *Age differences in neuropsychological performances among healthy well-educated subjects.* Paper presented at the annual meeting of the American Gerontological Society, Washington, DC.

Yerkes, R. M., & Dodson, J. D. (1980). The relation of strength of stimulus to rapidity of habit formation. *Journal of Comparative and Neurological Psychology, 18,* 459–482.

Yesavage, J. A. (1983). Imagery pretraining and memory training in the elderly. *Gerontology (Basel), 29,* 271–275.

Yesavage, J. A. (1984). Relaxation and memory training in the elderly. *American Journal of Psychiatry, 141,* 778–781.

Yesavage, J. A., & Rose, T. L. (1983). Concentration and mnemonic training in elderly with memory complaints: A study of combined therapy and order effects. *Psychiatry Research, 9,* 157–167.

Yesavage, J. A., Rose, T. L., & Bower, G. H. (1983). Interactive imagery and affective judgments improve face–name learning in the elderly. *Journal of Gerontology, 29,* 197–203.

Yesavage, J. A., Rose, T. A., & Spiegel, D. (1982). Relaxation training and memory improvement in elderly normals. *Experimental Aging Research, 8,* 195–198.

Yesavage, J. A., Westphal, J., & Rush, L. (1981). Senile dementia: Combined pharmacologic and psychologic treatment. *Journal of the American Geriatrics Society, 29,* 164–171.

Zarit, S. H., Cole, K. D., & Guider, R. L. (1981a). Memory training strategies and subjective complaints of memory in the aged. *Gerontologist, 21,* 158–164.

Zarit, S. H., Gallagher, D., & Kramer, N. (1981b). Memory training in the community aged: Effects on depression, memory complaint and memory performance. *Educational Gerontology, 6,* 11–27.

Zelinsky, E. M., Gilewski, M. J., & Thompson, L. W. (1980). Do laboratory tests relate to self-assessment of memory ability in the young and old? In L. W. Poon, J. L. Fozard, L. S. Cermak, D. Arenberg, & L. W. Thompson (Eds.), *New directions in memory and aging: Proceedings of the George A. Talland memorial conference* (pp. 519–550). Hillsdale, NJ: Lawrence Erlbaum.

Part IIIC

Designing programs for cognitive rehabilitation

32 Designing memory-therapy programs

Barbara A. Wilson

There are growing numbers of people whose lives have been extended through the application of increasingly sophisticated medicine and surgery, but whose memory functioning remains severely impaired. In many cases these impairments will be so bad that a normal life cannot be led; yet therapy, which might enable the severely memory-impaired person to return to the community, frequently is unobtainable. Many people who face such a predicament will consult doctors and other medical staff who, through lack of knowledge, believe that little or nothing can be done to alleviate some of the problems connected with memory impairment. At best, a psychological assessment of memory difficulties may be offered, but usually this is not followed up by advice on how to manage or, in some cases, overcome the problems that have been highlighted by the assessment.

A possible explanation for the existence of such a situation in the health services may have much to do with the lack of evidence to suggest that restoration of memory is possible. However, though I do not quarrel with the view that practically nothing can be done to restore memory functioning, I do want to claim emphatically that there is always something that can be done to improve the daily life of a memory-impaired person. At the same time as holding this view, I want to dissociate myself from the opinion that memory problems will disappear if the "right" drug or therapy is provided.

This chapter argues that it is possible, in a number of cases, to reduce the handicap caused by deficient memory functioning. It also discusses the identification of problems for treatment, strategies available to help the memory-impaired, how to select the most appropriate strategy, and evaluation of therapy. Arguments will be supported by reference to the theories, methodologies, and research findings from the disciplines of cognitive psychology, neuropsychology, and behavioral psychology.

Influence of cognitive psychology

Cognitive psychology has provided us with models of human memory that enable therapists to understand and to some extent explain the nature of memory functioning in their clients. Baddeley (1984) reported a case of a woman who attempted to commit suicide by inhaling carbon monoxide. She was left with a classic amnesic syndrome, but the psychiatrist treating her believed that her memory failures were due to hysteria. The psychiatrist's belief was based on a mistaken conception of the nature of human memory that did not include the distinction between primary and secondary memory. Had he been familiar with the current thinking, which was stimulated by the arguments of cognitive psychologists such as Baddeley (1982), the woman might have received more appropriate treatment at an earlier stage.

Cognitive psychologists have also tried to explain why the human amnesic syndrome occurs. The three main theoretical frameworks are constructed by (1) those who regard amnesia as an encoding deficit (Butters & Cermak, 1975), (2) those who argue that amnesia is due to a storage problem (Meudell & Mayes, 1982), and (3) those who suggest that it is due to a retrieval deficit (Warrington & Weiskrantz, 1970).

These theories have implications for treatment. If encoding strategies are faulty, then we can induce deeper levels of processing in our patients, using methods similar to those developed by Craik and Lockhart (1972) and Cermak (1975). Although encoding-deficit theories prove inadequate for explaining the amnesic syndrome, they may nevertheless explain, to some extent, less severe memory failures. The same can be said of storage and retrieval deficits (Baddeley, 1982). Few of our patients, after all, will suffer from a pure amnesic syndrome.

Cognitive psychology can inform us about the learning abilities of amnesic patients and thus help us to design memory-therapy programs. We know, for example, that procedural learning is relatively intact in many of the amnesic patients studied (Brooks & Baddeley, 1976; Milner, Corkin, & Teuber, 1968; Starr & Phillips, 1970). Thus, the ability to learn motor skills, mazes, jigsaws, and perceptual tasks is not severely impaired in these people. Some paired-associate learning tasks, such as those involving semantic or phonological relationships, also are learned without great difficulty (Warrington & Weiskrantz, 1970, 1982; Winocur & Weiskrantz, 1976). This knowledge is potentially very important in memory therapy. If a patient can learn certain skills, this might enable him or her to remain at home rather than live in an institution. If it is possible to learn some associations, providing there is a logical link between two items, then therapists possibly can manipulate the situation in order to promote learning. For example, visual imagery as a mnemonic aid often fails to benefit people with severe memory problems (Cutting, 1978; Jones, 1974), but the technique might be more useful if we ensure a relationship between the two stimuli. This can be illustrated by the story of a patient at Rivermead Hospital who was taught one visual-imagery technique, the method of loci. He used the rooms of his house as the locations and could learn the correct responses if there was a semantic association (e.g., "Kitchen–steak"), but not if the response was arbitrary (e.g., "Kitchen–uncle").

Influence of neuropsychology

Neuropsychology contributes toward memory-therapy programs in three ways. First, it helps us to understand the organization of the brain. The concept of cerebral asymmetry, for example, has a role to play in selecting appropriate therapeutic strategies. If a memory-impaired person has primarily left-hemisphere damage and verbal-memory deficits, we can select strategies involving the use of the right hemisphere and visual-memory skills. Similarly, patients with severe frontal-lobe damage may be expected to respond differently to memory therapy than patients without frontal-lobe damage. Wilson (1985), for example, in a study of amnesic patients with and without unilateral frontal-lobe damage, demonstrated that there were differences between the two groups in procedural learning tasks, and Baddeley and Wilson (1985) showed differences in autobiographical memory between amnesic patients with and without frontal-lobe damage.

The second way in which neuropsychology can influence rehabilitation is through the knowledge it provides about specific disorders. Thus, management of memory problems in head-injured patients probably will be different from treatment for those with Alzheimer's disease. With the former group, the therapist may introduce a range of external aids and teach some mnemonic strategies to the patients and their families. Slow improvement will be expected for some time, and there will be less need to adapt the intervention procedures with the passage of time. In contrast, Alzheimer patients may, initially, be taught some mnemonic strategies, but as the disease progresses, the memory techniques and aids will need to be simpler, involving environmental changes to an increasingly greater degree (Wilson & Moffat, 1984a), reality orientation (Holden & Woods, 1982), and reminiscence therapy (Merriam, 1980). Having provided this example, it is perhaps timely to point out here that the *nature* of the memory deficit will almost always be more important in memory therapy than the *cause* of the deficit, even though they often are closely related. The recommendation is, therefore, that therapists take account of each individual patient's diagnosis without letting that diagnosis dictate the intervention strategy.

The third important contribution made by neuropsychology to rehabilitation is in the area of assessment. In order to design an effective treatment program, we need to know about the patient's neuropsychological status. This will include the general level of current intellectual functioning, the type and severity of the memory disorder, and the presence or absence of perceptual, reasoning, language, and planning problems. The degree to which these areas are affected will influence the design and procedure of a program of therapy. If severe general intellectual impairment is present, certain treatment approaches will be precluded. Perceptual problems, such as face-recognition difficulties or unilateral neglect, may require the adaptation of available aids or techniques. The severity of the memory impairment will also influence the type of therapeutic intervention selected.

Influence of behavioral psychology

Although the neuropsychology assessment procedures referred to earlier are important, they do not provide us with sufficient information for designing memory-therapy programs. They need to be complemented by behavioral-assessment techniques. These include direct observation, questionnaires, rating scales, self-monitoring, and simulated observations (Hay, 1982). Behavioral assessment differs from the standardized assessment procedures in several ways. A behavioral investigation samples behavior in a particular situation, rather than regarding a response as a sign of some underlying disorder. For example, a behavioral assessment might focus attention on the number of times an amnesic patient repeats a question, and a count would be taken of the repeated question in a given period of time. Neuropsychological assessment, on the other hand, is more likely to decide that poor performance on delayed recall is evidence of amnesia, that is, a sign of a memory disorder.

A behavioral assessment usually means observing a problem behavior in many situations and under different conditions, such as time of day, place, and presence or absence of certain staff or relatives; neuropsychological assessment typically will be conducted on one or two occasions only. As Mischel (1968) indicated, a conventional assessment is concerned with what a person *has,* whereas a behavioral assessment is more concerned with what a person *does.*

The relationship between assessment and treatment is much stronger when adopting a behavioral approach, and it is sometimes difficult to separate the two. For further discussion of this topic, the reader is referred to Ciminero, Calhoun, and Adams (1977). In memory therapy, both kinds of assessment are important. Behavioral-treatment strategies have proved useful in several areas of rehabilitation (Ince, 1978; Wilson, 1981a), including memory therapy (Wilson & Moffat, 1984b). Several different techniques have been used, including modeling, chaining, and shaping. In all cases, however, it is necessary (1) to be specific about the problem behavior and the aims of the therapy, (2) to measure the frequency or severity of the problem, and (3) to monitor the effectiveness of the intervention strategy. The most important contribution of the behavioral approach to treatment is contained in the structure it provides for designing treatment programs. These are flexible and can be adapted to a wide range of individuals and a variety of problems.

Behavioral psychology has also given us a number of single-case experimental designs with which to evaluate the effectiveness of treatment. Many professionals (including some psychologists) are reluctant to accept that good research can be carried out with individuals or small groups of subjects. Nevertheless, the single-case and small-*N* approaches are gaining ground. These designs are invaluable tools for the rehabilitation therapist, avoiding many of the problems inherent in large-group designs. With the latter, studies usually are described in terms of the average or mean response of each group under each condition. Such information tells us little about individual variations (which are common); nor do we learn how many individuals improved, remained the same, or deteriorated. Large-group studies highlight statistical rather than clinical significance and often are not helpful for the therapist who wants to know if a particular treatment will help a particular patient. Furthermore, group studies typically involve a small number of measurements (such as pretreatment and posttreatment levels); so we do not know the *pattern* of changes throughout the intervention period. In contrast, single-case designs allow us to tailor the treatment to the individual, to obtain a stable baseline before introducing treatment, to monitor progress, and to adapt the treatment procedure if necessary. Several designs are in use, but probably the most flexible and adaptable is the multiple-baseline-across-behaviors design. There are many good references available for single-case designs, including Hersen and Barlow (1976) and Kazdin (1982).

There are two major criticisms advanced by opponents of single-case designs: The first is that it is difficult to know how far procedures that are successful with one patient will be successful with another; the second points to the difficulty of obtaining stable baselines when a patient either is continuing to show some recovery or is showing variation from day to day. As mentioned earlier, the first criticism can also apply to group studies, particularly when the group is inclined to be heterogeneous. In such a case we cannot be certain that group results are typical of any one individual within the group. However, generalizations are more likely to be possible within a group that is homogeneous. Similarly, it is more likely to be possible to generalize from one individual to another when they appear to share a number of characteristics. However, in both group and single-case studies, the possibility of generalization should never be assumed, and those that are claimed should be supported by several successful replications. Where difficulties are experienced in obtaining stable baselines, it might be appropriate to wait until stability in this respect can be achieved. However, there is some disadvantage in delaying treatment, because optimum periods for introducing certain stages of treatment might be missed, and therapists are likely to experience anxiety during such intervals. A better approach might be to introduce treatment with an unstable baseline and use statistical procedures to determine if there is a significant difference in performance before and after treatment. Although statistics are used less frequently in single-case studies than in group studies, there are occasions when statistical intervention is indicated. There are several statistical procedures suited to single-case designs (e.g.,Edgington, 1982; Hersen & Barlow, 1976; Kazdin, 1982).

Identification of problems for treatment

Designing treatment programs will be aided considerably once we are informed by the three disciplines discussed earlier. Initially we need to decide what it is that we are going to treat. Although the patient might want us to improve his or her memory, or relatives might request memory training, these are not suitable goals for the therapist embarking on a program of treatment. A more promising start will be made if we can isolate some specific problem encountered by the memory-impaired person and aim to reduce this problem, or find the best way for the individual to bypass the problem. Memory-impaired people are not, as a rule, troubled by their inability to learn paired associates or reproduce complex designs, although many studies on improving recall in amnesic patients have used only such experimental material, with real-life, practical problems being ignored. This is regrettable, as there is no evidence to support the notion that practicing strategies for learning experimental material presented in the laboratory or clinic can be generalized to the learning of everyday material outside the laboratory or clinic (Wilson & Moffat, 1984a).

In order to find out more about everyday problems, the memory therapist can interview the patient, the relatives, and any staff working with the patient. These interviews can be followed up by questionnaires and checklists. In many cases, patients will not be aware of the extent of their memory problems. A questionnaire study conducted with head-injured patients, orthopedic controls, and their relatives (Sunderland, Harris, & Baddeley, 1984) showed that many of the head-injured patients were not good at evaluating their memory problems. A recent study carried out at Rivermead with a mixed group of memory-impaired people found that although some patients had reasonable insights into their problems, many others did not (Wilson, 1986). Parkin (1984) discussed differences in insight among amnesic patients with differing etiologies.

Direct observation is also likely to provide useful information on the nature of everyday memory probems. These observations may be carried out in natural settings, such as the patient's home, or in occupational-therapy or simulated situations (such as a mock office or shop).

Standardized assessment procedures have a part to play, although they are limited as to the information they can provide about the nature, severity, and extent of everyday problems. What we can learn from the conventional tests is whether or not additional cognitive handicaps are present and the patient's level of general intellectual functioning. One assessment tool that may prove useful is the Rivermead Behavioral Memory Test (Wilson, Cockburn, & Baddeley, 1985). This test is a bridge between the standardized, conventional tests and behavioral assessment. Thus, it is administered and scored in a standardized manner, but it includes material and items analogous to situations encountered in everyday life. There are 12 subtests that attempt to assess such skills as remembering an appointment, learning a short route, and remembering to deliver a message. The test aims to predict which people are likely to experience everyday memory problems, to specify the nature of those problems, to identify areas for treatment, and to monitor change over time. Four alternative versions are available so that practice effects through repeated testing can be eliminated.

Having identified many of the problems faced by a memory-impaired person, the therapist must next decide which of these problems are to be tackled in the treatment program and how many are to be tackled at once. There are no clear-cut answers to these questions. Among other factors, the therapist will be influenced by the patient's future plans or future placement. A patient who is likely to remain in long-term care will possibly need to remember the way to the bathroom and the names of a few fellow patients and staff. The patient who hopes to return to work will be more concerned to remember written material and appointments. Another influential factor will be the nature of the complaints cited by relatives and staff. A patient who is constantly getting into the wrong bed or repeating the same question over and over again will cause stress and frustration to others, and such problems may have priority in treatment. Of course, the patient's wishes are also very important. Some patients will be so unaware of their difficulties that they will have no desire to do anything about their memory problems. Others will be painfully aware and may have strong views as to which problem should be tackled first. Whether or not they will *remember* their views on other occasions is another matter.

The number of problems treated at any one time will depend on the patient's intellectual level, the levels of perception, concentration, reasoning, or other cognitive skills, degrees of insight and motivation, the presence or absence of physical or sensory handicaps, the involvement of other staff and relatives, the setting in which the memory therapist works, and the amount of time available.

Strategies available to help the memory-impaired

Memory performance can be improved in numerous ways. Drugs, for example, can (under certain circumstances) improve retention of material; rote learning is commonly used by students, actors, and others; rhymes are sometimes employed to remember information (e.g., how many days in each month); a kitchen timer will remind the cook that it is time to check the oven. Harris (1978, 1984) describes some of these methods. Not all of the techniques available can be applied successfully to brain-damaged people or to confused elderly people. Nevertheless, there are several strategies that can be considered. These include the following:

Environmental adaptations that reduce the need to remember. These involve such techniques as labeling doors and positioning material so that it will not be easily forgotten.

External aids. Harris (1984) subdivides these into (1) cuing devices for accessing internally stored information and (2) systems for storing information externally. The former category includes alarm clocks and kitchen timers (which remind us to do something). The latter category includes notebooks, diaries, and computers. External aids frequently are the most useful kinds of memory aids for the memory-impaired person. Moffat (1984) and Wilson and Moffat (1984b) discuss their use with brain-damaged people. Harris (1980) describes the extent of their use by groups of students and housewives.

Internal strategies. Again, Harris (1984) subdivides these into two groups: (1) the naturally learned strategies and (2) artificial mnemonics. Naturally learned strategies are not usually thought of as memory *aids,* because they are used by all of us without thinking. For example, if asked to recall a list of unrelated words, many people recall the last two or three words first, before going back to the words presented earlier. Most people, of course, have not heard of the primacy and recency effects, but realize, nevertheless, that they are likely to forget rapidly the items presented last. Artificial mnemonics may be further subdivided into visual and verbal mnemonics. Visual methods include the method of loci and face–name associations. Verbal methods include alphabetical searching and first-letter cuing. More detailed descriptions of these and other methods are provided by Moffat (1984), Wilson and Moffat (1984a), and Wilson (1986).

Rehearsal and repetitive practice. In many cases, simply repeating the same information over and over again is not helpful for the memory-impaired person, although the expanded-rehearsal method employed by Landauer and Bjork (1978) may be useful for amnesic patients. In this method, a piece of information is presented, and the subject is tested after a very brief delay, and then again after a slightly longer delay. The interval is gradually increased as learning proceeds.

Memory games and exercises. In many rehabilitation centers the only treatment for a memory disorder may be frequent exposure to games such as Kim's game or Pelmanism (and memory tests such as recalling lists of words). There is little evidence that exercising memory in this manner leads to any improvement in memory functioning, although it may be of some indirect assistance. For example, patients and relatives often think it is helping, and this may increase morale and motivation. Furthermore, Harris and Sunderland (1981) argue that mental exercise during a critical period of neural regeneration may conceivably enhance recovery. At present, this is not usually attempted, because therapists wait for a stable baseline.

Reality orientation and reminiscence therapy. Reality orientation (RO) is a process by which attempts are made to teach or maintain awareness of time, place, and person in confused individuals. It is usually a continuous process whereby staff or relatives remind the confused person of time, place, and company. A commentary on what is happening in the patient's immediate environment is also provided. Signposts and other cues help the person to remain aware of surroundings. Classroom RO refers to treatment sessions that usually (but not always) are included as a supplement to 24-hour RO. These sessions are held typically for half an hour to an hour each day, with one or two therapists attending. Also, encompassed in RO is a respect for the individuality, dignity, and autonomy of each confused person at all times. For those readers wishing to know more about RO the work of Holden and Woods (1982) is recommended.

There has been a tendency in recent years to recognize the importance of the patient's past life. Reminiscence therapy is a procedure whereby old photographs, songs, and objects from earlier times are used to stimulate discussion. Merriam (1980) reported some therapeutic success with this method. Baddeley and Wilson (1986) suggest that it is probably more important for confused patients to establish and maintain *who* they are than *where* they are.

Both RO and reminiscence therapy may prove to be useful in the treatment of other memory-impaired people who share certain characteristics with the confused elderly. Some head-injured patients are, for example, disoriented in time and place and may have poor autobiographical memory (Baddeley & Wilson, 1986). Similar manifestations may be found in those suffering from carbon monoxide poisoning, anoxia following cardiac arrest, encephalitis, or other disorders affecting the brain.

Selecting appropriate strategies for individuals

Given the number and variety of techniques available, how does the therapist decide which of these to choose for each individual person? Several factors will influence the decision. The nature of the memory problems selected for treatment may preclude some strategies. For example, RO will be unnecessary for someone with a pure amnesic syndrome who makes use of calendars, diaries, and notebooks, who is not confused, and whose goal is to find the way around a new neighborhood. The assessments conducted will provide information on cognitive strengths and weaknesses, which may further reduce the number of potentially useful strategies. Thus, an aphasic patient will be unlikely to benefit from first-letter mnemonics, and a patient with acquired dyslexia will be limited in the ability to use notebooks as memory aids. The overall level of intellectual functioning may also be an influential factor. Other impairments need to be considered. For people with severe physical handicaps, many of the external aids will be inappropriate. The same is true for blind people. Those who are very depressed or anxious may require treatment for these problems prior to, or in conjunction with, memory therapy. If a patient is receiving speech, occupational, or physical therapy during the period of treatment, then it may be possible to involve other therapists in the memory treatment. One of the common memory problems at Rivermead is failure to remember how to transfer safely from a wheelchair to an ordinary chair (or to a bed or toilet). Combining forces with other therapists can help in such a situation.

The patient's own personal preferences also need to be taken into account. An amnesic patient described by Wilson (1982) was enthusiastic about first-letter mnemonics and made use of this strategy in certain situations. Another amnesic patient showed considerable anger whenever visual-imagery strategies were used. He said, each time these were introduced to him, "Where's the logic in that!" Because of his disapproval of visual imagery, these methods were not recommended to his relatives on discharge.

Bearing all these aspects in mind, there are several ways therapists can decide on which strategy to use for a particular patient or particular memory problem. The first question to answer might be whether to carry out individual or group treatment. There are advantages and disadvantages with both. Usually, individual treatment is preferable because it is then possible to tailor therapy to each patient's needs, pace, and style. It is also possible to adjust the treatment according to progress (or lack of progress) and to focus on any specific problems that might arise. Evaluation of progress is easier with individuals. At Rivermead, individual treatment sessions for inpatients typically last 90 min each day for 5 days per week, for a period of 4 or 5 weeks. Day patients usually attend for 2 or 3 days per week, also for sessions lasting 90 min. All patients have some memory training in occupational therapy in addition to their psychology sessions. However, it is not always possible to provide a one-to-one situation in occupational therapy; so the patient spends a greater or lesser part of the session working alone.

The main disadvantage of individual treatment is, of course, the amount of time that it takes. For the relatively small gains made, the cost of intensive professional help may be considered unjustifiable. In some cases it might be possible to use volunteer helpers and relatives to carry out the treatment, with supervision from a psychologist or other memory therapist. Group treatment has obvious advantages in terms of time and cost. It may also have indirect therapeutic value in that patients often are reassured by seeing others with similar (or worse) memory problems. It is not uncommon for amnesic people to think that they are "going crazy," and the reassurances given to them are quickly forgotten. Group treatment can sometimes reduce this fear. Furthermore, as the problems faced by group members differ to some extent, the participants can be both givers and receivers of help. Being able to give advice, suggestions, and support to peers may also be beneficial for morale and motivation. Group activities can be designed to ensure that each member of the group will succeed at some memory task, and this may also boost morale in front of their peers. Given that memory-impaired people experience considerable failure, it is no bad thing to build in elements of success whenever possible.

Obviously, group treatment has the disadvantage that attention is not focused exclusively on the particular problems of the individual. It is also difficult to evaluate the effectiveness of such treatment. One study that looked at the effectiveness of group training on memory functioning in patients with acquired brain damage was carried out by Wilson, Cooper, and Kennerley (1983). There were 20 patients in that study; half received 3 weeks of daily treatment in a memory group, followed by 3 weeks of treatment in a problem-solving group where reasoning tasks were set for the group to solve. The remaining patients received group problem-solving treatment first and group memory treatment second. There were some gains made by many of the patients with regard to everyday memory functioning, as assessed by the Rivermead Behavioral Memory Test (RBMT) described earlier. However, no significant differences emerged between training in a memory group and training in a problem-solving group. Nevertheless, 11 people showed greater improvement with group memory training, 5 showed greater improvement following training in the problem-solving group, and 4 showed no change in functioning with either group.

In recognition of the fact that both approaches have their different strengths, both are tried at Rivermead whenever possible, with patients receiving one individual session and one group session each day. This is obviously demanding in terms of time, but, as indicated earlier, it is sometimes possible to enlist the help of volunteers or relatives to supplement the professional staff.

The 3-week syllabus of the Rivermead memory group has been described by Wilson and Moffat (1984b). Many other tasks, activities, and arrangements for memory groups are possible, and further research on the effectiveness of these for different patient groups should be encouraged. Apart from RO studies, little research on group work appears to have been carried out.

The remainder of this section on appropriate strategies for patients concerns ways of selecting such strategies for individuals. One way is a systematic trial of each possible strategy in turn for a given problem. For example, if the problem is inability to learn people's names, then the therapist can begin by trying repeated practice, then face–name association procedure, then first-letter cuing, and so on. This is not likely to be the preferred method of selecting a strategy, because it is time-consuming and because of the development of interference effects. Material presented in one treatment session (particularly if it is presented several times) is likely to interfere with material presented in a later session. The amnesic patient's tendency to make prior-list intrusions has, of course, been known for some time (Weiskrantz, 1978). It is perfectly acceptable to compare the effectiveness of different methods, such as rehearsal versus visual imagery, and visual imagery versus motor movements. This can be accomplished by a matched-pairs design in which the names (or other material) to be learned are put randomly into two or more groups, depending on the number of strategies that are to be compared. The different treatments can be introduced at the same time. For example, one name from the visual-imagery condition, one from rehearsal, and one from motor movements can be presented in the first session; another three names can be presented in the second session, with the order of memory strategy being balanced across sessions. Descriptions of this approach with brain-damaged people have been provided by Wilson (1986).

A different way of selecting a treatment strategy is to attempt to treat the underlying deficit. If memory failures occur because of impaired attention, then attention training will be the method of choice; if the failures are due to storage deficits, then an attempt to ensure that proper encoding takes place will be appropriate; if the problem is one of retrieval, then improving the ability to retrieve information will be an appropriate goal. This approach, which owes its framework to certain theoretical principles developed in the field of cognitive psychology, has an obvious appeal: If it brings success, then many, if not all, of the problems faced by the memory-impaired patient will disappear or will be markedly reduced. However, there is little evidence that treating the presumed underlying deficit is effective. Attention training, for example, is seen by some as the underlying deficit in head-injured patients with memory problems (Trexler, 1982; Wood, 1984). Yet, as Wilson and Moffat (1984a) point out, there is only limited evidence for the view that impaired attention follows brain damage. Neither is there much evidence to suggest that generalization occurs from artificial attention training to real-life tasks. I do not mean to imply that attention training is never appropriate. Indeed, there is no doubt that some patients do have impaired attention, and a proportion of these may benefit from attention training. However, it should not be assumed that memory problems result from impaired attention in any given group of patients, such as those who are head-injured. Careful definition of the kind of attention disorder, for example, focused attention, divided attention, or sustained attention (Wilson & Moffat, 1984a), should be carried out, together with careful individual assessment of the disorder and proper evaluation of the intervention strategy.

Similar arguments can be made for treating memory problems as disorders of storage or retrieval. I have already argued that neither storage nor retrieval problems can explain the human amnesic syndrome, although improving the storage or retrieval process may help some memory-impaired people. A recent piece of research (Wilson, 1986) compared the effectiveness of two methods to improve recall of newspaper stories. Eight severely head-injured patients took part in the study, and the two methods used were rehearsal and PQRST, which stands for preview, question, read, state, and test; see Robinson (1970) for a full description. The times spent under the two conditions were equated. In delayed free recall, significantly more was retained under the PQRST condition than under the rehearsal condition. These results were interpreted as evidence for deeper processing in the PQRST condition (i.e., improving storage). Furthermore, in response to questions about the passages, more correct answers were supplied under the PQRST condition than under rehearsal. This finding suggested that PQRST provided better retrieval cues than did rehearsal. Thus, the PQRST procedure appeared to aid both storage and retrieval. Although all the patients had marked memory deficits, they were not as severely amnesic as those suffering from the human amnesic syndrome, thus indicating that whereas tackling storage and retrieval may help some memory-impaired people, it may prove difficult to apply to others.

Whereas the approaches described earlier were influenced by theoretical principles developed within the field of cognitive psychology, the next approach to the selection of an appropriate strategy to be discussed here has been influenced by certain theories within the field of neuropsychology. This approach is based on an attempt to use intact areas of the brain to compensate for damaged areas. Thus, in patients with left-hemisphere damage, the therapist can make use of right-hemisphere skills. Wilson (1981b) attempted this in the treatment of a man who had a left-temporal-lobe tumor removed. This man had severe verbal-memory problems, but was not dysphasic. He particularly wanted to remember the names of staff and neighbors with whom he came into regular contact. A visual-imagery program was designed that made use of his intact (or at least less damaged) right hemisphere and his normal visual memory. He learned the names of 10 people successfully when using imagery, but learned only one name when using verbal rehearsal. A similar study with a mildly aphasic man was reported by Wilson and Moffat (1984a).

If the right hemisphere can be used to compensate for verbal-memory problems, then perhaps the left can be used to compensate for non-verbal-memory or visual-memory problems. Some patients with right-hemisphere damage and topographical memory loss find this out for themselves. A patient at Rivermead who had suffered right-side cerebrovascular damage, for example, said, "I could never remember where the ward was until I told myself, 'Look for No Entry signs and go in the next entrance.' "

It is open to question how adaptable this approach of using intact areas of the brain may be. Most patients with memory problems do not have unilateral damage. It can be assumed that for these people, other parts of the brain can be utilized. For example, for pure amnesics with bilateral temporal damage, there are still the frontal, parietal, and occipital areas that can be used to help overcome the problems. Clinical experience suggests that such pure "temporal" amnesics can indeed compensate for their deficits with external aids to a much greater degree than amnesic patients with frontal-lobe damage. However, little systematic research has been conducted, although Hirst (1985) reported interesting differences between frontal amnesics and others with regard to (1) how they viewed their memory functioning and (2) the use made of strategies to aid recall. Again, the problem remains that many memory-impaired people have diffuse brain damage, and for these people, using intact areas of the brain is impracticable. Like the previous approaches, this one may be useful for a small group of patients, but will not hold as a general rule.

One way of selecting a treatment strategy that we find useful at Rivermead for a number of patients is to use a series of questions that probe each person's general intellectual level and the nature of the memory problems. The first question is, Does the patient have severe general intellectual impairment? If the answer is yes, then the methods of choice will be (1) RO, (2) reminiscence therapy, and (3) environmental restructuring. The assumptions here are that those with severe intellectual handicaps will be unlikely to benefit from internal memory aids and that most external aids will be lost or ignored.

If the answer to this first question is no, then the second question follows: Is the memory deficit material-specific? If yes, then we ask, Is it a verbal- or non-verbal-memory deficit? For verbal-memory problems, visual-imagery procedures are recommended, together with external aids. This is an instance of using intact skills (i.e., visuo-spatial skills) to compensate for damaged skills (in this case, impaired verbal-memory skills). If the problem is a nonverbal, material-specific disorder, then verbal mnemonics are recommended, together with an attempt to turn nonverbal tasks into verbal tasks (e.g., using verbal descriptions for places, shapes, faces, etc.). External aids should also have an important part to play.

If the problem is not material-specific, then we ask if it is modality-specific. This question is included because there are some people who experience difficulties with verbal *and* nonverbal material in one modality (such as the visual modality) but not in another (such as the auditory modality). For example, some right-hemisphere-stroke patients have difficulties remembering what they see, irrespective of whether this is written material, faces, or shapes; they are better at remembering what they hear, such as speech, music, and other nonverbal sounds. In these cases, patients may be suffering from unilateral neglect, and the procedures used to reduce neglect (Weinberg et al., 1979) can be tried. Alternatively, therapists can encourage patients to turn visual tasks into auditory tasks and also investigate the use of external aids, particularly tape recorders, dictaphones, timers, and alarms. In other cases, patients may have problems remembering what they hear (speech or nonverbal sounds), while remembering better what it is they see (written words or other visual material). Such patients are likely, in many cases, to have language problems that will require speech therapy. Alternatively, therapists can recommend that patients attempt to turn the auditory tasks into visual tasks. This can sometimes be accomplished by mental imagery or by writing/drawing the material to be remembered. Again, external aids can be used, and among these perhaps the most helpful are notebooks, lists, noticeboards, photographs, maps, and diagrams. These questions are tackled in diagrammatic form by Wilson and Moffat (1984b).

Most memory-impaired people will fall into categories revealed by the previous questions. The only group still to be discussed comprises the global amnesics with little or no general intellectual deficits: those known to have the human amnesic syndrome. These people, few in number, are likely to find internal strategies difficult to use, although often it is worth investigating whether or not such strategies can be used (Wilson, 1982). I have known three global amnesics with high I.Q. scores who were able to use first-letter mnemonics to a limited degree. Nevertheless, the most useful kind of aids for these people are the external aids. Because their intelligence is relatively unimpaired, frequently they can make efficient use of such aids. Procedural-learning tasks can also be learned with relative ease by pure amnesics and by many other memory-impaired people. "Procedural learning" is a term used to cover a wide range of skill learning. The feature that these various skills have in common is that it is not necessary to remember having completed them before in order to actually do them. Thus, we demonstrate how to ride a bicycle by riding it, not by remembering where and how we learned to do so. If a way could be found to describe procedures for other memory tasks, then memory rehabilitation would take a large step forward. It is possible to teach amnesic patients people's names by means of motor movements (Wilson, 1986), and we know that motor skills often are intact in these people (Brooks & Baddeley, 1976). We also know that some paired-associate learning tasks are quickly learned by people with amnesia (Warrington & Weiskrantz, 1982). Motor movements for names aim for some kind of logical relationship, usually a phonological similarity; for example, pretending to mix by using a stirring movement has been used for the name "Mick," and a mime of a barber at work has been used for "Barbara." However, at present we still have a long way to go in capitalizing on the amnesic patient's procedural-learning skills in order to help overcome everyday problems.

Evaluation of memory-therapy programs

Some doctors, psychologists, and therapists believe that evidence for the effectiveness of memory-therapy techniques can be obtained only through large-scale studies. Unfortunately, rigid adherence to this belief can result in failure to recognize that evaluation of memory therapy can also be achieved through single-case studies. For instance, in a recent and largely favorable review of a book on the management of memory problems (which contained several reports of single-case studies), the reviewer (Neary, 1984) complained that many of the strategies described in the book had not been properly evaluated and that the examples cited concerning success and failure were therefore anecdotal. It is my view that the reviewer missed the point that all intervention programs for brain-damaged and elderly people have to be evaluated *on an individual basis.* The results of a large-group study may not be particularly applicable to an individual patient whose situation, responses, and needs may be very different from those of the subjects in the experimental sample. The argument I wish to promote is that academics, researchers, and therapists should recognize that one of the ways of extending our knowledge of the effectiveness of treatments, and thereby extending our understanding of theory, is to be receptive to a range of methodologies, including studies that aim to evaluate the effectiveness of treatment for the individual patient.

Our studies of treatment for individuals have been assisted and illuminated by techniques and approaches that have been developed in the field of behavioral psychology. Thus, at least some of the reports that Neary (1984) considered to be anecdotal were, on the contrary, evaluated in minute detail through behavioral-treatment programs and/or single-case experimental designs.

If memory-therapy programs follow the same format as behavior-modification programs, then evaluation is built in. A behavior-modification program usually proceeds in the following stages:

1 Specification of the behavior to be changed
2 Definition of the goals or aims (usually both immediate and long-term aims are described)
3 Obtaining baselines
4 Deciding on appropriate treatment
5 Planning the treatment
6 Beginning the treatment
7 Monitoring and evaluating progress
8 Changing the procedure if necessary

Provided that each stage has been properly carried out, measurements will be obtained that usually will allow the therapist to determine if the treatment has been effective, has resulted in no change, or has been detrimental to the patient.

Table 32.1 *A.H.'s program*

1. Specify behavior	Inability to learn people's names.
2. State aim	To teach A.H. the name of one member of the staff (Janet).
3. Obtain baseline	On four occasions, Janet was introduced to A. H., and he was asked her name 2–3 min later. He never remembered correctly.
4. Decide on treatment	An expanded rehearsal strategy was selected (Landauer & Bjork, 1978).
5. Plan treatment	As A.H. could not remember Janet's name after 2 min, it was decided to present the stimulus (Janet), then test after 1, 2, 4, and 8 min, and so on. The intervals would be filled with other memory activities (e.g., recall of Rey Osterreith figure and questions about past life). If A.H. failed the rehearsal, times would be reduced, and testing would begin with the interval prior to his failure.
6. Begin treatment	Treatment started. A.H. was seen three times each week. The test sessions ended when his hospital transport arrived.
7. Monitor and evaluate progress	A.H. was able to retain Janet's name for 32 min on two occasions.
8. Change procedure if necessary	It was hoped that treatment could be extended outside the clinical psychology sessions. Unfortunately, however, A.H. was discharged.

An example of a memory-therapy program designed along these lines is illustrated in Table 32.1. The patient, A.H., was a 42-year-old man with severe amnesia and other cognitive problems resulting from carbon monoxide poisoning.

A summary of A.H.'s improvement can be seen in Figure 32.1. This is presented in the form of an ABAB design in which A = baseline and B = treatment. Following initial baselines (A), the expanding-rehearsal method was introduced. The second (and third) A phases refer to the second (and third) treatment sessions. Because the sessions were to some extent dependent on the time of arrival of transport, the number of baseline measurements varied.

The program appeared to be working, but it was not possible in the time allowed to ensure that A.H. learned Janet's name permanently. On his discharge, the method was explained to the staff caring for him at the referring hospital. Other examples of behavioral-therapy programs for memory improvement can be found in Wilson and Moffat (1984b) and Wilson (1985).

There are other ways in which therapists can evaluate treatment with individual patients. The simplest are straightforward before-and-after measurements. Although simple to organize, they can lead to difficulties in interpretation. If a series of memory tests is given before and after memory therapy, and if improvement occurs, then it is unclear how far this is due to natural recovery and how far it is due to the effects of treatment. If there are no alternate forms of the test available, then a practice effect may be a further confounding factor. If alternate

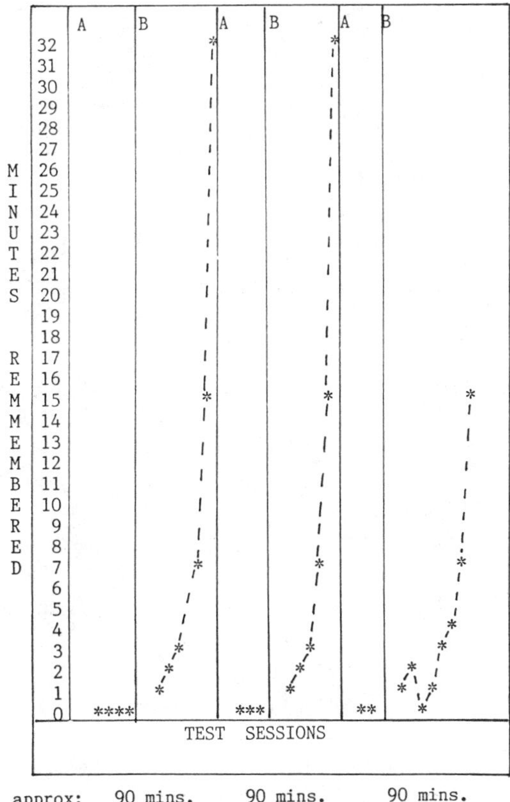

Figure 32.1. Summary of A.H.'s improvement.

forms are available, then they may not be of equivalent levels of difficulty, and this also may confuse the issue (although with the RBMT described earlier, we know that the parallel forms of the test are not significantly different from each other).

If the therapist is interested in comparing two or more treatment approaches, then it is possible to use the method referred to earlier, namely, a matched design. It is important to ensure that the materials to be used in the two conditions are equally easy/difficult for the patient to remember and that the same amount of time is spent learning the material under each condition. Some examples of this approach can be found in Wilson (1986); one of these examples involved K. J., who demonstrated pure amnesia, a high I.Q., and no other identifiable cognitive deficits. PQRST and rehearsal strategies were used in an attempt to aid his recall of current news items. Neither helped his delayed free recall, which was always nil, but in response to questions about the stories, he retained significantly more

Table 32.2 *Percentages of questions answered correctly after PQRST method and rehearsal alone*

	PQRST		Rehearsal	
Test session	Immediate recall (%)	Delayed (30-min) recall (%)	Immediate recall (%)	Delayed (30-min) recall (%)
1	75	50	25	0
2	75	50	100	25
3	100	50	75	25
4	75	75	75	50
5	75	50	75	0
6	25	0	50	25
7	100	50	25	0
8	75	50	75	0
Mean	77.7	47.1	62.5	15.6

after a delay with the PQRST material than with the rehearsal material. The difference in immediate recall was not significant. See Table 32.2 for a summary of the results.

Perhaps the best way of evaluating treatment is to use one of the single-case experimental designs described earlier. Figure 32.1 illustrated an *ABAB* or reversal design. Although simple designs, *ABAB* designs are limited in practice for three main reasons: First, it is not always possible to revert to baseline conditions. Once a piece of information has been thoroughly learned, for example, the patient cannot ''unlearn'' it. Second, sometimes a return to baseline conditions is unacceptable because it is unethical. If, for example, we taught a paraplegic patient to remember to lift himself from his chair every 10 min in order to prevent pressure sores developing, then we should not return to a situation in which pressure sores would be likely in order to prove a scientific point. Third, often it is impracticable to return to baseline conditions. For example, if we have taught a dementing patient to find his own bed by use of signposts, then no one would thank us for removing the signposts and thereby causing the patient to disturb other patients again.

The number of situations in which reversal designs can be used in clinical practice probably is limited, but the multiple-baseline designs are much more flexible and adaptable. Examples of multiple-baseline-across-behaviors designs in memory therapy have been provided by Wilson (1981a, 1982, 1986). A multiple-baseline-across-settings design was used by Carr and Wilson (1983), and a multiple-baseline-across-subjects design was described by Wilson and Moffat (1984a).

Loftus and Wilson (unpublished manuscript) used a multiple-baseline-across-behaviors design in the treatment of a 43-year-old Korsakoff patient: T.B. Three problems were selected for treatment: (1) remembering short routes around the rehabilitation center, (2) remembering newspaper articles, and (3) remembering

Table 32.3 *Baseline measures on three of T. B.'s memory problems*

Problem	Procedure	Score
1. Routes	T. B. was instructed: "Take me to the workshop/canteen/office, etc."	1 point if he took the most direct route (max. 10 points)
2. Newspaper articles	Article read to T. B., who was asked for immediate and delayed (20 min) recall.	Scoring system adapted from the Wechsler Memory Scale (max. 20 points)
3. Names of staff	Photographs of staff were shown one at a time, with names provided. Following presentation of 10 photographs, T. B. was asked for immediate and delayed (20 min) recall.	1 point for each correct name (max. 10 points)

names of staff at the center. The baseline procedure can be seen in Table 32.3. T.B.'s ability to remember his way around the rehabilitation center improved with rehearsal. No improvement occurred during baseline conditions with regard to newspaper articles or to remembering the names of staff. For one session, extra rehearsal was used for both newspaper articles and names, but with little or no effect. A PQRST strategy was then introduced for the newspaper articles, and the face–name association procedure was used to teach the names of staff.

Figure 32.2 illustrates that the routes improved with practice, that PQRST helped considerably with newspaper articles, and that the face–name association procedure made a dramatic difference to T. B.'s learning of the names of staff.

The point of the multiple-baseline designs is that by staggering the introduction of treatment, we can see whether or not improvement is directly related to the intervention strategy. If it is, then there will be a direct relationship between improvement and introduction of treatment. If something other than treatment is responsible for improvement, either all the problems will change simultaneously or there will be no direct relationship between changes and intervention strategies.

Possible ways forward in memory therapy

It is unlikely that any of the memory-therapy strategies and programs described in this chapter will make large differences in the quality of the everyday lives of the memory-impaired people who participate in them. However, memory-impaired people have been neglected for too long, and I would argue that treatment of their problems should be considered a matter of urgency. The point I wish to stress here is that more effective strategies may be developed in the long term if we have the determination to pursue evaluation of present practices in a scientific manner. At the present time in the history of memory therapy, we should take the line that *anything* that will improve the lives of the memory-impaired, however slight, should be pursued with vigor and resourcefulness.

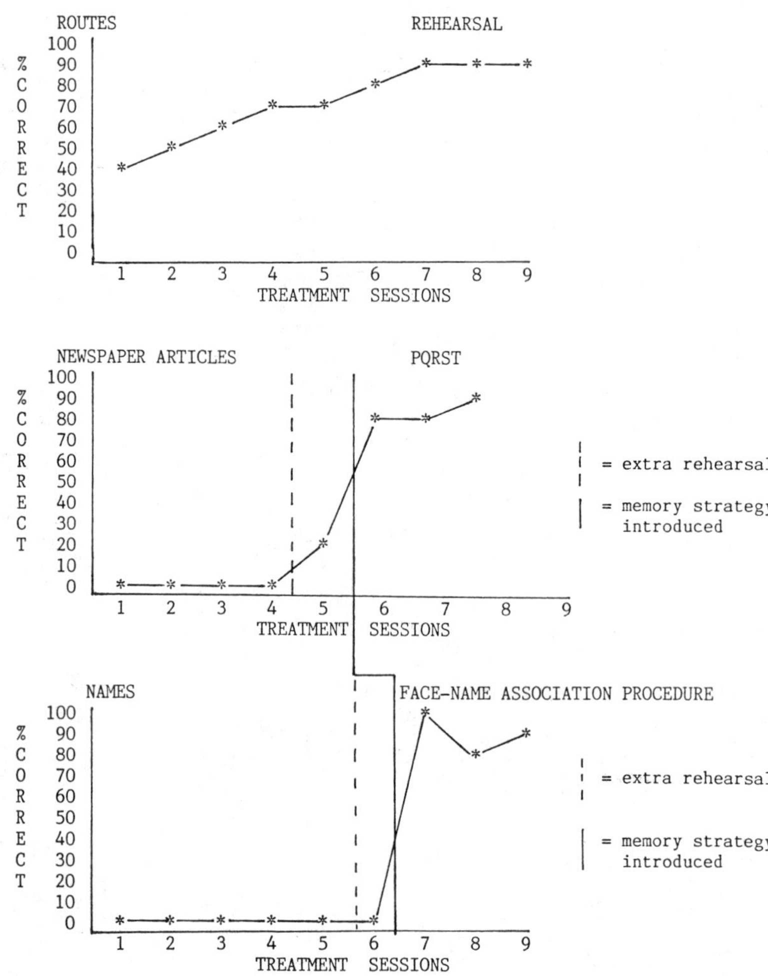

Figure 32.2. A multiple-baseline-across-behaviors design to evaluate T.B.'s memory-therapy program.

A program that is properly augmented by research will almost certainly achieve wider understanding of the problems faced by the memory-impaired. This may include increased appreciation of the nature of their disorders and the drawing of more subtle distinctions between treatments for different diagnostic groups and different individuals. We can expect better management of our patients' problems, which may involve improvements in restructuring their environments in order to reduce memory load. We can certainly improve our selection procedures concerning the appropriate usage of rehearsal and other techniques. More knowledge about the kinds of prompts or cues to use, how often to use them, and how best to fade them can be gained through persistent practice and evaluation. We still have much to learn about shaping, chaining, modeling, and other behavioral techniques as adjuncts to memory therapy. Much of the literature on visual imagery, for example, suggests that amnesic patients are not helped by this procedure. However, such failures may result from presenting patients with too much material at any one time. Certainly, the studies reported by Wilson (1986) indicate that visual imagery is potentially useful for many severely amnesic patients as long as only one piece of information is taught at any one time. Here, then, is an example of a specific area that is worthy of further investigation.

Much further progress can be made in improving generalization of the procedures we would have our patients learn. This includes generalization across subjects, across behaviors, and across settings. How far generalization across subjects can proceed is not easy to answer on the basis of large-group studies. Although such investigations sometimes are useful for comparing different treatments, particularly when order and interaction effects are expected, it is perhaps too easy to obtain significant results with large-group studies – even when a substantial minority of the subjects do not show the desired effect or are actually made worse by the intervention procedure. Provided the majority show a fairly good response, then significant results can almost be guaranteed. How does the therapist interpret such findings with regard to an individual patient? Simply adopting a process of trial and error on the basis of such findings may indeed be harmful to the patient.

Small-group studies are sometimes more helpful, because significant results usually are obtained only when all (or almost all) the subjects show the desired effect. If an individual patient shares the characteristics of those in the small-group study, it is likely that similar effects can be produced for that patient. In general, brain-damaged people show as many individual differences as any other group, and we have to take these into account when designing treatment programs. However, given a sufficient number of properly evaluated memory-therapy programs to consider, we should be able to predict with some accuracy which strategies will generalize across subjects.

Generalization across behaviors occurs in a situation in which a strategy taught to help with one problem is used to help with another. For example, if a patient is taught PQRST for newspaper articles and uses it to learn a poem, then generalization has occurred. No studies have been reported investigating how far such generalization occurs, although in many, if not most, cases, *spontaneous* generalization is rare. Because this is such an important concept for treatment, deliberate efforts should be made to build this kind of generalization into programs, as is being done with some mentally handicapped people (Carr, 1980).

Generalization across settings occurs in a situation in which a strategy taught in one setting is used in another. For example, if an electronic memory aid is used by a patient in the rehabilitation center and is then used at home, generalization has occurred. Again, there are no research findings on this topic, but this kind of generalization also is unlikely to occur spontaneously in the majority of memory-therapy programs. It must also follow that we should make this an essential part of treatment; see Wilson (1986) for further discussion of this topic.

Finally, there is perhaps one area above all others in which memory therapists should concentrate their efforts: how to make everyday memory tasks more like procedural-learning tasks, which most memory-impaired people can learn with comparative ease. Once we have achieved this, then our contribution to memory-therapy programs will have increased considerably.

References

Baddeley, A. D. (1982). Implications of neuropsychological evidence for theories of normal memory. *Philosophical Transactions of the Royal Society, London B, 298,* 59–72.

Baddeley, A. D. (1984). Memory theory and memory therapy. In B. Wilson & N. Moffat (Eds.), *Clinical management of memory problems.* London: Croom Helm.

Baddeley, A. D., & Wilson, B. A. (1986). Amnesia, autobiographical memory and confabulation. In D. Rubin (Ed.), *Autobiographical memory* (pp. 225–252). Cambridge University Press.

Brooks, D. N., & Baddeley, A. D. (1976). What can amnesic patients learn? *Neuropsychologia, 14,* 111–122.

Butters, N., & Cermak, L. (1975). Some analyses of amnesic syndromes in brain damaged patients. *Hoppocampus, 2,* 377–409.

Carr, J. (1980). Imitation, discrimination and generalisation. In W. Yule & J. Carr (Eds.), *Behavior modification for the mentally handicapped.* London: Croom Helm.

Carr, S., & Wilson, B. (1983). Promotion of pressure relief exercising in a spinal injury patient: A multiple baseline across settings design. *Behavioral Psychotherapy, 11,* 329–336.

Cermak, L. S. (1975). Imagery as an aid to retrieval for Korsakoff patients. *Quarterly Journal of Studies of Alcoholism, 34,* 1110–1132.

Ciminero, A. R., Calhoun, K. S., & Adams, H. E. (Eds.). (1977). *Handbook of behavioral assessment.* New York: Wiley.

Craik, F. I. M., & Lockhart, R.S. (1972). Levels of processing: A framework for memory research. *Journal of Verbal Learning and Verbal Behavior, 11,* 671–684.

Cutting, J. (1978). A cognitive approach to Korsakoff's syndrome. *Cortex, 14,* 485–495.

Edgington, E. S. (1982). Nonparametric tests for single-subject multiple schedule experiments. *Behavioral Assessment, 4,* 83–91.

Harris, J. E. (1978). External memory aids. In M. M. Gruneberg, P. E. Morris, & R. N. Sykes (Eds.), *Practical aspects of memory* (pp. 172–179). Academic Press: New York.

Harris, J. E. (1980). Memory aids people use: Two interview studies. *Memory & Cognition, 8,* 31–38.

Harris, J. E. (1984). Ways of improving memory. In B. A. Wilson & N. Moffat (Eds.), *Clinical management of memory problems.* London: Croom Helm.

Harris, J. E., & Sunderland, A. (1981). A brief survey of the management of memory disorders in rehabilitation units in Britain. *International Rehabilitation Medicine, 3,* 206–209.

Hay, L. R. (1982). Teaching behavioral assessment to clinical psychology students. *Behavioral Assessment, 4,* 35–40.

Hersen, M., & Barlow, D. H. (1976). *Single case experimental design strategies for studying behavior change.* New York: Pergamon.

Hirst, W. (1985, June). *Use of mnemonic in patients with frontal lobe damage.* Paper presented at the International Neuropsychological Society's annual conference, Copenhagen.

Holden, U. P., & Woods, R. T. (1982). *Reality orientation: Psychological approaches to the confused elderly.* London: Churchill Livingstone.

Ince, L. P. (1978). *Behavior modification in rehabilitation.* Springfield, IL: Charles C. Thomas.

Jones, M. (1974). Imagery as a mnemonic aid after left temporal lobectomy: Contrast between material specific and generalised memory disorders. *Neuropsychologia, 12,* 21–30.

Kazdin, A. E. (1982). *Single case research designs.* London: Oxford University Press.

Landauer, T. K., & Bjork, R. A. (1978). Optimum rehearsal patterns and name learning. In M. M. Gruneberg, P. E. Morris, & R. N. Sykes (Eds.), *Practical aspects of memory* (pp. 625–632). New York: Academic Press.

Loftus, M., & Wilson, B. *Memory therapy with a Korsakoff patient: A multiple baseline design.* Unpublished manuscript.

Merriam, S. (1980). The concept and function of reminiscence: A review of the research. *Gerontologist, 20,* 604–608.

Meudell, P., & Mayes, A. (1982). Normal and abnormal forgetting. In A. W. Ellis (Ed.), *Normality and pathology in cognitive functions.* New York: Academic Press.

Milner, B., Corkin, S., & Teuber, J. L. (1968). Further analysis of the hippocampal amnesic syndrome: A 14 year follow-up study of H.M. *Neuropsychologia, 61,* 215–234.

Mischel, W. (1968). *Personality and assessment.* New York: Wiley.

Moffat, N. (1984). Strategies of memory therapy. In B. Wilson & N. Moffat (Eds.), *Clinical management of memory problems.* London: Croom Helm.

Neary, D. (1984). Review of clinical management of memory problems. *Journal of the Royal Society of Medicine, 77,* 994.

Parkin, A. J. (1984). Amnesic syndrome: A lesion-specific disorder? *Cortex, 20,* 479–508.

Robinson, F. P. (1970). *Effective study.* New York: Harper & Row.

Starr, A., & Phillips, L. (1970). Verbal memory in the amnesic syndrome. *Neuropsychologia, 8,* 75–82.

Sunderland, A., Harris, J. E., & Baddeley, A. D. (1984). Assessing everyday memory after severe head injury. In J. E. Harris & P. Morris (Eds.), *Everyday memory, actions and absentmindedness* (pp. 191–206). New York: Academic Press.

Trexler, L. (1982). *Cognitive rehabilitation, conceptualization and intervention.* New York: Plenum Press.

Warrington, E. K., & Weiskrantz, L. (1970). Amnesic syndrome: Consolidation or retrieval? *Nature, 228,* 628–630.

Warrington, E. K., & Weiskrantz, L. (1982). Amnesia: A disconnection syndrome? *Neuropsychologia, 20,* 233–248.

Weinberg, M. A., Diller, L., Gordon, W. A., Gerstman, L. J., Liebermann, A., Larkin, P., Hodges, G., & Ezrachi, O. (1979). Training sensory awareness and spatial organization in people with right brain damage. *Archives of Physical and Medical Rehabilitation, 60,* 491–496.

Weiskrantz, L. (1978). A comparison of hippocampal pathology in man and other animals. In *Functions of the septo-hippocampal system. Ciba Foundation Symposium* (Vol. 58). Amsterdam: North Holland.

Wilson, B. A. (1981a). A survey of behavioral treatments carried out at a rehabilitation centre for stroke and head injuries. In G. Powell (Ed.), *Brain function therapy.* Aldershot, UK: Gower Press.

Wilson, B. A. (1981b). Teaching a patient to remember people's names after removal of a left temporal lobe tumor. *Behavioral Psychotherapy, 9,* 338–344.

Wilson, B. A. (1982). Success and failure in memory training following a cererbral vascular accident. *Cortex, 18,* 581–594.

Wilson, B. A. (1985, June). *What is different about frontal amnesia?* Paper presented at the International Neuropsychological Society's annual conference, Copenhagen.

Wilson, B. A. (1986). *Rehabilitation of memory.* New York: Guilford Press.

Wilson, B. A., Cockburn, J., & Baddeley, A. D. (1985). *The Rivermead Behavioral Memory Test.* Reading, UK: Thames Valley Test Co., 22 Bulmershe Rd.

Wilson, B. A., Cooper, Z., & Kennerley, H. (1983, December). *An investigation of the effectiveness of group training on memory functioning in adults with acquired brain damage.* Paper presented at a meeting of the Society for Research in Rehabilitation, London.

Wilson, B.A., & Moffat, N. (1984a). Rehabilitation of memory for everyday life. In J. Harris & P. Morris (Eds.), *Everyday memory, actions and absentmindedness* (pp. 207–234). New York: Academic Press.

Wilson, B. A., & Moffat, N. (Eds.). (1984b). *Clinical management of memory problems.* London: Croom Helm.

Winocur, G., & Weiskrantz, L. (1976). An investigation of paired-associate learning in amnesic patients. *Neuropsychologia, 14,* 97–110.

Wood, R. L. (1984). Attention training. In B. A. Wilson & N. Moffat (Eds.), *Clinical management of memory problems.* London: Croom Helm.

33 Management of memory problems in a hospital setting

Nadina B. Lincoln

Management techniques used in hospitals will vary according to the type of hospital ward and the clinical diagnoses of the patients. Different programs are used on acute general medical wards, rehabilitation wards, and long-stay wards. Different approaches are taken according to whether an impairment is one that is likely, to some extent, to show improvement (stroke or early head injury), to remain static (longer-term head injury), or to deteriorate (multiple sclerosis and dementia). Most of the previous literature has reported studies based on rehabilitation or geriatric wards. These will be considered in this chapter, but most emphasis will be placed on approaches that might be used on general medical wards, as there have been few published reports on the training of memory in this setting.

The studies considered are those that were designed for real-life memory problems, as opposed to investigations of the ability to learn experimental material. The former studies fall into two main categories. On geriatric or long-stay wards, the main approaches used are reality orientation, environmental modification, and reminiscence therapy. In a rehabilitation setting, training in specific memory strategies, such as visual imagery (Glasgow, Zeiss, Barrera, & Lewinsohn, 1977; Wilson 1981, 1982), PQRST (Glasgow et al., 1977), and first-letter cuing (Wilson, 1982), is more often used. These strategies may be carried out with individuals or in groups (Wilson & Moffat, 1984a).

Management approaches

Settings

Long-stay wards. Reality orientation (RO) is the most widely reported and most commonly used technique for rehabilitation of people who have suffered memory loss. It is designed to teach or maintain awareness of time, place, and person in confused, usually elderly, people. This may be 24-hour RO, in which all staff–

patient interactions are designed to promote awareness of time, place, and person, or classroom RO, in which specific group sessions are held several times a week to supplement the 24-hour RO (Holden & Woods, 1982).

Some studies that have evaluated the effectiveness of RO have yielded encouraging results, but the clinical significance of the behavior changes observed may not be great. When considering evaluations of RO, one must realize that RO is not a set technique but a collection of general principles. Its application will therefore vary between different centers. Most studies have been of formal or classroom RO, rather than informal 24-hour RO, which may be the more important. However, despite these problems, we now have quite a number of published investigations, which should enable us to draw some overall conclusions. The main conclusion is that RO programs have an effect that is statistically significant. Most studies have found an improvement in verbal orientation (Brook, Degun, & Mather, 1975; Citrin & Dixon, 1977; Hanley, 1981; Harris & Ivory, 1976; Johnson, McLaren, & McPherson, 1981; Woods, 1979). However, two studies (Barnes, 1974; Holden & Sinebruchow, 1978) have not shown even these beneficial effects. In the case of the Holden and Sinebruchow study (1978), this may, to some extent, reflect the lack of specificity of the assessment technique used, whereas Barnes (1974) used subjects in the most advanced stages of intellectual decline. Few studies have found any associated improvement in other areas of cognitive function. Only Woods (1979), in a study that compared RO with a social-therapy control group and an untreated control group, found that the RO group improved on various aspects of memory, as measured on the Wechsler memory scale, more than did either control group. Similarly, there have been few reports of improvements in general behavior. However, Brook and associates (1975) reported a positive change in the behavior of moderately, but not severely, demented patients. They found that withdrawn patients began to mix well on the ward, became talkative, and engaged in rational conversation. They also reported that almost all cases of incontinence began to show signs of improvement.

In a review of RO, Powell-Proctor and Miller (1982) stressed that the benefits are small and do not generalize widely and reliably to other aspects of behavior. Despite the cost in time and effort of achieving these results, they did point out that RO can be treated as a stepping-stone to developing more effective intervention programs with an often neglected group of patients. It also seems that many of the features of informal RO can be incorporated into management procedures on all wards where there are memory-impaired patients.

Rehabilitation wards. The approach usually used on rehabilitation wards has been to apply various mnemonic techniques to help patients overcome specific practical problems. Both internal and external strategies have been used, and only applications of these to real-life memory problems will be considered in this chapter.

Types of problems

Names. The most common problem to have been treated using a mnemonic strategy is that of remembering people's names. An early study of this problem was by Glasgow and associates (1977), who used a face–name association method, though without success. However, more encouraging results have been obtained using visual imagery. Wilson (1981) taught a patient with severe memory problems to remember the names of 10 staff members in a rehabilitation unit using visual images for names.

Subsequent studies on visual imagery for names have also reported success (Wilson, 1982; Wilson & Moffat, 1984a). Another strategy, suggested by Powell (1981), is to use motor coding. Thus, a name such as Mr. Bird might be learned by associating the person with an appropriate action symbolizing that name. There is one case report of an amnesic, severely head-injured patient using this method to learn the name of his physiotherapist (Wilson & Moffat, 1984a): The name "Anita" was learned by association with a headshaking movement, which acted as a cue for "a neater way of doing her hair."

Timetables. In many rehabilitation units, patients have a daily timetable for attendance at therapy sessions. Although these are in written form, memory-impaired patients may need training to refer to them. Fowler, Hart, and Sheehan (1972) described the use of a portable timer for a head-injured man. He used this as a prompt to refer to his timetable card, and after several weeks the auditory signal was removed. In another study, an alarm watch was used that "bleeped" every hour to remind a patient with Alzheimer's disease to look at his daily program (Kurlychek, 1983). A peg-rhyming method has also been described (Davenport & Hall, 1981) for prompting daily self-care activities with a severely head-injured patient who was taught the "one is a bun, two is a show, . . . etc." peg list, and then each stage in his morning routine was linked with one of the peg words.

Lists. Lists of words often are investigated as experimental material, but there are few occasions in daily life when one has to remember such lists. The most common instance is a shopping list, but most patients are able to circumvent this problem by writing down the items. One problem that may arise is that a patient may forget to refer to the list. Hussian (1981) described the use of a self-instructional statement to help solve this problem. An elderly forgetful woman was taught to use statements (e.g., "I'll go into one of the shops along the way, whenever I forget all five items that I came for, and refer to my list.") to remind her to use her shopping list. However, mnemonic techniques have been used when a written list has not been appropriate. Wilson (1982) used a first-letter mnemonic to teach a man 10 items of shopping. He was able to recall the 10 items once he was told that the first letters of the 10 items made the words "Go shopping.'' However, this may not be practical if a person has to learn a new mnemonic on each shopping trip.

Texts. Another problem that has been tackled is recall of texts, newspaper articles, and stories. The technique usually used is the PQRST method, which was applied by Glasgow and associates (1977) to assist the verbal-memory disorder of a severely head-injured woman. This method consists of five stages:

P	Preview	Briefly skim the material to learn the general content.
Q	Question	Ask key questions about the content.
R	Review	Read actively with the goal of answering the questions.
S	State	Repeat or rehearse the information that has been read.
T	Test	Test oneself by answering the questions that have been developed.

This was found to result in superior recall compared with a rehearsal condition or the subject's own preintervention strategy. Wilson (1984) used the technique to stop a patient who repeatedly asked the same questions. This man continually asked ''Why have I got a memory problem?'' The patient wrote from dictation a summary of his illness, operation, resultant problems, and prognosis. The PQRST technique was then followed, with the patient selecting key questions that by the end of 3 weeks he was able to answer. However, although he obtained 100% correct responses when the therapist asked the questions, he still repeated the original question several times a day.

Another study reported the use of semantic-elaboration techniques in conjunction with visual imagery as a preliminary stage of treatment for a similar problem (Malec & Questad, 1983) for a man who sustained a traumatic head injury in a motorcycle accident. The first stage of treatment consisted of teaching the patient a series of words by putting them into a simple story (semantic elaboration). After the patient had made up a story, he was asked to make a mental picture of the story's content, paying particular attention to the words to be remembered. This latter strategy was reported to be more helpful for him. The second stage of treatment was to reinforce memory for the words, getting the patient to ask himself questions that were related to the stories he had made up. This procedure was evaluated by comparing three baseline assessments and one assessment after treatment. Although orientation improved during the baseline period, performance on other memory tasks did not. Comparison of pretreatment and posttreatment assessments showed changes on measures of memory, but only minimal improvements in other cognitive abilities. The extent to which this improved his daily life skills was not assessed.

Although other problems have been treated using various strategies, these have not been sufficiently numerous to enable us to draw any overall conclusions. The specific training studies reviewed here indicate that the most successful strategies are visual imagery for the recall of names, alarms for recall of timetables, and PQRST for the recall of texts. However, these conclusions are based on relatively few case reports; clearly, further investigations are needed. There is also the problem that ineffective treatments are rarely reported, and so there is a risk of getting an unrealistically optimistic impression of therapeutic success. Nevertheless, these techniques have been used successfully to deal with clinical problems and therefore should be tried.

Memory groups

The group activities described by Wilson and Moffat (1984b) consist of opportunities to practice using mnemonic strategies. Much of this practice is carried out by means of memory games. These differ from the traditional approach of practicing remembering because strategies for remembering are discussed in relation to each game. For example, the Rivermead group play a game called "Mrs. Brown went to town," in which the first person says, "Mrs. Brown went to town and bought a bar of soap" (or some other item). The second person repeats this and adds a second item. Each successive person repeats the previous items and adds an item of his or her choice. As a therapy activity, this is combined with an explanation of different strategies that might be used to play the game. For example, if the items are soap, flour, lemons, sausages, eggs, and meat, a first-letter mnemonic can be constructed: "Six fat ladies struggled to eat more." Or an example using the method of loci (Figure 33.1) might be images of the following:

soap	in the bath
flour	in the bedroom
lemons	rolling down the stairs
sausages	sitting round the dining-room table
eggs	lined up on the living-room mantlepiece
meat	a joint of beef asleep in the dog's basket in the kitchen

Wilson, Cooper, and Kennerley (1983) evaluated the effectiveness of these group activities to aid memory using 20 subjects who were inpatients at Rivermead Rehabilitation Centre. They were aged 13 to 63 years (mean, 31.9 years; SD, 15 years); 12 were men, 15 had received severe head injuries, 4 had suffered cerebrovascular accidents, and 1 was post-encephalitic. Two initial assessments were made in weeks 1 and 2 to establish their pretreatment performances. Group A then received 3 weeks of memory training, which included playing memory games, discussing coping strategies, introduction to internal strategies and external aids, and practice in their use. Group B received 3 weeks of problem-solving, which included verbal and nonverbal tasks designed to be like those used by the memory group, but not including special techniques for improving memory; these included games of logic, word games, and attainment tests. On week 5, assessments were repeated, and group A then attended problem-solving sessions for 3 weeks, while group B attended the memory sessions. Assessments were then repeated immediately after treatment and 1 year later. The assessments at each

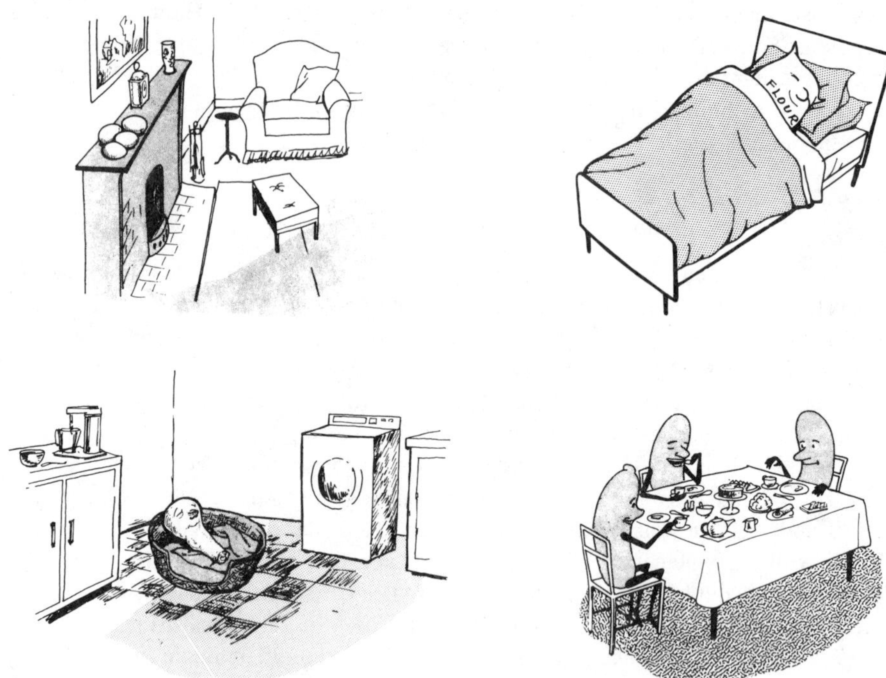

Figure 33.1. Example of use of method of loci to remember items on a shopping list.

stage included prose recall (Wechsler, 1945), digit span, paired-associate learning (Randt, Brown, & Osborne, 1980), the Rivermead Behavioural Memory Test (RBMT) (Wilson, Cockburn, & Baddeley, 1985), a modification of the Kapur and Pearson (1983) rating scale, and an adapted version of the Harris (1980) questionnaire on the use of memory aids. The results showed that improvement occurred in both groups. Eleven subjects improved more after memory training, five improved more after problem-solving training, and four did not change. Although more subjects improved after memory-group training, the difference did not reach significance. However, the most important finding was that memory skills, as assessed by the RBMT, improved following group treatment. Of all the tests, the RBMT had the most similarities to the problems of everyday life functioning, and so the gains on the RBMT may be clinically significant. These gains were maintained at 1-year follow-up, although no further gains in everyday memory functioning occurred between the posttreatment assessment and 1-year follow-up for the majority of patients.

Environmental modifications

Environmental modifications have been included in studies conducted on geriatric wards, as well as studies in rehabilitation centers. Hanley (1981) described the use of signposts in conjunction with active orientation training in the management of ward disorientation. Eight elderly female demented patients on two wards of a long-stay psychogeriatric unit were studied. In the first experiment, using *ABABA* designs, the effect of orientation training was evaluated. This consisted of showing patients areas of the ward that they were unable to locate, describing those areas verbally, and coaching each patient to repeat the names of the areas. After a 5-month follow-up period, large signposts were introduced on the ward, and the effects of introducing the signs and the effects of the combination of signs and ward training were evaluated using single-case designs. Signposts alone were not generally effective in assisting patients to find their way through a fixed route, but in combination with prior ward-orientation training, or, more especially, accompanying ward-orientation training, improvements were effected and maintained fully at 3-month follow-up. Replication of these findings with two disoriented residents of an old people's home supported these conclusions, as did a further study by Gilleard, Mitchell, and Riordan (1981), but in the latter, signposts alone had some beneficial effect, which was further enhanced by training.

Other environmental modifications that have been suggested include painting the lavatory doors a different color from all other doors (Harris, 1980). This was found to reduce incontinence in one geriatric unit. Pictorial instructions have been used to help an aphasic woman remember how to transfer from her wheelchair to her bed (Wilson, 1984). Another example is to rearrange material so that physical proximity between items will act as a reminder. For example, simply placing a chart indicating whether or not tablets had been taken by the side of the tablet bottle, instead of in a different room, helped one woman keep track of whether or not she had taken her tablets (Lincoln, 1984).

Environmental modifications have the advantage that they are relatively easy to carry out in virtually any environment. However, their effectiveness remains to be evaluated.

Frequency of reported memory problems: A questionnaire study

The treatment of memory problems in a hospital setting depends on the problems that occur, and these may not be the same as those observed in people's homes. In an investigation of memory problems experienced by stroke patients (Tinson & N. B. Lincoln, unpublished data), all patients who were admitted to two general hospitals in Nottingham with a diagnosis of stroke were registered. All those who were under 80 years of age were given a subjective memory questionnaire (Sunderland, Harris, & Baddeley, 1983) 1 month after the stroke. This questionnaire consisted of a series of 28 questions on the frequency of events such as forgetting people's names, losing items around the house, and getting lost. Of the 119 stroke patients admitted to hospital, 47 were still in hospital and able to complete the questionnaire 1 month later. They were aged 39 to 80 years (mean, 68.7 years; SD, 8.8 years). Twenty-six patients had suffered left-

Table 33.1. *Percentage of patients in hospital reporting memory problems*

	Patients		Patients' relatives	
Item	Stroke (n = 47)	Orthopedic (n = 13)	Stroke (n = 39)	Orthopedic (n = 12)
13. Finding a word that is on the tip of one's tongue	40	15	33	0
6. Forgetting when it was that things happened	23	8	36	8
10. Rambling on about unimportant or irrelevant things	21	0	20	0
28. Repeating to someone something or asking the same question twice	21	0	23	0
1. Forgetting where things have been put	19	8	26	8
8. Forgetting things that one has been told	19	0	33	0

hemisphere stroke, and 17 had suffered right-hemisphere stroke; this information was missing for 4 patients. The patients' relatives were asked to complete an equivalent questionnaire about the memory problems that they had noticed in the patients. Replies were available for 39 of the 47 patients. In addition to the stroke patients, we studied a group of orthopedic controls. These patients were aged 40 to 80 years and had been admitted to hospital 1 month previously as a result of injury or for an operation. Only 13 of the 126 controls were still in hospital for this assessment; so the results on the control group are rather limited. These patients were aged 40 to 80 years (mean, 61.0 years; SD, 11.4 years), and all were on acute orthopedic wards.

The proportion of stroke patients who experience memory problems is generally low. If we consider events occurring more than once a week as a problem, then according to the stroke patients, difficulties arose for more than 15% of them on only seven questions. These are shown in Table 33.1. If we consider as problems only those events that occur daily, then the questions for which most problems occurred were questions 1, 10, and 13, and these were reported by 7% of patients.

Despite the small number of controls that were still in hospital at 1 month following injury or operation, the same events were among the most frequently occurring in non-brain-damaged patients (i.e., questions 1, 6, and 13). These patients also reported forgetting what had just been said when talking to someone (Q16). However, there were significantly fewer reports of memory problems among the control patients.

It might be expected that relatives would notice more problems than would patients. Results from the relatives' versions of the questionnaire were available for 39 of the stroke patients in hospital and 12 of the controls. Problems that occurred more than once a week for more than 15% of the stroke patients were reported for 19 of the 28 questions, but for none of the questions for control patients.

If we consider only those things that occur daily as problems, then the most commonly reported problems observed by relatives of stroke patients were on questions 6 (18%), 13 (15%), and 16 (15%). This is still a significant proportion, and it suggests that these patients did have difficulties with memory, but not all of them were fully aware of the difficulties that were occurring. These results pertain to patients in hospital, but if we consider outpatients as well, these same difficulties were the ones most commonly reported by stroke patients and most often observed by relatives. Control patients rarely reported any memory difficulties occurring more than once a week, but even in this group these same questions covered the events most likely to occur.

Thus, it seems that there was consistency in terms of those memory problems that occur most frequently among both inpatients and outpatients, but our stroke patients experienced difficulties more frequently than did the orthopedic controls. These problems have also been reported to occur in head-injured patients (Sunderland, Harris, & Baddeley, 1983, 1984) and in normal elderly subjects (Sunderland, Watts, Baddeley, & Harris, 1986). However, the latter study by Sunderland and associates (1986) raises the question of the validity of these subjective measures with elderly subjects. Because most of our subjects, both patients and relatives, were elderly, the accuracy of their observations may be low. Nevertheless, in terms of selecting problems for treatment, their subjective impressions of items that were forgotten may be as important as the items that were actually forgotten.

This consistency in the problems experienced by stroke patients and head-injured patients gives us an indication of which difficulties need to be treated. A similar approach, described by Wilson (1984), is to ask relatives or staff to fill in a checklist about events that have happened in a given period of time. Wilson presented a list of 28 items, based on those used by Sunderland and associates (1983), recorded at the end of each treatment session each day for 2 weeks.

Practical considerations in memory therapy

The choice of treatment strategy for many memory problems will depend on the setting in which treatment is to be carried out. There are some practical considerations when conducting memory therapy on hospital wards. The first limitation is the number of staff. On general medical wards, large numbers of staff may be involved with any one patient. Memory therapy is not likely to be a common treatment, and it would be impractical to try to train all staff in a consistent approach to each patient, considering the resources we have available. This problem, to a lesser extent, arises on rehabilitation or long-stay wards. However, in these settings, the length of stay for any one patient is likely to be much longer, and so it is more feasible to train the staff. Also, memory problems are likely to be common on these wards, relative to other conditions, and therefore to assume higher priority.

One possible means of circumventing the problem of adequate staffing when working on general wards is to involve other patients. Because other patients will see the subject patient almost all of the time, they can be more readily available than any member of staff. However, the length of their own involvement may be unpredictable. We have, on occasion, used other patients as "checkers" to see that programs have been carried out, or as providers of relatively simple information. For example, we provided a calendar of the tear-off variety for a patient who had difficulty remembering the date. The staff were supposed to ensure that the previous day's page was torn off first thing each morning; because that did not happen, we asked one of the other patients on the ward to check that this was done each day. Volunteers might fulfill similar roles, provided that a treatment program were amenable to being carried out at convenient times of the day.

A second practical difficulty arises when memory problems are assigned a low priority for treatment. On medical wards, medical treatments are going to be more important for those who are acutely ill. Memory training quite reasonably must be given low priority. Consequently, even when time is available, memory programs may tend not to be carried out because the reason for their low priority may not be made explicit. This should not apply to the same extent on rehabilitation or geriatric wards.

Treatment approaches on a general medical ward

Despite practical limitations, there are many ways we can help overcome some of the memory problems that occur in hospitals. Some methods are very general and can be applied in any hospital; others are more suited to a rehabilitation setting.

In a survey of the management of memory disorders in rehabilitation units in Britain, Harris and Sunderland (1981) found that there was considerable variation in approaches to treatment. The most commonly used overall strategy was to attempt to teach patients ways of coping with (or learning to overcome) the particular everyday problems of which they specifically complained. More rarely, the approach involved giving training on memory tasks generally, so that practice would improve a patient's memory overall and therefore help overcome certain practical everyday problems. This latter strategy was used by 12 of the 22 respondents to the survey questionnaire. The most commonly used technique was the provision of external aids in the form of notebooks, diaries, and electronic prompters. More surprisingly, the next most popular method involved the use of memory games and laboratory-type memory tasks. This provided repetitive practice and seemed to be based on the assumption that memory responded like a "mental muscle" and that exercising it on one task would strengthen it for use on other tasks, so that any improvement on artificial games would be expected to generalize to the requirements of everyday life. Although, as Harris and Sunderland (1981) pointed out, this seems to be too simple and over optimistic, apparently there have been no controlled trials of repetitive training on memory tasks and its effect on general memory performance. Clearly, such studies are needed before we discard this approach as inappropriate. The better-evaluated approaches, such as reality orientation and the provision of internal memory aids, did appear in the list of techniques used and therefore have been adopted in at least some rehabilitation units in Britain.

Environmental modifications

Designing the hospital environment to put the fewest demands on memory may help some patients to cope. It is likely to help patients with milder deficits to a greater extent, as well as patients who are showing recovery from their deficits, which makes this a particularly appropriate approach to use on general wards. There are several features of wards that can be changed to overcome some of the common difficulties suggested earlier. Most wards have clocks, but in many cases a clock cannot be seen from a patient's bedside; also, clocks can stop, and often they are not put right. On our rehabilitation ward, patients are encouraged to bring their own alarm clocks, to be put where they can most easily be seen. In hospitals, there are rarely clues as to the date. A glance out of the window will sometimes indicate the season, but in many of our hospitals, all that is visible is another building. Calendars can be helpful, but they need to be large, explicit, and automatic. If these are not available, an alternative is to use display calendars and cross off each day with a wide, felt-tip marker. At least patients can see at a glance whether it is the beginning, middle, or end of the month, even if they cannot see the exact day.

There can be many clues in the ward routine that can indicate the time of day or the day of the week if the ward routine is made explicit. Patients usually are not told at what times coffee, tea, and meals are served; they simply arrive when they arrive. Drug rounds are carried out at approximately set times. Consultant ward rounds are on a given day of the week. If the times of these events were clearly indicated to patients, they might be able to use them as environmental cues.

All members of our staff wear name badges showing name and position. However, name badges are small and difficult to read, and the name does not always correspond to the name by which the person is actually called. It is not much help being able to read that the badge says Mrs. Walker if the person is always called Marion. A badge indicating the used name would be more helpful, and of course it should be in large print.

Different uniforms signify different posts and responsibilities. For example, in Britain, the blue-check dress is worn by a qualified nurse, and the green uniform by an occupational therapist. If the patients had this information in diagrammatic or written form, they would at least have a better chance of remembering it and

Table 33.2. *Summary of test results for J.H.*

General intellectual abilities: WAIS		
Information	13[a]	
Comprehension	7[a]	
Similarities	11[a]	
Digit Span	10[a]	
Vocabulary	11[a]	
Block Design	10[a]	
Picture Arrangement	6[a]	
Object Assembly	7[a]	
Memory		
Wechsler Logical Memory I[b]		4[c]
Wechsler Logical Memory II		4[c]
Frontal-lobe functions		
Word fluency	Score 5[c]	
Modified card sorting	Categories 4[c]	
	Errors 20[c]	
	Perseverative errors 35%	

[a]Age-scaled scores.
[b]Followed by 30-min delay before Logical Memory II.
[c]Below average.

would be better able to know who is helping them with different aspects of their treatment.

None of these environmental changes is going to solve big problems, but at least we might give those patients with mild difficulties a better chance and help to boost their shattered self-confidence.

How the environment may affect a patient's abilities is illustrated by the case of J.H., a 54-year-old man who had right hemiplegia and mild dysarthria as a result of a stroke. At the time he was referred for treatment, he was living in a residential unit, where the aim was for him to achieve sufficient independence to live on his own. However, after months in the unit, he still was not carrying out domestic tasks, such as making himself tea or going out, and he was independent only in basic self-care skills, such as washing and dressing. Baseline records of his activities of daily living showed a slight change over 4 weeks, but he was not carrying out all activities necessary for independent living. Formal testing showed that he had marked memory problems (a summary of test results is shown in Table 33.2). He was considered to be a suitable candidate for intensive memory training and therefore was transferred to our stroke unit. The plan was to have a 2-week baseline period, with no special memory therapy, and then 4 weeks of intensive memory therapy. During the 2 weeks of postadmission baseline, he showed marked improvements in activities of daily living, presumably as a result of the change in environment. His progress is shown in Figure 33.2. The

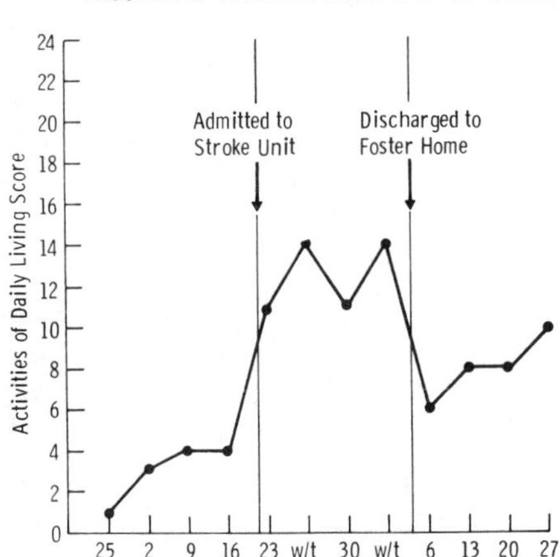

Figure 33.2. Progress of J.H. in activities of daily living.

assessment used is shown in Table 33.3. Our unit differed from the unit where he had been in two respects: (1) We had a planned program of activities for each day. (2) Because most of these patients had recently suffered strokes, most of them were improving, whereas in his previous unit there had been many long-stay residents who were not expected to change. Whether or not these were the crucial features we have no way of telling. However, it seems that the change in environment produced the desired effect; no specific memory-training program was needed. After discharge, monitoring of his abilities continued, and he has managed to live independently since then.

General ward management policies

Although the limitations of RO have already been described, there are several features of informal or 24-hour RO that can be incorporated into the management of patients with memory problems in other settings. Disorientation in regard to time, person, and place often occurs in the early stages of recovery from head injury and early after a stroke or a confusional state. RO should therefore be tried on general medical and surgical wards to see if it helps alleviate the problems of these patients. Because these people are likely to recover to some extent without specific intervention, evaluation of the effectiveness of such a procedure is likely to be difficult. However, this recovery may help to encourage staff to participate in such a policy and make them more likely to be involved in specific retraining programs that might be introduced later. It has been found that RO compliance is low, and behavior change among ward staff does not occur as

Table 33.3. *Assessment of activities of daily living*

Please record which activities Mr. Harrison did in the week beginning. . .	Yes	No
Mobility		
Did he:		
Walk round outside		
Walk over uneven ground		
Cross roads		
Climb stairs		
Get in and out of a car		
Travel on public transport		
Kitchen		
Did he:		
Make himself a hot drink		
Take hot drinks from one room to another		
Make a hot snack		
Do the washing up		
Domestic		
Did he:		
Go shopping		
Do any housework		
Wash small items of clothing		
Do a full wash		
Manage his money when out		
Leisure		
Did he:		
Go out alone socially		
Read newspapers or books		
Write a letter		
Use the telephone		
Do any gardening		
Drive a car		
Visit friends		
Go for a walk		
Go to church/pub/club		

expected (Hanley, 1981); so any policy change of this type will need to be carefully monitored.

Individual treatment programs

In some cases, environment and overall ward policies are not sufficient, and programs must be devised for dealing with specific memory problems. The advantage of treating patients in the hospital is that they are available for a large proportion of the day. Any treatment that requires direct involvement of a therapist can be carried out intensively.

External aids can be introduced as part of a ward rehabilitation program, and patients can be trained in their use. It will then be possible to identify the most successful and acceptable aid for a given patient before discharge. Individual timetable cards help alert the patient to the date and time, as well as ensure that the patient attends the planned session, provided the patient consults the timetable; if not, then behavioral-treatment methods may be used to train the patient to refer to the timetable. One might, for example, use regular prompting by staff and then systematically fade this out. Patients may also be trained to use notebooks in this way. Some patients with additional perceptual or physical problems find notebooks inconvenient. A stroke patient with verbal-memory problems was too embarrassed to make notes while talking to people; so instead he used a small cassette recorder usually used for dictating letters. He would dictate the conversation to his cassette while talking to people, and then play it back to himself later to remind him what the conversation had been about. He also used this method when talking on the telephone. He would turn the cassette on before answering the phone, and then repeat the relevant bits of conversation back to the caller, thus recording it on the tape.

A second advantage of treating patients while they are in the hospital is that one can investigate the effectiveness of different mnemonic strategies before applying them to deal with practical problems. Although guidelines are available (Wilson, 1984; Wilson & Moffat, 1984a) for matching strategy to patient, this is not always successful. One must try different strategies systematically to see if any will assist the patient, so that when the patient is discharged home and encounters new problems as a result of memory impairment, one already has some clear guidelines as to which strategies are likely to be most helpful. We devised such an investigation for a stroke patient, T.J., and it was carried out daily by his wife, following written instructions. We adapted the paired-associate learning task of Randt and associates (1980). The four versions of the task were modified to include four unrelated pairs of words and two related pairs. Baseline recordings were made in nine consecutive sessions, and it was intended that a maximum of three sessions per day would be attempted. In session 10, a visual-imagery strategy was introduced for list 1, and cards were drawn to illustrate pairs of words. This was repeated in sessions 13, 16, and 19. In session 12, a motor-coding strategy was introduced for list 3 and repeated in sessions 15, 18, and 21. The instructions were that a maximum of three sessions would be carried out on any day. However, because of their enthusiasm for his treatment, T.J. and his wife carried out more sessions on some days. This produced marked improvement in his performance for those lists that were repeated on the same day. Results from these sessions were therefore excluded from the analysis, resulting in two baseline sessions and three treatment sessions for each list. The results are shown in Figure 33.3. They indicate that motor coding had no observable beneficial effect. Both visual imagery and rehearsal seemed helpful, though it is possible that introduction of visual images for list 1 facilitated learning of list 2 by encouraging T.J. to produce his own images. T.J. did not report using visual imagery for list 2, but he

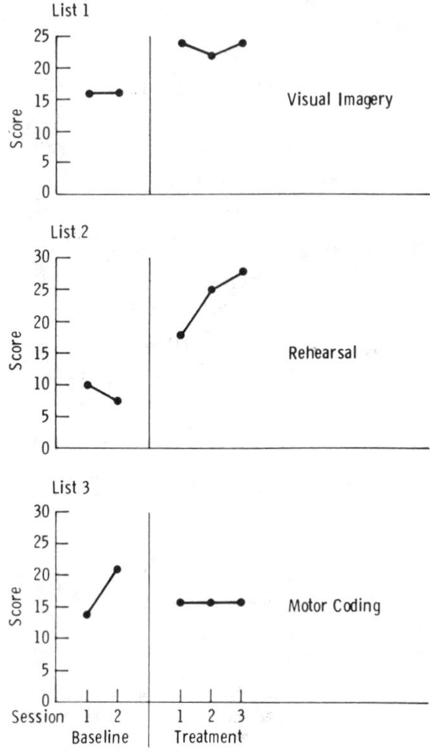

Figure 33.3. Evaluation of mnemonic strategies with T.J.

did feel that this technique had been the most helpful and was keen to apply it to more practical difficulties. This method was useful in identifying strategies that would be most helpful to T.J.

There are certain items of biographical information that a person will need to know on returning home that can be taught in advance of discharge. Sometimes the items may be identified after a weekend at home, whereas in other cases it is fairly predictable which things it is necessary to teach. For example, we taught a stroke patient the names of his wife and family using the visual-imagery technique described by Wilson (1981). Another head-injury patient, H.H., found that she was worried about going out shopping for fear she could not find her car again, as she would forget the number on her license plate. She would not be able to telephone her husband to ask him, because she could not remember the telephone number either. Although she could have written this information in a notebook, she felt it important to be able to remember these things without having to look them up, and she worried that she might lose a notebook. We used a

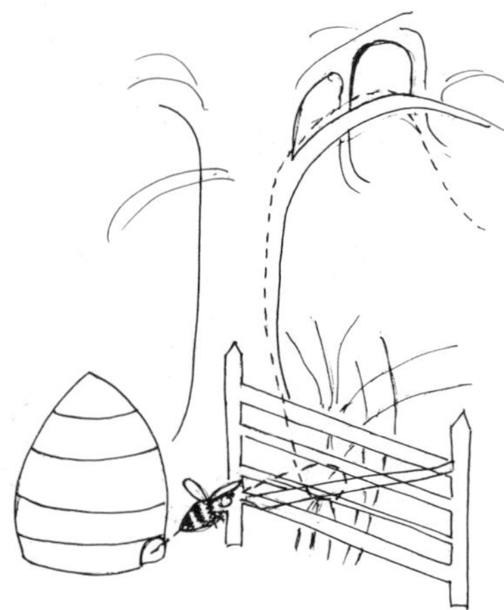

Figure 33.4. Visual image of a telephone-number story for H.H.

first-letter mnemonic to help her recall her car number (NRC 99P): "Naughty rabbits catch double-line [99 derived from the rhyming peg list 'one is a bun'] pneumonia." This nonsensical sentence she found easy to remember because it was so ridiculous. We used the rhyming peg method to generate a story for her to remember her phone number: "A bee came out of its hive (5) and went toward a gate (8), but found its way blocked by sticks (6), so instead flew upward through the branches of a tree (3), which were shaped like a door (4)." We also had a sketch that reminded her of the story (Figure 33.4). Teaching patients this kind of background information can help boost their confidence so that they will be able to cope once discharged from the hospital. It may also enable them to identify problems that can be tackled as soon as they occur, rather than waiting for several months in the hope of getting better before discussing the difficulty.

In the hospital it is also possible to devise methods for overcoming difficulties in practical activities of daily living. We designed a training procedure to help a lady who had difficulty with dressing because she forgot the sequence of actions required. She could perform each action correctly, but would get in a muddle by doing things in the wrong order and not completing one action before starting the next. For example, she would put her hemiplegic arm through the sleeve of her blouse and then try to put the blouse around her back without first ensuring that her entire arm was in the sleeve. We tried a written list of instructions to follow, but she would read several items on the list and then try to do them all, omitting some stages. We therefore tape-recorded the instructions and included a signal to stop the tape in order to carry out each instruction. She would then have to turn the tape recorder on again to receive the next instruction.

Visual strategies can also be introduced for daily activities, as in the case of A.W., a 36-year-old housewife who suffered a head injury in a car accident. She

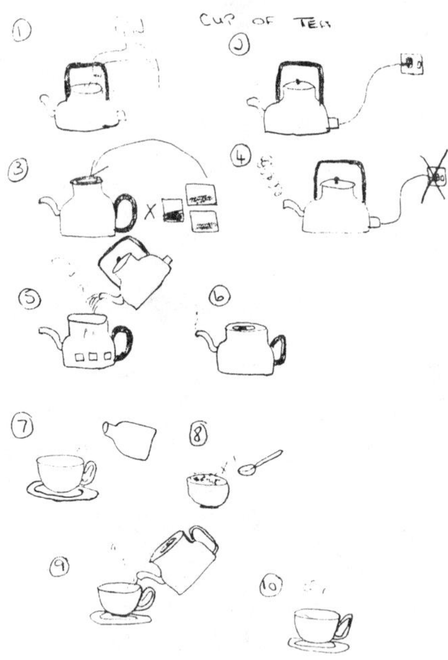

Figure 33.5. Visual instructions for making tea for A.W.

found cooking meals for her family difficult because she could not remember what to do. If she used a recipe, she would forget the instructions between reading them and carrying them out. Also, recipe books do not usually include simple cooking, such as making a cup of tea and preparing scrambled eggs on toast. On formal testing, her verbal memory was found to be impaired, but her visual memory was within the average range. The chosen method was therefore to use visual strategies by drawing out the sequence of tasks in pictures (an example is shown in Figure 33.5). She was then able to prepare a meal from these pictures, rather than from a written recipe. As she progressed, she was able to tackle more ambitious meals.

Although memory-training programs can be carried out directly in the home, there are advantages to beginning treatment while in the hospital. If the problems are severe, lengthy hospitalization is likely, and most treatment will be carried out on a rehabilitation or geriatric ward. If the problems are mild, it is still worth modifying the environment to assist memory-impaired patients to cope. This also provides an opportunity to investigate different strategies and to circumvent problems in daily life skills.

Conclusion

There are large numbers of people who can benefit from memory-therapy programs in hospitals; yet these programs are rarely applied. The survey by Harris and Sunderland (1981) showed that some attempts are being made to increase such programs, but these are few relative to the enormous scope of the problem. The most widely used ward-based technique is RO. This is probably fairly widespread within geriatric and psychogeriatric hospitals, but there is likely to be considerable variation in its quality and intensity. Many elderly people with dementia do not get any treatment for their memory problems (Moffat, Chapter 34, this volume). The rehabilitation units use some memory-training procedures with neurological and head-injury patients. The approaches used are general memory stimulation and, to a lesser extent, training in specific strategies. Even in these settings, evaluation of treatment techniques using single-case designs is a rarity, and progress, in terms of establishing the effectiveness of different procedures, is slow. Many memory-impaired people are admitted to medical and surgical wards, but on most of these wards, memory therapy does not form part of the rehabilitation program. Although many recover spontaneously, much could be done in the early management of patients on these wards to reduce difficulties resulting from memory impairment.

The patients who have received treatment for memory problems have been mainly those suffering from dementia, stroke, or head injuries. However, there are other conditions associated with memory impairment, such as multiple sclerosis (Jambor, 1969; Staples & Lincoln, 1979), that are equally in need of such treatment. A change in expectations throughout the medical and paramedical professions is needed so that the treatment of memory problems, using proven techniques, can become an integral part of the rehabilitation of all memory-impaired patients.

References

Barnes, J. (1974). Effects of reality orientation classroom on memory loss, confusion and disorientation in geriatric patients. *Gerontologist, 14,* 138–144.

Brook, P., Degun, G., & Mather, M. (1975). Reality orientation, a therapy for psychogeriatric patients: A controlled study. *British Journal of Psychiatry, 127,* 42–45.

Citrin, R. S., & Dixon, D. N. (1977). Reality orientation: A milieu therapy used in an institution for the aged. *Gerontologist, 17,* 39–43.

Davenport, M., & Hall, P. (1981). Speech therapy. In C. D. Evans (Ed.), *Rehabilitation after severe head injury.* London: Churchill Livingstone.

Fowler, R., Hart, J., & Sheehan, M. (1972). Prosthetic memory: An application of the prosthetic environment concept. *Rehabilitation Counseling Bulletin, 15,* 80–85.

Gilleard, C., Mitchell, R. G., & Riordan, J. (1981). Ward orientation training with psychogeriatric patients. *Journal of Advanced Nursing, 6,* 96–98.

Glasgow, R. E., Zeiss, R. A., Barrera, M., & Lewinsohn, P. M. (1977). Case studies on remediating memory deficits in brain damaged individuals. *Journal of Clinical Psychology, 33,* 1049–1054.

Hanley, I. G. (1981). The use of signposts and active training to modify ward disorientation in elderly patients. *Journal of Behavioral Therapy and Experimental Psychiatry, 12,* 241–247.

Harris, C. S., & Ivory, P. C. B. (1976). An outcome evaluation of reality orientation therapy with geriatric patients in a state mental hospital. *Gerontologist, 16,* 496–503.

Harris, J. E. (1980). We have ways of helping you remember. *Concord, The Journal of the British Association for Service to the Elderly, 17,* 21–27.

Harris, J. E., & Sunderland, A. (1981). A brief summary of the management of memory disorders in rehabilitation units in Britain. *International Rehabilitation Medicine, 3,* 206–209.

Holden, U. P., & Sinebruchow, A. (1978). Reality orientation therapy: A study investigating the value of this therapy in the rehabilitation of elderly people. *Age and Ageing, 7,* 83–90.

Holden, U. P., & Woods, R. T. (1982). *Reality orientation, psychological approaches to the confused elderly.* London: Churchill Livingstone.

Hussian, R. A. (1981). *Geriatric psychology: A behavioral perspective.* New York: Van Nostrand Reinhold.

Jambor, K. (1969). Cognitive functioning in multiple sclerosis. *British Journal of Psychiatry, 115,* 765–775.

Johnson, C. H., McLaren, S. M., & McPherson, F. M. (1981). The comparative effectiveness of 3 versions of classroom reality orientation. *Age and Ageing, 10,* 33–35.

Kapur, N., & Pearson, D. (1983). Memory symptoms and memory performance of neurological patients. *British Journal of Psychology, 74,* 409–415.

Kurlychek, R. T. (1983). Use of a digital alarm chronograph as a memory aid in early dementia. *Clinical Gerontologist, 1,* 93–94.

Lincoln, N. B. (1984). Future developments. In B. A. Wilson & N. Moffat (Eds.), *Clinical management of memory problems.* London: Croom Helm.

Malec, J., & Questad, K. (1983). Rehabilitation of memory after craniocerebral trauma: Case report. *Archives of Physical Medicine and Rehabilitation, 64,* 436–438.

Powell, G. E. (1981). *Brain function therapy.* Aldershot, UK: Gower.

Powell-Proctor, L., & Miller, E. (1982). Reality orientation: A critical appraisal. *British Journal of Psychiatry, 140,* 457–463.

Randt, C. T., Brown, E. R., & Osborne, D. P. (1980). A memory test for longitudinal measurement of mild to moderate deficits. *Clinical Neuropsychiatry, 2,* 184–194.

Staples, D., & Lincoln, N. B. (1979). Intellectual impairment in multiple sclerosis and its relation to functional abilities. *Rheumatology and Rehabilitation, 18,* 153–160.

Sunderland, A., Harris, J. E., & Baddeley, A. D. (1983). Do laboratory tests predict everyday memory? A neuropsychological study. *Journal of Verbal Learning and Verbal Behavior, 22,* 341–357.

Sunderland, A., Harris, J. E., & Baddeley, A. D. (1984). Assessing everyday memory after severe head injury. In J. E. Harris & P. E. Morris (Eds.), *Everyday memory, actions and absentmindedness* (pp. 181–206). New York: Academic Press.

Sunderland, A., Watts, K., Baddeley, A. D., & Harris, J. E. (1986). Subjective memory assessment and test performance in the elderly. *Journal of Gerontology, 41,* 376–384.

Wechsler, D. (1945). A standardized memory scale for clinical use. *Journal of Psychology, 19,* 87–95.

Wilson, B. A. (1981). Teaching a patient to remember people's names after removal of a left temporal lobe tumor. *Behavioral Psychotherapy, 9,* 338–344.

Wilson, B. A. (1982). Success and failure in memory training following a cerebral vascular accident. *Cortex, 18,* 581–594.

Wilson, B. A. (1984). Memory therapy in practice. In B. A. Wilson & N. Moffat (Eds.), *Clinical management of memory problems.* London: Croom Helm.

Wilson, B. A., Cockburn, J., & Baddeley, A. D. (1985). *The Rivermead Behavioural Memory Test.* Thames Valley Test Company, 22 Bulmershe Road, Reading, Berks., England, RG1 5RT.

Wilson, B. A., Cooper, Z., & Kennerley, H. (1983). *An investigation of the effectiveness of group training on memory functioning in adults with acquired brain damage.* Paper presented at a meeting of the Society for Research in Rehabilitation, London.

Wilson, B. A., & Moffat, N. J. (1984a). Rehabilitation of memory for everyday life. In J. E. Harris & P. E. Morris (Eds.), *Everyday memory, actions and absentmindedness* (pp. 207–234). New York: Academic Press.

Wilson, B. A., & Moffat, N. J. (1984b). Running a memory group. In B. A. Wilson & N. J. Moffat (Eds.), *Clinical management of memory problems.* London: Croom Helm.

Woods, R. T. (1979). Reality orientation and staff attention: A controlled study. *British Journal of Psychiatry, 134,* 502–507.

The talk that I gave on how to cope with memory problems improved steadily across the group sessions, as did some of the other talks. It was felt that the experience of running each session helped to improve the quality of the presentation and the handout. The following information was included in this talk.

The talk on memory problems began by distinguishing the development and nature of memory complaints associated with dementia from those that might be due to aging, a sensory problem, depression, an acute confusional state, or other forms of brain damage. This was followed by an outline of the likely causes of the memory loss in Alzheimer's disease and the type of memory impairment expected, together with consideration of any preserved memory abilities. Examples of the kinds of everyday memory problems associated with dementia were described and sometimes were confirmed by the carers present at the group meeting. Then some useful tips for carers were described, covering the following areas: memory aids; reality orientation; tips about communication; reducing distractions; maintaining a routine and keeping things in the same place; limiting the available choices when the patient or dependent is dressing or eating; dealing with dependents who lose and hide things; wandering behavior; making use of residual memory. It was emphasized that the memory problems of the dependent, such as repetitive questioning, can place considerable strain on the carer. However, it was suggested that carers need not add to their own strain by attributing the same level of distress to their dependents, because a severe amnesic may no longer possess good insight and may not be upset by his or her own memory failures.

The overall results from the evaluation of the relatives' support groups were encouraging: There appeared to be a strong trend for the carers in these groups to show greater reductions in their GHQ scores than did the relatives in the control condition.

The relatives' support group has now become an established part of the psychogeriatric service at each site, with an ongoing joint monthly outing for the carers once they have completed the initial 10-Week course.

Generally, I like to include carers in a relatives' support group before setting up home-based training with them. In this way it is hoped that carers will gain an appreciation of what dementia is and the limitations of what can be done to help. This can be important; as Jeffrey and Saxby (1984) have argued, families should be allowed to make preparations and adjustments for the future, and retraining programs may overburden them or might mislead them into overoptimism about what can be achieved.

Additional advantages of waiting until after a family has been in a relatives' support group are that the carer and I will have become better acquainted, and further opportunities to work with the patient may have arisen. I am responsible for the running of the memory-therapy group that now meets at the same time as the relatives' support group. This was designed to offer a positive intervention with the dependents, rather than simply providing a sitting-in service or a holding operation for the patients while the carers attended the relatives' support group.

34 Home-based cognitive rehabilitation with the elderly

Nicholas J. Moffat

Strain on those caring for the elderly

Although there has been an emphasis on the development of day-hospital and community provisions, there is little evidence that such facilities provide an alternative to hospital care or relieve the strain on the carers, which is the main reason for referral (Greene & Timbury, 1979). It is well recognized that there is severe strain on carers, and there are deleterious effects on their health. Gilleard (1984) reported that on the General Health Questionnaire (GHQ) (Goldberg, 1978), 73% of persons caring for patients attending a geriatric or psychogeriatric day hospital probably were suffering from some degree of psychiatric disturbance. The reported level of distress among those caring for psychogeriatric patients was only just higher than the level for those caring for geriatric patients (Table 34.1).

Gilleard also noted that there was no significant difference between the two groups of carers in regard to the numbers of problems reported. However, the nature of the problems did distinguish between the two groups. In general, the geriatric patients experienced greater impairments of mobility, which have been shown to be reasonably well tolerated by carers (Isaacs, 1971). This group of carers also described significant levels of behavioral disturbance and/or communications problems, although these were less frequent than those reported by people caring for psychogeriatric patients. These behavioral and communications problems are particular sources of strain for carers.

However, other studies did not find a relationship between the severity of disturbed behavior and the burden on carers (Greene, Smith, Gardiner, & Timbury,

Britain has been described as a country that has concentrated on the provision of community services rather than hospital services for the elderly, particularly the elderly infirm. Compared with many other European countries, the level of institutional provision in England is much lower, with only 27 beds per 1,000 population over 65 years of age, compared with much higher figures in The Netherlands (133.4), Sweden (83.3), and Denmark (78.2) (Thom, 1981).

Table 34.1 *Distress among those caring for the elderly*

Condition	Geriatric sample (n = 127)	Psychogeriatric sample (n = 54)
No distress (GHQ < 4)	33% (n = 42)	15% (n = 8)
Distress (GHQ = 5–8)	21% (n = 26)	20% (n = 11)

Source: Adopted from Gilleard (1984).

Table 34.2. *Ten most highly rated topics from the Needs Questionnaire*

1. Information about dementia	6. Coping with one's own depression
2. Coping with memory problems	7. The role of the occupational therapist
3. Problems experienced by carers	8. Emotions experienced by carers
4. Coping with behavior problems	9. Activities for one's dependent
5. Coping with one's own anxiety	10. Role of the psychogeriatrician

1982; Zarit, Reever, and Bach-Peterson, 1980). Greene and associates (1982) did find that the personal distress of the carer was related to the severity of the apathy and withdrawal of the patient, and the carer's negative feelings concerning the patient were related to the degree of disturbance of the patient's mood. A detailed description of the coping strategies used by the carer in response to the problems of the patient is beyond the scope of this chapter. However, it is of note that generally the level of cognitive functioning is not related to the degree of burden (Gilhooly, 1984; Greene et al., 1982; Zarit et al.,(1980). This seems a rather surprising finding given the high frequency with which memory problems are reported by carers, as well as their expressed need for help in coping with memory problems (Table 34.2). Thus, almost all of the carers for the dementia patients, and three-quarters of the carers for the geriatric patients, reported occasional or frequent forgetfulness by their patients (Gilleard, 1984). Among the most frequently reported memory problems were asking repetitive questions, losing things, and forgetting what day it was (Zarit et al., 1980). Attempts to help with each of these problems are described later, but first we describe a study that was aimed at identifying and meeting the needs of carers, including helping them to cope with the memory problems of their elderly charges.

Relatives' support groups

In an attempt to provide an appropriate service for the carers for dementia patients in East Dorset, a Needs Questionnaire was constructed and used to establish the priority of needs (Trigg, 1984). There was significant agreement

Table 34.3. *Average ratings of usefulness of talks and contact (1–5) by the carers in each support group*

Talk	Site 1	Site 2		Average
		Group 1	Group 2	
1. Day hospital and activities	4.4	4.0	4.0	4.13
2. Coping with memory problems	3.8	4.3	4.8	4.3
3. Incontinence and medication	4.0	5.0	4.8	4.6
4. Dementia	3.8	4.8	5.0	4.53
5. Coping with behavior problems	4.6	5.0	4.8	4.6
6. Safety and independence	4.0	4.5	4.3	4.27
7. Problems and emotions of carers	4.2	—	4.9	4.65
8. Coping with one's own anxiety	4.4	4.7	5.0	4.7
9. Coping with one's own depression	4.5	—	5.0	4.75
10. Long-term and short-term care	—[a]	—	4.9	4.9
11. Role of the social worker	—	4.0	—	4.0
12. Allowances and helpful organizations	—	4.7	—	4.7
Contact with other carers	4.8	4.0	4.7	4.5
Contact with staff	4.8	4.2	4.2	4.4
Handouts	4.5	—	—	4.5
Overall rating of usefulness of group	4.8	4.4	5.0	4.7

[a] *Indicates no responses given.*

among the 17 carers interviewed with regard to the perceived needs ($p < .01$), and they placed information about caring for themselves as the highest priority. However, when carers were directly asked to rank-order six aspects of needs, caring for themselves was placed last, behind information on (1) caring for their relatives (patients, dependents), (2) what services were available, (3) old age and dementia, (4) access to services, and (5) social contact. It appears that the carers were reluctant to be seen to place high priority on caring for themselves, but that this was nevertheless an important need. From the interview data, the 10 most highly rated topics were used as the basis for the relatives' support groups (Table 34.2).

Relatives support groups were then formed for the carers who had been interviewed, with each group having 10 weekly meetings. Each meeting had a speaker for approximately 20 min, with the remainder of the hour devoted to discussion of the topic presented. There were slight differences in the contents of the groups run at different sites (both psychogeriatric services in East Dorset catering to dementia patients). Following the end of each meeting, the feedback given by the carers was generally very positive (Table 34.3). Furthermore, there was a non significant trend for those carers who had attended the relatives support group to show greater reductions in their expressed need for information, compared with the control condition. This suggests that the group was providing at least some the information the carers had identified as needs.

The group carries out memory exercises, some of which are similar to those described by Moffat (1984a) and Wilson and Moffat (1984a, 1984b), and these have been adapted to suit the memory difficulties of patients with dementia.

Holding separate meetings for carers and for dependents allows for clarity of purpose in the meetings. The carers are there to receive help and support with the burden of coping; the dependents are receiving some help for their memory problems. This policy overcomes some of the difficulties cited by Zarit, Zarit, and Reever (1982) about involving both carers and dependents in the same group.

Zarit and associates (1982) randomly allocated senile dementia patients, together with their carers, to one of three conditions: a didactic memory-therapy group involving visual imagery, a problem-solving group dealing with everyday memory difficulties, and a waiting-list control condition. Each condition lasted for 3.5 weeks, with each group meeting for 90 min twice per week. There was no lasting benefit for the patients following any of the training conditions, perhaps because mnemonic strategies are of little value with dementia patients (Yesavage, 1982).

Furthermore, the carers in the Zarit study (1982) did not benefit from the didactic or problem-solving groups, but in fact became significantly more depressed, whereas those in the control group did not. Part of the reason why relatives became more depressed may have been because they had unrealistic expectations about the treatment groups and only later realized the severity of their dependents' problems. Thus, two-thirds of the carers stated that they had changed their understanding of their dependents' problems following the group sessions, with one-third of the carers stating that they wished they had not gained this insight. The enforced exposure to their dependents' problems may have disrupted an apparently common coping strategy of psychologically distancing or ignoring dependents' problems (Gilhooly, 1980; Johnson & Catalona, 1982), without offering an alternative coping style. There was some indication that the carers valued the opportunity to meet other carers, and apparently a relatives' support group was formed as a consequence of the study. The potential value of such a relatives' group has already been discussed, but another aspect of the study worth following up was the positive, but nonsignificant, trend for the carers in the problem-solving group to report fewer memory and behavior problems over time and to indicate less distress when the problems did occur.

It may be that some of these practical suggestions can be systematically investigated to determine their efficacy. There have been a few reports of direct training involving carers that have provided some optimism for the development of this type of intervention.

Involvement of carers in the treatment of the elderly

The involvement of the carer in home-based therapy can vary from minimal (in which the therapist works with the patient in the home) to moderate (involving the carer in ensuring that exercises are carried out, but without involving the carer in the exercises) to maximal (with the carer acting as the main therapist, possibly supported by outsiders).

Haley (1983) suggested that in addition to offering to carers for the elderly information about dementia and about the care provisions available, they might also be taught to apply behavior-modification techniques to overcome specific problems. Thus, he described how an 87-year-old woman with a moderate level of dementia was taught to reduce her anxiety about being left on her own for more than 20 min. First, she was taught to relax. Then the family left her with a message board explaining where they had gone. A kitchen timer was set for 20 min, and a reward was offered if she had remained quiet until the timer rang. After initial success at this baseline time interval, the family gradually increased the duration on the timer until she could be left alone for 50 min. Apparently this improvement made the situation more tolerable for the family.

Repetitive questions

Haley also commented that a colleague had reduced a patient's repetitive questioning by reinforcing gradually increasing time intervals during which the identified questions had not been asked. We have successfully replicated this procedure with a woman with mild dementia who exhibited repetitive behavior before admission to hospital. The various repetitive questions observed during her admission to hospital were significantly reduced by reinforcing increasing time periods without such inappropriate utterances. The improvements were maintained when she was transferred to another hospital. She was later discharged to a residential home near her relatives.

An alternative approach to deal with repetitive utterances is to acknowledge their occurrence and assist the person in answering his or her own questions. Thus, a severely head-injured man was encouraged by his wife to use first-letter cuing whenever he repeatedly asked her a question (e.g., "What is the name of the person we met last night?"). He needed to carry a card with the letters written down, which also highlighted the first letters of the names he regularly could not recall. This seemed to reduce the frequency of repeated questioning and also considerably lessened the strain experienced by his wife.

A further approach to management is to make use of residual abilities and to reduce the memory load by providing a suitable prosthetic environment (Lindsley, 1964).

Losing things around the house

Although losing things around the house may be an infrequent problem for normal elderly people (Abson, 1984; West, Chapter 30, this volume), this has emerged as a frequent issue in the memory-therapy groups we use with dementia patients. In order to lessen this problem for a man with presenile dementia, two forms of external memory aids were used (Moffat, 1984b). First, he was taught to use a large, brightly colored bag in which to keep his pipe and other possessions. Observations were carried out by the family to determine where he usually left his bag. Then a flow chart was constructed that indicated the most likely places to search. The chart was placed on the wall in the kitchen and contained a card to take with him while searching any room. This was to remind him what he was doing, because he sometimes forgot why he had gone into a particular room. If the search of a room was unsuccessful, he returned to the kitchen, replaced the card in the appropriate slot, and proceeded to the next location on the flow chart. The family noted a reduction in his repeated questioning and were relieved of the irritation this had caused. The system was not without drawbacks, in that sometimes he would search part of the house before discovering that his bag was next to where he had been sitting.

Davies and Binks (1983) provided a detailed account of the practical techniques they developed to help a 31-year-old Korsakoff patient and his wife cope with his memory deficits. Many of the strategies they used would seem suitable for use with older brain-damaged patients and their families. These authors produced a prompt card for him that was similar in size to a credit card. On one side the hospital address was written, followed by the words ''Mr. F has a profound memory disorder. Please help him to make the most of his memory in the ways listed on the other side of this card.'' Side two contained the following recommendations:

> Speak slowly and directly to him.
> Get him to make notes in his book, and remind him to use it.
> Write down important dates and addresses for him, and get him to check them.
> Ask him to repeat back messages to you in his own words.

Copies of the card were then distributed by the family to those with whom he came in regular contact. In addition, a leaflet entitled ''Making the most of your memory'' was produced for him. Efforts were made to ensure use of the prompt card and notebook by role-play, and encouragement was given to pursue appropriate activities, such as woodwork, walking, and one-to-one conversations.

At follow-up 1 year later, the notebook, prompt card, and leaflet were still being used. At this stage, a further leaflet was produced entitled ''Managing your memory''; it gave advice about putting things into memory, using associations and repetition, as well as advice about getting things out of memory, using recognition, guessing, or asking others to give prompts. His wife was taught to encourage the use of these strategies.

The use of clear instructions to help a family cope with and, to some extent, overcome an acquired problem is further illustrated in the following study using a single-case experimental design.

Retraining of dysgraphia

Mr. D is an intelligent man in his late sixties who lives at home with his caring wife. He appeared to have suffered cerebral anoxia following a myocardial infarction 9 months before he was referred for therapy. He had been seen by speech and occupational therapists, who reported no real recovery. The main problem was severe dysgraphia for letters and numbers, with otherwise a reasonably intact receptive and expressive ability, including reading and spelling. He also showed a marked dyscalculia, although he could recall most of his arithmetic tables. He had considerable difficulty in dressing and in managing simple constructional tasks. This was confirmed by testing, because he had scaled scores of zero on the Wechsler Block Design, Picture Arrangement, and Object Assembly subtests (Wechsler, 1958). In addition, he showed evidence of ideomotor and ideational apraxia and finger agnosia. His memory was moderately impaired. Overall, his presentation was similar to that seen in Gerstmann's syndrome.

He was keen to overcome his dysgraphia, and he spent much of his time at home attempting to write his name, of which he could write only the first three letters. A structured program was set up for him that he could follow at home, aided by his wife and supported by my visits every 2 weeks.

The order in which the letters would be relearned was chosen on a semirandom basis. A balance was achieved between his desire to relearn particular letters in order to write certain words and an even distribution of common letters across the training, so that interest would not decline once he had mastered his most popular letters. The letters were learned one at a time, with, on average, 3 days to practice each letter. This provided a multiple-baseline design across behaviors, which in this case was letters.

The plan involved spacing out the practice each day using the method described by Landauer and Bjork (1978) and recently applied to the memory-disordered by Schacter, Rich, and Stampp (1985). A practice session of writing a given letter in uppercase was followed by a predetermined retention time. Mr. D then tested his ability to write the letter; if necessary, he added further practice before starting the next retention interval. The duration of retention was roughly doubled each time, starting at 5 min and extending to 4 hours, with a final test the next day. Thus, if he started at 10 a.m., his last retention test that day would be taken at 5:45 p.m. The timer in the cooker acted as the reminder for the time periods, and a manual set out the tasks for the next 2 weeks, and the responses were recorded in the manual.

The manual also contained two repeating sections, one of them being a probe test in which Mr. D attempted to write each of the letters to dictation, every 3 days. The other feature was that every time he practiced an additional letter, he should write down any words he could compose using the letters he could write. This made use of his intact and rich vocabulary and increased his interest in the task. It also helped to practice the letters he had learned as well as the one he was currently practicing, which, it was presumed, might help to maintain the ability to write the letters he had already learned.

The results of this training are shown in Figure 34.1. Mr. D learned the letters in the sequence taught, with no evidence of any generalization or spontaneous recovery. He learned to write in uppercase and could not write lowercase characters. He maintained this level of functioning for 12 months, during which he

Results of probe test every third training session

Order in which letters were retrained (starting with J)	1	4	7	10	13	16	19	22	25	28	31	34	37	40
J	√	√	√	√	√	√	√	√	√	√	√	√	√	√
O	√	√	√	√	√	√	√	√	√	√	√	√	√	√
H	√	√	√	√	√	√	√	√	√	√	√	√	√	√
N	X	X	X	X	√	√	√	√	√	√	√	√	√	√
D	X	X	√	√	√	√	√	√	√	√	X	√	√	√
E	X	X	√	√	√	√	√	X	√	√	√	√	√	√
A	X	X	√	√	√	√	√	X	X	√	√	√	√	√
B	X	X	X	√	√	√	√	√	X	√	√	√	√	√
L	X	X	X	X	√	√	√	√	√	X	√	√	√	√
F	X	X	X	X	√	√	√	√	√	√	√	√	√	√
P	X	X	X	X	√	√	√	√	X	X	√	√	√	√
I	X	X	X	X	X	√	√	√	X	√	√	√	√	√
I	X	X	X	X	X	√	√	√	√	√	√	√	√	√
C	X	X	X	X	X	X	√	X	X	√	√	√	√	√
M	X	X	X	X	X	X	X	√	√	X	√	√	√	√
V	X	X	X	X	X	X	X	X	√	√	X	√	√	√
S	X	X	X	X	X	X	X	X	X	X	√	√	√	√
G	X	X	X	X	X	X	X	X	X	X	√	√	√	√
V	X	X	X	X	X	X	X	X	X	X	√	√	√	√
R	X	X	X	X	X	X	X	X	X	X	√	√	√	√
L	X	X	X	X	X	X	X	X	X	X	√	√	X	√
K	X	X	X	X	X	X	X	X	X	X	X	√	√	√
Q	X	X	X	X	X	X	X	X	X	X	X	√	X	√
Y	X	X	X	X	X	X	X	X	X	X	X	X	X	√
W	X	X	X	X	X	X	X	X	X	X	X	X	X	√
X	X	X	X	X	X	X	X	X	X	X	X	X	X	√

TICK = correct Cross = incorrect

Thick border = start of training for each letter
Left of border = baseline
Right of border = training and follow-up

Figure 34.1. Multiple-baseline retraining dysgraphia.

used his writing ability to deal with his correspondence, including domestic finance and personal letters. He then decided to teach himself to write in lowercase. With the help of his wife, they followed the original method of practicing one letter at a time using an expanded rehearsal procedure. In this way he relearned all of the lowercase characters and can now use the appropriate mixture of uppercase and lowercase letters in his writing.

These results suggest that the training was beneficial and could not be attributed to spontaneous recovery. However, it is difficult to judge whether or not the expanded rehearsal procedure was necessary, because the learning of one item at a time may have provided sufficient structure to allow learning to take place. Certainly Schacter and associates (1985) suggest that limiting the amount of information to be remembered at any one time may be an important requirement of the spaced-retrieval approach. Even if the expanded rehearsal method does add to treatment efficacy, the appropriate spacing of intervals has not been determined in this study. A further example of the application of the expanded retrieval procedure is given in the following single-case study involving retraining of word retrieval for a woman with mild dementia.

Retraining of word retrieval in dementia

One of the features of dementia may be some form of disturbance of language functioning. Although there have been varying reports about the type of language disorder present, one of the more consistently reported features, particularly at the early stages of dementia, is impairment of naming ability (Appell, Kertesz, & Fisman, 1982; Barker & Lawson, 1968; Ernst, Dalby, & Dalby, 1970). The cause of the dementia appears to play only a small part in determining the type of naming deficit (Overman, 1979), but the severity of dementia has been found to be related to the difficulty of confrontation naming (Skelton-Robinson & Jones, 1984).

Although there have been reports that verbal cuing has beneficial effects on naming ability for dysphasic subjects (Rochford & Williams, 1963), only limited success has been reported for verbal cuing with dementia patients (Skelton-Robinson & Jones, 1984). This may be consistent with the suggestion by Rochford (1971) that dysphasics show a linguistic deficit, whereas dementia patients suffer from an object-recognition problem. However, Bayles (1982) failed to find visual agnosia problems in her sample of dementia patients, and Skelton-Robinson and Jones (1984) found that even verbal definitions of the words did not help to correct errors in naming made by dementia patients, suggesting that the recognition of the object was not the primary deficit.

Wiegel-Crump and Koenigsknecht (1973) were interested in whether naming difficulties could be attributed to a deficit in the lexical store itself or to a deficit in the retrieval of items from that store. They gave subjects repeated practice on certain items and reported improvement in recall on both practiced and unpracticed items. The gains in picture naming were substantial, because the items could not be recalled prior to training, but after 6 therapy sessions, 61% were correctly named, with 74% after 12 sessions, and 84% correctly named following 18 therapy sessions. Furthermore, the mean latency for a response decreased from 24.4 sec to 3.3 sec for practiced items, and from 23.6 to 9.33 sec for unpracticed items. Although generalization of training was demonstrated, there was no attempt to measure the maintenance of treatment effects. When Patterson, Morton, and Purrell (1983) investigated the benefits of repetitive practice on word finding by aphasics, they found that the benefits were not maintained. This would be consistent with a number of studies that have not found rote rehearsal to be an effective memory-therapy procedure (Brooks & Baddeley, 1976), despite its popularity as a treatment technique (Harris & Sunderland, 1981). In order to investigate whether or not the efficacy of treatment and maintenance could be improved, an alternative rehearsal procedure was attempted using the optimal rehearsal pattern of test and then practice.

Case study of retraining nominal dysphasia

Miss S is an "intelligent" spinster in her late fifties who lives alone in an immaculate flat. She has shown gradual mental deterioration over several years and has been diagnosed as suffering from Alzheimer's disease. She retains good insight, but has severe impairment of verbal memory, with evidence of generalized intellectual impairment. The most noticeable deficit is a marked and stable nominal dysphasia. When tested on naming tasks, she insisted on writing down the names of any objects she could not recall, together with verbal definitions of the words and/or suitable drawings. She appeared to consult these notes regularly and to practice the items in between the test sessions, which were conducted at least 2 weeks apart. She did not appear able to retain a correct name for more than a few minutes. Furthermore, attempts to provide prompts were generally unsuccessful. The provision of the first letter, and, if necessary, subsequent letters, did not help, even when all letters but the last were provided. The same appeared true when the appropriate phonemes were spoken to her. When given a choice of three words, one of which was correct, she sometimes was able to eliminate the inappropriate alternatives and hence make the correct choice. Occasionally she immediately recognized the correct word, but on most occasions she was unable to do so. Following the five-session baseline period (Figure 34.2), a retraining program was implemented.

All of the assessment and training sessions were carried out in her own flat. The decision to maintain a home-based service in this case was based on the following factors: (1) She lived alone, and so visits to her flat enabled us to check that she was looking after herself adequately. (2) Training in her own home, often using her objects as the items to remember, might reduce the need for generalization from practiced items to everyday objects, and from one setting to another. (3) A patient aide (untrained helper attached to the community psychiatric nurse) could carry out the training, under supervision. This person could visit Miss S as part of her calls on other patients living in the area. The idea was that Miss S could be seen during the middle of the day, when the patient aide was not busy with her normal duties of getting patients washed and dressed or providing assistance with other chores, such as at mealtimes. The primary aim was to lessen the

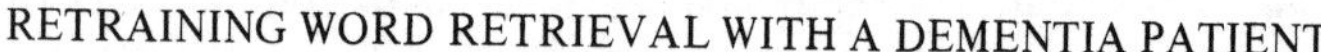

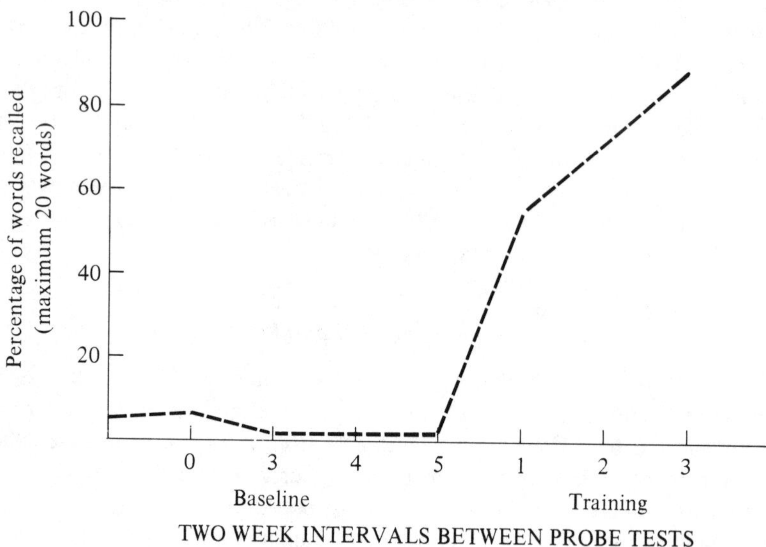

Figure 34.2. Retraining word retrieval with a dementia patient.

disruption to her routine, because her continued survival on her own might become threatened by any alterations to her established routine.

Pilot work with Miss S showed that she could retain the name of an object for only a few minutes. Therefore, the expanded rehearsal procedure was used during training, in which the name for a picture was practiced, and retention was checked after 2 min. Then, if she correctly named the object, the next retention interval was doubled (or, if incorrect, the time interval was halved). It was hoped that this technique might overcome some of the limitations of rote rehearsal already mentioned.

A multiple-baseline design across behaviors (pictures) was used so that an item was trained to the criterion of successful recall before adding an extra item to the training. A probe test of the full 20 items was also given every three sessions in order to check for specific and generalized improvements in naming ability. The latency of recall was measured, in addition to the number of items correctly recalled.

The results show a rapid improvement in naming ability following the introduction of training, and that improvement was not confined to the items taught (Figure 34.2). In addition, the mean latency of response for the correctly named objects decreased from approximately 30 sec after three sessions of training to 23.6 sec after a further three sessions, and it was down to 8.5 sec by the ninth training session. There was evidence of specific training effects in that the first few words were recalled only following their specific training, and once learned, they were always recalled immediately. Furthermore, the sessional records indicated that learning was taking place. Thus, as each new word was introduced, the number of errors at the various retention intervals decreased across training sessions. The evidence for generalization is strong in that by the third session only three words had been taught, and yet the majority of the 20 pictures were correctly named on the probe test. The evidence for generalization is consistent with the findings of Wiegel-Crump and Koenigsknecht (1973). The training also produced maintenance of learning, because the probe tests were conducted several days after the last training session. This was an improvement over the results of Patterson and associates (1983), and it may have been due to the alternative rehearsal procedure used in this study, despite the apparent similarity between rote and expanded rehearsal.

There were many weaknesses in the methodology of this study, but the results were sufficiently promising to warrant more thorough investigation, and this method may provide a relatively simple strategy for assisting word retrieval in dsyphasic and dementia patients. It is also refreshing to observe the maintenance and generalization of treatment effects in cognitive rehabilitation.

Another simple procedure that has shown not only specific effects but also generalization with patients suffering from dementia is reality orientation.

Reality orientation

A full review of the studies on reality orientation is outside the scope of this chapter and is available elsewhere (Holden & Woods, 1982; Moffat, 1986a; Powell-Proctor & Miller, 1982). Although most of the research on reality orientation has been conducted with inpatients, recent studies have involved day-hospital patients, and several studies have mentioned the possibility of involving relatives with the treatment.

Our own work has included a study of five day-hospital patients with dementia, using a modified form of reality orientation that incorporated both a method of reducing prompts with learning (Glisky, Schacter, & Tulving, in press) and an expanded-interval rehearsal procedure (Schacter et al., 1985). The results showed improvement in verbal orientation for four of the five patients. During the 6 weeks of the main study, the patients were given training on 22 items using a multiple-baseline design. Improvements in free recall were noted on 17 items (77%) following the introduction of training, with little evidence of spontaneous improvement prior to the onset of training for any given item. Furthermore, the process of change across training sessions often involved a gradual reduction in the number of prompts required within any given time interval, and then a systematic increase in the length of the retention interval. In addition, the ability to benefit from this type of therapy was found to be related to the level of baseline performance on the cognitive measures.

The scope of the investigation thus far has been limited. We have not explored generalization to the home environment, nor the maintenance of any gains from the therapy. However, we have carried out additional training with mildly impaired patients in their own homes that has enriched our understanding of the potential of this form of therapy.

Our experience of working with two typical patients is of interest: Both of these patients were concerned to remember the names of staff members at the respective day hospitals they visited. Photographs were taken of the relevant staff, and these pictures were available at home for practice. Each of these men was supported by a caring and capable wife who acted as therapist, backed up by myself at weekly home visits.

The first man had suffered a stroke and was embarrassed that he could not recall the names of the staff at the day hospital he attended several times a week. He wanted to tell his wife whom he had seen, and he wanted to be able to address these people by name. He gradually learned the names using the expanded rehearsal procedure, and he could recall almost all of them after a 4-month break from the day hospital, with no practice during the intervening period. The fact that he knew these people may have enhanced his learning of this task by providing semantic associations (Yesavage, Rose, & Bower, 1983).

He also wanted to remember a variety of other basic information, such as his own and other people's addresses. He was encouraged to learn these with the help of his wife, but without professional guidance, in order to determine if professional guidance is necessary. There was no improvement during the baseline period of 1 month. He then practiced one item at a time, using the expanded rehearsal procedure. Following 2 weeks of practice, he had learned the six main items by phasing in a new item every few days. The results (Figure 34.3) showed that learning took place in advance of the use of the expanded interval rehearsal, suggesting that learning in stages may have been responsible for much of the improvement. An additional consideration was that the items were not completely unrelated, so that learning one item may have helped learn another (e.g., recalling his doctor's name may have assisted recall of the doctor's address). These two items were taught at the same time to allow for generalization, without contravening the requirements of the multiple-baseline design.

The advantage of working with this family was that he and his wife were motivated, and their efforts were rewarded by gains once they used a structured method of practice. They were further reassured that his condition was reasonably stable and that improvements could be achieved despite the unlikelihood of further spontaneous recovery, given the time period since his stroke.

In contrast, the case of the second man illustrates the particular difficulties of working with patients with dementia, a generalized and progressive disorder. Some of the same problems to be discussed in relation to this man were also noted with the five patients reported earlier. This 63-year-old man had mild generalized brain damage attributable to Alzheimer's disease. He had a partial understanding of the nature of his condition and was anxious about his failings and his inability to carry out many tasks. He was initially enthusiastic about learning the names of the staff at the day center, but he had some reservations about his

	DATE OF PROBE TEST				
	29 March 1984	1 April 1984	3 April 1984	4 April 1984	11 April 1984
ADDRESS	✓	✓	✓	✓	✓
TELEPHONE NUMBER	X	✓	✓	✓	✓
NEIGHBOR'S NAME	X	X	✓	✓	✓
DOCTOR'S NAME	X	X	✓	✓	✓
DOCTOR'S ADDRESS	X	X	X	✓	✓
DAUGHTER'S ADDRESS	X	X	X	X	✓

Tick = correct
Cross = incorrect

Thick border = start of training for each item
Left of border = baseline
Right of border = training and follow-up

Figure 34.3. Retraining verbal operations using a multiple-baseline design.

ability to learn and about whether or not his wife would pressure him too much, together with a more general concern about the value of this "game" and whether or not it would help him overcome his illness.

Training to remember people's names began successfully, but was phased out in favor of relaxation training and counseling that helped him to reduce his general anxiety. The value of relaxation therapy with dementia patients has also been reported by Welden and Yesavage (1982). This case illustrates an important point regarding the need for a comprehensive service for mild-dementia sufferers. With dementia patients, there are many abilities that may be affected, and with a progressive disorder there are many and varied adjustments that may need to be made by the sufferer as well as the carer. The reduced mental abilities of the sufferer make it particularly difficult for that person to reason satisfactorily, and hence make such an appropriate adjustment. This process is made even more difficult by the changing pattern of deficits, requiring what may be termed a "mobile mourning" for the loss of abilities. Thus, cognitive rehabilitation needs to be concerned not only with the understanding and treatment of specific neuropsychological deficits but also with the psychosocial adjustment of the brain-damaged person and the family as well as ways of helping them to cope with these problems (Moffat, 1986b).

Utilization of community services in cognitive rehabilitation

There appear to be numerous possible benefits associated with home-based treatments. First and foremost, "the elderly almost invariably express preference for home based training" (Garland, 1985). Therefore, performance at home may yield a more accurate assessment of functioning, because the person may be adversely affected by the unfamiliar hospital environment. Assessment in the home may also be necessary because the intervention is specific to the home. For example, consider the case of a woman who, as the result of a traffic accident, not only suffered severe memory problems but also lost her husband. She wanted to return home and look after her children. She partially recognized the risks involved, in that she might forget to turn fires off, or might leave doors unlocked.

In order to help her to cope, notes were pinned up around the house reminding her what to do. This included memoboards on which she could jot things down as they occurred to her (e.g., for shopping), as well as fixed lists to remind her to lock up and turn off the fires before going to bed. Social work and other professional agencies were organized to provide regular contact to check on how she was coping, with further advice being sought from me if necessary.

Second, even when the task can be learned in another environment, as in the case of the man learning to write again, there is likely to be more time available for practice at home, and convenient times can be found for study that might not coincide with those available at the hospital. I should not wish to imply that learning is commensurate with the amount of time spent practicing, but practice can be spaced out, as described for the expanded-retention-interval technique.

A third consideration is that visiting a person at home may be less disruptive to family life than having the person come to the hospital. Many carers for patients with dementia complain that persuading the dependent to attend the day hospital causes them considerable stress, which often outweighs the relief gained from having the break. An additional point that carers often raise is that the dependent cannot recall what he or she has been doing at the hospital. This may cause distress for the family, with the carer possibly not being able to provide suitable cues about what has gone on. The problem may be compounded by the apparently frequent lack of regular consultation between day-hospital staff and family members.

In contrast, there can be close involvement of the family members in any home-based treatment. Obviously it is crucial to understand something of the dynamics of the family in order to decide whether or not to offer such an approach. In some families it would be unacceptable for a son or daughter to be acting as co-therapist, because this might imply a complete reversal of roles, with the daughter now giving her mother or father home practice, rather than the converse, which once was the norm in the family. The aim is to provide a relaxed and nonthreatening approach to the material, trying to avoid a teacher–pupil type of relationship. Many families possess the right qualities and can relate to one another in a natural, warm, and concerned manner, involving the sharing of humor. This is undoubtedly true in some cases, but the special circumstances of the particular carers must be taken into consideration. Many of the carers are themselves elderly and may be suffering ill-health. They may be experiencing considerable stress as a result of caring, and they have the responsibility of caring all the time, unlike professionals, who have a time-limited commitment. Also, there may be a conflict of interests, as with daily living skills, where the carer may find it easier to help the person (for reasons of time saved and reduced frustration), while recognizing the conflicting aim of trying to maintain or retrain the patient's independence in such tasks. Preferably, involvement of the carer as a therapist should be considered only when both the carer and the dependent are in agreement with the treatment plan, and where adequate support can be provided.

Finally, the nature of the problem selected for training can also make a difference regarding the acceptability and success of a treatment program. If the patient is able to identify a problem that the family also agrees to work on, then training may proceed smoothly. If the carer identifies problems that the patient does not recognize, such as repeated questioning, then a more gradual approach may be necessary. Systematic observations at the baseline period, as, for example, with the man who lost things around the house, can lead to increased understanding of the problem and can be of help in monitoring the success of treatment.

The various models of home-based intervention need to be clearly defined and evaluated in terms of treatment outcome, relative cost of providing care, and the effects on the family.

In some conditions, such as myocardial infarction, the patient may be managed at home just as well as in the hospital (Mather et al., 1971). However, the provision of such a home-care service, with specially appointed community staff, may not result in a reduced need for hospital beds (Rowley, Hampton, & Mitchell, 1984). In a similar way, Wade, Langton-Hewer, Skilbeck, Bainton, and Burns-Cox (1985) did not find any advantage in a home-care service for stroke patients. In fact, the rate of admission to hospitals was slightly higher in the group using the home-care service than in the control service. Furthermore, the patients did not show any greater emotional adjustment, nor the relatives any greater reduction in stress, following participation in the home-care service as compared with the control (outpatient) service.

One of the reasons that the home-care services mentioned earlier have not proved particularly effective is that they appear to have followed the traditional model of "doing things to" the patient, simply applying the treatment at home rather than in the hospital. Inevitably, the total amount of therapist contact per week for a given number of patients is likely to be less in a home-care setting than in a hospital setting because of the therapist's traveling time between homes and the restriction to seeing one patient at a time. The limited amount of direct treatment time can be illustrated by reference to studies of stroke patients. On average, speech therapists (David, Enderby, & Bainton, 1982), physiotherapists, and occupational therapists (Wade, Skilbeck, Langton-Hewer, & Wood, 1984) each offer a patient no more than 30 hours treatment time during the 6 months (or more) following the stroke. For any one individual, this represents an average of 11 min of treatment time per working day from each of the services offered, which in most cases will be only a select few of those potentially available.

There appear to be several alternatives to the therapist conducting individual sessions at home: First, volunteers or therapy assistants can be trained to provide specific skills or can offer general therapeutic intervention, which in some cases can be equally effective as professionally trained intervention (David et al., 1982). Clear lines of responsibility and the availability of consultation may be important for voluntary workers, and this may be available from within a voluntary organization, or by establishing links with appropriate professionals. A further advantage of working with voluntary organizations is that many of them already offer a wide variety of services to the elderly, such as stroke groups, day centers, and visiting the elderly in their own homes.

Second, community staff who already work with the elderly can be taught specific skills and supervised when carrying out treatment programs. The addition of specific skills to their repertoire of abilities may be welcomed, because some professional groups, such as "health visitors," feel that in their work with the elderly they have "no useful frame of reference from which to make a meaningful, relevant and satisfying contribution" (Luker, 1981).

Third, computerized training can be set up in the patient's home. The advantage of this is that the patient can work with the computer at convenient times, and as often as desired. The programs can be written so that they will alter the level of difficulty according to past performance and provide feedback about performance, and they can store the results of a session on a disk (Skilbeck, 1984). The computerized training can then be supervised via the telephone to discuss progress. With the use of a modem, programs can be downloaded to the family for their use, with information sent back from the patient's computer to the main office to monitor progress. This type of contact has recently been set up at the Burden Unit at Bristol. A more typical arrangement may consist of home visits by the therapist, or of outpatient appointments, at which the data disk can be inspected, and any alterations needed can be made to the program itself, or the type of program can be changed. This procedure is illustrated by Bracy (1983), who writes his own programs and has now made these commercially available (Bracy, 1985). Another commercially available set of software for cognitive rehabilitation is that written by Gianutsos and Klitzner (1984). These two sets of programs cover a range of areas for training. The set of programs aimed at teaching mnemonic strategies (Einstein Corporation, 1983) may be suitable for use with young healthy subjects (Geiselman, McCluskey, Mossler, & Zielun, 1984), but in our experience they appear to be inappropriate for older subjects, particularly those with severe memory impairments. Furthermore, program listings often are featured in the publication *Cognitive Rehabilitation*, which is aptly aimed at the therapist, the family, and the patient. Writing one's own software is not that difficult, and we have prepared our own programs, including some that incorporate the method of expanded rehearsal.

A fourth alternative is to use carefully constructed therapy manuals that provide clear guidelines for the patient and therapist, who may be a member of the family. We have prepared training manuals for word retrieval, dysgraphia, and expanded rehearsal practice for memory, as outlined earlier. In addition, we have adapted specific cognitive-rehabilitation approaches that we had been using in the hospital, compiling manuals and materials for the family to follow at home. These packages cover the retraining of visual neglect (Weinberg et al., 1977), sensory awareness (Weinberg et al., 1979), and the use of a block-design training package (Diller, Ben-Yishay, Gerstman, Goodkin, Gordon, & Weinberg, 1974; Diller & Gordon, 1981) as part of our overall therapy approach.

We believe that any form of home-based therapy must begin by providing adequate training for the family in how to carry out the therapy. In our own work we start by giving a clear introduction to the training materials and manuals. The therapist then demonstrates their application with the patient. We often have a therapist and another staff member role-play particular problems that may arise in therapy, illustrating how to cope. We then involve the relative as therapist and provide suitable guidance until we are satisfied that the relative and patient have properly understood the tasks. We then allow them to carry out training in between our regular (usually weekly) visits. The training manuals include sessional record forms, so that these can be reviewed and progress can be charted.

Our experience with these training packages has thus far been positive, in that they have been well received by families, and in some cases worthwhile therapeutic gains have been achieved. We have had minor problems involving some families moving on to the next level of task difficulty before fully consolidating performance at the current level. In future evaluations of this work we hope to include measures of the learning and maintenance of the skills of the relative as therapist, as well as outcome measures for the performance of the patient. A good example of the evaluation of these factors is contained in a study of training spouses to improve the functional speech of aphasic patients, carried out by Diller and associates (1974). They found positive improvements in the behaviors of patients and spouses following training, although generalization of the spouse's training from the experimental to the home environment was somewhat limited. It was suggested that aspects of the enduring relationship between the family members, such as dominance of one partner, may have an important bearing on the ability of families to carry on with the therapy in their own homes.

The overall aim of our home-based approach to cognitive rehabilitation is for the therapist to work closely with the whole family and to act in a supportive role to help them overcome or come to terms with the problems.

We still have a great deal to learn about the needs of the families of the cognitively impaired and how to meet these needs in an effective and acceptable way. However, there is increasing interest in providing cognitive rehabilitation for the elderly, and it is hoped that this will have some positive effects on the quality of life of the memory-impaired and their families, perhaps by involving the families with the training.

References

Abson, V. (1984). *Where did I put It? Do old age and IQ predict the frequency with which objects are mislaid?* Paper presented at a British Psychological Society conference, London.

Appell, J., Kertesz, A., & Fisman, M. (1982). A study of language functioning in Alzheimer patients. *Brain and Language, 17,* 73–91.

Barker, M. G., & Lawson, J. S. (1968). Nominal aphasia in dementia. *British Journal of Psychiatry, 114,* 1351–1356.

Bayles, K. A. (1982). Language function in senile dementia. *Brain and Language, 16,* 265–280.

Bracy, O. L. (1983). *Computer based cognitive rehabilitation.* Paper presented at the annual meeting of the International Neuropsychological Society, Mexico City.

Bracy, O. L. (1985). *Psychological software services,* P.O. Box 29205, Indianapolis, IN 46229.

Brooks, D. N., & Baddeley, A. (1976). What can amnesic patients learn? *Neuropsychologia, 14,* 111–122.

David, R. M., Enderby, P. M., & Bainton, D. (1982). Treatment of acquired aphasia: Speech therapists and volunteers compared. *Journal of Neurology, Neurosurgery and Psychiatry, 45,* 957–961.

Davies, A. D. M., & Binks, M. G. (1983). Supporting the residual memory of a Korsakoff patient. *Behavioral Psychotherapy, 11,* 62–74.

Diller, L., Ben-Yishay, Y., Gerstman, L. J., Goodkin, R., Gordon, W., & Weinberg, J. (1974). *Studies in cognition and rehabilitation in hemiplegia* (Rehabilitation Monograph No. 50). New York University Medical Center.

Diller, L., & Gordon, W. A. (1981). Rehabilitation and clinical neuropsychology. In S. B. Filskov & T. J. Boll (Eds.), *Handbook of clinical neuropsychology.* New York: Wiley.

Einstein Corporation (1983). *MemoryTrainer* (computer software package). Los Angeles: Einstein Corp.

Ernst, B., Dalby, A., & Dalby, M. A. (1970). Aphasic disturbances in presenile dementia. *Acta Neurologica Scandinavica, Suppl. 43,* 99–100.

Garland, J. (1985). Adaptation skills in the elderly, their supporters and carers. *British Journal of Medical Psychology, 58,* 267–274.

Geiselman, R. E., McCluskey, B. P., Mossler, R. A., & Zielun, D. S. (1984). An empirical evaluation of mnemonic instruction for remembering names. *Human Learning, 3,* 1–8.

Gianutsos, R., & Klitzner, C. (1984). *Computer programs for cognitive rehabilitation* (computer software package). Bayport, NY: Life Science Associates.

Gilhooly, M. L. M. (1980). *The social dimensions of dementia.* Paper presented at the British Psychological Society annual conference, Aberdeen.

Gilhooly, M. L. M. (1984). The impact of care-giving on care-givers: Factors associated with the psychological well-being of people supporting a dementing relative in the community. *British Journal of Medical Psychology, 57,* 35–44.

Gilleard, C. J. (1984). Problems posed for supporting relatives of geriatric and psychogeriatric day patients. *Acta Psychiatrica Scandinavica, 70,* 198–208.

Glisky, E. L., Schacter, D., & Tulving, E. M. (in press). Learning and retention of computer related vocabulary in amnesic patients – methods of vanishing cues. *Journal of Clinical and Experimental Neuropsychology.*

Goldberg, D. (1978). *Manual of the General Health Questionnaire.* London: NFER–Nelson.

Greene, J. C., Smith, R., Gardiner, M., & Timbury, G. C. (1982). Measuring behavioral disturbances of elderly demented patients in the community and its effects on relatives: A factor analytic study. *Age and Ageing, 11,* 121–126.

Greene, J. G., & Timbury, G. C. (1979). A geriatric psychiatry day hospital service: A five year review. *Age and Ageing, 8,* 49–53.

Grundy, E., & Arie, T. (1982). Falling rate of provision of residential care for the elderly. *British Medical Journal, 284,* 779–802.

Haley, W. E. (1983). A family-behavioral approach to the treatment of the cognitively impaired elderly. *Gerontologist, 23,* 18–20.

Harris, J. E., & Sunderland, A. (1981). A brief survey of the management of memory disorders in rehabilitation units in Britain. *International Rehabilitation Medicine, 3,* 206–209.

Holden, U. P., & Woods, R. T. (1982). *Reality orientation: Psychological approaches to the confused elderly.* London: Churchill Livingstone.

Isaacs, B. (1971). Geriatric patients: Do their families care? *British Medical Journal, 4,* 282–286.

Jeffrey, D., & Saxby, P. (1984). Effective psychological care for the elderly. In I. Hanley & J. Hodge (Eds.), *Psychological approaches to the care of the elderly.* London: Croom Helm.

Johnson, C. L., & Catalona, D. J. (1982). *A longitudinal study of family supports to impaired elderly.* Paper presented at the 35th annual scientific meeting of the gerontological society of America, Boston.

Landauer, T. K., & Bjork, R. A. (1978). Optimal rehearsal patterns and name learning. In M. M. Gruneberg, P. E. Harris, & R. N. Sykes (Eds.), *Practical aspects of memory,* (pp. 625–632). New York: Academic Press.

Lindsley, O. R. (1964). Geriatric behavioral prosthetics. In R. Kastenbaum (Ed.), *New thoughts on old age,* (pp. 41–60). New York: Springer.

Luker, K. A. (1981). The role of the health visitor. In J. Kinnaird, J. Brotherston, & J. Williamson (Eds.), *The provision of care for the elderly.* Edinburgh: Churchill Livingstone.

Mather, H. G., Pearson, N. G., Read, K. L. Q., et al. (1971). Acute myocardial infarction: Home and hospital treatment. *British Medical Journal, 3,* 334–338.

Moffat, N. J. (1984a). Strategies of memory therapy. In B. A. Wilson & N. J. Moffat (Eds.), *Clinical management of memory problems.* London: Croom Helm.

Moffat, N. J. (1984b). Memory therapy with the elderly. In S. Simpson, P. Higson, R. Holland, J. McBrien, J. Williams, & L. Henneman (Eds.), *Facing the challenge.* London: British Association for Behavioral Psychotherapy.

Moffat, N. J. (1986a). *Cognitive rehabilitation of acquired brain damage.* Unpublished PhD dissertation, University of Birmingham.

Moffat, N. J. (1986b). Coping with brain damage in the family. In J. Orford (Ed.), *Coping with disorder in the family.* London: Croom Helm.

Overman, C. A. (1979). *Naming performance in geriatric patients with chronic brain syndrome.* Paper presented at a meeting of the American Speech and Hearing Association, Atlanta.

Patterson, K., Morton, J., & Purrell, J. (1983). Facilitation of word retrieval in aphasia. In C. Code & D. J. Muller (Eds.), *Aphasia therapy.* London: Edward Arnold.

Powell-Proctor, L., & Miller, E. (1982). Reality orientation: A critical appraisal. *British Journal of Psychiatry, 140,* 457–463.

Rochford, G. (1971). A study of naming errors in dysphasic and in demented patients. *Neuropsychologia, 9,* 437–443.

Rochford, G., & Williams, M. (1963). Studies in the development and breakdown of the use of names. *Journal of Neurology, Neurosurgery and Psychiatry, 25,* 377–381.

Rowley, J. M., Hampton, J. R., & Mitchell, J. R. A. (1984). Home care for patients with suspected myocardial infarction: Use made by general practitioners of a hospital team for initial management. *British Medical Journal, 289,* 403–409.

Schacter, D. L., Rich, S. A., & Stampp, M. S. (1985). Remediation of memory disorders: Experimental evaluation of the spaced retrieval technique. *Journal of Clinical and Experimental Neuropsychology, 7,* 79–96.

Skelton-Robinson, M., & Jones, S. (1984). Nominal dysphasia and the severity of senile dementia. *British Journal of Psychiatry, 145,* 168–171.

Skilbeck, C. (1984). Computer assistance in the management of memory and cognitive impairment. In B. A. Wilson & N. J. Moffat (Eds.), *Clinical management of memory problems.* London: Croom Helm.

Thom, W. T. (1981). Housing policies. In J. Kinnaird, J. Brotherston, & J. Williamson (Eds.), *The provision of care for the elderly.* Edinburgh: Churchill Livingstone.

Trigg, A. (1984). *Evaluation of a structured support group for relatives of patients with dementia.* Dissertation for the diploma in clinical psychology, British Psychological Society, Leicester.

Wade, D. T., Langton-Hewer, R., Skilbeck, C. E., Bainton, D., & Burns-Cox, C. (1985). Controlled trial of a home care service for acute stroke patients. *Lancet* (Feb. 9, pp. 323–326).

Wade, D. T., Skilbeck, C. E., Langton-Hewer, R., & Wood, V. A. (1984). Therapy after stroke: Amounts, determinants and effects. *International Rehabilitation Medicine, 6,* 105–110.

Wechsler, D. (1958). *The measurement and appraisal of adult intelligence* (4th ed.). Baltimore: Williams & Wilkins.

Weinberg, J., Diller, L., Gordon, W. A., Gerstman, L. J., Lieberman, A., Lakin, P., Hodges, G., & Ezrachi, O. (1977). Visual scanning training: Effect on reading related tasks in acquired right brain damage. *Archives of Physical Medicine and Rehabilitation, 58,* 479–486.

Weinberg, J., Diller, L., Gordon, W., Gerstman, L. J., Lieberman, A., Lakin, P., Hodges, G., & Ezrachi, O. (1979). Training sensory awareness and spatial organisation in people with right brain damage. *Archives of Physical Medicine and Rehabilitation, 60,* 491–496.

Welden, S., & Yesavage, J. A. (1982). Behavioral improvement with relaxation training in senile dementia. *Clinical Gerontologist, 1,* 45–49.

Wiegel-Crump, C., & Koenigsknecht, R. A. (1973). Tapping the lexical store of the adult aphasic: Analysis of the improvement made in word retrieval skills. *Cortex, 9,* 410–417.

Wilson, B. A., & Moffat, N. J. (Eds.). (1984a). *Clinical management of memory problems.* London: Croom Helm.

Wilson, B. A., & Moffat, N. J. (1984b). Rehabilitation of memory for everyday life. In J. Harris & P. Morris (Eds.), *Everyday memory, actions and absentmindedness.* New York: Academic Press.

Yesavage, J. A. (1982). Degree of dementia and improvement with memory training. *Clinical Gerontologist, 1,* 77–81.

Yesavage, J. A., Rose, T. L., & Bower, G. H. (1983). Interactive imagery and affective judgments improve face–name learning in the elderly. *Journal of Gerontology, 38,* 197–203.

Zarit, S. H., Reever, K. E., & Bach-Peterson, J. (1980). Relatives of the impaired elderly: Correlates of feelings of burden. *Gerontologist, 20,* 649–655.

Zarit, S. H., Zarit, J. M., & Reever, K. E. (1982). Memory training for severe memory loss: Effects on senile dementia patients and their families. *Gerontologist, 22,* 373–377.

35 Memory retraining: Everyday needs and future prospects

Herbert F. Crovitz

Several themes appear and reappear in the work presented in this Part III: (1) the question of the types and characteristics of elderly subjects, (2) theoretical process questions, and (3) an emphasis on practical everyday memory.

Three themes

1. Types and characteristics of elderly subjects. Yesavage, Lapp, and Sheikh (Chapter 31, this volume) suggest that the elderly perform poorly when using visual imagery and often are anxious when using new techniques in testing situations. These authors emphasize the roles of affect, depression, mood-specific effects, and medications in learning and memory processes. Barbara Wilson (Chapter 32, this volume) emphasizes the selection of appropriate strategies for use by particular individuals. Nadina Lincoln (Chapter 33, this volume) discusses these problems as they appear in the general hospital setting. Nick Moffat (Chapter 34, this volume) discusses them at home, where cognitive rehabilitation interacts with the unmet needs of relatives caring for the confused elderly. Apparently it is sometimes necessary to supply external aids for such people. There is growing emphasis on the potential usefulness of well-designed external aids.

I am reminded of a man who suffered from senile dementia of the Alzheimer's type. His daughter-in-law noticed him pushing a silent vacuum cleaner back and forth on a rug. "No, Bill," she said, as she plugged the vacuum cleaner in, so that it started working. How did he interpret her saying "No"? His immediate response, anyway, was to *unplug* the cord and resume pushing the vacuum cleaner back and forth.

2. Theoretical process questions. Lars Bäckman (Chapter 28, this volume) asked why healthy young adults seldom need the kinds of contextual support that the elderly do, and he invoked the concept of spontaneous recoding. Sherry Willis (Chapter 29, this volume) questioned whether or not training improvements

This work was supported by the Medical Research Service of the Veterans Administration.

reflect remediation of age-related decline in cognitive functioning. Or does training result in new learning for elderly people who had experienced no prior decline in the ability or skill being trained? There is growing interest in how skills generalize.

3. A third theme is the emphasis on practical everyday memory. Bäckman (Chapter 28, this volume) mentioned memory for real-life situations, such as television shows. Robin West (Chapter 30, this volume) discussed strategies for enhancing performance on such practical memory tasks as coping with names and faces, spatial learning, remote memory, autobiographical memory, and miscellaneous everyday activities needing prospective memory: grocery lists, finding objects, keeping up with planned activities, and maintaining attention. Yesavage, Lapp, and Sheikh (Chapter 31, this volume) modified mnemonics for the use of the elderly, because the usual devices may be too complicated or may not address practical problems. Wilson (Chapter 32, this volume) likewise emphasized the need to identify and focus on everyday memory problems.

Perhaps the core question raised by the preceding chapters on cognitive enhancement in everyday contexts is this: What are the appropriate memory-training methods for people with memory deficits to use in their everyday lives? It is clear that many different memory disorders exist, varying along such dimensions as severity and permanence, and corresponding to such distinctions as verbal versus figural. Some elderly people may have chronic memory problems, such as the transient problems sometimes seen in young adults shortly after suffering accidental closed-head injury. Such people may have transient amnesias. So far as everyday memory is concerned, they may have a retrograde amnesia in which they cannot recall incidents that occurred before the head injury and loss of consciousness. They also may have an anterograde amnesia in which they are unable to recollect new material when they try to learn it. Both these deficits usually resolve themselves, as does the inability they may have to give a consecutive account of the past few days, that is, to recall incidents from their recent everyday lives and arrange them in the correct space and time contexts (Crovitz, Horn, & Daniel, 1983; Schacter & Crovitz, 1977).

We all know the disadvantages of abnormally poor new-learning ability, and we may see patients who want us to clarify what specific methods will assist them to learn the specific kinds of things on which they do poorly. Clues to some ways to proceed can be found in the work of Pressley, Heisel, McCormick, and Nakamura (1982) and McDaniel and Kearney (1984).

Three interesting methods

Several chapters in this Part III provide information about three possibly important methods for memory enhancement: (1) visual-imagery mnemonics, (2) expanded retrieval, and (3) transformation of everyday memory into procedural memory.

1. The first method is visual-imagery mnemonics. Wilson and Poon (Chapter 27, this volume) worked with an amnesic patient who showed considerable anger

whenever visual-imagery strategies were tried. "Where's the logic in that?" he asked. Yesavage, Lapp, and Sheikh (Chapter 31, this volume) found that the elderly are poor at using visual imagery and described their pretraining method in the use of visual imagery and the elaboration of encoding. Several authors have tried teaching names using imaginative transformation of the name into an image that can be pictured or into an action that can be performed. In my own work on visual-imagery mnemonics (Crovitz, 1979a, 1979b; Crovitz, Harvey, & Horn, 1979) it became clear that some people with memory deficits may need excessive amounts of time for processing the requirements of the task, and some success may result from letting people do the interactive-imagery-mnemonics task by picturing one thing with another thing in any way they like. Young people often are comfortable with relating one thing with another in bizarre ways, whereas older people often are more comfortable making more plausible associations between things. Improvements in making some sort of imagery encoding available to people will no doubt continue, and some people would be well advised to add it to their bag of tricks. The difficulty I see with expecting widespread use of such a method is that the basic methodology of imagery mnemonics has been around for about two thousand years (Yates, 1966), but almost nobody in the modern everyday world likes it or uses it, except perhaps to write articles or books about it. Of course, the whole point of mnemonics was historically determined at its outset: to do covertly the kinds of things forgetful people in a literate society might do overtly – write things down instead of trying to memorize them, and then refer to one's notes when they have slipped one's mind.

2. The second method is concerned with practice or rehearsal in one form or another. Willis (Chapter 29, this volume) discussed training through facilitating one's cognitive strategies: the pattern-description rules of reasoning and rotation-practice tasks of space. West (Chapter 30, this volume) also discussed the usefulness of practicing mental-rotation tasks. Lincoln (Chapter 33, this volume) suggested that a controlled trial is needed before abandoning repetitive practice for learning material.

Then we come to spaced rehearsal (Bjork, 1979; Landauer & Bjork, 1978). Moffat (Chapter 34, this volume) talked about spaced rehearsal that showed some evidence of speeding up and generalizing, and he described a lovely choice for deciding on its retention intervals (if correct, double it; if wrong, cut it in half). There is no doubt that expanding the interval between tests is a powerful technique, at least for rather short time periods. I have used it to teach names to amnesics, using an overly simple method. To role-play: Were I an amnesic trying to learn the name of our leader, I would be told to intercollate his name with expanded numerals, as "Lennie Poon, one; Lennie Poon, one, two; Lennie Poon, one, two, three; Lennie Poon, one, two, three, four," and so on. I recall an elderly gentleman with an inability to remember names who practiced a name through the equivalent of " . . . nineteen, twenty, Lennie Poon," and he was so delighted that he was able to get that far, and then remember the name 5 and 10 min later, that he was willing to bet money he would never forget the name. In fact, he could not recollect it after practicing a second name the same way.

In contrast to my overly simple expanded retrieval method for learning a name, an article with an excellent method has recently been published by Schacter, Rich, and Stampp (1985). Its method is complex, and it should be studied by all of us. This article apparently establishes the validity of the spaced-retrieval method for name learning by memory-disordered patients, and it should be replicated and extended. Schacter and associates (1985) suggested that patients may need explicit help in recognizing everyday situations in which spaced retrieval might be helpful in regard to memory failures, and we should try to design and implement spaced-retrieval techniques for patients.

Another rehearsal method I have played with, which some patients have found useful, uses kinesthetic-motor encoding rather than verbal encoding. The "10-finger-exercise mnemonic" can be used for storing number strings with spaced retrieval. Imagine that the 10 fingers represent numbers, with 1 assigned to the little finger of the left hand, 2 to the ring finger of the left hand, and so on through 9 to the ring finger of the right hand and 0 to the little finger of the right hand. A four-digit number for a money machine in a bank or a seven-digit telephone number can be represented by the corresponding finger series, and some people have practiced the set of appropriate finger presses and can later retrieve it. Such a rehearsal method as this 10-finger-exercise mnemonic comes rather close to procedural-memory tasks, which we consider next. As pianists know, after enough practice, the fingers "know" the sequence.

Future work might profit from trying to understand what general and specific cognitive skills can benefit from various types of practice and how such practice generalizes.

3. The third method, proceduralizing everyday memory, has yet to be investigated. Wilson (Chapter 32, this volume) and West (Chapter 30, this volume) noted that procedural-memory tasks can be learned more or less normally by pure amnesics and by many other memory-impaired people. Wilson said we should concentrate our efforts on understanding how to make everyday memory tasks more like procedural-learning tasks. Would our contribution to memory therapy be increased considerably thereby?

Let us consider typical procedural-memory tasks. The one that has been studied most in experimental psychology is the pursuit-rotor task. Normals and amnesics may get better with practice on keeping the point of a stylus on a disk that circles swiftly in a rather erratic path. For a brilliant book on the methodology and theories covering 50 years of work on the pursuit rotor, see Eysenck and Frith (1977). Recently, there was been a focus on the towers-of-Hanoi problem, which does not require much apparatus. Cohen (1985) and others have studied it using five rings of increasing sizes arranged on one of three pegs. The goal is to recreate their order on a different peg, moving only one ring at a time, and never putting a larger ring on top of a smaller one.

The good news is that some people with serious memory disorders can practice doing the towers-of-Hanoi and, with practice, can get better and better at it, making fewer wrong moves, and they may in a few days attain perfect performance on it. Eventually, when we sit such people down in front of the apparatus, we see such people solving the five-disk version in the minimum 31 moves, whereas these people had once taken 100 moves, more or less. This is evidence that these people have learned the moves and perhaps even have learned the more abstract procedural rules.

The bad news is that the same patients may be unable to recall that they ever practiced the procedure. When we ask such people if they remember coming to the laboratory and practicing, they may deny they have ever seen the silly game before. This is evidence that these people do not recall that they practiced. They have a gap in autobiographical memory. They know how to do it, but they do not know that they have spent time doing it.

Forgetting the source of knowledge

This raises the difficult question of what constitutes normal memory ability and what parts of it can be lost. In an analogous case, we taught amnesics of one sort or another to study hidden-figure picture puzzles. Crovitz, Harvey, and McClanahan (1981) had investigated perceptual learning versus autobiographical amnesia in a group of neurosurgical patients, all of whom on a second day attained the perception of figures within difficult picture puzzles in less time than was needed to perceive the figures at initial study. Some of the patients were still in the amnesia period following severe head injury, and their scores indicated normal perceptual learning. However, questioning about practice on the first testing day disclosed autobiographical amnesia (i.e., inability to recall the testing session in which the unusual pictures were first inspected). The method developed by Crovitz and associates (1981) was then used by us to study autobiographical amnesia (Daniel, Weiner, & Crovitz, 1983) and perceptual learning (Daniel, Crovitz, & Weiner, 1984) after electroconvulsive therapy (ECT).

All too similarly, patients with verbal-memory disorders can be taught a list of words such as the "airplane list" (Crovitz, 1979a). The method consists of reading a bizarre story to patients, the story being built up around a list of mnemonic-chained words (the response word of pair n is the stimulus word for pair $n + 1$). Some time later, they may have autobiographical amnesia for the learning episode, but they can be given retrieval cues and came up with some of the forgotten words. However, when asked how they come up with the right words, they deny that they have ever learned them, but rather state that the words are "logical" or that they are "just guessing." Crovitz (1979a) developed this method for differentiating between learning verbal material and amnesia for the practice session, using patients with alcoholic Korsakoff's disease and closed-head injury. This method was then used to investigate verbal learning in the presence of autobiographical amnesia associated with ECT (Daniel, Crovitz, Weiner, & Rogers, 1982). A reanalysis of this study related postictal electroencephalogram (EEG) suppression to autobiographical amnesia (Daniel, Crovitz, Weiner, Swartzwelder, & Kahn, 1985).

The situation in which one knows and at the same time does not know how one knows is an old problem. The concepts that are necessary to understand this state of affairs are related to the terms *source amnesia* and *divided consciousness.* The key concepts embedded in this topic have a long history within psychology (about 100 years). Alfred Binet and others began a tradition of demonstrating that in such states as hypnosis, anesthesia, and distraction, people may fail to recall the source of information that they can be shown to possess. Some important references are Binet (1890, 1896), Hilgard (1977), Evans (1979), and Robinson (1982).

These concepts have recently been related to computer memory by Lisa West (private communication), a graduate student in psychology at Duke University. In her theory, procedural memory is intact in amnesics: Although they cannot easily "search" for memories, they can "dump" memories when presented with an external cue, namely, the stimulus that brings them to the memory location they cannot search for and find by themselves.

Within experimental cognitive psychology, Jacoby and Dallas (1981), and then Jacoby and Witherspoon (1982) with respect to perceptual learning, and Graf, Squire, and Mandler (1984) with respect to completion of word stems, have carried out studies indicating that people who are given words to remember may, after a delay, be unable to recall them. Nonetheless, it is easy to show that the material still exists in memory. For example, when they are asked to complete three-letter stems, producing any word they like, they tend to retrieve the words with those three-letter stems that were on the forgotten list. Recently, I tried an adaptation of the Graf-Squire-Mandler method with a patient who had undergone bilateral temporal-lobe neurosurgery. The first two words on the list were *rival* and *caviar.* The patient forgot the list, but when asked to think of any words that began with *riv* and *cav,* he completed the stems with the low-associate-value words *rival* and *caviar,* which had been on the "forgotten" list. I should mention that there had been six more words on the list, and this patient completed their stems with words that were not on the list. Worse still, when asked after each stem was completed whether or not that word had been on the list, she said that it had been. To make a bad story worse, when the patient made words out of three-letter stems that had not been on the list at all, she also said that those words had been on the list.

The awful practical problem is that even when people are able to be cued to dump information they have forgotten, it simply seems like a guess, separate from their everyday memory. Future work should try to discover how to revive the space–time context of dumped information. Alternatively, there may be conditions under which perceptual sequelae of forgotten information can be used to generate "guesses" that are trustworthy enough. All this means that more research is needed.

Is retrieval cuing desirable or feasible?

In a book on the first century of experimental psychology, Cofer (1979) summarized the current state of affairs in learning and memory from his point of view: "Although much forgetting may be due to inadequate initial learning," he said, it seemed likely that forgetting will increasingly be construed as a failure of retrieval in the light of the significance of retrieval cuing (Tulving, 1983). He argued that an important prospect for the future is afforded by the possibility that a technology of retrieval cuing might be developed. If it is, it may be useful for the elderly and others, including us. Readers of this volume may be the people who are in a position to develop such a technology, because they will have the right training and the right talents, and some of them will encounter the right sorts of cases.

So far as everyday memory is concerned, applying this idea of retrieval cuing to everyday memory failures necessitates a listing of the *specific* types of everyday memory failures experienced by people in various categories. Up to the present, subjective self-report questionnaires usually have been used to study complaints of everyday memory failures.

Studies of memory complaints by normal college students have tended to appear in the literature on cognitive psychology: Herrmann and Neisser (1978), Herrmann (1979, 1982), and Broadbent, Cooper, Fitzgerald, and Parkes (1982). Questionnaires also have been used to study memory complaints in normal elderly subjects (Squire, Wetzel, & Slater, 1979; Zarit, 1981; Zelinski, Gilewski, & Thompson, 1980). Cordoni (1981) tried to bridge studies of memory complaints in college students and in the elderly. He used a modified version of the Herrmann-Neisser Inventory of Memory Experiences to assess retrospective judgments of the frequency of a set of types of everyday real-world forgetting events. He added ratings of how uncomfortable each event would make the subject feel and how much effort the subject would be willing to invest to improve performance on each event. Subjects were 150 college students (mean age = 18.7, range = 17–22; mean years of education = 13.06, SD = 0.94) and 150 elderly volunteers recruited from the Duke Aging Center subject pool (mean age = 72.3, range = 65–97; mean years of education = 15.02, SD = 2.90).

College students and elderly subjects did not differ significantly with respect to their estimates of the frequency of forgetting. With respect to ratings of bothersomeness and willingness to work at improving memory performance, ratings were significantly lower for the elderly than for the college students (i.e., the elderly sample was less bothered by memory failures and were less willing to invest effort toward improving memory). Comments made in an open-ended section of the survey suggested that the elderly volunteers believed in the inevitability of loss of memory with age, tended to expect little of themselves, and were grateful that they were not as bad off as they believed their peers to be. It should be emphasized that these well-educated elderly subjects were merely elderly; they did not have serious memory disorders.

Everyday-memory failure is a significant problem for large numbers of patients. The development of memory-retraining techniques that will be useful in daily activities may result from an understanding of the exact types of forgetting that occur and an assessment of the degree to which some of these exceed and are different in type from normal everyday forgetting experiences.

Subjective beliefs and retrospective judgments depend on metamemory and judgmental processes, which may be quite separate from memorial processes. Finally, even if the retrospective self-assessments of everyday memory function are accurate, the question can be raised of what use they are in rehabilitating a disordered memory.

Recently, an interesting idea has appeared in the neuropsychology literature with regard to understanding everyday memory demands in brain-damaged patients. A number of investigators called for careful analysis of the information-processing demands of daily life – an inventory of mental "activities of daily living." Accordingly, with regard to everyday memory functioning, we (Crovitz, Cordoni, Daniel, & Perlman, 1984) had subjects keep memory diaries in which notations of forgetting experiences were made *immediately* whenever they were noticed in everyday living for a 1-week period. We hypothesized that this diary method provided more objective information about actual everyday forgetting experiences than is provided by retrospective self-assessment questionnaires in which complaints are based on a patient's long-term memory.

The literature on measurement of memory complaints led us to attempt to measure actual everyday forgetting episodes outside the laboratory in groups of undergraduates, healthy old people, and neuropathological patients. For a period of 7 days, they were asked to *immediately* write down every instance of noticing that they had forgotten anything, along with details concerning what they realized they had forgotten, and how they came to recognize that they had forgotten something. Types of forgetting, their frequency (mean = 25 episodes per subject per week), and types of real-world cues that served as reminders that forgetting had occurred were analyzed (Crovitz et al., 1984). No age differences were found, but the sample size was too small for a meaningful age analysis in this diary study. Such on-line real-time memory diaries, in which notes about forgetting are made immediately when they are noticed, avoid some of the problems of diaries that are filled out later, even a short period later, when people may have forgotten what really happened (Morris, 1984; Reason & Lucas, 1984; Sunderland, Harris, & Baddeley, 1983; Sunderland, Harris, & Gleave, 1984).

This was followed by work by Crovitz and Daniel (1984), who made a listing of the gists of 1,000 consecutive episodes of forgetting recorded in the earlier study (Crovitz et al., 1984). They found that about half of the 1,000 episodes of forgetting could be reduced to a set of 33 gists, and half the forgetting episodes concerned the forgetting of intended actions (e.g., "I forgot to make a phone call." "I forgot to take medicine."). We suggested that from such memory diaries and such derived lists, sets of retrieval cues (e.g., a sign asking, "Do you need to make a phone call?") might be constructed as a type of external aid to be used in studies of the prevention of forgetting in specific groups with memory complaints.

After all this excursion into mnemonic and rehearsal and questionnaire and diary methods, we seem to have ended where we began – with the realization that external aids such as notes and reminders and manuscripts may be sensible alternatives for people who, for one reason or another, have learned that they cannot trust their everyday memory ability.

In line with a tradition that has developed on the heels of certain other occasions, I would like to end with a commemorative limerick, composed by a committee whose contributors included Lewis Petrinovich:

Anna Thompson aged with rapidity,
Exchanging memory for serendipity.
Yet she clearly made the grade,
Employing her external aid,
And acquired functional validity.

References

Binet, A. (1890). *On double consciousness.* Chicago: Open Court.

Binet, A. (1896). *Alterations of personality.* New York: Appleton.

Bjork, R. A. (1979, October). *Retrieval practice.* Paper presented at the Conference on Developmental and Experimental Approaches to Memory, Ann Arbor.

Broadbent, D. E., Cooper, P. E., Fitzgerald, P., & Parkes, K. R. (1982). The Cognitive Failures Questionnaire (CFQ) and its correlates. *British Journal of Clinical Psychology, 21,* 1–16.

Cofer, C. (1979). Human learning and memory. In W. Hearst (Ed.), *The first century of experimental psychology* (pp. 323–370). Hillsdale, NJ: Lawrence Erlbaum.

Cohen, N. (1985). *Preserved learning in medial temporal amnesia.* Paper presented to the 13th annual meeting of the International Neuropsychological Society, San Diego.

Cordoni, C. N. (1981). *Subjective perceptions of everyday memory failures.* Unpublished doctoral dissertation, Duke University.

Crovitz, H. F. (1979a). Memory retraining in brain-damaged patients: The airplane list. *Cortex, 15,* 131–134.

Crovitz, H. F. (1979b). Presentation-time limits on memory retrieval. *Cortex, 15,* 37–42.

Crovitz, H. F., Cordoni, C. N., Daniel, W. F., & Perlman, J. (1984). Everyday forgetting experiences: Real-time investigations with implications for the study of memory management in brain-damaged patients. *Cortex, 20,* 349–359.

Crovitz, H. F., & Daniel, W. F. (1984). Measurements of everyday memory: Toward the prevention of forgetting. *Bulletin of the Psychonomic Society, 22,* 413–414.

Crovitz, H. F., Harvey, M. T., & Horn, R. W. (1979). Problems in the acquisition of imagery mnemonics: Three brain-damaged cases. *Cortex, 15,* 225–234.

Crovitz, H. F., Harvey, M. T., & McClanahan, S. (1981). Hidden memory: A rapid method for the study of amnesia using perceptual learning. *Cortex, 17,* 273–278.

Crovitz, H. F., Horn, R. W., & Daniel, W. F. (1983). Interrelationships among retrograde amnesia, post-traumatic amnesia, and time since head injury: A retrospective study. *Cortex, 19,* 407–412.

Daniel, W. F., Crovitz, H. F., & Weiner, R. D. (1984). Perceptual learning with right unilateral versus bilateral electroconvulsive therapy. *British Journal of Psychiatry, 145,* 394–400.

Daniel, W. F., Crovitz, H. F., Weiner, R. D., & Rogers, H. J. (1982). The effects of ECT modifications on autobiographical and verbal memory. *Biological Psychiatry, 17,* 919–924.

Daniel, W. F., Crovitz, H. F., Weiner, R. D., Swartzwelder, H. S., & Kahn, E. M. (1985). ECT-induced amnesia and postictal EEG suppression. *Biological Psychiatry 20,* 344–348.

Daniel, W. F., Weiner, R. D., & Crovitz, H. F. (1983). Autobiographical amnesia with ECT: An analysis of the roles of stimulus wave form, electrode placement, stimulus energy, and seizure length. *Biological Psychiatry, 18,* 121–126.

Diller, L., & Gordon, W. A. (1981). Interventions for cognitive deficits in brain-damaged adults. *Journal of Clinical and Consulting Psychology, 49,* 822–834.

Evans, F. J. (1979). Contextual forgetting: Posthypnotic source amnesia. *Abnormal Psychology, 88,* 556–563.

Eysenck, H. J., & Frith, C. D. (1977). *Reminiscence, motivation, and personality: A case study in experimental psychology.* New York: Plenum Press.

Graf, P., Squire, L. R., & Mandler, G. (1984). The information that amnesic patients do not forget. *Journal of Experimental Psychology: Learning, Memory, and Cognition, 10,* 164–178.

Harris, J. E., & Morris, P. E. (Eds.). (1984). *Everyday memory, actions and absentmindedness.* New York: Academic Press.

Harris, J. E., & Wilkins, A. J. (1982). Remembering to do things: A theoretical framework and an illustrative experiment. *Human Learning, 1,* 123–136.

Heaton, R. K., & Pendleton, M. G. (1981). Use of neuropsychological tests to predict adult patients' everyday functioning. *Journal of Consulting and Clinical Psychology, 49,* 807–821.

Herrmann, D. J. (1979). *The validity of memory questionnaires as related to a theory of memory introspection.* Paper presented to the British Psychological Association.

Herrmann, D. J. (1982). Know thy memory: The use of questionnaires to assess and study memory. *Psychological Bulletin, 92,* 434–452.

Herrmann, D. J. (1984). Questionnaires about memory. In J. E. Harris & P. E. Morris (Eds.), *Everyday memory, actions and absentmindedness* (pp. 133–151). New York: Academic Press.

Herrmann, D. J., & Neisser, U. (1978). An inventory of everyday memory experiences. In M. M. Gruneberg, P. E. Morris, & R. N. Sykes (Eds.), *Practical aspects of memory* (pp. 52–60). New York: Academic Press.

Hilgard, E. R. (1977). *Divided consciousness: Multiple controls in human thought and action.* New York: Wiley.

Jacoby, L. L., & Dallas, M. (1981). On the relationship between autobiographical memory and perceptual learning. *Journal of Experimental Psychology: General, 110,* 306–340.

Jacoby, L. L., & Witherspoon, D. (1982). Remembering without awareness. *Canadian Journal of Psychology, 36,* 300–324.

Kahn, R. L., Zarit, S. H., Hilbert, N. M., & Niederehe, G. (1975). Memory complaint and impairment in the aged: The effects of depression and altered brain function. *Archives of General Psychiatry, 32,* 1569–1573.

Landauer, T. K., & Bjork, R. A. (1978). Optimum rehearsal patterns and name learning. In K. M. Gruneberg, P. E. Morris, & R. N. Sykes (Eds.), *Practical aspects of memory* (pp. 625–632). New York: Academic Press.

McDaniel, M. A., & Kearney, E. M. (1984). Optimal learning strategies and their spontaneous use: The importance of task-appropriate processing. *Memory & Cognition, 12,* 361–373.

Morris, P. E. (1984). The validity of subjective reports on memory. In J. E. Harris & P. E. Morris (Eds.), *Everyday memory, actions and absentmindedness* (pp. 154–172). New York: Academic Press.

Oddy, M., Humphrey, M., & Uttley, D. (1978). Subjective impairment and social recovery after closed head injury. *Journal of Neurology, Neurosurgery, and Psychiatry, 41,* 611–616.

Pettinati, H. M., & Rosenberg, J. (1984). Memory self-ratings before and after electroconvulsive therapy: Depression- versus ECT-induced. *Biological Psychiatry, 19,* 539–548.

Pressley, M., Heisel, B. E., McCormick, C. B., & Nakamura, G. V. (1982). Memory strategy instruction with children. In C. J. Brainerd & M. Pressley (Eds.)., *Progress in cognitive development. Vol. 2: Verbal processes in children.* New York: Springer-Verlag.

Reason, J., & Lucas, D. (1984). Using cognitive diaries to investigate naturally occurring memory blocks. In J. E. Harris & P. E. Morris (Eds.), *Everyday memory, actions, and absentmindedness* (pp. 53–70). New York: Academic Press.

Robinson, D. N. (1982). Cerebral plurality and the unity of self. *American Psychologist, 37,* 904–910.

Schacter, D. L., & Crovitz, H. F. (1977). Memory function after closed-head injury: A review of the quantitative research. *Cortex, 13,* 150–176.

Schacter, D. L., Rich, S. A., & Stampp, M. S. (1985). Remediation of memory disorders: Experimental evaluation of the spaced-retrieval technique. *Journal of Clinical and Experimental Neuropsychology, 7,* 79–96.

Squire, L. R., Wetzel, C. D., & Slater, P. C. (1979). Memory complaint after electroconvulsive therapy: Assessment with a new self-rating instrument. *Biological Psychiatry, 14,* 791–801.

Sunderland, A., Harris, J. E., & Baddeley, A. D. (1983). Do laboratory tests predict everyday behavior? A neuropsychological study. *Journal of Verbal Learning and Verbal Behavior, 22,* 341–357.

Sunderland, A., Harris, J. E., & Gleave, J. (1984). Memory failures in everyday life following severe head injury. *Journal of Clinical Neuropsychology, 6,* 127–142.

Tulving, E. (1983). *Elements of episodic memory.* New York: Oxford University Press.

Wilson, B., & Moffat, N. (1984). Rehabilitation of memory for everyday life. In J. E. Harris & P. E. Morris (Eds.), *Everyday memory, actions and absentmindedness* (pp. 207–233). New York: Academic Press.

Yates, F. A. (1966). *The art of memory.* University of Chicago Press.

Zarit, S. H. (1981). Affective correlates of self-reports about memory of older people. *International Journal of Behavioral Geriatrics, l,* 25–34.

Zelinski, E. M., Gilewski, M. J., & Thompson, L. W. (1980). Do laboratory tests relate to self-assessment of memory ability in the young and old? In L. W. Poon, J. L. Fozard, L. S. Cermak, D. Arenberg, & L. W. Thompson (Eds.), *New directions in memory and aging: Proceedings of the George A. Talland memorial conference* (pp. 519–544). Hillsdale, NJ: Lawrence Erlbaum.

Subject index

Author index